Thieme

ENT—Head and Neck Surgery: Essential Procedures

Juergen Theissing, MD
Professor Emeritus
Department of Otorhinolaryngology,
Head and Neck Surgery
Nuremberg Hospital
Nuremberg, Germany

Jochen A. Werner, MD
Professor and Chairman
Department of Otorhinolaryngology,
Head and Neck Surgery
Phillips University Marburg
Marburg, Germany

Gerhard Rettinger, MD
Professor and Chairman
Department of Otorhinolaryngology,
Head and Neck Surgery
University Hospital Ulm
Ulm, Germany

With contributions by

Florian Hoppe, MD
Professor and Chairman
Department of Otorhinolaryngology,
Head and Neck Surgery
Clinical Center Oldenburg
Oldenburg, Germany

Claudia Rudack, MD
Professor and Leading
Senior Physician
Department of Otorhinolaryngology,
Head and Neck Surgery
University of Münster
Münster, Germany

943 illustrations

Thieme
Stuttgart · New York

Library of Congress Cataloging-in-Publication Data

Theissing, Jürgen.
[HNO-Operationslehre. English]
ENT-head and neck surgery : essential procedures / Juergen Theissing, Gerhard Rettinger, Jochen A. Werner ; with contributions by Florian Hoppe, Claudia Rudack ; [translators, Grahame Larkin, Terry Telger ; illustrators, Emil Wolfgang Hanns and Rose Baumann].
p. ; cm.
"Authorized, revised translation of the 4th German ed."--T.p. verso.
Includes bibliographical references and index.
ISBN 978-3-13-148621-9 (alk. paper)
1. Otolaryngology, Operative. I. Rettinger, Gerhard. II. Werner, J. A. (Jochen A.), 1958- III. Title.
[DNLM: 1. Face--surgery. 2. Ear--surgery. 3. Neck--surgery. WE 705 T376h 2010a]
RF51.T54 2010
617.5'1059--dc22 2010019020

This book is an authorized, revised translation of the 4th German edition published and copyrighted 2006 by Georg Thieme Verlag, Stuttgart, Germany. Title of the German edition: HNO-Operationslehre. Mit allen wichtigen Eingriffen.

Translators: Grahame Larkin, MD, East Sussex, UK; Terry Telger, Fort Worth, TX, USA

Illustrators: Emil Wolfgang Hanns and Rose Baumann, Schriesheim, Germany

Cover design: Thieme Publishing Group
Typesetting by medionet Ltd, Berlin
Printed in India by Gopsons Papers Ltd, Noida

ISBN 978-3-13-148621-9 1 2 3 4 5 6

Important note: Medicine is an ever-changing science undergoing continual development. Research and clinical experience are continually expanding our knowledge, in particular our knowledge of proper treatment and drug therapy. Insofar as this book mentions any dosage or application, readers may rest assured that the authors, editors, and publishers have made every effort to ensure that such references are in accordance with **the state of knowledge at the time of production of the book.**
Nevertheless, this does not involve, imply, or express any guarantee or responsibility on the part of the publishers in respect to any dosage instructions and forms of applications stated in the book. **Every user is requested to examine carefully** the manufacturers' leaflets accompanying each drug and to check, if necessary in consultation with a physician or specialist, whether the dosage schedules mentioned therein or the contraindications stated by the manufacturers differ from the statements made in the present book. Such examination is particularly important with drugs that are either rarely used or have been newly released on the market. Every dosage schedule or every form of application used is entirely at the user's own risk and responsibility. The authors and publishers request every user to report to the publishers any discrepancies or inaccuracies noticed. If errors in this work are found after publication, errata will be posted at www.thieme.com on the product description page.

Foreword

Writing a surgical textbook is, in many ways, like building a house. There must be a strong foundation, high quality materials, a highly motivated workforce, and the appropriate decorations. In *ENT—Head and Neck Surgery: Essential Procedures*, Professors Theissing, Rettinger, and Werner used previous editions of their textbook since 1971 as their foundation. The substantial combined experience of the authors provided excellent building materials. They were obviously highly motivated to do this book in English in order to expose their techniques to a broader audience than was possible in the German language editions. Once their house was completed, they decorated it with the highly detailed, yet remarkably clear, line drawings, essential for guiding the reader through every step of the surgical procedures.

The book is a pure surgical atlas without patient photos or references to distract the reader. While the names of some of the instruments and the procedures will not be known to the readership, still they will seem familiar thanks to the illustrations. I think of this as being similar to seeing a Mercedes in England with the steering wheel on the right-hand side. It will seem a bit different, but you will still recognize the fine lines of the exterior and the luxurious interior.

The noble purpose of medical writing, whether it be in an online journal or a multivolume textbook, is sharing our knowledge and experience with others in the medical community. The process of lifelong learning reflects the essence of what being a physician means, and the application of this knowledge to the well-being of our patients defines us.

Even today, in the era of the highest technology, textbooks still play an important role in education. The expectation of the reader is that a textbook will be an immediate source of comprehensive, authoritative, well-organized, and clearly written information. *ENT—Head and Neck Surgery: Essential Procedures* certainly meets these expectations.

Eugene N. Myers, MD, FACS, FRCE Edin (Hon)

Preface

The purpose of *ENT–Head and Neck Surgery: Essential Procedures* is not to provide an exhaustive listing of every common surgical technique but to present only a selection of those proven surgical interventions that are important for both the practicing otolaryngologist and the beginner in a clear and concise manner. The individual steps of each respective surgical procedure are outlined consistently to facilitate easy reference. Indications, contraindications, informed consent, complications, rules, tips and tricks, and notes on postoperative care are highlighted to draw the reader's attention to these matters of practical importance. The anatomic, functional, and clinical aspects required for an understanding of the procedure are presented at the beginning of each chapter. Conversely, elaborate or rarely used procedures that by their very nature are reserved for a small group of surgeons are mentioned only insofar as they may shed light on fundamental questions pertaining to the indication or informed consent.

All important further developments of surgical techniques have naturally been given the space they deserve. Functional endoscopic/microscopic paranasal sinus surgery and the entire spectrum of ENT plastic reconstructive surgery warrant special mention in this regard. Endoscopic/microscopic laser tumor surgery and the modern techniques of glottis expansion are covered, as are the classic and modified partial resection of the larynx and the techniques of radical, modified radical, and selective neck dissection and thyroid surgery. Modern developments in ear surgery, transplants and implants, cochlea implants, bone-anchored prothesis, and laser procedures have been included. Special emphasis was placed on richly illustrating the text with figures. Here we would like to extend our great thanks to Emil Wolfgang Hanns for his excellent work.

Given the task defined, the literature cited can hardly be exhaustive. Aside from standard references we have included only a few specialized publications we feel are important.

The editors take special pleasure in noting that *ENT–Head and Neck Surgery: Essential Procedures,* which has been available in several editions in the German-speaking countries since 1971, will now publish in English. We would like to thank Georg Thieme Verlag including Mr. Albrecht Hauff and his coworkers, especially Mr. Stephan Konnry and Ms. Anne Lamparter, for the generous design of the book and their support in realizing the project.

Juergen Theissing
Gerhard Rettinger
Jochen A. Werner

Contents

1 General Preparations for Surgery

Indication and Operative Planning

The most important principle in any medical intervention is "nil nocere"—do no harm. Surgical operations inevitably involve risks, thus making it particularly imperative to follow this maxim when operating. Initially, there must always be a convincing indication for the operation, and this indication can only be reached once exact preoperative investigations have been completed. It should critically weigh up the possible outcomes against the stress of an operation as well as its risks, while also taking into account an assessment of the patient's general state of health, the severity of the disorder, and any possible treatment alternatives. The surgeon's own technical and personal abilities and the preconditions for adequate postoperative care must also be included in all deliberations.

The operation will be all the more straightforward and expeditious if preoperative planning of the surgical approach has been based on an exact and detailed assessment.

Legal Prerequisites and Informed Consent

Every medical intervention requires the *legally binding consent* of the patient or their legal representative. To exercise their right to decide, patients must be thoroughly informed about the nature and severity of their disorder and about the risks and possible outcome of the proposed procedure, as well as about possible alternatives and their prospects. The informed consent procedure should be conducted in a suitable manner, taking into account the severity of the disorder and the mental condition of the patient as well as their level of understanding. Particularly *high demands* should be placed on the extent of the informed consent when dealing with interventions that are *not absolutely necessary* from a medical point of view, such as cosmetic operations (an external rhinoplasty, for example). On the other hand, a patient who is already in a life-threatening situation, where intervention cannot be delayed and for which there is no alternative form of treatment, should not be put under even more stress with a list of the most extreme risks, which would normally have no influence on the decision reached by any reasonable person.

Surgical operations must not be undertaken against the expressly declared will of the patient. Borderline situations may arise, however: for example, in a case of an otherwise treatable underlying disorder when asphyxia occurs after the patient has initially declined a tracheotomy. The question of whether the unconscious patient would have changed their mind when faced with mortal danger remains unanswered.

Tacit approval may be assumed for an absolutely urgent operative intervention in an unconscious patient. If the operation allows a certain degree of delay, an application will need to be submitted for a court-appointed guardian to give permission to operate. The next of kin may be interviewed to ascertain the assumed will of the patient; this does not, however, replace a formal informed consent.

An informed consent must *specify the exact definition of the planned intervention and also briefly list the risks and possible outcomes discussed*. It must also confirm the consent for the intervention with the signatures of the parent/legal representative and the physician undertaking the informed consent procedure. Consent forms designed as operation information leaflets, which both explain the procedure and also provide a written account of any possible consequences and complications it may have, are very useful. They do not, of course, release the physician from the duty of offering a personal discussion. For the purposes of documentation, therefore, it is recommended that the most important risks should also be recorded on the form in writing.

Patients must be allowed *sufficient time for consideration* between receiving the information and the operation; time during which they may also change their mind. The timeliness of an informed consent should be assessed according to circumstances: urgent cases with unpredictable outcomes will be dealt with differently than planned interventions. As a rule, therefore, the informed consent should be obtained at the time the indication is defined. For interventions with low or nonserious risks, an informed consent procedure on the day before the operation will allow the patient sufficient time to reach a rational decision regarding the pros and cons. For interventions associated with serious risks and consequences, obtaining informed consent on the evening before the operation, or even on the day of the operation itself, is no longer regarded as adequate.

For day-case interventions, when the surgeon sees patients for the first time on the day of the operation, informed consent obtained on the day of surgery for simple operations will still be regarded as timely if it is made quite clear to patients that they are still free to choose, and have the option to decline consent even at such short notice. Adherence to an adequate time interval between obtaining informed consent and performing the operation must be documented on the consent form by an entry stating the actual time. It should be specifically borne in mind, however, that it is no longer possible to obtain a legally effective informed consent after premedication has been administered or after sedation.

An informed consent obtained on the day of surgery for major outpatient operations associated with considerable risks is not regarded as timely.

With regard to day surgery, patients should be made aware that after local anesthesia with premedication, or after operations under general anesthesia, their *ability to react and their decision-making ability* may be *temporarily impaired.* Patients should therefore refrain from activities such as driving, bicycling, or walking on roads; operating dangerous machinery; or making important decisions until the after-effects have definitely worn off. A recent decision by the German Federal Court of Justice even requires the treating physician to take suitable measures to ensure that patients do not leave the premises unnoticed after an operation and attempt to drive themselves home while their fitness to drive is severely diminished.

The patient's right to self-determination allows them to forego a comprehensive informed consent. A general blank waiver, however, is invalid. A waiver can only be valid if the patient is, on the one hand, able to discern and is, on the other hand, aware of the necessity of the planned intervention and knows that it generally involves risks. A certain amount of basic information should therefore be provided for the consent procedure and this should be set out in writing, together with the waiver of any further information and the actual consent.

Patients whose knowledge of the language used locally is not adequate should receive the informed consent through a translator as intermediary. This intermediary should also sign the consent form and confirm that the translation into the foreign language was conducted truthfully and conscientiously.

Operations on minors always require the consent of a parent or guardian; whether or not both parents/guardians need to sign depends ultimately on the severity of the intervention and the risks involved.

Informed consent usually needs to be obtained from adolescents between the ages of 14 and 18 years, together with their parents.

The legal representative (carer) should be involved during the informed consent of patients who are not competent; the guardianship court may need to be notified in cases where the operation is not absolutely urgent.

Rules, Tips, and Tricks

The legal validity of informed consent for an operation is also always subject to the fulfilment of the following preconditions:

- Proficiency of the operating surgeon in undertaking the recommended procedure and availability of adequate personnel resources.
- Precautions guaranteeing asepsis of the room, staff, and equipment.
- Availability of the required surgical instruments and ancillary equipment (anesthetic apparatus, suction, lighting).
- Provisions for emergency situations, intubation set and anesthetic apparatus, emergency instruments, monitor, emergency medications.
- Adequate postoperative monitoring by nursing staff with medical supervision.

General Pre-assessment and Preparation

Rules, Tips, and Tricks

A specific *medical history* should always be taken, even before minor operations under local anesthesia:

- Indications of clotting abnormalities in the patient's history or that of the family.
- Hypertension, cardiac arrhythmias, coronary heart disease, infarction, heart defect.
- Disposition to thrombosis or embolism.
- Hepatitis, HIV.
- Any known drug allergies, especially to local anesthetics.
- Regular medication.
- Problems during previous operations or general anesthesia.
- Diabetes mellitus.

General physical examination with emphasis on heart, lungs, abdomen, extremities, blood pressure.

Basic laboratory tests: hemoglobin, erythrocyte count, white blood count, thrombocytes, PTT and INR or bleeding and clotting times.

Further tests are usually required for *operations under general anesthesia*, depending on the patient's age and general condition, and ECG and chest radiograph may also be indicated.

Operations associated with a risk of bleeding will require blood grouping and possibly the precautionary ordering of cross-matched erythrocyte concentrates or arrangements for autologous blood.

As a rule, autologous blood is considered appropriate for an elective operation with a probability of at least 10% of requiring transfusion.

Prerequisites for autologous blood donation are a hemoglobin level >12.5 g/dl and a hematocrit >33 %. Cardiac risk patients should be excluded. Age does not necessarily restrict the indication; the procedure is usually successfully applied at ages between 14 and 75 years. Cancer patients are not suitable for providing autologous blood because of the possible delay in surgery and their chronic anemia. A focus of infection with possible hematogenous seeding is also a contraindication. Autologous blood donations may be given at weekly intervals 4–6 weeks before the operation, depending on requirements, with the final session being 1 week before surgery. Unused autologous blood units must not be used for allogenic transfusion.

Daily oral iron should be administered from the start of autologous donation until the hemoglobin has reached a normal value after the operation.

Platelet aggregation inhibitors (e.g., acetylsalicyclic acid [aspirin]) should be discontinued at least 3 days before elective operations; order a bleeding time test (normal 2–5 minutes).

Discontinue warfarin and administer vitamin K until INR has returned to normal. After blood clotting has reached normal values, anticoagulate with heparin, with a target PTT value of 50–60 seconds.

Thrombosis Prophylaxis

No authoritative evidence-based studies are currently available on the effectiveness of anticoagulation for thrombosis prophylaxis for operations in the ENT region, especially with regard to short operations. Except for high-risk patients, however, short ENT operations such as tonsillectomy are regarded as extremely low-risk procedures with respect to a thromboembolic event. In all ENT operations the decision regarding heparinization will have to be reached for each individual case. Typical risk factors that should be taken into consideration are:

- Obesity.
- Age over 40 years.
- Varicose veins.
- Previous history of a thromboembolic event.
- Long operating time.
- Immobility.
- Cancer.
- Heart disorder.
- Infection.
- Pregnancy and lactation.
- Oral contraceptives, high-dose estrogen.
- Smoking.

All surgical patients should generally be supplied with compression stockings, and early postoperative mobilization is the aim.

2 Local Anesthesia

Topical Anesthesia

Indications

- In the region of the ear: paracentesis, polypectomy.
- In the region of the nose: polypectomy, turbinate surgery, endoscopy and maxillary antral lavage, as a supplement in maxillary sinus surgery, septal resection.
- In the region of the mouth: prior to tonsillectomy, for excision biopsies.
- In the region of the nose, throat and larynx: for indirect laryngeal surgery or nose–throat operations and for tracheobronchoscopies and esophagoscopies.

Dosage

Rules, Tips, and Tricks

Application is either by spray, drop instillation, painting on, insertion of swabs or pledgets soaked in the local anesthetic.
Lidocaine is the local anesthetic commonly used.
Lidocaine spray (e.g., Xylocaine spray, maximum dosage 20 puffs of 10 mg each). *Note:* Lidocaine 4 % solution, maximum dosage 5 mL = 200 mg, is too concentrated for the tracheobronchial system.
All maximum dosages refer to a healthy adult with a body weight of approximately 70 kg.
The duration of effect is approximately 10–20 minutes.

Manipulations in the region of the pharynx and larynx during topical anesthesia cause increased salivation, which decreases the effect of the anesthesia. A premedication is particularly important to reduce salivation, to lower the reflex threshold, and for sedation.

Side Effects

Side effects usually arise as a result of overdosage.

Symptoms

- *Mild side effects:* agitation, dizziness, light-headedness; relieve the effects by stopping administration of anesthetic (remove swab, rinse out).
- *Severe side effects* (considerable overdosage, rarely as a result of metabolic disturbances in the liver or problems of renal excretion): additional central nervous or cerebral irritation with convulsions, cardiovascular symptoms with fall in blood pressure, reduction in myocardial contractility and asystole.

Therapy

Rules, Tips, and Tricks

- Discontinue the anesthetic.
- Ensure oxygen supply (give oxygen), secure airways or intubation and artificial respiration.
- Short-acting barbiturate in small doses (50–150 mg) for convulsions; consider inducing a short-acting relaxant.
- Treat circulatory failure by placing the patient in the Trendelenburg position and administering a plasma expander such as orciprenaline (drip infusion 5–10 ampoules of 0.5 mg in a 500 mL solution, drip rate of 15–30 drops/minute).
- For bradycardia, administer 0.5–1 mg atropine IV.
- For asystole, commence standard resuscitation measures.
- For allergic reactions or allergic shock, administer steroids 500–1 000 mg, epinephrine 0.1 mg, possibly repeat (1 mL 1:1 000 dissolved in 9 mL 0.9 % saline, of which 1 mL is given).

2

Infiltration and Regional Anesthesia

Dosage

We prefer prilocaine and lignocaine for regional and infiltration anesthesia; maximum (adult) dose: 400 mg prilocaine with 600 mg epinephrine; 200 mg lidocaine with 500 mg epinephrine.

For tonsillectomy, the dose of 200 mg lidocaine should not be significantly exceeded, even with the addition of epinephrine.

Addition of a Vasoconstrictor: Epinephrine

The dose is not uniform when added to local anesthetics. Usually *5 drops of the 1:1 000 solution* are regarded as the *maximum dose*. One drop in 10 mL of local anesthetic fluid corresponds to an epinephrine concentration of 1:200 000.

During *surgery of the ear*, the concentration for achieving an adequately bloodless surgical field, while still observing the maximum dose, is higher, i.e., up to 1 drop of the 1:1 000 solution in 1 mL of local anesthetic or physiological saline solution for infiltration during general anesthesia; the amount of solution for infiltration is thus limited to 3–5 mL.

In extremely rare cases, infiltration anesthesia in the region of the nose or septum or in the periorbital region can result in impaired vision, which is presumably caused by reflex vascular spasms following transfer of epinephrine-containing infiltration solution. The concentration of epinephrine administered for these areas must therefore be low. Inadvertent intravascular application must be definitely excluded by aspiration before infiltration.

Contraindications for the Addition of Epinephrine

- Anesthesia in the region of end arteries, for example, the tip of the nose.
- Narrow-angle glaucoma.
- Paroxysmal tachycardia or high-frequency absolute arrhythmia, thyrotoxicosis.
- The simultaneous use of cyclopropane and halothane anesthesia (possible cardiac arrhythmias), yet no expressed contraindication for enflurane (Ethrane) anesthesia.
- Relative contraindication for arteriosclerosis, severe hypertension, and diabetes mellitus.

Side Effects

The side effects from infiltration and regional anesthesia result essentially from overdosage of the local anesthetic or the vasoconstrictor, or from inadvertent intravascular injection. Allergic reactions to the more recent local anesthetics are rarely seen nowadays; if present, they are more likely to be the result of a para-group allergy to the preservative methylparaben which is added to the anesthetic solution.

Symptoms

- *Central nervous system*: signs of stimulation such as sudden restlessness, dizziness, tinnitus, nystagmus, fine tremor of the extremities, tonic-clonic convulsions, or signs of depression such as respiratory depression.
- *Cardiovascular system*: signs of stimulation such as tachycardia, increase in blood pressure or signs of depression such as bradycardia, fall in blood pressure or asystole.

Therapy

See topical anesthesia.

Premedication

Rules, Tips, and Tricks

- Premedication: atropine and pethidine, and for special sedation promethazine.
- Timely IM application 30–45 minutes before the start of the operation, or in emergencies IV 5 minutes before surgery.
- Benzodiazepine is also suitable for premedication. This may also be administered orally, as may atropine, with a correspondingly longer latency.
- Administer premedication before local anesthesia too.
- The adverse effect on fitness to drive should also be borne in mind, even if only atropine has been administered.
- Venous access is generally recommended even for local anesthesia, except for minor operations. Any benzodiazepine already administered may be topped up intraoperatively via the IV access if sedation is inadequate.

Dosage

- *Atropine:* 0.01 mg/kg body weight IM. Watch out for glaucoma, tachyarrhythmia.
- *Pethidine:* 1 mg/kg body weight.
- *Promethazine* (for longer lasting operations): 25–50 mg (e.g., Atosil 0.5–1 ampoules) for adults. Watch out for postural hypotension on sitting up.
- *Dimenhydrinate* (as a suppository) or *triflupromazine* (10–20 mg) may be administered 2 hours before the start of the operation to deal with nausea.

3 General Anesthesia for ENT Surgery

General Aspects

Anesthesia for ENT operations entails some special features, which both anesthetist and surgeon must consider:

Rules, Tips, and Tricks

- Correct positioning, especially of the arms (take care not to cause injury to the brachial plexus).
- Secure endotracheal tube and hose connections in particular, given that they are only accessible with some difficulty after the surgical site has been draped.
- The siting of the anesthetic machine and venous access should be discussed with the surgeon, as should the positioning of the endotracheal tube: orotracheal or nasotracheal; in the corner of the mouth or over the middle of the lip, depending on the operation.
- Changes in the position of the head, reclination, or insertion of the tongue depressor can result in displacement or kinking of the endotracheal tube; correct if necessary.
- Avoid addition of epinephrine with halothane or cyclopropane anesthesia.
- Intubation may be made more difficult by facial deformities, receding lower jaw, tumors of the tongue and larynx regions, or inflammatory swellings of the epiglottis and glottis regions; nevertheless, in many cases intubation is still possible using an emergency tube or by fiber-optic assisted intubation. Today, a preliminary tracheotomy under local anesthesia and intubation via the tracheostoma is only indicated in exceptional cases.
- Even though endotracheal intubation still represents the safest way to secure the airways during general anesthesia, the *laryngeal mask* is gaining in importance, especially for adenoidectomies and tonsillectomies. It does not always guarantee absolute protection against aspiration and its exact positioning sometimes produces problems (air insufflation of the stomach); high ventilation pressures, e. g., due to obesity or chronic obstructive bronchitis, also present limitations. However, it has the definite advantages of less traumatization of larynx and trachea, in addition to the good tolerability during the recovery phase and the lower incidence of broncho- and laryngospasms.
- Despite its inherent problems, such as the lack of protection against aspiration, mucosal dehydration, and the risk of barotrauma, *superimposed high-frequency jet ventilation* offers concrete advantages in larynx and tracheal surgery on account of its minimal space requirements and the best possible view for the surgeon, with barely perceptible movements of the surgical field due to breathing.

Special Considerations

Surgery of the Ear

- *The supply of nitrous oxide should be interrupted when the graft is being inserted*, otherwise the graft can balloon away from the ossicles.

Surgery of the Nose

- Ensure reliable inflation of the tube cuff, *pharyngeal suction before extubation.*
- Await the return of the protective laryngeal reflex.
- Considerable blood loss is no rarity.
- Consider controlled hypotension.
- Slightly elevated upper body and head.
- Secure the nasal tamponade with a suture and external splinting to prevent its slipping should mask ventilation be necessary.

Surgery of the Mouth and Pharynx

- Avoid kinking of the tube when inserting the tongue depressor.
- Do not extubate until after hemostasis has been secured, the trachea has been suctioned, and the protective laryngeal reflex has returned.

- Postoperatively, place the patient in the lateral decubitus position.

Rules, Tips, and Tricks

Post-tonsillectomy hemorrhage:

- Have a large-bore suction catheter ready during intubation, and remove swallowed blood via a nasogastric tube prior to intubation.
- Intubate with slightly elevated upper body and head, perform bronchoscopy for aspiration (initially with a flexible endoscope via the endotracheal tube), consider volume fluid replacement and blood transfusion.
- *Peritonsillar abscess, abscess of the floor of the mouth*: difficult intubation in the presence of trismus, although trismus does partially relax during the induction of anesthesia. *The possibility of mask ventilation should be ensured before inducing paralysis.*
- *Deep abscess of the mouth floor and tongue abscess can cause significant intubation problems*, so here too do not induce paralysis unless mask ventilation is ensured. Consider an incision from outside without intubation.

Surgery of the Larynx for Endolaryngeal Operations

- Administer an antitussive agent, consider cortisone before extubation.
- *Microlaryngoscopy, small endotracheal tubes* up to a maximum of 28 Fr, protect the tube with aluminum foil when using laser or use special laser-resistant tubes.
- Injector ventilation during microlaryngoscopy, ensure correct position of the laryngoscope, careful monitoring of oxygenation.

4 Postoperative Management

- Detailed operative notes should be kept, reporting the operative findings, the procedures performed, and the course of the operation. The notes should provide details about the time of surgery and any medications given or implants inserted, as well as listing a postoperative prescription plan (analgesics, antibiotics, infusion, thrombosis prophylaxis, etc.), even for minor operations.
- Order any removed tissue or wound swabs to be examined.

Postoperative Monitoring

- After *general anesthesia* the patient should be monitored *in the recovery room*, or on the *intensive care unit* if indicated.
- Special nursing-care observations are required even after *local anesthesia*.
- Patients who are particularly at risk are those who might bleed into the throat or aspirate after surgery of the nose, paranasal sinuses, or mouth, and those with stenoses in the region of the airways or with obstructive sleep apnea (pulse oximetry).
- Postoperative ward round.

5 Reconstructive Plastic Surgery of the Face

Basic Principles

General Remarks

Plastic surgery of the face has two main objectives: it should correct *dysfunctions* and restore or improve the *aesthetics* of the face. Apart from addressing malformations, plastic reconstructive procedures are required to revise scars, resurface skin and soft-tissue defects, or correct deformities after trauma or tumor surgery. Operations to maintain or improve function are not feasible without incisions and the subsequent formation of scars. Sometimes function and aesthetics contradict each another in reconstructive plastic surgery. It requires experience, detailed knowledge, and careful planning to achieve the intended improvement of function with a minimal loss of aesthetics. Obviously, aesthetics play an essential role, especially when the face is involved.

Before undertaking plastic surgery of the face, therefore, the following general rules should always be kept in mind:

Rules, Tips, and Tricks

- Before each operation: analyze the alteration exactly, document all findings, and undertake thorough planning.
- Provide the patient with comprehensive information; the use of photographs can be helpful.
- Avoid making any unduly optimistic statements about the planned procedure; carefully enquire about the patient's expectations and weigh them up against what is technically possible.
- Never correct more than what has been stated in the informed consent.
- Take the patient's age into consideration; given the increased rate of hypertrophic scar formation in children and adolescents, be cautious with operations that do not necessarily need to be undertaken at this age.
- Be patient when doing revision surgery: allow an adequate period of time to elapse after the previous operation, usually 9–12 months; *do not yield* to understandable pressure from the patient.
- Do not play down an aesthetically unsatisfactory result to the patient, given that an inadequate result is not necessarily the surgeon's fault.
- Analyze residual deformities and discuss subsequent measures for improvement with the patient.

Adhering to these rules will help avoid many disappointments. Nevertheless, results that are not completely satisfactory are unavoidable in certain cases, even for experienced surgeons; the dynamic processes involved in wound healing and scar formation are only partially predictable and are subject to individual variation. Achieving results that are largely predictable requires a detailed knowledge of the basic principles of the procedures used in plastic surgery and of established operative techniques for the face.

Surgical Anatomy of the Skin

Plastic surgery of the face is, in the first instance, surgery of the skin. **Figure. 5.1** depicts the topographic *architecture of the skin*. The skin (cutis) is made up of two layers: the epidermis and the dermis (corium). The epidermis consists of a superficial keratinized layer and a deep nonkeratinized layer, which is responsible for the color of the skin as a result of its content of melanocytes. The dermis bears the vascular and nerve supply of the skin and is rich in elastic and collagen fibers. This fiber content is responsible for the elasticity of the skin and its ability to retract. Both types of fibers are reduced in advanced age, which is why aged skin is loose and prone to form wrinkles.

The superficial part of the dermis is interdigitated with the epidermis (papillary bodies), rendering horizontal movement of these two layers with respect to one another impossible. Any shifting of the skin, therefore, always takes place at the level of the subcutaneous fat layer (subdermis), which separates the skin from the underlying structures (muscle, bone). The subdermis is well developed in some areas of the face, thus giving shape to these areas (e.g., the cheek), but is completely lacking in others (e.g., the eyelids or the anterior surface of the ear).

Hairs, sebaceous glands, and sweat glands are found as *skin appendages*, partly in the subdermis and partly in the dermis. It is important in plastic surgery to bear in mind that the epithelial components of the dermal appendages run through both epidermis and dermis.

The hairs of the head and the eyebrows grow at an oblique angle to the skin surface. This should be kept in mind when directing the scalpel (the plane of incision should be parallel to the hair follicle). Wound healing may be influenced by, among other things, the content of sebaceous glands in the skin. Visible scars may develop around sutures in areas rich in sebaceous glands (above all on the nose, and in adolescents in general) as

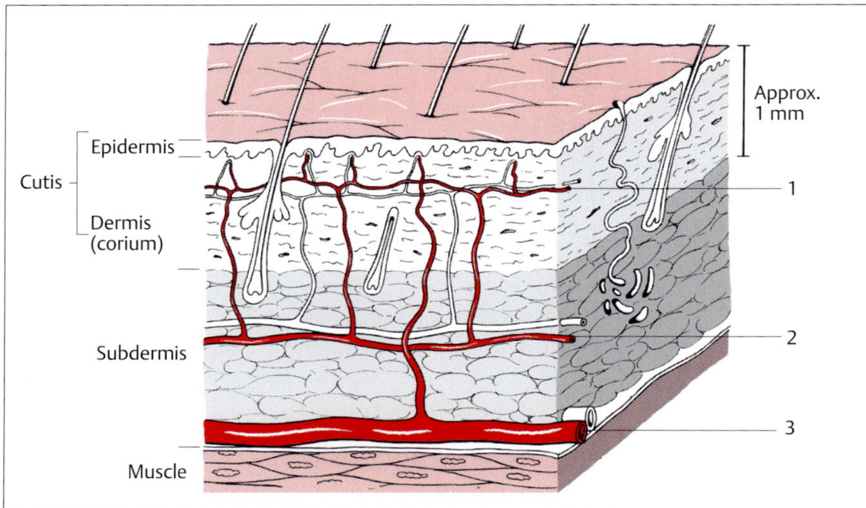

Fig. 5.1 Surgical anatomy of the skin. As a rough size comparison, the thickness of the cutis is given as 1 mm.
1 Vascular plexus in the papillary layer of the dermis.
2 Vessel coursing in the subcutaneous layer.
3 Axial artery over the muscular fascia.

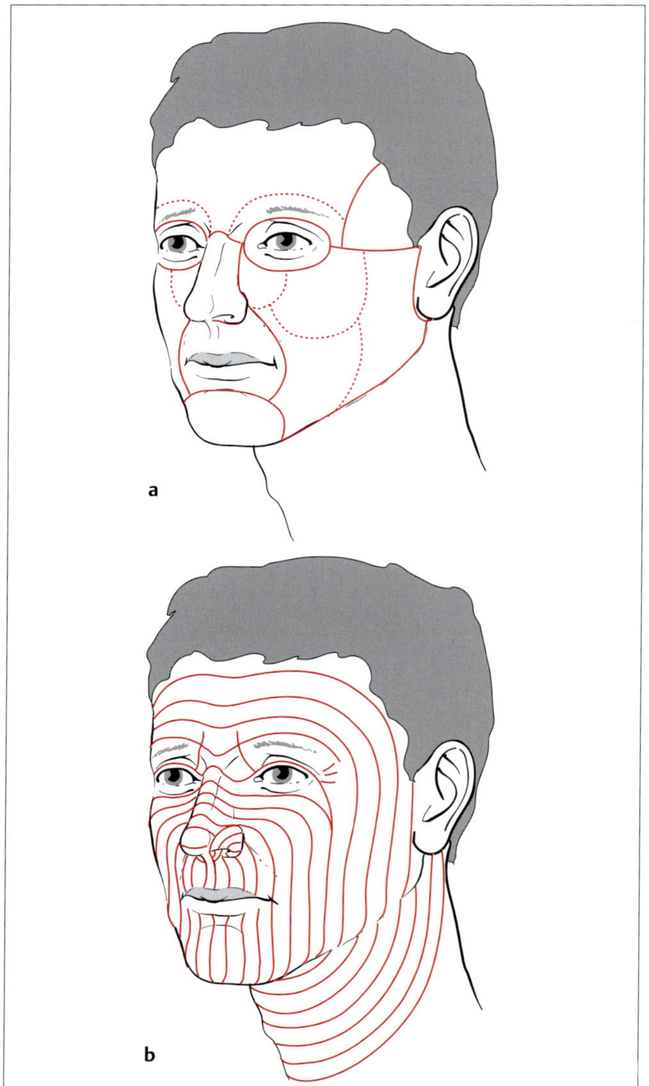

Fig. 5.2a, b Aesthetic units (see text for explanation of illustration) (**a**) and relaxed skin tension lines (**b**).

a result of epithelialization of the puncture marks by injured glands.

Knowledge of the vascular supply of the skin is of fundamental importance for reconstructive plastic surgery, especially in designing skin flaps for defect coverage.

The vascular plexus within the papillary body of the dermis may be supplied by two routes (**Fig. 5.1**):

- From the *subdermal vascular plexus*, which runs in the subdermis and is ubiquitous. *Random pattern flaps* are supplied by these vessels.
- From a *specific artery* (with accompanying vein). These arteries usually run over muscles, parallel to the surface of the skin, and give off vertical vessels (in addition to the vessels from the subdermal plexus) to the skin. It is possible to raise skin flaps on these arteries which are considerably longer than random pattern flaps. Owing to the special position of the artery along the axis of the flap's pedicle, these flaps are known as *axial pattern flaps* or *arterial flaps*. Typical examples of such arteries are the superficial temporal artery ("temporal flap") and the supratrochlear artery ("[para-]median forehead flap", see **Fig. 5.36**).

Aesthetic Units and Relaxed Skin Tension Lines (RSTL)

Aesthetic units are defined regions of the face which should, whenever possible, be reconstructed in their entirety during reconstructive surgery. On the other hand, the restoration of a structure with the aid of adjacent tissue must not be undertaken at the expense of destroying the aesthetic unit of the donor site. The aesthetic units of the face are the frontal, supraorbital, orbital, infraorbital, nasal, zygomatic, buccal, labial, and mental units (**Fig. 5.2a**). Some regions, such as the nose, are further divided into subunits (see **Fig. 5.35**).

When making incisions or revising scars on the face, it is essential to respect the "relaxed skin tension lines" (RSTL, **Fig. 5.2b**) and the wrinkle lines of the skin. Whereas the RSTL correspond to the spontaneous course of wrinkles after relaxation of the skin, the wrinkle lines are oriented perpendicular to the direction of the fibers of the facial muscles. RSTL and wrinkles lines are more or less identical, although they run differently in some regions (glabella, lateral epicanthus, lateral nasal wall). Incisions on the face should correspond to the direction of the RSTL (less wound tension, rapid wound healing, minimal scar formation) or, when creases are present, follow the wrinkle lines ("hide the scar within the skin crease").

Rules, Tips, and Tricks

Always consider the RSTL when making skin incisions on the face. If the wounds are predetermined, orientate the subsequent scars in the direction of the RSTL by advancement of the skin.

Instruments

The instruments must be adapted to the special requirements of plastic surgery. This means that the tips of forceps or the jaws of needle holders should be suitably small, although the handles must be large enough to be manageable. The following instruments have been proven useful:

- *Needle holders*: Instruments with flat jaw surfaces for holding the needle or suture are preferable. With textured jaw surfaces, the very fine suture material that is often used can either pass through the grooves, making it impossible to grasp, or be crushed and thus lose its tensile strength.
- *Forceps*: Adson or Adson–Brown forceps for plastic surgery have fine tips to allow tissue to be grasped precisely and securely. Nevertheless, despite this reduced tissue traumatization, only the subcutaneous tissue should be grasped, whenever possible.
- *Scissors*: One rounded and one pointed, curved pair of scissors are usually adequate.
- *Hooks/retractors*: Fine single skin hooks are very useful and can be inserted through the skin without leaving scars. This allows the skin to be moved or held without the crushing action of forceps. Retractors with more prongs are used for extensive mobilization, but should then only grasp the subcutaneous tissue.
- *Scalpel blades*: Usually a small, curved blade (No. 15) is used. For mobilization of larger skin areas to cover defects, especially in the area of the neck and chest, a correspondingly larger curved blade (No. 10) is used. For fine, angulated skin incisions, e.g., for scar revisions, a pointed blade (No. 11) is used.
- *Bipolar coagulation forceps*: Targeted bipolar coagulation is an essential guarantee for good hemostasis with minimal tissue damage. It is indispensable for plastic surgery of the face.
- *Further aids*: A ruler and a pair of dividers, as well as templates made of sterile material, are suitable for preoperative and intraoperative planning. In special cases, e.g., for sutures in the area of the free alar margin, the use of loupes is helpful.

Suture Material

Only atraumatic needle/suture combinations are suitable for plastic surgery of the face. Absorbable braided suture materials based on polyglycolic and polylactic acid (e.g., Vicryl) are used for subcutaneous sutures. These have a half-life (time until reduction of the tensile strength to 50%) of 10–12 days. Polylactic acid is broken down into CO_2 and H_2O. Complete absorption, however, is only achieved after approximately 9 months. The absorption time of a thread is determined by its size, among other factors, so the times stated above are therefore average values. The required thickness of subcutaneous sutures depends primarily on the tension required to achieve approximation of the wound edges.

Skin sutures are placed using monofilament, nonabsorbable synthetic strands made out of polyamide (e.g., Ethilon, Supramid) or polypropylene (e.g., Prolene). These sutures have a high tensile strength, skin irritation is minimal, and they have no "wick effect" (infiltration of bacteria into deeper skin layers).

A suture size of 4/0 or 3/0 is usually chosen for subcutaneous sutures. Skin suturing for the face should be undertaken with a maximum suture size of 5/0, even better 6/0. The *suture size* is stated according to the American system (USP) or the European system (metric) (**Table 5.1**).

Cutting *needles* of various lengths and forms are suitable. Needles in the form of an arc of a circle (e.g., ⅜ circle) are used for superficial sutures. Semicircular or even more strongly curved needles are used for deep sutures, especially for sites with restricted access. The various manufacturers use different terminology for the needle shapes, so there is no universally valid nomenclature.

Wound Healing and General Wound Management

Wound Healing

Wound healing proceeds in several phases. The wound surface is initially covered with a fibrin net, and after 24 hours the epidermis begins to close over the wound. Wounds that are surgically closed have already achieved epithelial coverage, preventing the infiltration of pathogens. This epithelial layer does not yet provide the wound with any tensile strength, however. The necessary stability is only achieved with the production of collagen fibers, mainly by dermal fibroblasts. Scar maturity as a result of increased collagen turnover (collagen production and

Table 5.1 Terms for the main suture sizes

Average strand diameter (mm)	Size (metric)	Size (USP)
0.07	0.7	6/0
0.1	1	5/0
0.15	1.5	4/0
0.2	2	3/0
0.3	3	2/0

breakdown) takes several months and is not complete for more than 1 year. The visible sign of this is the paling of the previously red scar.

Given that only the production of collagen results in a visible scar, it must be contained within limits by correct wound management.

Wounds must
- not be under tension,
- not have any cavities.

If increased collagen production is induced by dehiscence of the wound edges, reduction of the wound surface by contraction will occur and the surface will be covered by a thin, functionally inferior, epithelial layer. This form of *secondary healing* results in considerable deformity of the surrounding tissue and should be avoided on the face.

General Wound Management

Wounds managed by suturing do not require any special covering, since—as stated above—the epithelial layer is closed after 24 hours. Exceptions are compression dressings required to avoid a subcutaneous hematoma after extensive undermining, or dressings to relieve tension. Larger epithelial defects, which are to be resurfaced at a later stage, may be managed temporarily with a synthetic or biological *skin substitute*. A compression dressing is often inadequate for hematoma prophylaxis of deep wounds. It is preferable in such cases to insert a soft drain or a suction drain.

Sutures on the face should be removed as early as possible, i.e., usually after 5–6 days. The timing depends on two factors:

- *Location of the suture*: In skin rich with sebaceous glands, such as the tip of the nose, epithelialization of the puncture hole occurs early from injured glands, resulting in unsightly scars. For this reason, sutures in this area should be removed by 5 days after surgery or even earlier.
- *Wound tension*: Skin sutures should never be placed under tension. The necessary relief of tension should always be achieved by subcutaneous sutures. In certain cases this may not be possible; if so, skin sutures should be left for a correspondingly longer time and possible cosmetically unfavorable scar formation must be accepted.

Suture Techniques

Standard Suture Technique

Primary wound closure usually involves a subcutaneous suture and a skin suture (**Fig. 5.3**). The subcutaneous suture is placed in such a way that the knot is buried in the depths of the tissue (**Fig. 5.3a**). The skin margins are then re-approximated with an interrupted suture (**Fig. 5.3b, c**).

Rules, Tips, and Tricks

The prerequisites for correct suturing are as follows.
- The wound edges must be of equal length at skin level. "Dog-ears" develop from incongruities and can be removed by the excision of Burrow triangles or by other techniques (**Figs. 5.4** and **5.5**).
- Wound edges with differing depths may be brought to the same level by skin excision and skin advancement (**Fig. 5.6**).
- Entry and exit holes in the skin should lie at the same distance from the wound edge (**Fig. 5.3b**).
- The depths of the entry and exit holes of the suture in the area of the wound must be equal (otherwise distortion of the wound edge will result) (**Fig. 5.3b**).

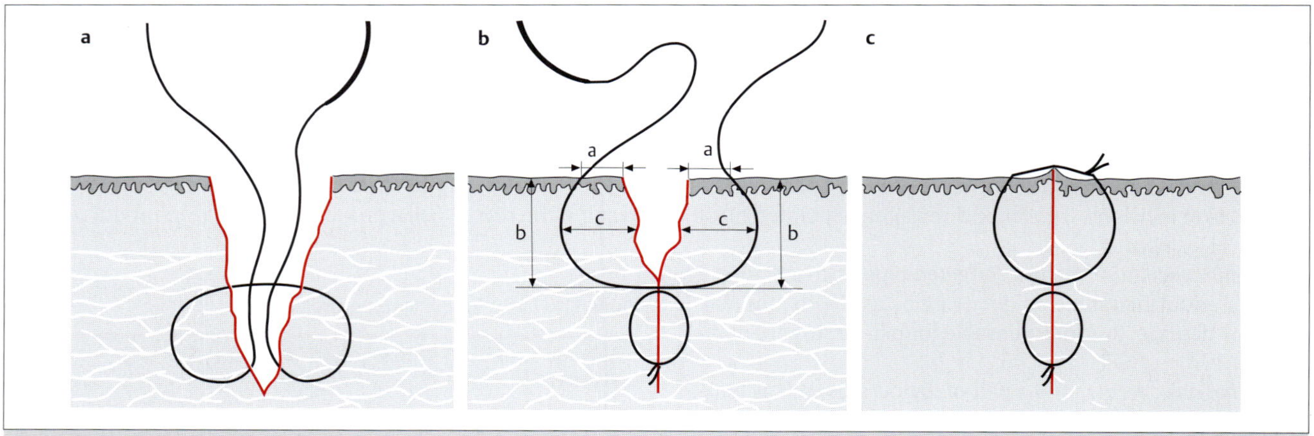

Fig. 5.3a–c Standard suture technique.
a Subcutaneous suture with buried knot.
b Suture in place
Note: Needle entry and exit holes must be the same distance from the wound edge (a), the depths of the entry and exit bites are the same (b). To achieve the desired eversion of the wound edges, the suture bites must grasp more subcutaneous tissue in the depths than at the surface (c > a).
c Wound closure completed.

- The skin knots must not be pulled too tight, otherwise scar constriction will develop (postoperative swelling of the wound must be taken into consideration).
- The ends of the sutures must be left long enough for their easy removal, but must be cut short enough to prevent them from interfering with the adjacent sutures.
- When suturing is completed, the wound edges should be checked. The epithelium should not be rolled in, but should be everted outward (**Fig. 5.3c**).

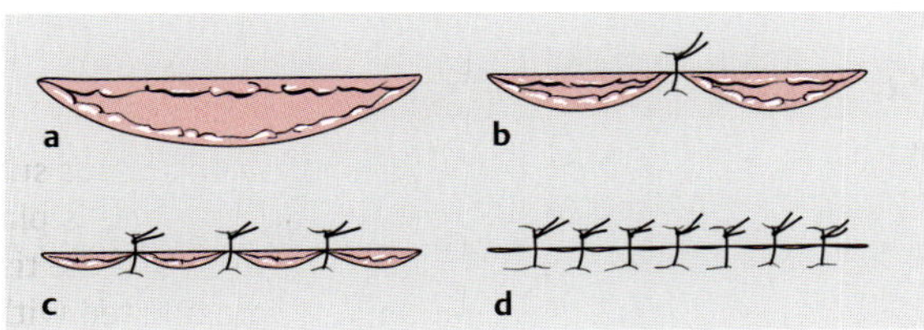

Fig. 5.4a–d Equalizing wound edges of differing lengths by "halving" (for differences in length up to ca. 5 mm).
a Short upper and long lower wound edge.
b First suture placed in the middle of the wound.
c Two further sutures, each at half the distance.
d Further sutures, each in the middle, distribute the excess skin equally along the whole length of the wound.

Special Suture Techniques

Subcuticular Suture

Surgical Principle

The special advantage of this suture is that usually only one entry and one exit hole are required. This avoids epithelialization of the puncture holes, especially in areas where the skin is rich in sebaceous glands.

Surgical Technique (Fig. 5.7)

The needle first enters the skin near one extremity of the wound and exits in the wound intradermally. The suture is then passed in a horizontal dermal plane at exactly the same level on alternating sides of the wound to the far end. The needle then exits the skin at the far end of the wound. The approximation of the wound edges is achieved by mild traction on the suture ends, which are then secured with sterile surgical tape to avoid inadvertent removal.

Rules, Tips, and Tricks

- This technique should only be used for wound surfaces which are well adapted at the subcutaneous level.

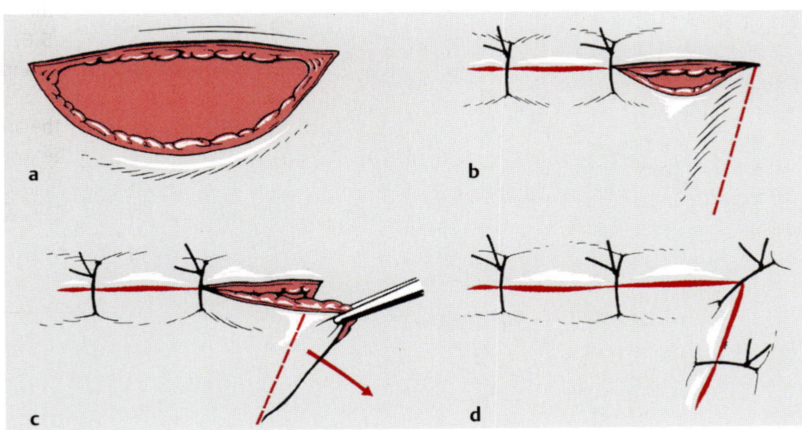

Fig. 5.5a–d Excision of a Burrow triangle (dog-ear) for differences in length >5 mm.
a Initial situation.
b Planning an auxiliary incision (broken line).
c Shortening the lower wound edge by creating an equilateral triangle and excision of the overlapping area of skin.
d Wound closure.

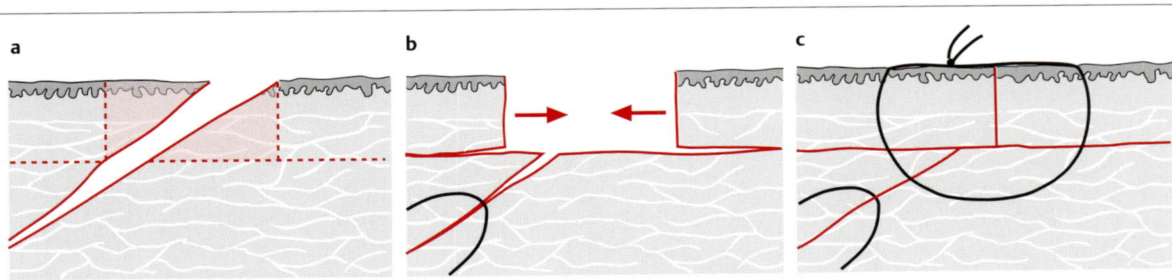

Fig. 5.6a–c Equalizing wound edges of unequal height.
a Oblique course of a laceration with a shorter and a longer wound surface. The parts of skin to be excised are marked, as is the area for undermining along the plane of subcutaneous fatty tissue.
b Closure of the subcutaneous wound and central advancement of the mobilized wound margins.
c Wound closure.

- Good results are achieved above all in sites where the suture line lies in a natural skin line (e. g., a neck crease).
- With longer wounds, bring the suture out once though the skin after approximately 3–4 cm. If necessary, repeat after the same distance (removal of the suture is thus considerably facilitated).
- Longer suture lines with a potential risk of wound infection should be secured by transcutaneous interrupted sutures (the whole suture line will then not need to be opened up should fluid collection develop).
- This suture is less suitable for wounds with a significant curvilinear course, which would result in distortions.

Vertical Mattress Suture (Donati Suture)

Surgical Principle

The advantage of the mattress suture is its safer re-approximation of wound edges with different depths, e. g., at the alar base or the nasolabial region. This suture everts the wound edges and helps avoid “furrowlike” scar formation (e. g., on the lip, see **Fig. 5.38b**). It also gives the suture additional stability.

Surgical Technique (Fig. 5.8)

The suture is inserted perpendicularly approximately 4 mm from the wound edge, carried down to the subcutis and then brought out of the wound on the opposite side at the same distance from the cut edge. It is then reinserted as a mattress suture 1 mm from the wound edge and passed intradermally across to the opposite side, where it is again brought out at the same distance from the wound edge. The stitch is pulled just tight enough to evert the wound edges slightly.

Rules, Tips, and Tricks

Each one of these sutures can result in the production of four stitch marks. This technique should therefore only be used in the facial region when absolutely necessary. As an alternative, a modified half-buried (Allgöwer) mattress suture can be used (**Fig. 5.9**).

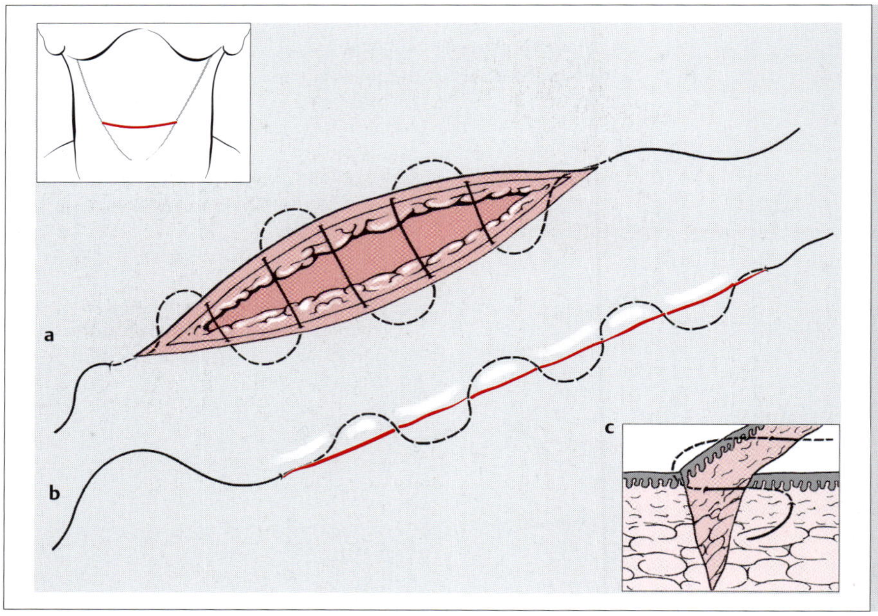

Fig. 5.7a–c Subcuticular suture (e. g., horizontal neck wound).
a Running subcuticular suture.
b Approximation of the wound edges after pulling tight the ends of the suture.
c Course of the suture within the level of the dermis.

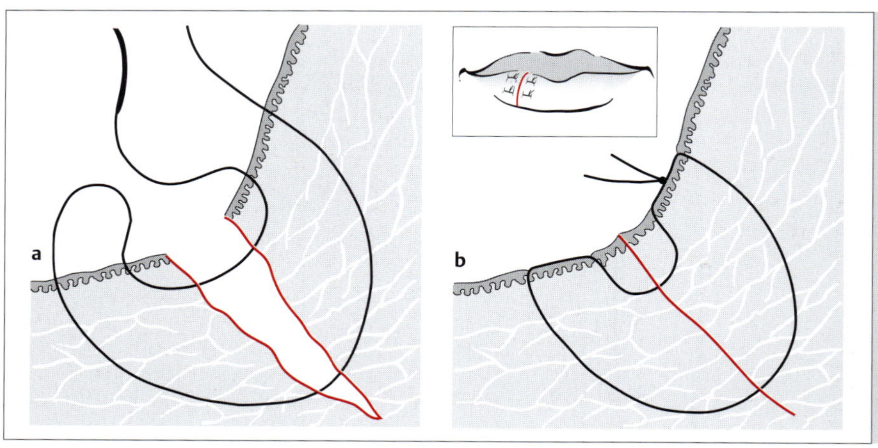

Fig. 5.8a, b Vertical mattress suture (e. g., lower-lip wound).
a Commence with entry and exit sites away from the wound (far–far technique) and continue with subcutaneous passage of the suture. The depths of the entry and exit holes must be equal.
b Wound closure.

Continuous (Running) Suture

Surgical Principle

The area of usage of this suture corresponds to that of the interrupted suture, but it can be sewn faster with longer wounds. Good results can be expected above all in areas of thin and readily mobile skin with few sebaceous glands. The eyelids in particular, and the skin of older people in general, have these properties.

Surgical Technique (Fig. 5.10)

After an interrupted suture has been placed and tightened, the thread is not cut but continued diagonally to the direction of the wound. Entry and exit holes lie exactly opposite one another. In the subcutaneous tissue, entry and exit passage must be made at exactly the same distance from the skin surface. Finally a knot is tied, as with an interrupted suture.

Rules, Tips, and Tricks

The end of the suture should be held under slight tension by an assistant. On completion, the wound edges should be checked and, if necessary, everted.
Unlike the intracutaneous suture, this suture technique is also suitable for curvilinear wounds, in which case the stitches should be placed closer together.

Management of Soft-Tissue Injuries and Their Sequelae

Primary Management

The primary management of soft-tissue injuries of the face is decisive for later results. Wounds that are not adequately treated at this stage can be corrected later only with much time and effort, and then only to a limited degree.

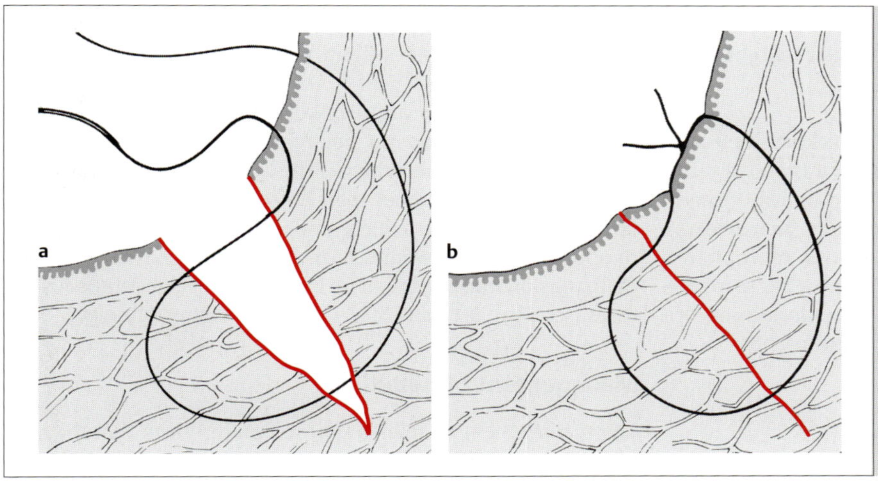

Fig. 5.9a, b Half-buried vertical mattress suture (Allgöwer stitch).
a The entry point is away from the wound, the suture passes in the depths of the wound to make an intracutaneous exit on the opposite side of the wound. Crossing back to the original side, the entry site is at the same intracutaneous level with a near exit site.
b Wound closure.

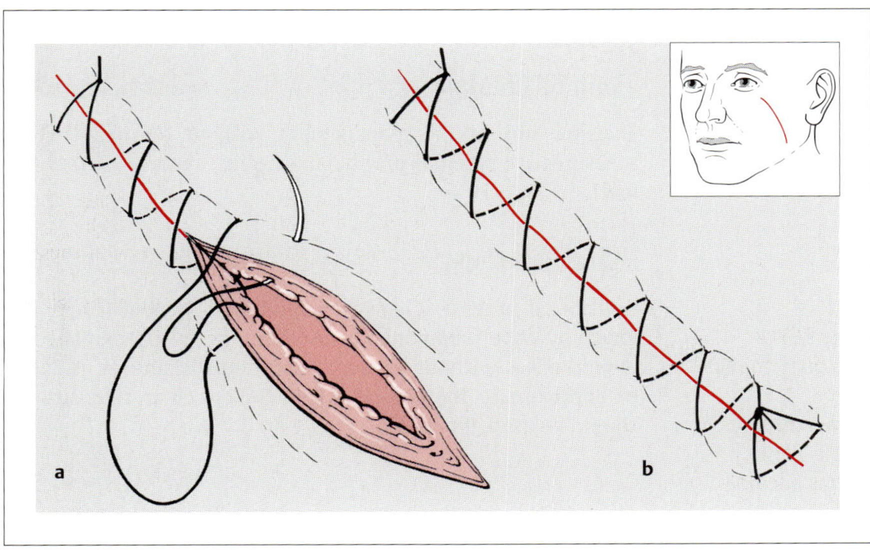

Fig. 5.10a, b Simple continuous over-and-over or running suture (e. g., cheek wound along RSTL).
a Passage of the suture after knotting at one end of the wound. Entry and exit sites are the same distance from the wound edge. The stitches are the same distance apart.
b Wound closure after knotting with the formation of a suture loop. Three suture ends remain after cutting the thread.

Diagnostic investigations (radiography, any required assessment by surgeons, neurosurgeons, ophthalmologists, maxillofacial surgeons, and others) must have been completed before any surgical treatment is undertaken, to enable management priorities to be set. Local wound management is the initial treatment for nonurgent bony injuries of the skull; the treatment of the fracture itself is undertaken at a later stage after swelling has resolved.

Primary Management of Facial Injuries

- Ensure adequate tetanus immunization.
- Check wounds for foreign bodies, consider cleansing and irrigation with physiological saline or hydrogen peroxide; remove embedded foreign bodies ("dirt tattoos") with a brush.
- Make conservative use of bipolar coagulation.
- Sparingly straighten any jagged wound edges, conservative skin excision (*no* formal wound excision).
- Re-approximate superficially avulsed epithelium with fibrin glue in a mosaic fashion.
- When faced with full-thickness defects, do not insert any sutures under tension (apply plastic reconstructive measures using transposition flaps from the adjacent area).
- Accurate suturing is essential in the region of the mucocutaneous junctions of skin and mucosa (free alar margin, lip, eyelid margin).

With *dog-bite injuries* there are usually full-thickness defects, commonly in the region of the tip of the nose. If it is only a gaping wound, then it may carefully cleaned and primarily closed in layers. Attempts should be made to reconstruct such defects early (within 24 hours after sterile dressing) with appropriate plastic reconstructive measures. Scar contracture after secondary healing requires generous excision and undermining of wound edges, which can enlarge the defect considerably.

Scar Revision

Scar revision may be indicated for functional reasons if severe contractures and distortions are present. In most cases, however, scar revision is indicated for cosmetically disturbing scars, which are not rendered invisible but may be made less conspicuous by surgical means.

Questions to Ask in the Preoperative Assessment of Scars

- Is it retracted, or thick and raised?
- Is it adherent to the undersurface, or mobile?
- What is the position of the scar relative to the RSTL?
- Is there distortion of adjacent tissue or functional impairment?
- How old is the patient? (There is a risk of hypertrophic scars or keloid formation in children and adolescents.)
- How "mature" is the scar? (Only a scar that has become pale is ready for revision.)

Hypertrophic scars develop as a result of increased skin tension. A scar that does not run along the RSTL, or the increased retraction of wounds in children and adolescents, can cause an increased production of collagen, resulting in reddish, lumpy scars that lie above skin level but do not extend beyond the boundaries of the original wound.

Keloids, on the other hand, are genuine neoplasms, which extend laterally beyond the boundaries of the original wound and into healthy tissue. They are more common in adolescents and dark-skinned individuals. The tendency to form keloids is often inherited. Areas of predilection are, among others, the posterior surface of the ear and the neck region. Since inconspicuous scars, hypertrophic scars, and keloids can coexist in the same patient, the existence of a "normal scar" (e.g., an appendectomy scar) in a patient is no sure indication for the absence of a disposition to keloid formation.

Standard Operative Techniques for Scar Revision

Small *retracted scars*, e.g., acne scars, are either excised or the affected area of skin is subjected to abrasion using a suitable laser procedure (CO_2, Er:YAG).

Slightly raised scars of less than 2 cm in length are planed down using a high-speed (up to 50 000 rpm) rotating brush or with a diamond fraise (dermabrasion). The operation is performed under local anesthesia and may be repeated at 4- to 6-week intervals.

Hypertrophic scars are excised, together with a margin of healthy tissue, if they do not regress spontaneously within 1 year. Wound tension, which is the cause of the increased production of collagen, must then be reduced. As a rule, the adjacent tissue must be widely undermined to make it possible to approximate the wound edges under minimal tension. The main tension must be taken up by absorbable subcutaneous sutures (see **Figs. 5.11** and **5.12** for scar revision technique).

Management of Keloids

The management of keloids is problematic, given that they are neoplastic growths initiated by injury to the dermis. Any skin incision made for scar revision will therefore induce the formation of new keloid substance.

Surgical Principle

Excision and wound management without tension. Further measures are taken as prophylaxis against recurrence (see below).

Surgical Technique

Excision, if necessary leaving behind a fine keloid fringe, followed by wide subcutaneous undermining to approximate the wound edges without tension. Subcutaneous sutures are used to approximate the wound edges. Subcuticular skin sutures should be used, if possible.

Rules, Tips, and Tricks

Before any scar revision, hypertrophic scars and keloids must be strictly distinguished. Intralesional injection of the revised wound with a steroid crystal suspension, followed by weekly repeat injections, has proved effective for keloids. In addition, pressure dressings should be applied for as long as possible (depending on the affected region). Postoperative radiotherapy is not generally used nowadays for these mostly adolescent patients. Should the resulting defect after excision of the keloid be too large for primary suture closure, then it may also be resurfaced with a full-thickness skin graft. Retro-auricular keloids (e. g., after otoplasty) in particular may be treated with a skin graft harvested from the groin.

The indication for the revision of keloid scars should be made with extreme caution and the patient should not be encouraged to be too optimistic about the prospects of success.

W-plasty

Surgical Principle

Converting a linear scar into a zigzag shape distributes the tensile forces in the region of the scar so that the scar line is optically "broken up." With scars running perpendicular to the RSTL (e.g., scars in the region of the cheek, see **Fig. 5.11**), part of the newly formed scar is redirected in a parallel fashion. At the same time retracted scars are corrected by resection and undermining.

Indications

Linear course of the scar perpendicular to the RSTL, step-offs ("trap-door deformity").

Surgical Technique (Fig. 5.11)

- Under local anesthetic, the zigzag skin incisions are marked with a pen, ensuring that the lines of either side interdigitate.
- The previously marked skin is scored with a pointed scalpel blade (No. 11). Blurring of the ink marks is then of no consequence.
- The scar is then excised with the scalpel, producing vertical incisional edges down to the subdermis.
- The area should be generously undermined and adapting subcutaneous sutures placed.
- The triangular skin flaps are repaired with fine sutures (6/0).
- A pressure dressing is applied for 1 week.

Rules, Tips, and Tricks

The triangular skin flaps should not be cut too small and should be raised from unscarred skin. The area of undermining depends upon the resulting defect: it should at least equal the width of the defect on either side. This undermining of the skin is the simplest method for dealing with skin tension. A few skin sutures for approximation are helpful before placing the definitive skin suture, so as not to misjudge each corresponding flap and be left with a superfluous triangle of skin at the end.

Alternatives

Unlike the regular M- or W-shaped scar formation after W-plasties, the geometric broken-line technique results rather in a scar that is broken up and rendered less conspicuous. For this purpose the wound edges are excised in various geometric forms (triangles, squares, quadrangles) (**Fig. 5.12**).

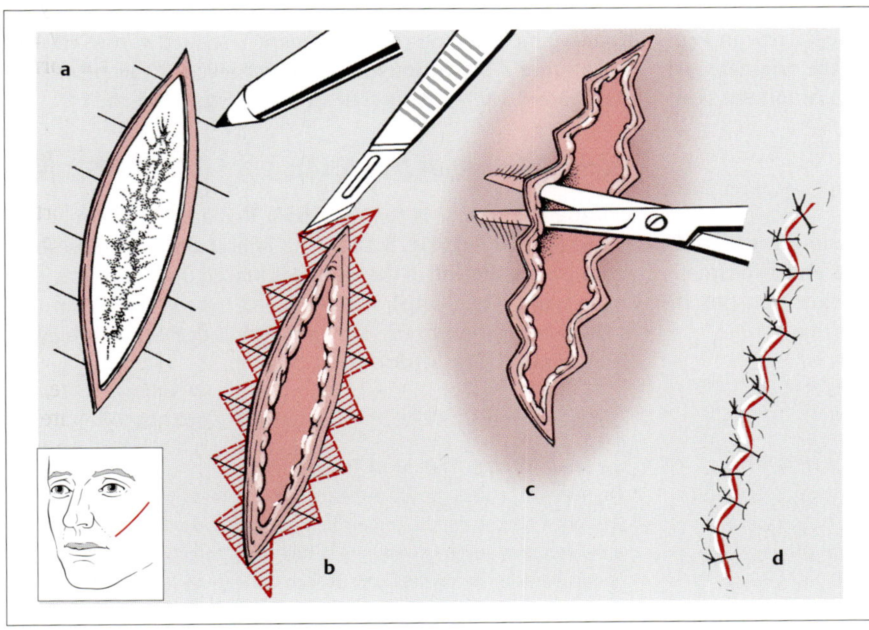

Fig. 5.11a–d Scar revision using W-plasty technique (e. g., cheek wound perpendicular to the RSTL).
a Elliptical incision around the contracted scar. Auxiliary lines indicate the tips of the zigzag line.
b The zigzag line is marked out and scored with the pointed scalpel. Note the incision along the wound edges where largely congruent surfaces are created. The scar has already been excised.
c Appearance after resection of the triangular areas. Undermining of the wound edges in the subcutaneous plane.
d Wound closure.

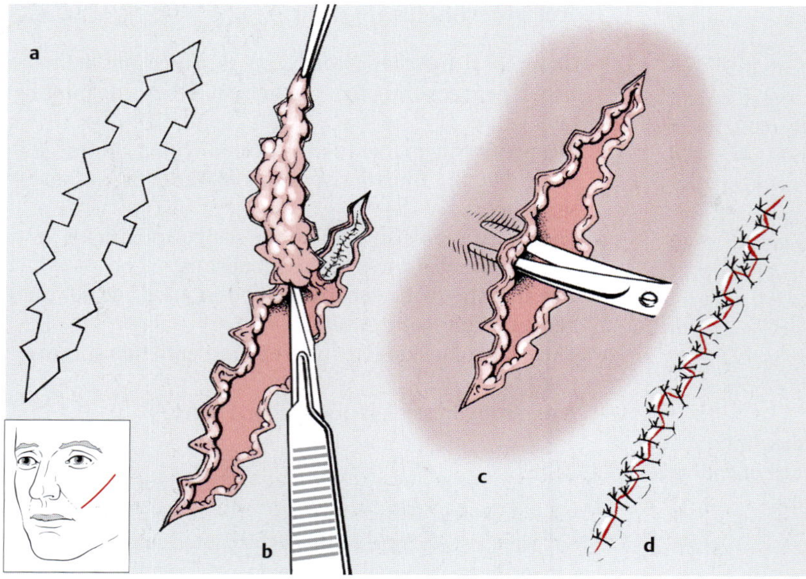

Fig. 5.12a–d Broken-line technique (e.g., cheek wound perpendicular to the RSTL).
a Marking the skin incision. Formation of identical geometric forms on either side of the scar (not mirror images).
b Excision of the marked skin areas down to the subdermis.
c Undermining of the wound edges.
d Wound closure.

Surgical Technique for Relieving Skin Tension

Z-plasty

Surgical Principle

A Z-plasty has three effects:

- Tension between the ends of the scar is relieved (a scar which is "too short" is lengthened).
- Two adjacent triangular skin flaps are exchanged.
- The original course of the scar is reorientated by up to 90°.

Indications

For any scar revision, it is above all the lengthening and transposition effect that is significant. The gain in length is achieved at the expense of the adjacent lateral tissue (see arrow in **Fig. 5.13**). Transposition is primarily desired when the original scar runs perpendicular to the RSTL (e.g., a vertical scar on the skin of the neck).

Surgical Technique (Fig. 5.13)

First, the existing scar is excised. Auxiliary incisions are placed to create lateral limbs at the end of the wounds and two triangles are elevated by undermining. The flaps are then transposed and inset by suturing in two layers.

Rules, Tips, and Tricks

- Maximal gain in length with reorientation of the scar by 90° is only achieved if the length of the lateral limbs corresponds to the length of the scar and they are at an angle of 60° to the scar (formation of equilateral triangles). If the course of the primary scar is different, preference should be given to a "multiple W-plasty").
- Undermining must be carried beyond the limits of the triangular flaps (shaded area in **Fig. 5.13a**) to allow suturing without tension.
- The mobility of the lateral skin should be taken into consideration when planning the operation (remember aesthetic units).
- The lateral limbs should lie more or less parallel to the prevailing RSTL.

V–Y Plasty

Surgical Principle

The technique achieves lengthening of the scar (without transposition) by linear advancement (e.g., ectropion of the lower eyelid, **Fig. 5.14**). The nomenclature comes from the initial V-shaped auxiliary incision and the subsequent Y-shaped suture closure. As with the Z-plasty, lengthening is achieved at the expense of the adjacent lateral tissue (see arrows in **Fig. 5.14a** and **c**).

Surgical Technique (Fig. 5.14)

Excision of the scar is followed by a V-shaped incision at one end of the wound (**Fig. 5.14a**). The lateral skin is undermined and the opposite end of the wound is placed under tension with a skin hook (**Fig. 5.14b**). The V-shaped incised flap is sutured in its new position to the lateral wound edges, thus achieving "lengthening" (**Fig. 5.14c**).

Rules, Tips, and Tricks

No new distortions should appear in the lateral regions of the wound; if necessary, the undermining should be extended. As with a Z-plasty, the auxiliary incisions should lie in the RSTL. Any resulting linear scars can be additionally broken up with a W-plasty.

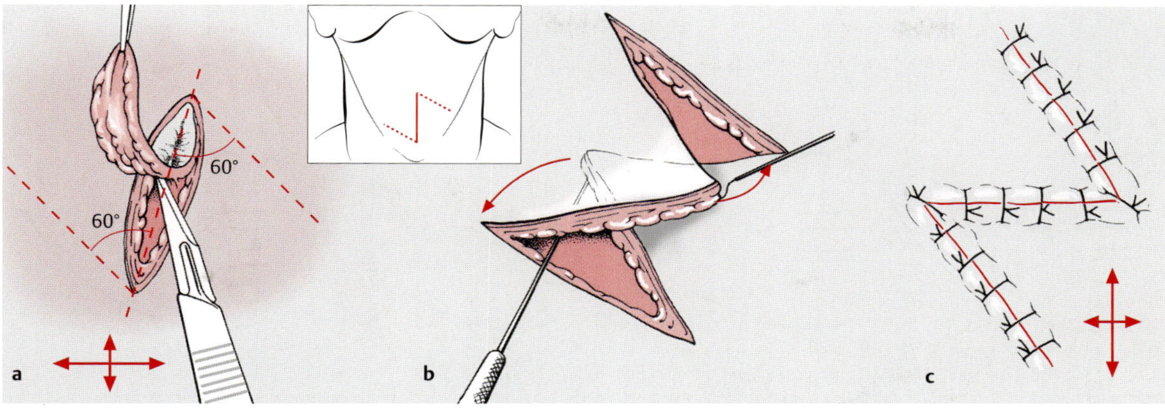

Fig. 5.13a–c Z-plasty (e.g., vertical scar on the neck).
a Scar excision; lateral limb incisions and area of skin undermining are marked.
b Transposition of the triangular areas of skin (generous undermining).
c Wound closure (crossed arrows indicate vertical lengthening at the expense of the adjacent lateral area.

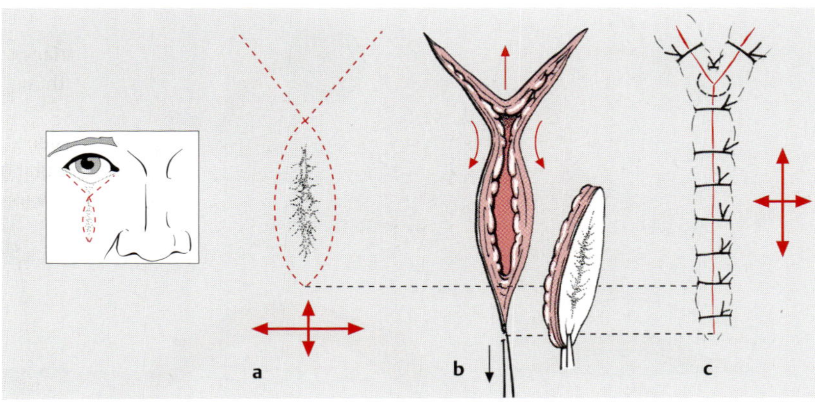

Fig. 5.14a–c V–Y plasty (e.g., ectropion of the lower eyelid caused by vertical scar contracture).
a Marking of the incision lines: elliptical incision around the scar, V-shaped auxiliary incision at one end of the wound.
b Resection of the scar area and undermining of the skin. The lower end of the wound is placed under tension.
c Y-shaped wound closure. The lengthening gained is marked by the dotted lines. (Crossed arrows indicate vertical lengthening at the expense of the adjacent lateral area.)

Scar Revision Techniques for Extensive and Adherent Scars

The simple excision and primary closure of *extensive scars* or other skin lesions (e.g., naevi) are often not possible. The resulting defect must then be resurfaced either with a flap or a skin graft (see below). Alternatively, the so-called *serial excision* technique may be employed (**Fig. 5.15**). This involves removing only a part of the area, with dimensions such that a primary wound closure is just about possible. This allows the skin lesion to be excised gradually in several sessions. Attention should be paid here to the *site* of the resulting scar, any potential *distortions* of the adjacent regions (e.g., the lower eyelid), and ensuring a sufficient interval between the individual excision sessions (2–3 months). Use of a subcutaneously inserted *tissue expander* can reduce the number of operations required.

Scars adherent to the undersurface cannot usually be closed directly after excision because of the lack of mobility of the adjacent skin. Here too, plastic reconstructive procedures using skin flaps or free grafts will be necessary. Because of their thickness, preference should be given to skin flaps to cover deep-seated defects.

Management of Soft-Tissue Defects

General Remarks

Soft-tissue defects can be managed with either *pedicle flaps* or *free grafts*. Pedicle flaps are attached to the adjacent tissue by a bridge of tissue, in which the feeding vessels run. They can also be freely transplanted when the *vascular pedicle* is connected to arteries and veins of the recipient site by microvascular anastomosis (vascular pedicle flaps). These flaps require a technically demanding procedure with a relatively long operating time, and are associated with an increased risk of flap necrosis. Usually other flap procedures are available to resurface defects of the head and neck region, which will achieve the desired result

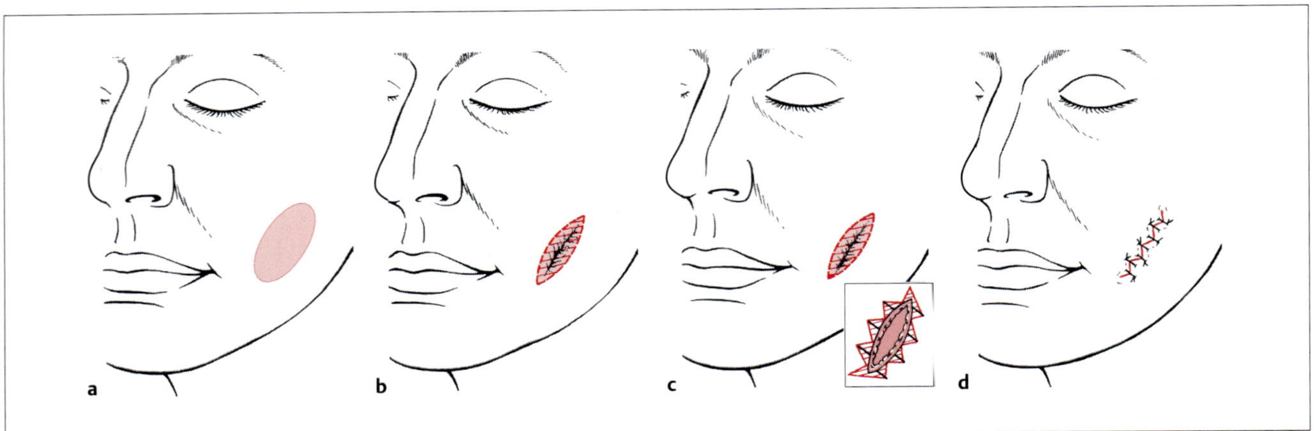

Fig. 5.15a–d Serial excision of an extensive skin lesion (e.g., naevus).
a Elliptical partial excision of the skin lesion and primary wound closure after undermining.
b Appearance of the residual lesion with a central scar. Elliptical incision is marked.
c Rearrangement of the wound edges with a W-plasty.
d Appearance after wound closure.

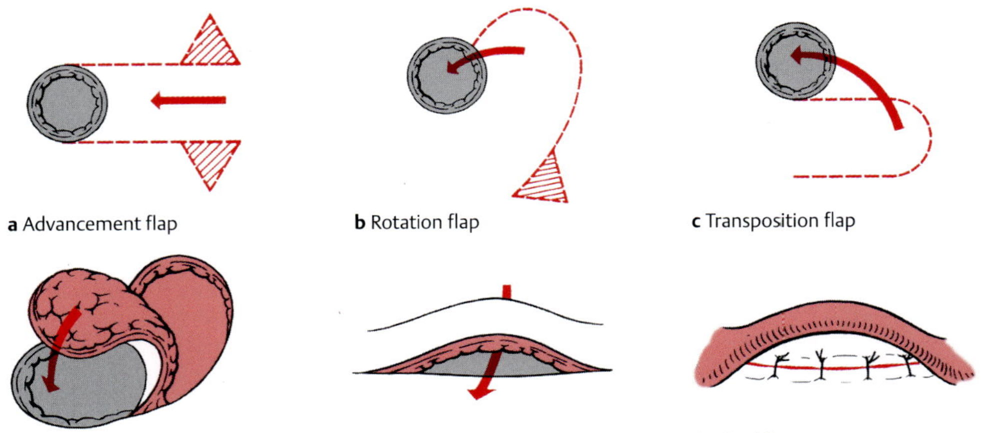

Fig. 5.16a–f Flaps with a continuous epithelial surface (see text).

with the greatest degree of safety. Because indications for their use in the facial region are limited, vascular pedicle flaps are not dealt with any further here.

Another possibility for facilitating the creation of skin flaps is to produce excess tissue in the vicinity of the defects by *skin expansion*; the excess skin created in this way is then recruited for the actual closure of the wound. For this purpose, silicone balloons are used as *tissue expanders*; they are implanted subcutaneously and connected to a port that also lies subcutaneously (see **Fig. 5.44a, b**). This port is punctured percutaneously and the balloon gradually filled with a physiological saline solution. The procedure requires a certain amount of preparation time and is not as easily employed in the region of the face as in other areas of the body.

Pedicle Flaps

Preliminary Remarks

Pedicle flaps are named according to the type of flap movement (linear advancement, rotation, transposition) and their pedicle. With regard to the pedicle. two groups are distinguished:

- Flaps with a continuous epithelial surface (**Fig. 5.16**).
- Flaps without a continuous epithelial surface (see **Figs. 5.22** and **5.23**).

In the following, a distinction will also be made within these two groups according to the type of flap movement.

Rules, Tips, and Tricks

Aspects regarding the planning of flaps:

- Size of the defect vs. size of the required flap (contracture causes a mobilized skin flap to become smaller).
- Vascular supply.
- Aesthetic unit of the donor site.
- The resulting scar (oriented according to the RSTL?).
- It is important to pay attention to the direction of the greatest gain in tissue length (line connecting the base of the flap and the furthest edge of the defect).

Size, Blood Supply, and Viability of Pedicle Flaps

As described above (p. 10), the skin is nourished by two different arterial systems. All over the body, the subdermal plexus is supplied by arteries of the subcutaneous layer. These are distributed randomly and allow the elevation of skin flaps of limited size (random pattern flaps). Since this type of flap needs to be nourished by the vessels in the remaining pedicle of tissue, they are dependent on a flap length-to-width ratio of 1:1. Because skin of the face has a better blood supply than other regions of the body, facial flaps may, however, be twice as long as they are wide (a length-to-width ratio of 2:1). This ratio can, however, only serve as a rough guide. The actual blood flow to the periphery of the flap depends on whether the perfusion pressure can overcome vascular resistance. This resistance may be high in a scarred or previously irradiated area, for example, so that widening the flap pedicle may indeed increase the number of afferent vessels, but not the perfusion pressure, because the feeding vessels belong to the same flow system.

If a random pattern flap is not large enough to cover a defect, its size may be enlarged by flap delay. For this purpose, the flap is initially incised and only partially (e.g., half) elevated. The flap is then reset. After 2–3 weeks the definitive flap elevation and transfer may be completed. However, scar formation will have already begun and this will limit the degree of modeling of the flap—it can no longer be so easily "folded." The delay phenomenon is not caused solely by an adjustment of the vessels in the flap pedicle to the interruption of the blood supply from the margins of the flap, or by an adaptation of the cells to oxygen deficiency; rather, it is due to a dilation of the shunt vessels caused by the autonomic nervous system. Flap delay is always recommended when the size of the flap exceeds a length-to-width ratio of 2:1, or if the skin is poorly vascularized.

Axial pattern flaps (arterial flaps) have a more extensive, defined arteriovenous system which allows a significant adjustment of the length-to-width ratio in favor of the length. These flaps are usually raised together with the subcutaneous fascia. The length of these flaps depends on the position of the feeding vessels, and the width depends on the dimensions of the defect to be resurfaced. In comparison with random pattern flaps, these flaps have the disadvantage of only being available in certain areas. Typical examples are the *paramedian forehead flap* (supratrochlear artery), the *cheek flap* (facial artery), the *temporal flap* (superficial temporal artery) and, as an important example of a pedicle flap from the chest region for covering defects in the region of the head and neck, the *deltopectoral flap* (branches of the internal mammary artery). Furthermore, these axial pattern flaps may be supplemented at their tip by a random pattern flap, resulting in flaps that receive their blood supply from two different systems.

The prerequisite for the successful coverage of a defect is the *viability* of the flap after its elevation. When the dimensions of the flap are borderline, as local conditions often dictate, additional risk factors, such as smoking, may put its viability at risk. This increased risk should be brought to the patient's attention. Pinpoint bleeding at the cut edges of a flap can be regarded as a sure sign of an adequate blood supply. Normal conditions prevail when, after a brief application of pressure to the flap, the skin first appears livid and then regains its normal color within seconds. The general information given in **Table 5.2** can of course only serve as a rough guide. If flap necrosis is anticipated, the flap should be immediately returned to the donor site, before a renewed transposition is undertaken after 3 weeks, thus taking advantage of the delay phenomenon.

Flaps with an Intact Epithelial Surface

Flaps of this type are summarized in **Fig. 5.16**.

Table 5.2 Assessment of flap viability

Color of the distal end of the flap	Time of assessment	Physiological substrate	Prognosis	Consequences
White	Immediately after mobilization of the flap	Reflex vasoconstriction	Viability not compromised	None
White	Ca. 30 min postoperatively	Capillaries empty of blood	Total or partial necrosis	Return flap to donor site
Livid	Up to approx. 24 h postoperatively	Low blood O_2	Limited viability	Re-assess after 24 h
Livid	>24 h postoperatively	Venous congestion	Total or partial necrosis expected	Return flap to donor site
Pink	30 min to 24 h postoperatively	Normal perfusion	Flap viable	None

Advancement Flap (Figs. 5.16 and 5.17)

The simplest type of linear skin advancement is the extensive undermining of the wound edges to close smaller, elliptical skin defects (**Fig. 5.17**). If there is a more significant degree of tension, then the contact area of the sutures may be enlarged by plastic disks or gauze pledgets (dental rolls) (**Fig. 5.18**). Advancement flaps which have been elevated on three sides (**Fig. 5.16a**) sometimes produce skin puckering or "dog-ears" at their base. These may be corrected by excising Burrow triangles (**Fig. 5.5**) or by Z-plasties. One special type is the V–Y plasty, which has already been discussed (**Fig. 5.14**).

Rotation Flap (Figs. 5.16b and 5.19)

This is the most commonly used type of flap. A prerequisite for its use is that the skin in the donor area must be sufficiently mobile to be able to cover the secondary defect primarily. Should the length of the flap be insufficient, then a limited extension can be achieved by a cutback. If the base of the flap becomes too narrow, however, there is a risk of flap necrosis.

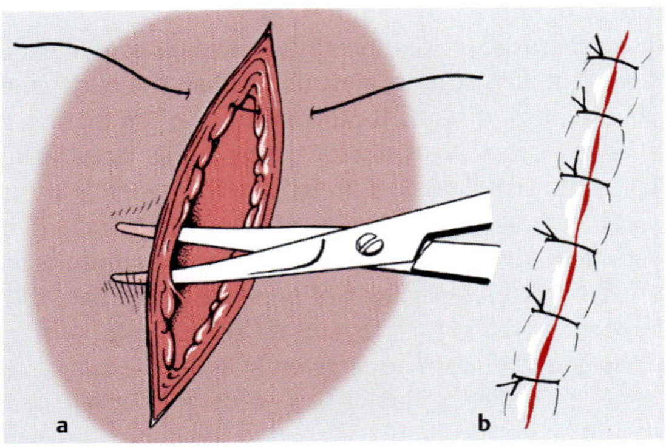

Fig. 5.17a, b Direct closure of an elliptical defect by skin advancement.
a Undermining of the skin around the elliptical defect. A deep suture has already been placed.
b Appearance after wound closure.

Special Forms

Rhomboid flaps are based on the geometrical concepts of Dufourmentel and Limberg, from whom they take their respective names. The planning and raising of the flaps are shown in **Fig. 5.20**. The following aspects should be borne in mind:

- A rhombus-shaped incision should be planned for the excision of skin lesions; with existing defects, consider the option of transforming them into a rhombus-shaped defect.
- The skin should be generously undermined.
- The RSTL and the direction of the greatest skin advancement should be taken into consideration.
- Rhomboid flaps are particularly suitable for donor sites with readily mobile skin (e.g., the cheek region).

Bilobed flaps consist of two flaps with a common base, with the first designed as a rotation flap and the second as a transposition flap (see below) (**Fig. 5.21**).

- The defect is first resurfaced with a rotation flap from an adjacent region with only poorly mobile skin.
- The resulting donor defect is covered with a transposition flap from a region with readily mobile skin.
- The elasticity of the skin is used to advantage: the first flap is slightly smaller than the defect, with the second flap being smaller again than the first.

Multiply lobed flaps are theoretically possible, but the option can usually be restricted to only two flaps. A typical usage is the resurfacing of a defect on the dorsum of the nose, with the primary flap recruited from the immediate vicinity and the second flap coming from the glabellar region.

Transposition Flap (Fig. 5.16c)

Transposition flaps have a partial bridge of tissue between recipient and donor site. The flap is swung into the defect across

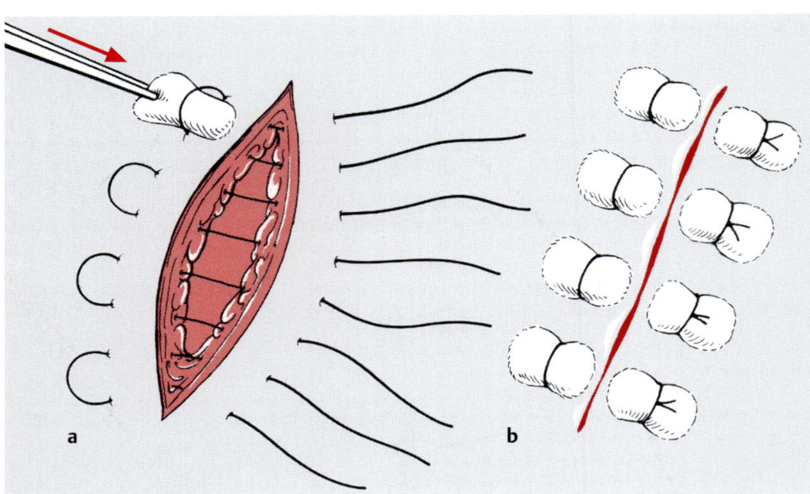

Fig. 5.18a, b Wound closure where the skin is under considerable tension.
a Strong U sutures are placed, with their contact area on the skin padded by dental rolls.
b Appearance after wound closure.

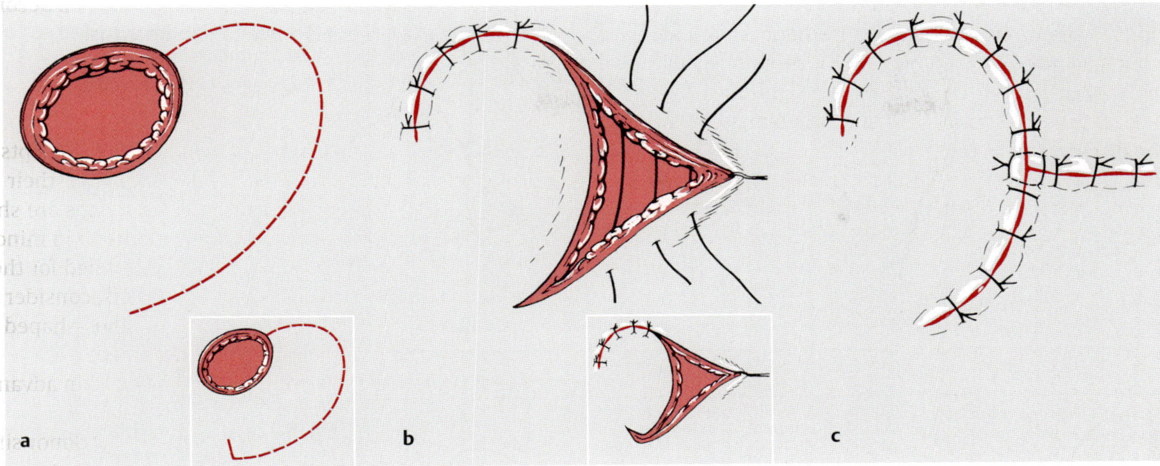

Fig. 5.19a–c Rotation flap.
a The skin flap immediately adjacent to the defect is marked. Inset: cutback made for localized lengthening of the flap pedicle.
b Flap is rotated into the defect. Sutures for closing the donor site have already been placed. Closure of the donor site is facilitated by elevating the corner of the wound with a skin hook inset.
c Appearance after wound closure.

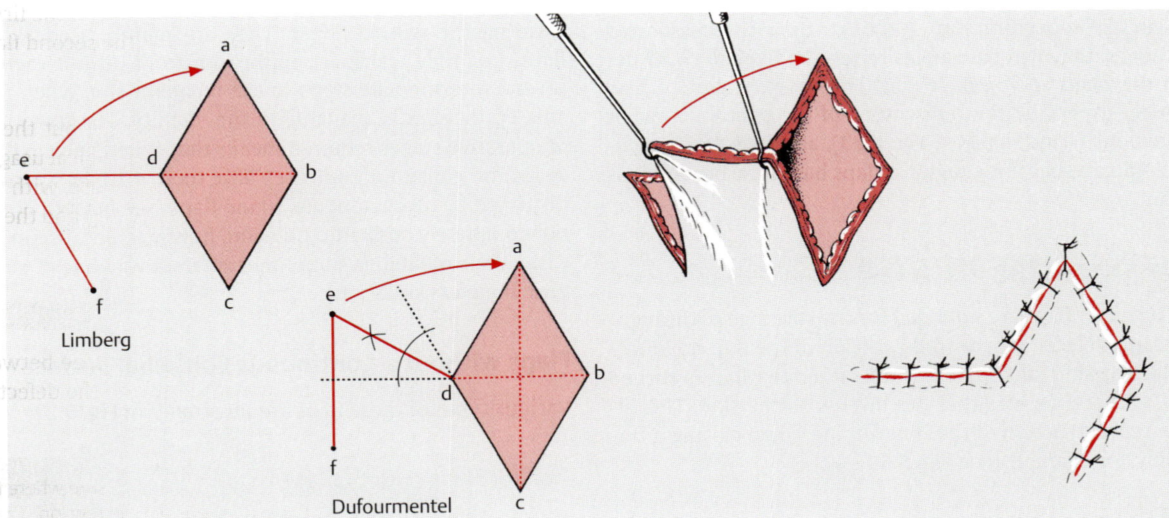

Fig. 5.20 Rhomboid flap for closure of a rhombus-shaped defect (abcd).
Limberg: The short diagonal b–d is extended; distance e–d = a–b; e–f parallel and equal to d–c.
Dufourmentel: d–e = Bisect the angle between the extension b–d and c–d; distance c–d = d–e; e–f parallel to a–c; distance e–f = c–d. Flap transposition and wound closure are identical for both techniques.

an intact surface of skin, so rotation of the pedicle by an angle of 90° or more is usually necessary. It should be kept in mind, however, that the more the flap is rotated the shorter it becomes. Because dog-ears may develop at the base of the flap, a second operation is often required for definitive management of the defect. The base of the flap may be contoured about 3 weeks after transposition by excision and thinning out. Transposition flaps are particularly suitable for resurfacing defects in the region of the nose (nasolabial flap, paramedian forehead flap, see **Fig. 5.36**).

The Z-plasty, a further example of a transposition flap, has already been mentioned (see **Fig. 5.13**).

Apart from these local transposition flaps, there are also regional flaps. The best known are Conley's chest flap and

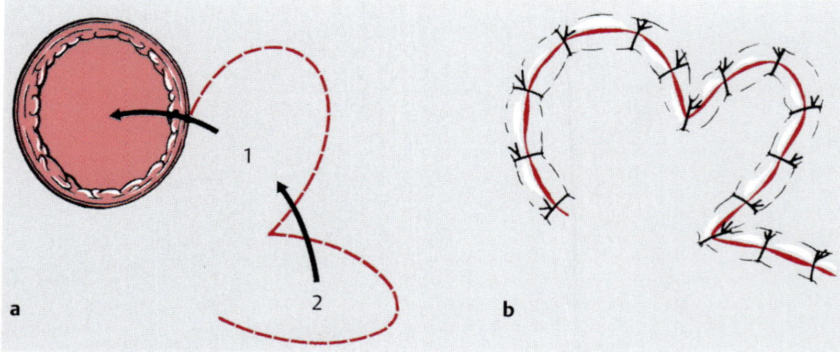

Fig. 5.21a, b Bilobed flap.
a The flaps 1 and 2 are marked out with different dimensions.
b Appearance after wound closure.

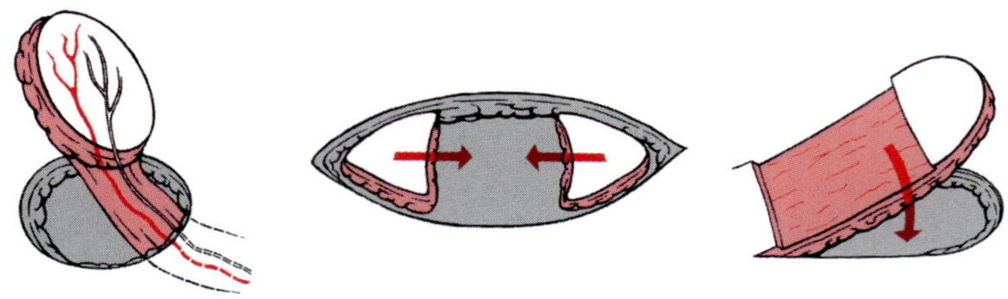

Fig. 5.22a–c Flaps without a continuous epithelial surface (see text).
a Island pedicle flap.
b Subcutaneous pedicle flap.
c De-epithelialized flap.

Bakamjian's deltopectoral flap. Although their base is located in the thorax, they can be used as long axial flaps to cover defects in the head and neck region. The development of new techniques—especially the rediscovery of the pectoralis major myocutaneous island flap (see **Fig. 5.23**), and free microvascular flaps—means that these regional flaps have now become less important.

Hinged Turnover Flap (Fig. 5.16d)

Hinged turnover flaps are intended for the coverage of through-and-through defects, where transposition of the flap no longer takes place at skin surface level, but rather the flap is turned over 180° around an axis that lies level with the skin. This allows the reconstruction of the inner lining when closing a tracheostomy, for example (see **Fig. 5.50**).

Bipedicled Flap (Fig. 5.16e)

Bipedicled flaps are now rarely used and are mentioned here only for completeness. The bilateral blood supply means that relatively long flaps may be raised, which can consequently overcome longer distances. The disadvantages, however, are the need for several operative sessions and the unfavorable scars, particularly in the area of the donor site. The temporary formation of a bipedicled flap is used together with a dislocation technique for exposure of the alar cartilage or the mucosal flap repair to close septal perforations (see Chapter 6).

Tubed Pedicle Flap (Fig. 5.16f)

Tubed pedicle flaps are initially raised as bipedicled flaps, but are then epithelialized on their undersurface by rolling in and suturing the wound edges. They are mainly used as distant flaps, i.e., they transport epithelium from distant regions via several intermediate steps to the recipient site, when no suitable epithelium is available in the vicinity. The large number of operative stages required means that tubed pedicle flaps are very time-consuming and they have therefore been more or less displaced by myocutaneous island flaps (see below). They have not completely sunk into oblivion, however, because in special cases their reliability sometimes offers a way out of an otherwise hopeless situation.

Flaps without a Continuous Epithelial Surface

Various types of these flaps are illustrated in **Fig. 5.22**.

Island Flaps (Fig. 5.22a)

These consist of an area of skin (island) corresponding to the size of the defect to be covered, and have a defined vascular pedicle. It is usual to leave a layer of connective tissue around the arteries and veins when dissecting the pedicle, to prevent injury to the vessels. These flaps usually have a longer feeding artery (e.g., supratrochlear artery, temporal artery, facial artery, see **Figs. 5.37** and **5.38**), which allows the formation of a long-segment pedicle, and consequently a longer reach.

Special Aspects of Island Flaps

- *Advantages* include the possibility of a one-stage approach and the avoidance of larger scars.
- One *disadvantage* is the prominence of the skin caused by the flap pedicle.

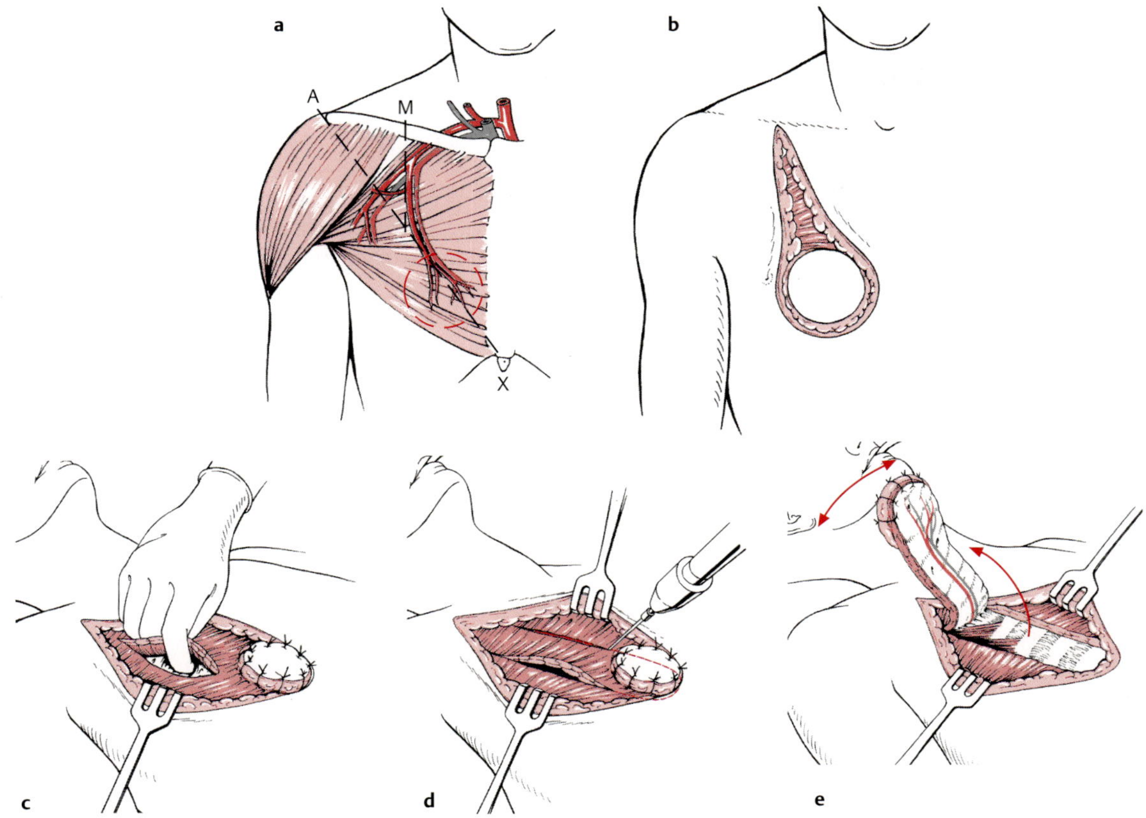

Fig. 5.23a–e Pectoralis major myocutaneous island flap.

a Concept of the flap and landmarks: acromion (A), xiphisternum (X), and midclavicular line (M) are marked. The skin island lies medial to the nipple. The thoracoacromial artery runs beneath the clavicle along the midclavicular line and then obliquely in a medial direction toward the xiphisternum.

b Skin incision commencing from the middle of the clavicle and extending around the skin island. Skin and fascia of the island are sutured together to avoid shearing movements. Pectoralis major has not yet been divided.

c Approximately 3 cm lateral to the assumed vascular pedicle, the pectoralis major muscle, together with its underlying fascia, is divided cranial to the skin island. The vascular pedicle can be dissected and palpated in the loose connective tissue.

d After identifying the vessels, the muscle is incised, together with the skin island by extending the medial muscle incision.

e The flap pedicle is mobilized as far as the clavicle. Pectoralis minor and the exposed ribs are visible. The arrow indicates the site of insertion for the skin island.

- Excessive restriction of blood flow to the flap by rotation or twisting of its pedicle is a *risk*.
- Dissection of the flap pedicle is *demanding and laborious*.

Special Form: Pectoralis Major Myocutaneous Island Flap

Surgical Principle

This flap consists of a skin island, the nutrient artery of which (the thoracoacromial artery) runs in or under a muscle pedicle (pectoralis major muscle). The flap pedicle therefore incorporates this muscle, and the size of the skin island can almost approach that of the palm of the hand. The donor site can be closed primarily.

Indications

The flap pedicle extends from the nipple to the clavicle and allows a large arc of action, reaching as far as the cheek region (**Fig. 5.23e**). Thus, for example, skin defects of the parotid region after radical parotidectomy can be treated, or defects of the floor of the mouth after tumor excision. The vascular supply of this flap is very good, allowing it also to be used for defects in irradiated areas. Because of its size, the flap is well suited for resurfacing larger defects, including full-thickness perforation defects of skin and mucosa, as well as for soft-tissue volume replacement (floor of the mouth, tongue). The very thick and muscular flap pedicle is a disadvantage and needs to be rotated at the clavicle at one level (when using the skin for an internal lining) or even at two levels (when used for external coverage of a defect).

Surgical Technique (Fig. 5.23)

- The course of the thoracoacromial artery is marked out (connecting line between a point immediately medial to the acromion and the xiphisternum) (**Fig. 5.23a**).
- The skin island medial to the nipple is marked (**Fig. 5.23a**).
- An incision is made around the skin island and the skin is divided over the vascular pedicle (alternatively, the muscle is exposed after mobilization of a deltopectoral flap) (**Fig. 5.23b**).
- After incision of the pectoralis major muscle by blunt dissection, the vascular pedicle is identified beneath the fascia (by palpation) (**Fig. 5.23c**).
- An incision is made around the muscle at the distal circumference of the skin island (the thoracoacromial artery runs between the undersurface of the pectoralis muscle and the fascia; inclusion of the fascia in the pedicle provides additional protection to the vessels).
- The muscle fascia is sutured to the skin margin (this avoids vascular damage by shear movements) (**Fig. 5.23c**).
- The muscle pedicle is dissected with division from the main muscle (preferably using an electric knife) approximately 3 cm lateral and medial to the palpable and visible vascular bundle (**Fig. 5.23d**).
- The flap is mobilized up to the clavicle (**Fig. 5.23e**).
- The arc of rotation includes the ipsilateral side of the neck and face (**Fig. 5.23e**).

Subcutaneous Pedicle Flaps (Fig. 5.22b)

Unlike island flaps, these flaps do not have a defined vascular pedicle and are supplied only via the subcutaneous tissue, which is dissected in two planes. They slide over the underlying tissue (sliding flap) and can close smaller defects in this way. An example of their use is the resurfacing of a defect in the region of the cavum conchae after the harvesting of a composite graft (Chapter 15).

De-epithelialized Flaps (Fig. 5.22c)

These are essentially transposition flaps, which are drawn through and under a skin bridge. The area lying beneath the bridge is de-epithelialized to avoid an additional second operative procedure (see Chapter 15). Because parts of the dermis remain at the base of the flap, it is possible for epithelial inclusion cysts to develop from any remaining skin appendages.

Free Skin Grafts

Preliminary Remarks

Skin grafts are freely transplanted tissue, have no feeding vascular pedicle, and consist only of skin, mucosa, fatty tissue, cartilage, bone, or similar tissues. A "composite graft" may be made of several types of tissue, such as cartilage and skin. Whereas the term "graft" refers to living tissue, "implants" are nonviable tissue, synthetic material, or similar substances. In everyday language, the term "transplant" is used without a clear distinction.

With firm material in particular (cartilage, bone, synthetic material and similar substances), a further distinction is made according to *origin*:

- Autograft = from the same individual.
- Allograft = from another individual of the same species.
- Xenograft = from another species.
- Alloplastic = inorganic.

Because grafts do not have their own blood supply, they depend upon the conditions prevailing at the recipient site for their nutrition. For the first 2 days they receive nutrients by diffusion; only after this phase does revascularization begin. After approximately 10 days the graft is firmly adherent to the recipient bed.

Special attention must be paid to the recipient site when planning free grafts. The basic requirement for successful grafting is a well-perfused wound bed, completely free of any infection. Fresh wounds are usually unsuitable for primary grafting, because the wound surface is uneven. Secondary coverage, after the formation of a flat layer of granulation tissue, is more favorable. Given that split-skin grafts are unable to level out depression, and full-thickness grafts and chondrocutaneous grafts (composite grafts) can do so only to a limited extent, deeper defects need to await the development of a sufficiently thick layer of granulation tissue.

The various skin grafts have their own specific properties, which need to be taken into account when planning the operation (**Table 5.3**).

Split-Thickness Skin Grafts (Fig. 5.24)

Split-thickness grafts are divided according to their thickness into *thin* (0.2–0.3 mm) and *thick* (0.4–0.5 mm) split-skin grafts. The thinner a graft is, the less demand it places on the blood supply of the recipient site. These grafts are harvested with the aid of a dermatome. A precondition for graft survival is good contact with the underlying surface. For this reason, split-thickness grafts should be scored in several places (to allow wound exsudate to drain) and should be secured to the wound surface with an appropriate dressing for 10 days (**Fig. 5.25**). The use of fibrin glue is helpful in obtaining good adaptation. The disadvantage of split skin is its tendency to contract, especially in the region of highly mobile skin. When split skin is used to cover periosteum, however, this effect is scarcely relevant. The grafted area can be enlarged threefold if the split skin is converted into a "meshed graft." For this purpose, the skin is passed over a foil through a cutting machine and transformed into a "skin net," which can be spread out much more widely than the original skin.

Donor sites suitable for providing split skin harvested with an electric dermatome are the inner and outer aspects of the thigh, the inner aspect of the upper arm, and the buttock.

Split skin is only rarely and exceptionally harvested from the face because of the unfavorable aesthetic results and the availability of other techniques. Split-thickness skin grafts are most

Table 5.3 Aspects to be considered when planning skin grafts

	Split-thickness graft	Full-thickness graft	Chondrocutaneous (composite) graft
Recipient site	• Heals even with poor vascular supply • Any defect size	• Good blood supply required • Any defect size	• Good blood supply required • Max. diameter of defect ca. 1.5 cm
Donor site	• Heals spontaneously • Possibly results in an area of scarring and discoloration	• Wound closure required • Scar usually inconspicuous • Size of the graft limited by the donor site	• Wound closure required (flap) • Scar usually inconspicuous
Properties of the graft	• Easier take • Contracts • Cosmesis usually unsatisfactory	• Takes well • Hardly contracts • Good cosmesis	• Takes in only ca. 80 % of cases • Hardly contracts • Good cosmesis

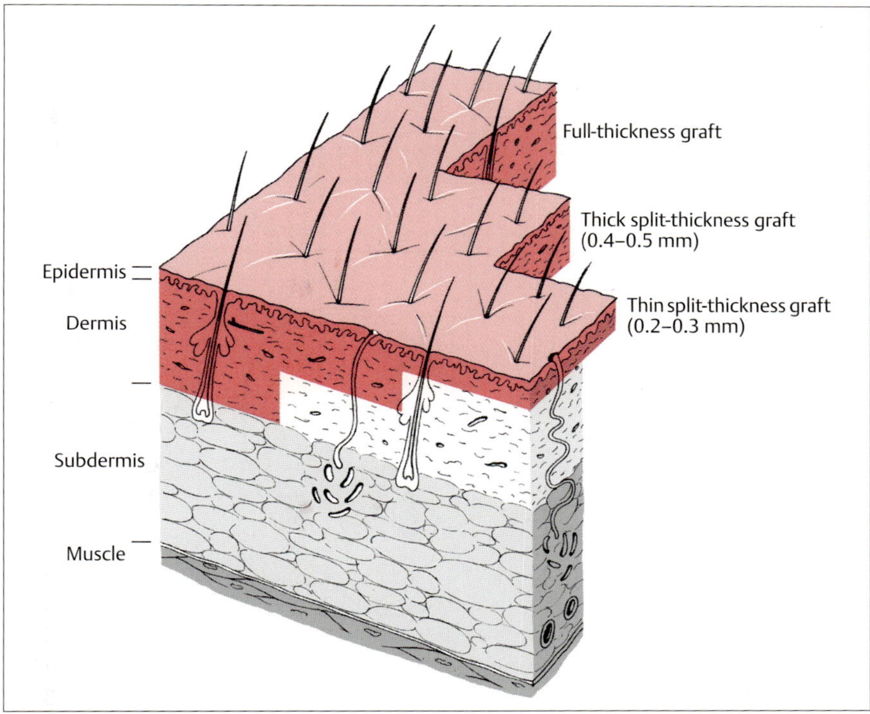

Fig. 5.24 Free skin grafts.

often used to epithelialize the auditory canal following the repair of stenoses.

Full-thickness Skin Grafts (Fig. 5.24)

Whereas split-thickness skin grafts include only sections of the epidermis and dermis, the *entire dermis* is used for full-thickness skin grafts. These grafts therefore have a thickness of around 1 mm. For its nutrition, the dermis must be in contact with the recipient site, so subcutaneous fat should not be left on the undersurface of the graft and must be carefully removed. This is best done by spreading the graft over a finger with the epidermis on the inside and cutting the fatty tissue away tangentially with curved scissors. Because of similarities in color and texture, the retroauricular, mastoid, and supraclavicular areas are particularly suitable as skin *donor sites* for the facial region. Smaller defects are often best managed with a strip of skin taken from the upper eyelid, especially in older patients. Regions that are more hidden (e. g., the retroauricular area) can be resurfaced with skin taken from the groin. Full-thickness skin grafts have only a slight tendency to contract and their thickness suits them for moderately deep-reaching defects. Because the donor site needs to be closed, the size of these grafts is limited above all by the possibility of mobilizing the skin to repair the donor site defect. The recipient area is managed in the same way as for split-thickness grafts (**Fig. 5.25**).

Composite Graft

A composite graft consists of different types of tissue. It is most often a *chondrocutaneous graft* (two- or three-layered) and less often a *chondromucosal graft* taken from the nasal septum. The cartilage component gives this graft its characteristic strength and form, making it particularly suitable for reconstructing

5

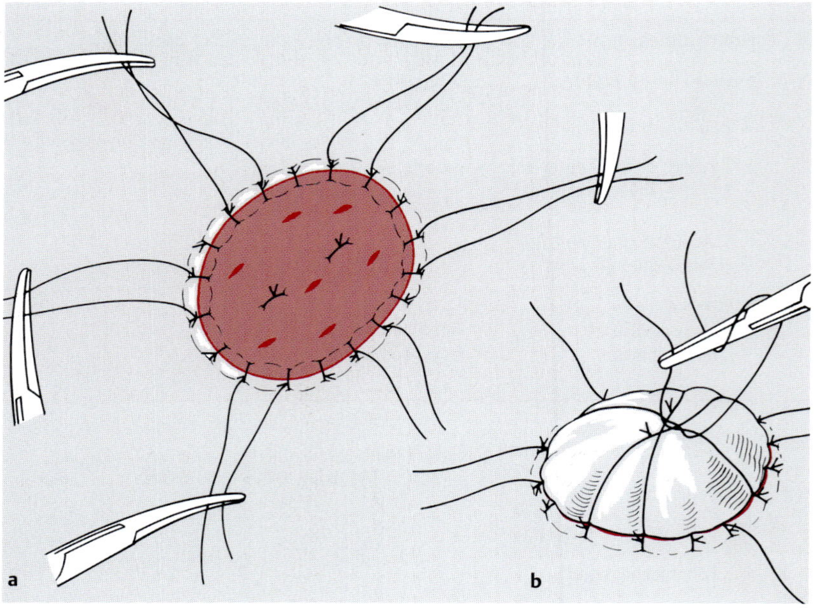

Fig. 5.25a, b Fixation of split-skin grafts.
a Split-skin graft is trimmed to size and sutured to the wound edge (needle is first passed through the graft and then through the wound edge). The sutures are left long at corresponding positions. Graft scored and quilted to the underlying wound bed with two deep sutures.
b After applying an ointment-impregnated mesh, the sutures that were left long are knotted over a gauze bolster.

complex structures. A composite graft, on the other hand, places special demands on the recipient site, because the attached cartilage prevents the skin or mucosa covering from having a broad contact with the underlying surface. The bradytrophic cartilaginous tissue tolerates this "deficient supply" well, whereas the epithelium is dependent on its nutrient supply coming from the wound edges. Since this contact surface is small, the size of a composite graft is limited to a maximum diameter of about 1.5 cm. Even when all precautions are taken, partial or total necrosis of the graft is not always avoidable (see **Table 5.3**).

The following aspects should be kept in mind:

- Maximum diameter of the graft approximately 1.5 cm.
- The skin or mucosa of the graft must not be crushed by forceps (this impairs nutrition by diffusion).
- The skin or mucosal component of the composite graft can contract (allow for this by forming overlapping skin/mucosa components).
- Even significant livid discoloration of the graft during the healing phase does not necessarily mean graft loss.

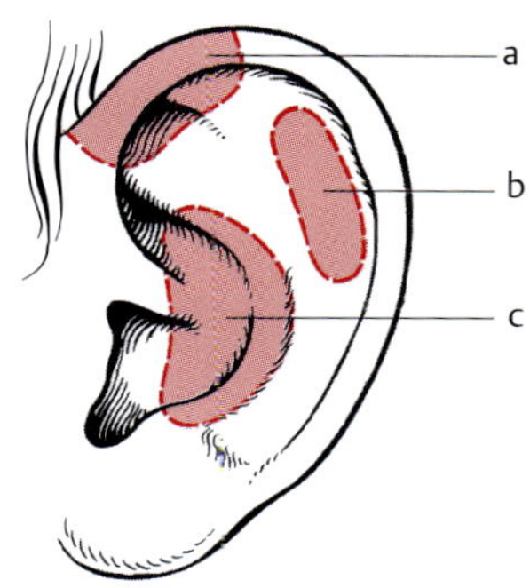

Fig. 5.26 Donor sites for chondrocutaneous composite grafts from the auricle (see text).

Figure 5.26 shows the most common donor sites for composite chondrocutaneous grafts from the auricle, which have the following properties:

- A graft with a *skin fold* (**Fig. 5.26a**) can be harvested from the anterior helical margin, e.g., for reconstruction of the nostril. The donor site on the auricle is repaired with a retroauricular pedicled transposition flap. The donor defect usually remains conspicuous.
- A *convex* graft, e.g., for the free alar margin, is taken from the antihelical fold (**Fig. 5.26b**). The resulting defect can be closed by undermining the skin, which leaves a slight residual deformity.
- Most commonly, a large chondrocutaneous graft is harvested from the concha (**Fig. 5.26c**). Depending on the required *concavity* of the surface, the graft is taken from the retroauricular or anterior surface. Management of the donor site after posterior harvesting is by direct suture, whereas closure after anterior harvesting is accomplished by a subcutaneous pedicle island flap. The technique is described in Chapter 15.

Plastic Reconstructive Operations in Various Regions of the Face

Preliminary Remarks

The operations described here can only be taken as examples of certain clinical constellations and represent only one of many options available for solving surgical problems. Since every case has its own peculiarities, an optimal therapeutic result can only be achieved with the knowledge of a broad spectrum of various techniques, allowing the surgeon to select the most favorable procedure for any individual case.

Forehead and Temple

The skin of the forehead has only a moderate degree of mobility. Thus, only defects of up to 3 cm in width can still be closed primarily after generous undermining, and suturing of the skin is only possible under tension. Round defects must first be converted by appropriate excision into elliptical wounds (**Fig. 5.27**). A W-shaped excision at the ends of the wound will reduce the surface of the required skin excision.

Defects of the frontotemporal region are managed with *rotation flaps*, with rhomboid flaps as described by Limberg and Dufourmentel being particularly suitable (**Fig. 5.28**).

Rules, Tips, and Tricks

Attention should be paid to the possible distortion of the eyebrows and eyelids when designing flaps in the forehead–temple region.

Full-thickness skin grafts survive on the forehead only when used to cover smaller defects, because of the reduced vascular supply of the galea aponeurotica, and *split-thickness grafts* are used only in exceptional cases because of their unfavorable cosmetic appearance.

Eyelids

Upper Eyelid

Minor distortions of the upper eyelid due to scars may be revised using V–Y or Z-plasties. Partial reconstruction of the upper eyelid may be accomplished by a *transposition flap* from the supraciliary region (**Fig. 5.29**). The upper eyelid is immobilized by temporarily closing the palpebral fissure with a suture. If the inner surface of the eyelid also needs reconstruction, then a *composite graft* taken from the septum may be used for full-thickness tarsoconjunctival repair.

Lower Eyelid

Narrow defects in the region of the lower eyelid are reconstructed with a *transposition flap* from the upper eyelid skin crease. This procedure is indicated where the upper eyelid shows age-related redundancy and for more laterally located defects. It leaves scarcely visible scars (**Fig. 5.30**). Larger and more medially situated defects which encroach on the cheek will require a *rotation flap* from the cheek (after Imre, **Fig. 5.31**). The base of the flap is located laterally and the incision is placed in the nasolabial fold to avoid conspicuous scars.

The following points should be observed when designing this flap:

- The laterally based flap must be raised strictly in the plane of the subcutaneous fatty tissue as otherwise there is a danger of injury to branches of the *facial nerve*.
- After rotation, the flap must be well secured with sutures to the bony undersurface (infraorbital rim) to avoid traction on the lower eyelid (danger of a *cicatricial ectropion*).
- *Excess skin* resulting from incongruities of the wound edges is compensated for either with a Z-plasty or by the excision of Burrow triangles.

As with the upper eyelid, full-thickness defects of the lower eyelid can also be reconstructed with chondromucosal grafts in the form of a full-thickness tarsoconjunctival repair. The lacrimal ducts must be kept in mind when dealing with defects of the medial canthal area.

Eyelid Surgery in Facial Paralysis

Paralysis of the orbicularis oculi muscle results in incomplete closure of the eyelid (lagophthalmus) and a loss of lower lid tone, with lower punctal ectropion and the danger of exposure keratitis from insufficient moisture to the corneal epithelium. Surgical management of this eyelid disorder is symptomatic: narrowing of the distance between upper and lower eyelid, i. e., *narrowing the palpebral fissure*, by tightening the lower eyelid and thus elevating the punctum after eyelid shortening.

Tarsorrhaphy (Fig. 5.32)

Upper and lower eyelids are incised vertically at their lateral margins and divided into a tarsoconjunctival and a musculocutaneous layer. After mobilization of the tarsoconjunctival layer of the upper eyelid using a vertical incision and excision of a corresponding part of the lower eyelid, the tarsus of the upper lid can be attached to the lower lid by a mattress suture. Additional tightening of the lower lid can be achieved by the excision of a lateral triangle. The skin edges are then re-approximated with sutures after adaptation of the wound surfaces.

Other plastic surgery procedures, such as a temporalis sling procedure, are also available to correct the sequelae of a facial palsy that is not merely transient. A simple method is the implantation of a metal weight into the upper eyelid, which closes the palpebral fissure passively; active opening is possible with the levator palpebrae (third cranial nerve, oculomotor nerve). Suitably shaped gold or platinum implants are secured onto the

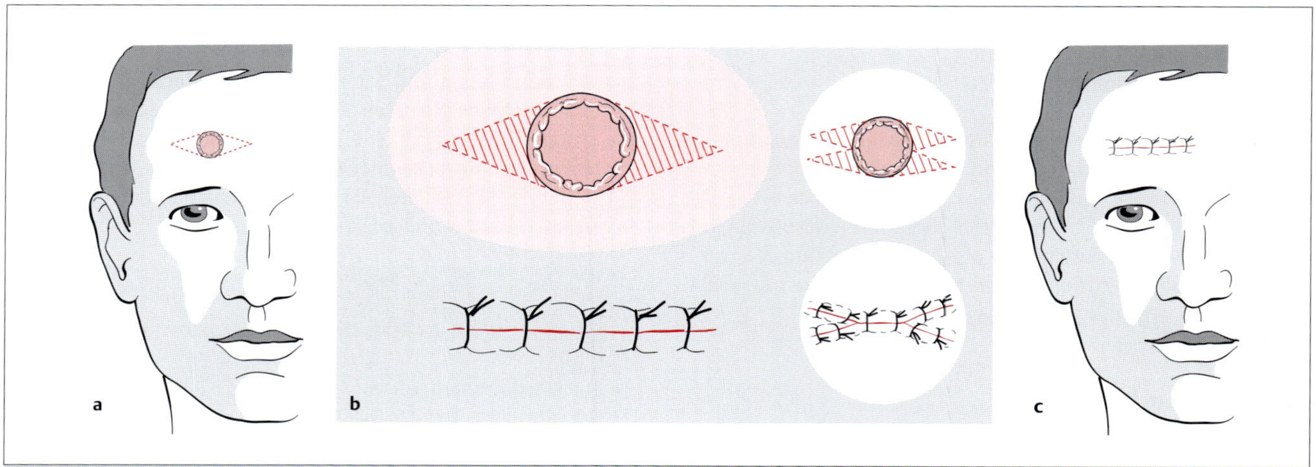

Fig. 5.27a–c Closure of a round defect after conversion into an elliptical defect (e.g., defect on the forehead).
a Elliptical excision of the defect and subcutaneous undermining.
b Modification of the ends of the defect by a W-shaped incision. This results in a shorter scar than after the elliptical excision.
c Appearance after wound closure.

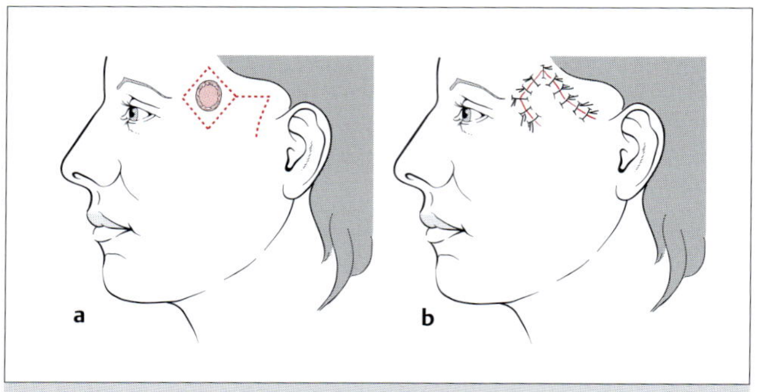

Fig. 5.28a, b Closure of a temporal defect with a rhomboid flap.
a Conversion of a round defect into rhombic defect by appropriate excision. The rhomboid flap is marked (see **Fig. 5.20** for planning).
b Appearance after wound closure. The donor defect closes itself almost automatically once the flap is transposed.

tarsus via a small skin incision. The disadvantage is that the effect of the weights is reduced on lying down, which may mean that it is still necessary to lubricate the eye at night.

Cheek

Because the skin of the cheek is highly mobile, smaller defects may be closed primarily after undermining the wound edges. The RSTL should be taken into consideration when planning incisions. *Rhomboid flaps* are also suitable in this region. For larger defects, particularly those situated medially at the junction with the nasal pyramid, an Esser *cheek rotation flap* is an option (**Fig. 5.33**). This flap is supplied by a broad caudal base. The incision line allows scars to be placed in a cosmetically favorable way in the infraorbital and pre-auricular regions. Here too, dissection must proceed strictly in the subcutaneous plane in order not to endanger branches of the facial nerve.

Medium-sized lateral cheek defects may be resurfaced with a medially based *bilobed flap* (**Fig. 5.34**). The inner lining for small perforating defects of the cheek is initially reconstructed with a *hinged turnover flap* to recruit external skin, after which the external defect is treated. Care should be taken here not to injure the excretory duct of the parotid gland (Stensen's duct). An injured duct should be reconstructed or re-implanted. More demanding reconstructive measures, e.g., using a pectoralis major myocutaneous island flap, are required for larger, full-thickness defects.

Nose

The aesthetic unit of the external nose is divided into several subunits, each requiring individual reconstruction (**Fig. 5.35**). This means that for defects involving several subunits, different management techniques should be planned for each individual subunit. In any one case, however, management will depend on the local conditions and above all on the aesthetic demands placed on the final outcome. Elderly people in particular tend to want a quick and less technically demanding reconstruction, in which case a free full-thickness skin graft could be perfectly adequate for defects that are not too large. Even healing by secondary intention is an alternative option in cases where distortions by scar formation are not to be expected. This danger arises more often on the alae and less over the dorsum of the nose.

The most important axial-pattern transposition flaps for partial reconstruction of the nose are the (para-)median or oblique forehead flap (supratrochlear artery) and the cranially or caudally based nasolabial flap (facial artery) (**Fig. 5.36**). The transposed skin of these flaps corresponds best in color and texture to the external skin of the nose. For full-thickness defects the best option is first to plan the reconstruction of the inner lining using tissue from the adjacent regions, and then to consider the options for the resulting larger skin defect. Using a

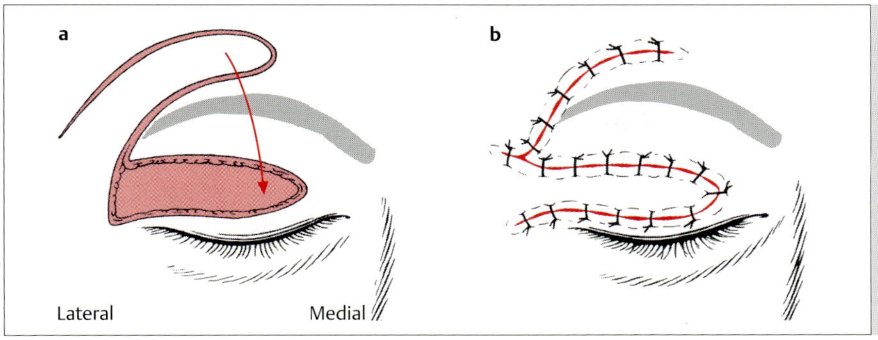

Fig. 5.29a, b Resurfacing a defect of the upper eyelid with a supraciliary transposition flap.
a Raising the flap after excising the area of skin to be replaced.
b Appearance after transposing and insetting the flap.

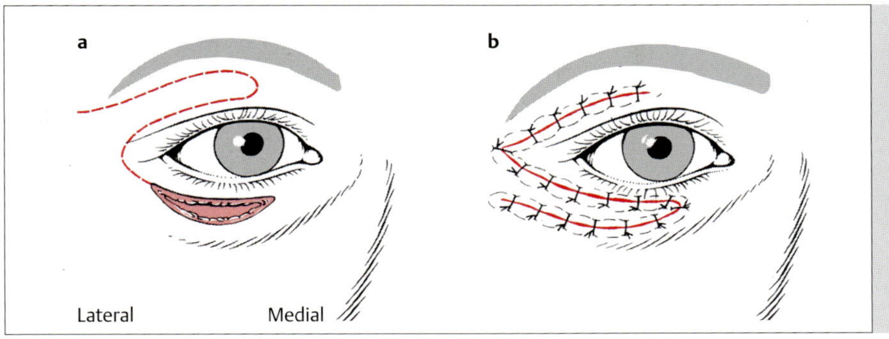

Fig. 5.30a, b Resurfacing a defect of the lateral lower lid with a transposition flap from the upper eyelid.
a Marking the lateral pedicle flap in the area of the upper-eyelid skin crease.
b Appearance after transposing and insetting the flap.

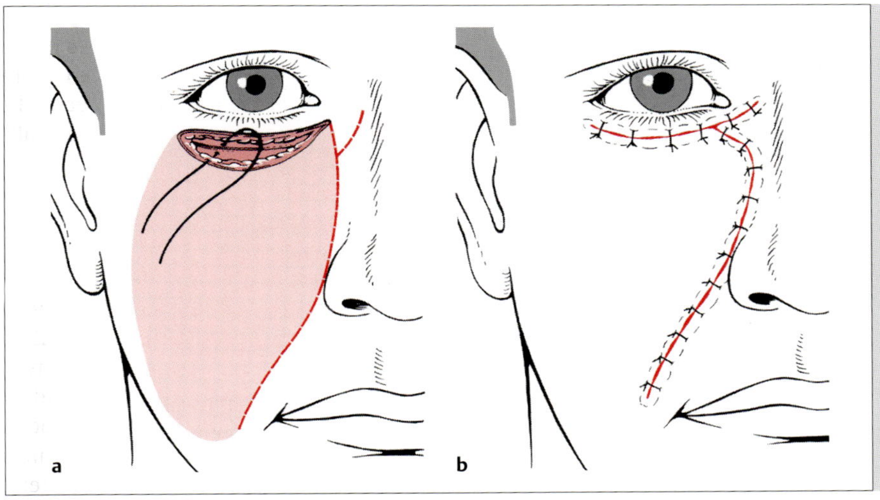

Fig. 5.31a, b Resurfacing an extensive defect of the lower eyelid with a rotation flap from the cheek.
a Raising the flap along the nasolabial fold with a relaxing incision at the level of the medial canthus. Wide undermining. Subcutaneous fixation of the flap to the bony undersurface (infraorbital rim) through a drill hole.
b Appearance after transposing and insetting the flap.

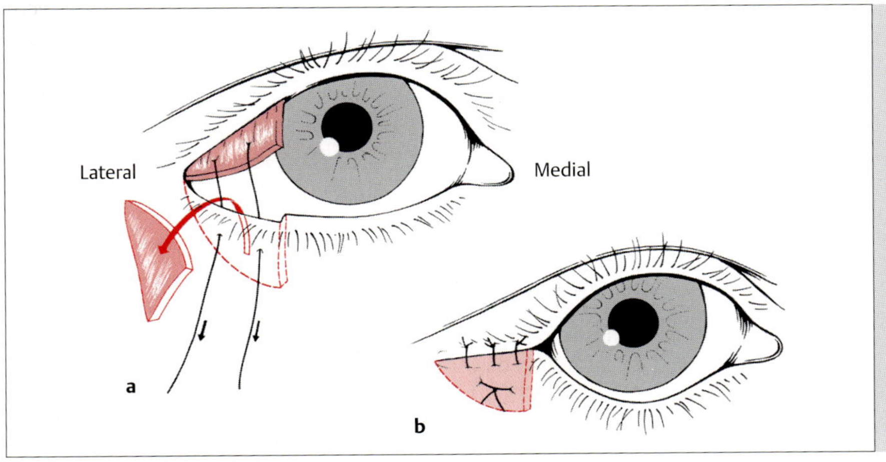

Fig. 5.32a, b Lateral tarsorrhaphy for lagophthalmos.
a Lateral separation of the upper and lower eyelids into their musculocutaneous and tarsoconjunctival layers. A vertical relaxing incision is made to transpose the tarsoconjunctival layer of the upper eyelid to the appropriately prepared defect of the lower eyelid.
b Fixation of the tarsoconjunctival component of the upper lid with mattress sutures. Skin sutures.

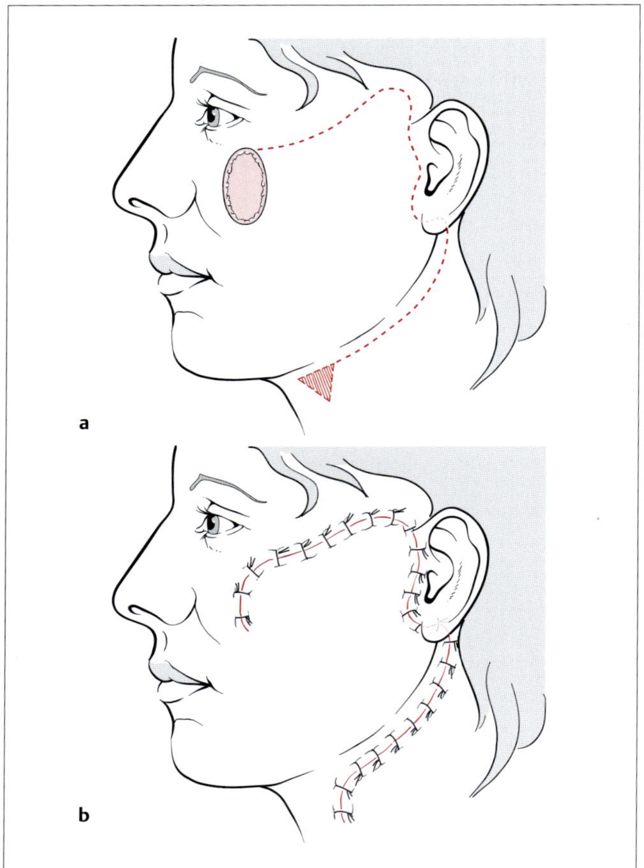

Fig. 5.33a, b Esser's cheek rotation flap to close a skin defect of the cheek.

a The flap is elevated with removal of a triangular area of skin at the base over the neck (Burrow triangle) to facilitate rotation. Care must be taken to extend the incision up to and behind the attachment of the ear. This diverts the traction to a cranial direction, thus avoiding ectropion of the lower eyelid.

b Appearance after rotation.

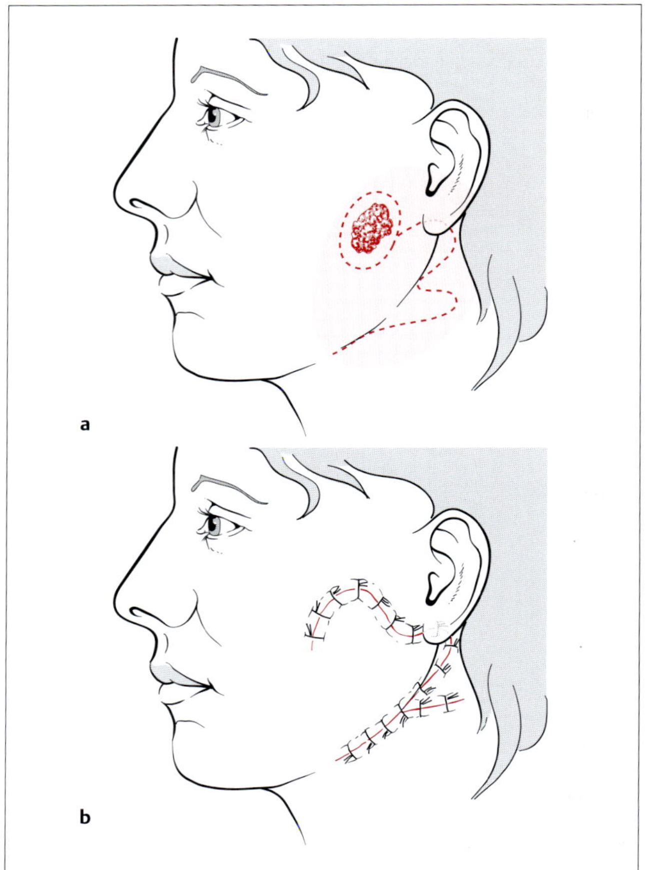

Fig. 5.34a, b Closure of a skin defect of the pre-auricular cheek with a bilobed flap.

a Circumferential incision of the tumor, elevation of the two flaps: a retro-auricular flap and one in the region of the neck. Extensive undermining (area marked).

b Appearance after insetting the flap.

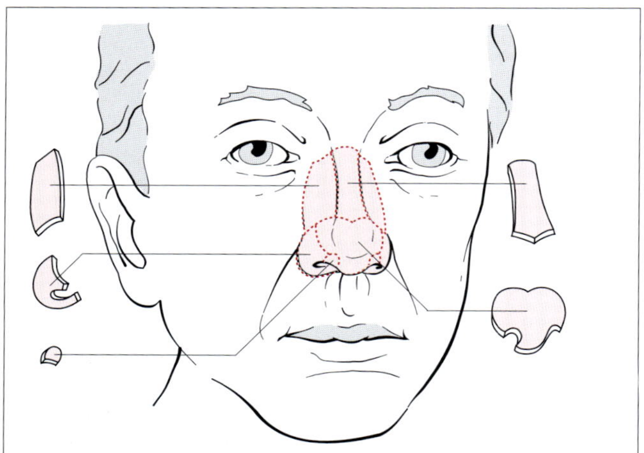

Fig. 5.35 Aesthetic subunits of the nose.
These subunits should be respected both during excision as well as during reconstruction. The unit formed by the tip of the nose and the columella is of particular importance for cosmesis.

template to measure the size of the defect is considerably more precise than relying on mere visual judgement (remember to calculate for skin contracture after excision at the donor site). Adequate flap length should also be considered: the greater the rotation of the pedicle of the transposition flap, the shorter the flap will become. Transposition under tension not only distorts the donor site bed but also endangers the vascular supply of the flap and its peripheral margins.

Management of Defects of the Nasal Dorsum and Lateral Sidewalls

Full-thickness skin grafts are effective in covering smaller defects, especially when the recipient site has a good blood supply. Island flaps from the forehead and cheek are also well suited, although their pedicles tend to elevate the skin tunnel (**Figs. 5.37** and **5.38**).

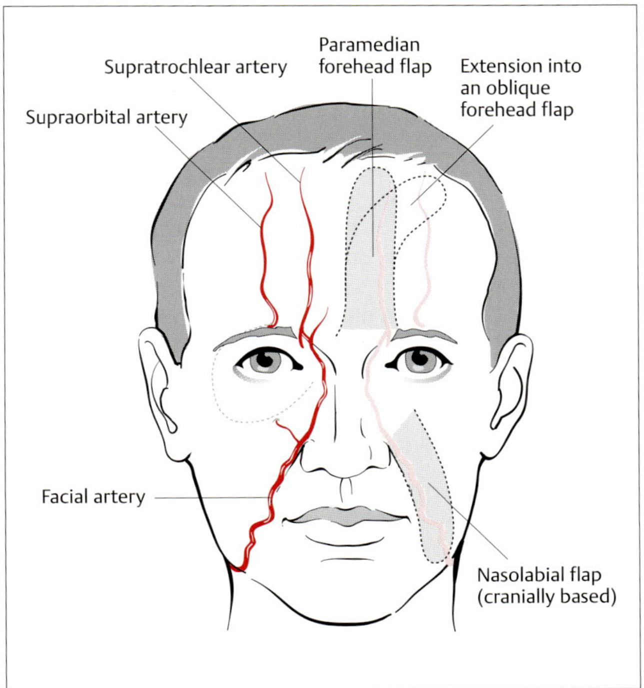

Fig. 5.36 Transposition flaps for reconstruction of the nose. The paramedian (oblique) forehead flap is based on the supratrochlear artery and is particularly suited for the dorsum of the nose, the tip and the columella. The nasolabial flap is based on the facial artery and is suited for the nostril and the inner lining of the nasal vestibule.

Skin defects in the region of the bony nasal pyramid and over the lateral side wall of the nose toward the medial canthus can be treated with a transposition–rotation flap from the glabellar region (**Fig. 5.39**).

Larger defects situated more caudally require the use of a (para-)*median forehead flap* (**Fig. 5.40**). If the lateral sidewall of the nose is also involved, it may be reconstructed independently as an aesthetic subunit using a cranially based nasolabial flap.

Midline Forehead Flap

Surgical Principle

This flap is supplied by the supratrochlear artery and can therefore be raised from the glabella to the hairline with a width of 3 cm. These unusually large dimensions are possible on account of its axial vascular supply.

Indications

Defects of the dorsum of the nose, the lateral sidewall of the nose and, as an oblique forehead flap, for reconstruction of the tip of the nose and the columella in particular.

Operative Planning

This applies to all types of flaps and is best approached systematically. The size and form of the donor site should be defined, as well as the required length and position of the "transport pedicle" to allow tension-free transposition:

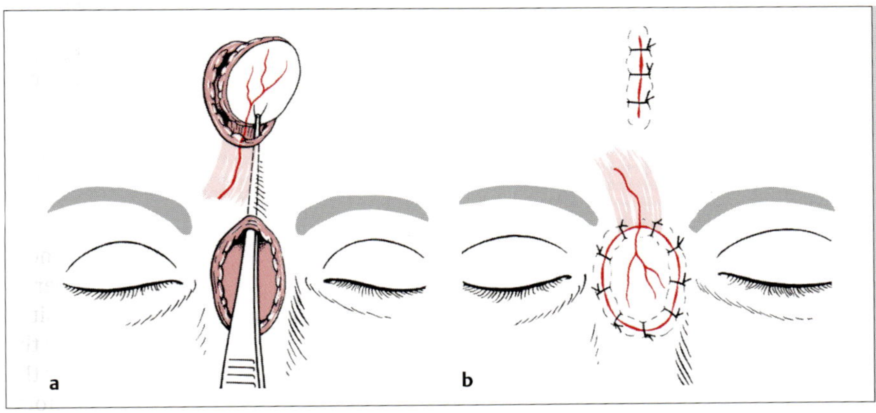

Fig. 5.37a, b Closure of a skin defect over the root of the nose with an island pedicle flap from the forehead.
- **a** The skin island is elevated, the subcutaneous pedicle of the flap is dissected together with the supratrochlear artery. A tunnel is formed to allow transposition of the skin island.
- **b** Appearance after transposition of the flap and wound closure.

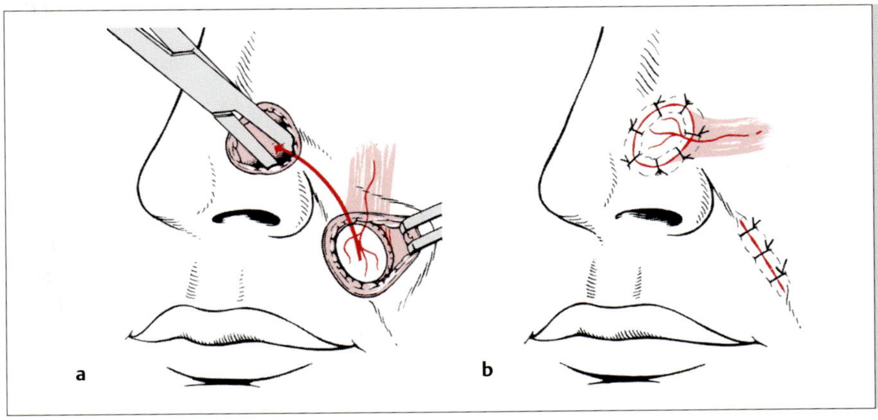

Fig. 5.38a, b Resurfacing a defect of the nostril with an island pedicle flap.
- **a** The skin island is incised in the region of the nasolabial fold and the flap pedicle and subcutaneous tunnel between the defect and the skin island are dissected.
- **b** Appearance after transposition of the flap and wound closure.

- The size and form of the defect are defined with the aid of a template (e.g., one made from the foil of a suture pack). The skin incision line should be kept approximately 2 mm away from the template to allow for contraction of the mobilized skin. The donor site should not cross the hairline. To be sure of recognizing the hairline, do not shave the hair but cut it short, if necessary.
- Once the paramedian position of the flap pedicle over the supratrochlear artery has been decided, the pivot point at the level of the eyebrows is then marked. Next, rotation of the flap is simulated using a strip of inelastic material (e.g., a roll of dressing gauze). It is important to ensure that the furthest wound edge of the donor site can reach the corresponding margin of the defect without tension. The greater this distance, the more obliquely the forehead flap must run in the direction of the lateral hairline of the forehead, and it must also be slightly curved (**Fig. 5.41**).

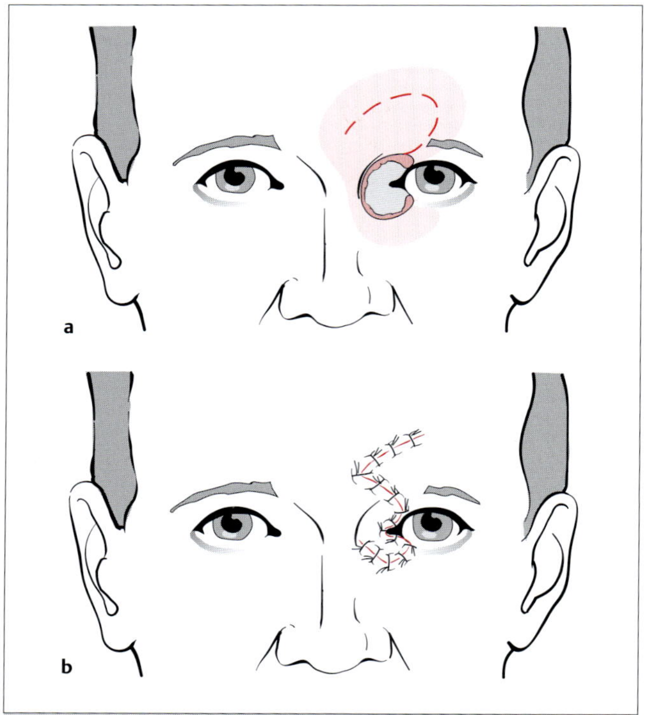

Fig. 5.39a, b Closure of a defect of the medial canthal region with a transposition–rotation flap from the forehead.
a Concept of the flap, which receives its blood supply from the supratrochlear artery of the ipsilateral side.
b Appearance after wound closure.

Surgical Technique (Fig. 5.40)

- Preparation of the recipient bed (trimming and undermining of the wound edges, cleaning of the wound bed).
- Planning and marking the flap.
- Incision around the flap (the incisions end at different levels at the glabella to facilitate rotation of the flap) (**Fig. 5.40a**).
- Elevation of the flap by developing the plane between the galea aponeurotica and the periosteum (pericranium).

- Care is needed when dissecting the flap pedicle: blunt dissection should be used to protect the vascular pedicle (the vessels lie immediately over the frontal muscle).
- The muscle should be more or less completely preserved (important for facial expression).
- The flap is rotation into the defect and fixed using two-layer sutures (**Fig. 5.40b**).
- The donor site is closed directly, after undermining the wound edges (**Fig. 5.40b**).

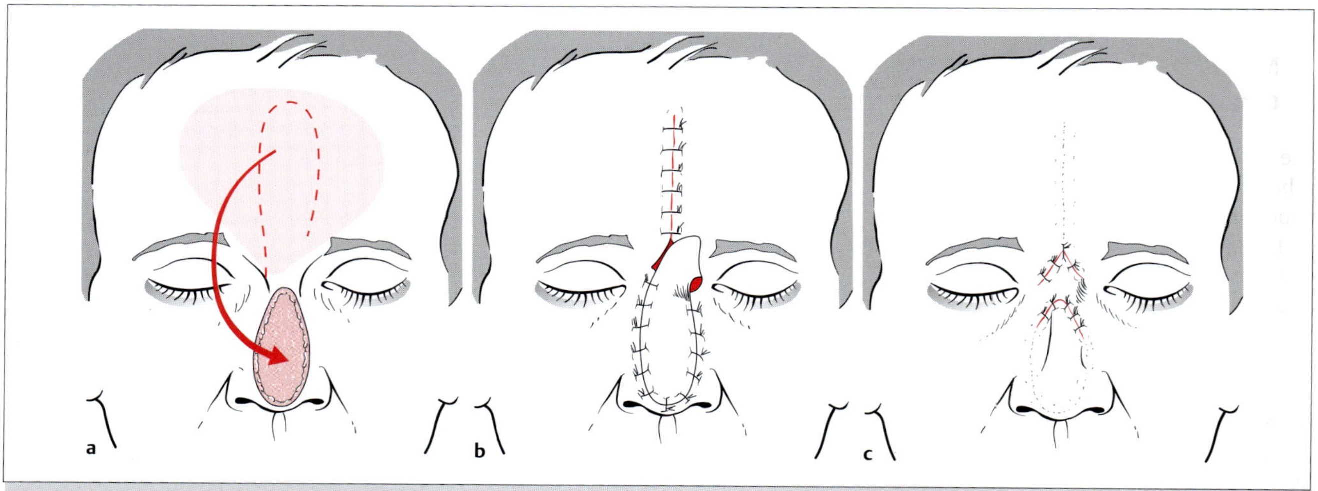

Fig. 5.40a–c Resurfacing of a defect on the dorsum of the nose and the tip of the nose with a midline forehead flap.
a The wound edges of the defect are trimmed and the planned incision line marked (the differing incision lengths facilitate rotation). The skin is undermined to allow closure of the donor defect.
b Transposition of the flap and primary wound closure. Temporary puckering of the flap pedicle.
c After the flap has healed in, the pedicle is revised and inset.

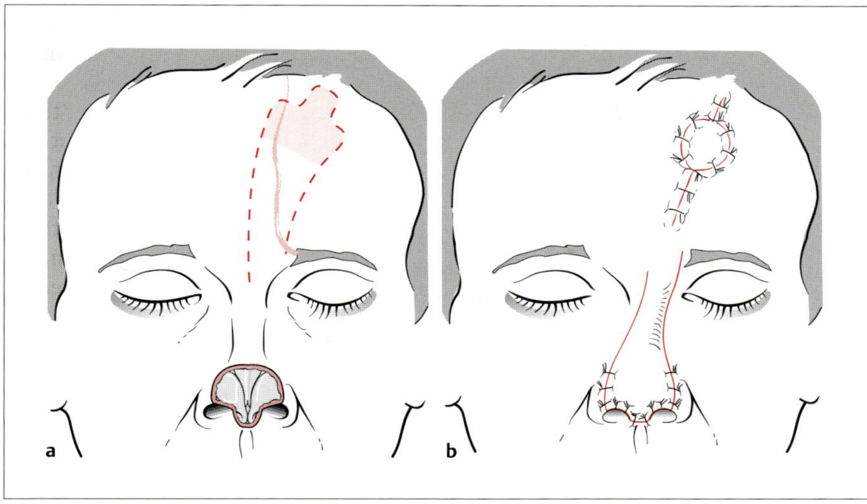

Fig. 5.41a, b Reconstruction of a defect of the nasal tip and columella with an oblique forehead flap.
a The wound edges of the recipient bed are trimmed, the cartilaginous framework is either preserved or reconstructed. The oblique forehead flap is marked, based on the supratrochlear artery. The actual resurfacing of the defect is accomplished by the distal shaded end.
b Appearance after transposition of the flap. The donor defect is partially closed primarily and partially covered with a retroauricular full-thickness graft.

- After the obligatory twisting of the flap pedicle, the viability of the flap should be checked.
- The exposed undersurface of the flap is covered with a sterile dressing (ointment-impregnated mesh).

Rules, Tips, and Tricks
Closure of the donor site is not possible without tension, but wound healing usually proceeds normally if a careful surgical technique is used. Cosmetically, the midline scar is hardly conspicuous. Closure of the donor site brings the medial borders of the eyebrows closer together. This is unavoidable and may be reversed by returning the flap pedicle to its original position after approximately 3 weeks (**Fig. 5.40c**). At that time it is advisable to take the opportunity of thinning out the flap, which will by now have healed in, to give it a better shape.

Management of Defects of the Nasal Tip and Columella

The tip of the nose and the columella are a common aesthetic subunit, which also includes the so-called "soft triangles" on the upper nostril rim (**Fig. 5.35**). Reconstruction of the columella is particularly difficult. It is best reconstructed as a unit, together with the nasal tip, using an oblique forehead flap (**Fig. 5.41**).

Before transposing the flap, the framework must first be reconstructed. Here, attention should be paid to placing the inner lining of the nostril rims as far caudally as possible to avoid cranial retraction after the flap has healed. The suture between forehead flap and vestibular skin should come to lie exactly at the nostril rim and not be everted outward by scar contracture.

It is essential to incise exactly around the donor site at the lateral region of the forehead. The use of a template is strongly recommended, and it is highly convenient if the patient has a receding hairline. The columella should be wide enough to allow it to be folded to form the membranous septum. The distal part of the flap, however, should not be thinned out too much to make it easy to shape, because it is in effect a random pattern flap and its blood supply is via the general vascular system of the skin. It is better to initially transpose "too much" material, which can then be thinned out and adjusted later (after 3–6 weeks), than to achieve an acceptable immediate result at the risk of developing necrosis of the flap tip.

Since the donor site is often too large for primary closure, a full-thickness skin graft taken from the retroauricular area should be anticipated (**Fig. 5.41b**). Prior stretching of the skin with the aid of a tissue expander is also an option (see **Fig. 5.44**).

Management of Defects of the Nasal Alae

Reconstruction of the Nasal Alar Margin with a Composite Graft

Surgical Principle

Reconstruction of the skin defect with simultaneous contouring of the nostril rim using a three-layered chondrocutaneous graft taken from the auricle.

Indications

Wedge-shaped defects of the alar margin with a maximum width of 1.5 cm.

Surgical Technique (Fig. 5.42)

- Excise the skin in the region of the defect to form clean, well-vascularized wound surfaces (**Fig. 5.42a, b**).
- Harvest a wedge-shaped composite graft from the helical attachment (make it as large as possible to allow later forming of the rim) (**Fig. 5.42c**).
- Close the donor site with a direct suture (**Fig. 5.42e**) or use a retroauricular transposition flap.
- Inset the composite graft without any step-off (**Fig. 5.42d**).

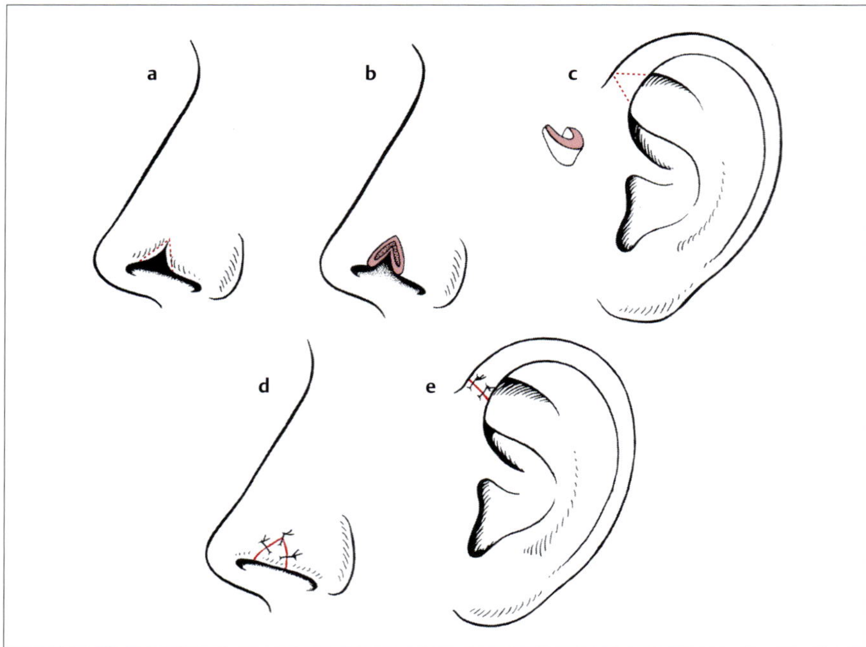

Fig. 5.42a–e Reconstruction of a triangular defect of the upper nostril rim with a composite chondrocutaneous graft from the auricle.
a Triangular defect with scarred edges.
b Wound edges are excised.
c The graft is harvested from the helix.
d The graft is slightly oversized when inserted.
e Primary closure of the donor defect on the crus helicis.

Rules, Tips, and Tricks

The cartilage should overlap the skin island laterally and be inserted into prepared "pockets" of the wound edges of the defect. This makes it easier to avoid step-offs. The skin fixation sutures should not be placed too close together, because nutrition of the skin is via the wound edges and not via the wound base. As with all free grafts, the operative site should be immobilized for 10 days. This may be achieved by providing support from medial with a loosely placed ribbon gauze pack impregnated with ointment (antibiotic ointment because of the length of time it has to be left in place) and an external dressing. Alternatively, the nostril can be left without a dressing if the operative site is covered with a U-shaped synthetic foil (e. g., silicone), which is secured to the nostril with two mattress sutures placed through the full thickness of the wall. Since the chondrocutaneous graft will shrink, it should be excised slightly larger than required. Despite this, the scars may still form step-offs at the wound edges, so the final aesthetic result does not always meet expectations. Unlike the otherwise technically demanding pedicle flaps, the chondrocutaneous graft is a direct and relatively simple procedure.

Complete Defects of the Nasal Alae

Surgical Principle

Full-thickness defects require reconstruction both of the inner lining of the nasal vestibule and of the nasal alae, with contouring of the nostril rim. The inner lining is formed by a two-layered composite graft taken from the auricular concha, which is able to form and stabilize the nasal ala with its concavity. At the same time its free margin lends the nostril the necessary contour. The external skin defect is then resurfaced with a suitable transposition flap (e. g., a cranially based nasolabial flap).

Indications

Complete full-thickness defects of the nasal ala with loss of the alar margin and inner lining, as often occurs after excision of skin tumors or secondary to trauma.

Surgical Technique (Fig. 5.43)

- First of all, the wound edges are trimmed; they should be free of scar tissue. They are also undermined to allow the cartilaginous component of the composite graft to be inserted into this "pocket."
- The composite graft is harvested from the anterior aspect of the auricular concha (ensuring concavity of the skin island) and the donor defect is closed with a retroauricular island flap (see Chapter 15).
- The chondrocutaneous graft is trimmed to slightly oversized dimensions and the overlapping cartilaginous edges are inserted into the prepared wound bed. The graft is secured with a few retention sutures, taking care to achieve exact symmetry with the contralateral side (**Fig. 5.43a, b**)
- The residual external skin defect may be reconstructed either with a cranially based nasolabial flap (one-stage procedure, **Fig. 5.43b, c**) or with an ipsilateral paramedian forehead flap (two-stage procedure), depending on its size.
- As with all free grafts, the operated site must remain untouched for 10 days.

Rules, Tips, and Tricks

- The position of the free margin of the composite graft must correspond exactly to the nostril rim of the contralateral side. This is best assessed by viewing from above.

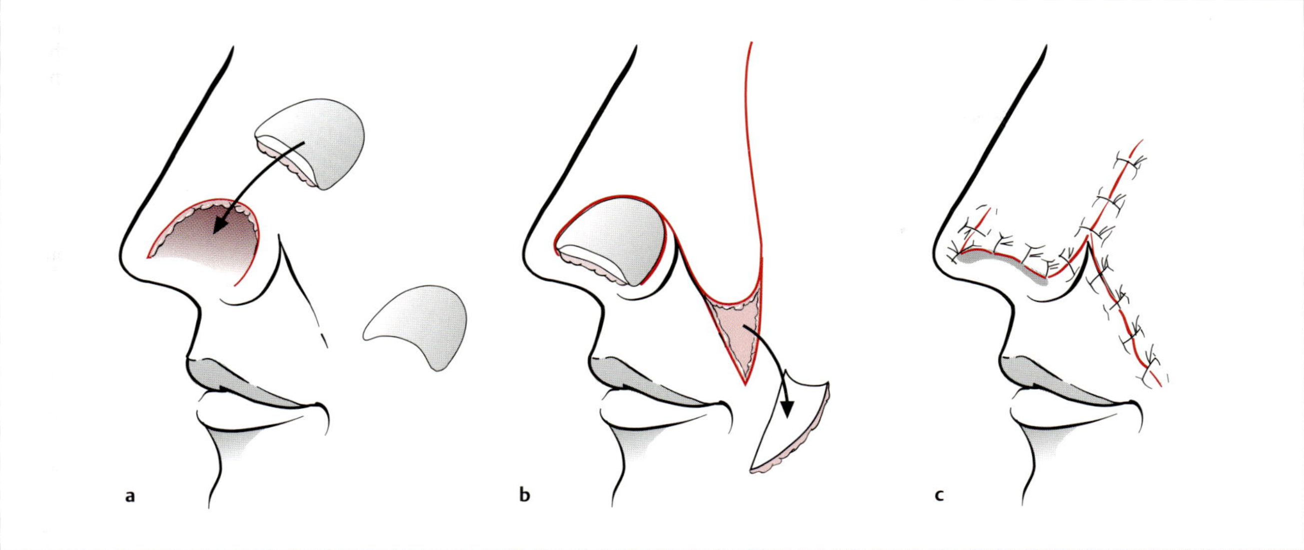

Fig. 5.43a–c Reconstruction of a subtotal defect of the nostril with a cranially based nasolabial flap.
a The wound edges of the full-thickness defect are trimmed. A composite graft from the anterior surface of the cavum conchae is inserted into the defect with the skin surface on the inside.
b After reconstructing the inner lining of the nostril, the skin defect is resurfaced with a cranially based nasolabial flap. The donor site is easily closed after excising a triangular area of skin, leaving the scar to lie inconspicuously in the nasolabial fold.
c Appearance after transposition of the flap and closure of the donor defect.

- When elevating the nasolabial transposition flap, one incision lies exactly within the nasolabial fold, while the parallel incision runs at the required distance down the skin of the cheek. If necessary, the flap may extend below the corner of the mouth. The skin of the cheek must be extensively undermined to achieve closure of the donor defect. This is done in the subcutaneous plane to protect the branches of the facial nerve. Excision of a distal triangle of skin will help closure (**Fig. 5.43b**). The final scar comes to lie exactly within the nasolabial fold (**Fig. 5.43c**).
- Minor irregularities of the flap pedicle may be corrected after 3 weeks, together with any necessary thinning of the flap.
- To achieve symmetry of the nostrils despite contracture of the composite graft, it is good practice to fit bilateral obturators for the vestibules, which should be worn at night for 6–9 months.

Total Nasal Reconstruction

Surgical Principle

Reconstructive surgery for total or subtotal loss of the nose can rely on a large number of procedures. Reconstructive flaps taken from forehead skin have generally proved reliable and effective. The procedure described here is based upon transposition of excess forehead skin gained from the implantation of a tissue expander. A sufficiently long flap for the simultaneous reconstruction of columella, nasal tip, and nasal alae is only obtainable by employing the principle of the oblique forehead flap. Male patients with a receding lateral hairline are therefore particularly suitable candidates.

Surgical Technique (Fig. 5.44)

- Incision above the hairline, dissection, and elevation of the skin (leaving the periosteum intact) and implantation of a 50-mL expander, e.g., with a remote valve (**Fig. 5.44a**).
- Adequate expansion of the skin (ca. 4–6 weeks); the recipient site is first prepared by reconstruction of the internal lining and the cartilaginous framework of the nose (**Fig. 5.44b, c**).
- As the central support column, the nasal septum can be reconstructed from residual septal cartilage or from costal cartilage (see Chapter 6). It is covered with the aid of nasolabial flaps, which also form the inner lining of the nasal vestibule. The inner lining is supplemented at the roof of the nose by a hinged turnover flap recruited from skin of the nasal dorsum. The supportive framework is supplemented by reconstruction of the alar cartilages using concave auricular cartilage.
- Incision and elevation of the trilobed oblique forehead flap (a broad base is important) and removal of the expander.
- Inset of the flap and primary closure of the donor site (**Fig. 5.44d**).
- After 3 weeks, division and relocation of the flap pedicle, and if necessary fine adjustments to the soft-tissue coverage.

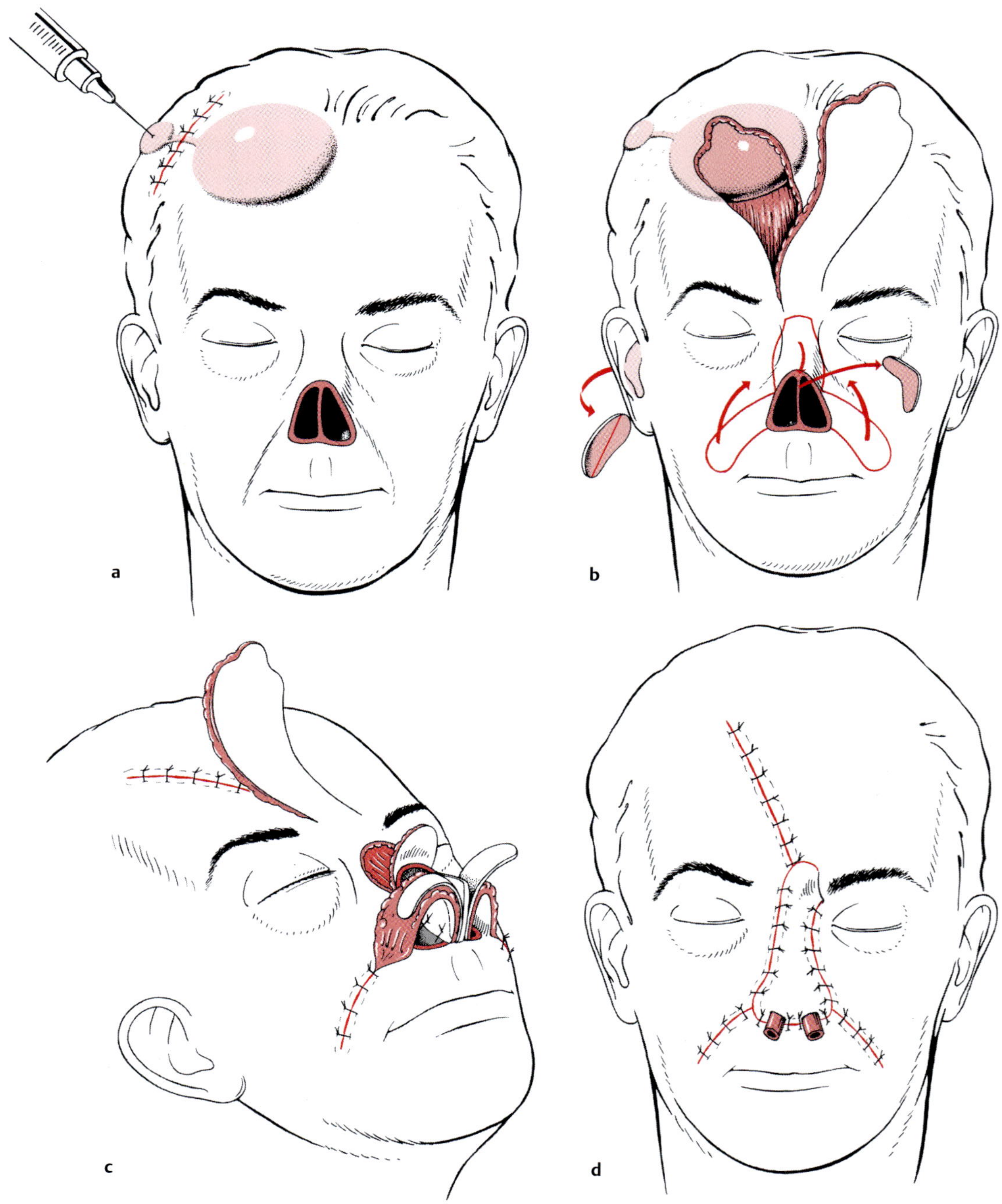

Fig. 5.44a–d Total nasal reconstruction with an oblique forehead flap after prior expansion of the donor skin with an expander (see text).
a After insertion of the expander.
b Elevation of the forehead flap. Septal cartilage is harvested to reconstruct the caudal septum. Auricular cartilage is harvested from the cavum conchae to be used for alar-cartilage reconstruction. Lining for the nasal vestibule is formed by nasolabial turnover flaps.
c Appearance after reconstruction of the nasal framework. The inner lining is supplemented by the turnover flap from the roof of the nose.
d Appearance after transposition of the flap, wound closure and packing of the vestibule with "breathing tubes."

Rules, Tips, and Tricks

To avoid furrowlike scars, the flap is best inset with everting sutures (see **Fig. 5.8**). As with alar reconstruction, it is advisable to fit bilateral obturators for the vestibules, to be worn at night for 6 months. The contours of the flap can be fine-tuned after 6 weeks by reopening the scar on one side at a time and thinning out the flap. Over-correction should be avoided, however, given that shrinkage of the soft-tissue coverage can be expected over the course of a year or more. This shrinkage may also produce a significant reduction in the length of the nose. When reconstructing the cartilaginous framework, care should therefore be taken to safeguard nasal length by inserting stable cartilaginous grafts, and to avoid small untreated defects of the inner lining before rotating the forehead flap into position.

Alternatives

The quality and vascular supply of the forehead flap as well as the stability of the cartilage grafts are decisive factors in the outcome of a total reconstruction of the external nose. If this cannot be guaranteed, or a multistage procedure is not acceptable to the patient, then a silicone nasal prosthesis should be considered. This can be attached using a skin adhesive, or anchored to spectacles or to bone screws/magnets.

Lips

Deformity of the Vermilion Caused by Scar Contracture

The conspicuous nature of the junction between vermilion lip and cutaneous lip (Cupid's bow) allows even minor irregularities to become clearly noticeable. It is therefore recommended to use dividers and possibly also loupes when undertaking corrective surgery in this region. Visual judgement does not necessarily guarantee a good aesthetic result.

Deformities from scar contracture are commonly found in patients with vermilion notching following cleft-lip repair. Here, the vermilion is drawn up into the skin of the upper lip (**Fig. 5.45**). Reconstruction involves separating it from the skin with a pointed blade. Excess tissue is excised according to the height of Cupid's bow and the wound repaired with fine skin sutures (6/0). A tension-free re-approximation of the wound edges will only be achieved if subcutaneous scar tissue is carefully excised before wound closure.

5

Minor Lip Defects

Minor lesions of the upper and lower lips up to a width of 1 cm may be treated by wedge excision followed by a three-layered closure. The slight shortening of the lip does not usually result in any functional impairment. A step-off can be avoided by a careful everting suture technique, possibly using a mattress stitch. Major lip defects, on the other hand, will require flap repair.

Central Defect of the Upper Lip

Surgical Principle

Medial advancement of the lip stumps resulting in a relative narrowing of the oral aperture.

Surgical Technique (Fig. 5.46)

- Resection of a central lesion of the upper lip, creating a full-thickness defect (**Fig. 5.46a**).
- Bilateral skin incision in the nasolabial folds up to the level of the piriform aperture.

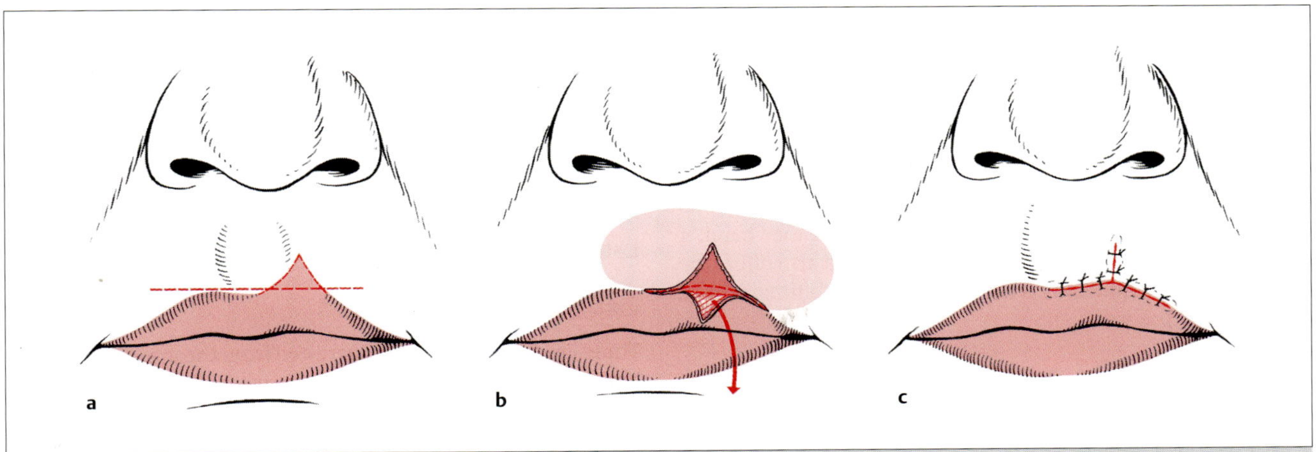

Fig. 5.45a–c Correction of a distortion of the vermilion border secondary to scarring.
a The vermilion border is contracted by a scar (notching after correction for cleft lip) superior to the corresponding level of the unaffected side into the upper lip skin.
b The excess vermilion is incised and turned down caudally. The skin is undermined in preparation for the primary closure.
c Skin closure after excision of the excess vermilion.

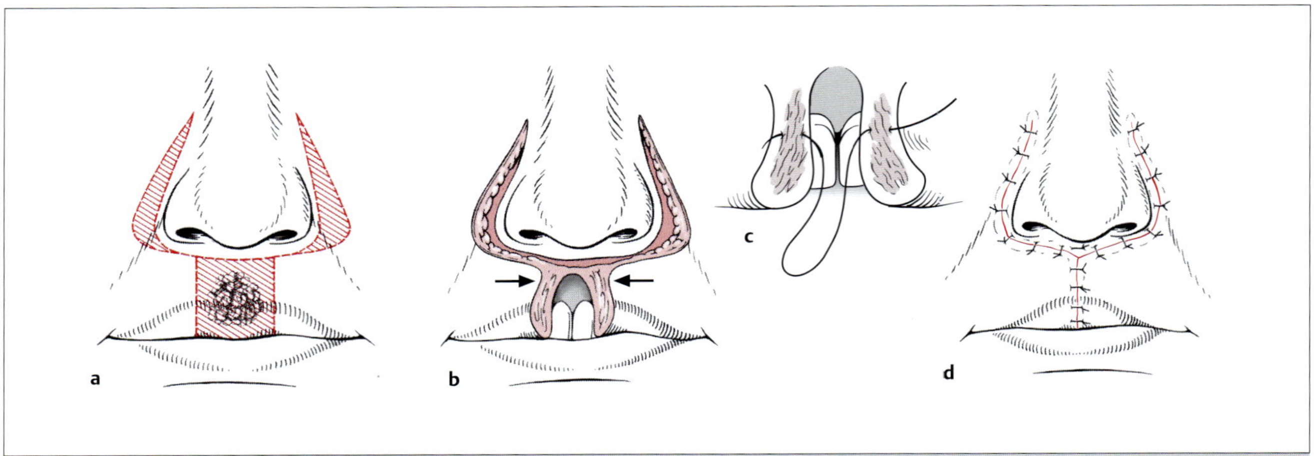

Fig. 5.46a–d Closure of a midline defect of the upper lip after excision of a lesion.
a Excision of the lesion, together with the mucosa. Para-alar auxiliary incisions (just skin) are marked.
b Medial advancement of the upper-lip stumps, while simultaneously closing the lateral defects.
c Wound closure, proceeding in three layers in the region of the lip from inside out.
d Appearance after reconstruction.

- Division of the mucosa in the labial sulcus.
- Undermining of the cheek skin and excision of a strip of skin and subdermis on either side from the lateral base of the nose (**Fig. 5.46b**).
- Three-layered suture repair of the lip stumps in the midline (mucosa–muscle–skin) (**Fig. 5.46b, c**).

Rules, Tips, and Tricks
An oral aperture which has been excessively narrowed may be widened at a further operation (see **Fig. 5.48d–f**).

Alternatives

A further option for closing central upper-lip defects is the Abbé flap (lip-switch flap, see also **Fig. 5.48**), with which a wedge-shaped upper-lip defect is replaced with a correspondingly sized segment of lower lip, pedicled on the labial artery. Unlike the technique described above, however, this procedure requires two sessions because the rotated vermilion connects both upper and lower lip in the midline. On the other hand, it avoids excessive narrowing the oral aperture and also offers the possibility of simultaneous reconstruction of the philtrum (e.g., with cleft lips).

Lateral Defect of the Upper Lip

Surgical Principle

Three-layered rotation flap recruited from the adjacent cheek region with secondary reconstruction of the vermilion.

Surgical Technique (Fig. 5.47)

- The flap is elevated in the region of the cheek, together with mucosa of the cheek (bearing in mind the duct of the parotid gland), parallel to the nasolabial fold (**Fig. 5.47a, b**).
- The width of the flap corresponds to the height of the defect (**Fig. 5.47c**).
- Reconstruction of the vermilion is undertaken after 6 weeks by a circumscribed de-epithelialization of the cheek flap with mobilization and advancement of the mucosa (**Fig. 5.47d**).

Rules, Tips, and Tricks
The flap should be as thick as possible along its free margin, to have as much volume as possible available for later reconstruction of the vermilion. The disadvantage of this technique is that there is no reconstruction of the oral sphincter, thus producing a functional deficit.

Lateral Defect of the Lower Lip

Surgical Principle

Three-layered rotation flap recruited from the upper lip, whereby the vermilion provides an adequate pedicle (labial artery). The vermilion is thus immediately reconstructed, with the oral aperture and oral commissure requiring secondary reconstruction.

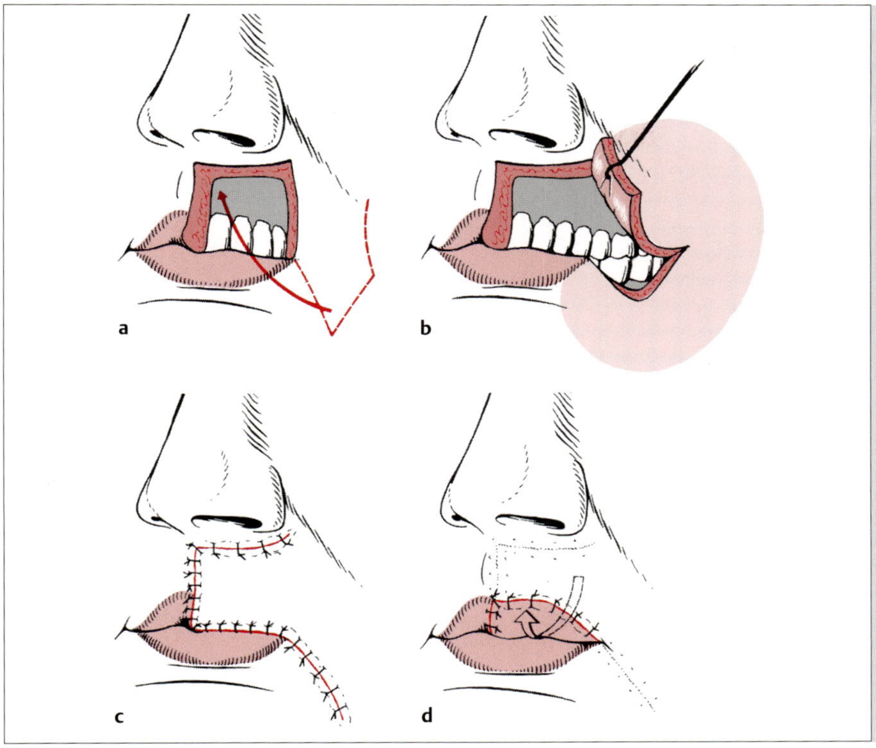

Fig. 5.47a–d Closure of a complete lateral defect of the upper lip with a cranially based three-layered cheek flap.
a Rhombic incision of a three-layered flap from the cheek (bear in mind the duct of the parotid gland!). The flap pedicle lies in the region of the nasolabial fold.
b Mobilization of the flap.
c Insetting the flap.
d Secondary reconstruction of the vermilion by mucosal advancement after de-epithelialization.

Surgical Technique (Fig. 5.48)

- The triangular flap is based centrally on the vermilion (**Fig. 5.48a, b**). Elevation begins at the vermilion border of the upper lip, with the distance to the corner of the mouth being slightly shorter than the length of the defect of the lower lip. The incision is extended as far as the nasolabial fold, from where it follows the fold down to the edge of the defect.
- Deep down, the muscle and finally the mucosa are gradually divided. This results in a flap that is roughly triangular in shape and based on the vermilion. This narrow bridge allows the flap to be easily rotated through 180°, so that the vermilion of the upper lip becomes the vermilion of the lower lip (lip switch) (**Fig. 5.48c**).
- The flap must be sutured from the inside out in three layers (mucosa, muscle, skin). It is usually possible to close the donor defect directly without undermining (mucosa, subcutaneous layer, skin).
- After 6 weeks the oral commissure, which initially appears rounded off, is widened. For this purpose, the desired width of the oral aperture is marked out (**Fig. 5.48d**) and the oral commissure is divided laterally. After circumscribed de-epithelialization, the adjoining mucosa of the inner aspect is mobilized (**Fig. 5.48e**) and turned outwards (**Fig. 5.48f**).

Rules, Tips, and Tricks

- The vermilion is the thin pedicle and must be very carefully protected. It is better to have a slightly thicker pedicle by maintaining a margin of skin than to thin it out too much. If the labial artery is divided, the flap is lost.
- Reconstruction using this flap (also known as the Estlander flap, vs. the Abbé flap, with which central defects can be reconstructed employing the same principle but using a lower-lip flap) has the advantage of not only preserving the vermilion, but also reconstructing the oral sphincter.
- The same principle can also be employed for central lower-lip defects. In this case, the central defect is first converted into a lateral defect by an auxiliary incision, running from the corner of the mouth parallel to the defect margin. This results in a rhombic, three-layered skin flap with a pedicle directed toward the tip of the chin, which is rotated to repair the central defect, leaving a triangular lateral defect.

Unilateral Defect of the Lower Lip

Surgical Principle

The defect is repaired with a large rotation flap, pedicled in the submandibular region. The vermilion is reconstructed at a second-stage procedure.

Surgical Technique (Fig. 5.49)

- Loss of half of the lower lip secondary to tumor excision (**Fig. 5.49a**).
- The flap is elevated across the middle of the chin in a submandibular direction.
- The mucosa in the labial sulcus is divided (**Fig. 5.49b**).
- The skin is undermined and a triangular area of skin is excised in the lateral corner of the mouth (**Fig. 5.49b**).
- The flap is rotated medially and sutured in three layers.

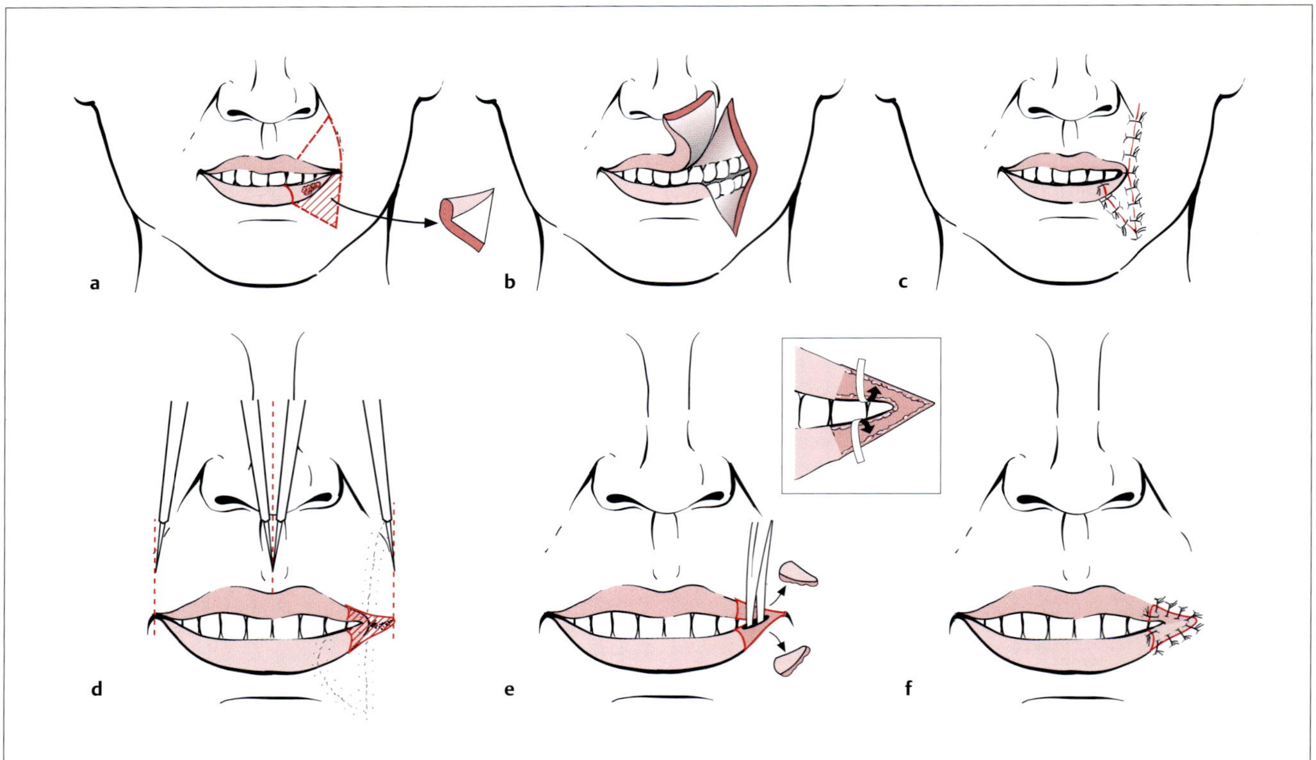

Fig. 5.48a–f Closure of a full-thickness defect of the lower lip with a pedicled lip-switch flap (Estlander flap).
a Lesion of the left lower lip, removed by wedge excision of skin and mucosa. The triangular flap on the upper lip is marked. The incision line of the flap runs, on the one hand, in the nasolabial fold down to the corner of the mouth and, on the other hand, from the attachment of the nostril to the vermilion border. This flap is based on the upper lip; it is essential to protect both the vermilion and the labial artery running within.
b Rotation of the flap around its vermilion pedicle (lip-switch).
c Mobilization of the adjacent skin and mucosa and direct closure. This results in a narrowed oral fissure and a rounded-off oral commissure.
d Secondary reconstruction of the oral commissure. The required distance to the middle of the lip is marked and the corner of the mouth is incised.
e Reconstruction of the vermilion in the oral commissure by circumscribed de-epithelialization and mobilization of the adjacent mucosa.
f Appearance after suturing.

- The vermilion is reconstructed after approximately 6 weeks by advancement of the adjacent mucosa over the corresponding de-epithelialized area of the rotation flap.

Rules, Tips, and Tricks

Large parts of the lower lip can be reconstructed using this technique. The required incision also allows regional lymph-node dissection if this is indicated. Any secondary mucosal defects which remain as a result of the reconstruction are left untreated for healing by secondary intention.

Neck

The technique for closing an epithelialized tracheostoma is described here as an example of plastic reconstructive procedures of the neck.

Tracheostoma Closure

Surgical Principle

Reconstruction of the anterior wall of the trachea using a hinged turnover flap. Suture repair of the sternocleidomastoid muscle avoids retraction of the sternal notch. Primary skin suture line is parallel to the RSTL.

Indications

Epithelialized tracheostoma. Respiratory capacity with stoma occluded must be sufficient (even under exertion).

Contraindications

Skin infection in the vicinity of the tracheostoma. Height of the lateral walls of the trachea too low, resulting in insufficient respiration after closure (tracheal stenosis, tracheomalacia).

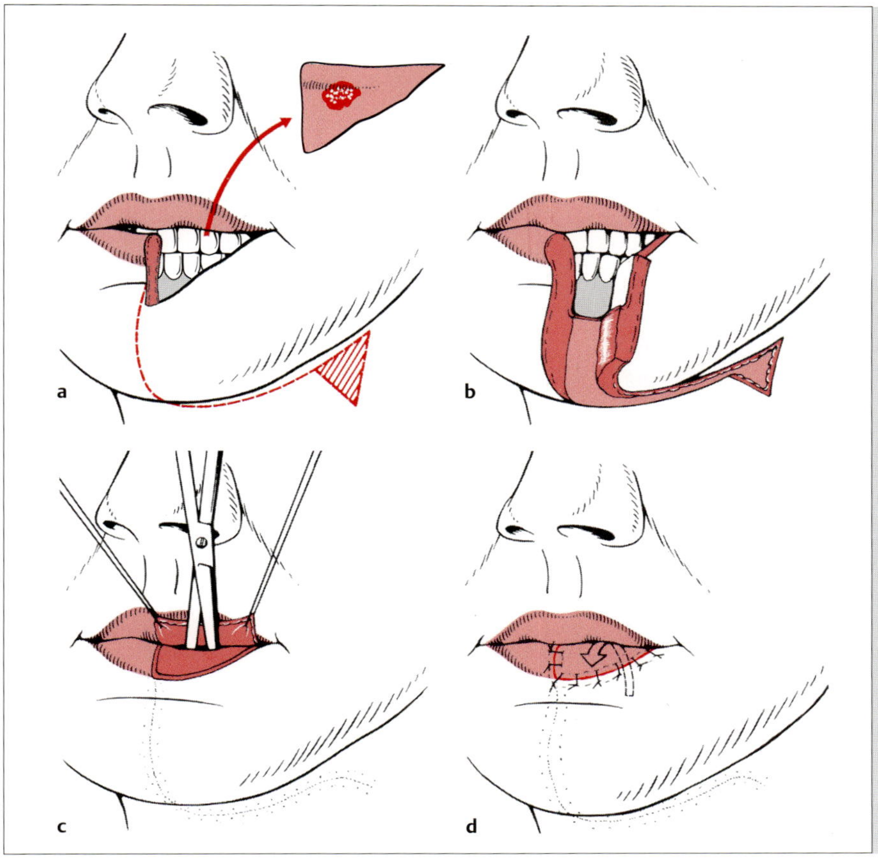

Fig. 5.49a–d Reconstruction of a unilateral defect of the lower lip with a submandibular pedicled rotation flap.
a Full-thickness three-layered unilateral defect after excision of a lesion. Skin incision and triangular excision are marked.
b Flap advancement after mobilization.
c Secondary reconstruction of the vermilion by de-epithelialization.
d Advancement of the oral mucosa to resurface the de-epithelialized area.

Surgical Technique (Fig. 5.50)

- The skin around the tracheostoma is incised asymmetrically in an elliptical curve (**Fig. 5.50a**).
- This leaves a rim of epithelium around the tracheostoma, which is elevated off the underlying tissue right up to the circular opening (**Fig. 5.50b**).
- The longer piece of skin is now flipped over 180°, hinged at the edge of the stoma as a turnover flap, and sutured to the adjacent margin of skin. These sutures are nonabsorbable and do not include the epithelium (**Fig. 5.50c**). This results in a reconstruction of the inner lining that is air- and watertight.
- To avoid too much skin retraction after a "deep tracheostoma," the adjacent margins of the sternocleidomastoid muscles may be sutured together (**Fig. 5.50d**).
- The residual skin defect is closed primarily in two layers after extensive undermining. The resulting scar comes to lie in the RSTL (**Fig. 5.50e**).

Rules, Tips, and Tricks

- The turnover flap required to reconstruct the inner lining needs an adequate pedicle. At this stage, therefore, the flap must be separated from the underlying tissue only just enough to make a turnover easily possible. The flap must then be able to reach the opposite skin margin without any undue tension (it must not be cut too short). The sutures should be inserted as close together as possible, or immediately adjacent to the lateral tracheostoma edge.
- The turnover flap should fit as exactly as possible into the defect of the anterior wall. If it is too long, it may be drawn in during inspiration. Additional stabilization can be achieved by the suturing of an onlay cartilage graft taken from the auricle, but this is not usually necessary.
- Adhesions of the skin to the anterior wall of the trachea secondary to scarring should be avoided, as they will result in distraction during swallowing. Apart from the muscle interposition, particular care should be taken to achieve an adequate subcutaneous gliding layer. The skin should therefore be mobilized immediately above muscle fascia level to leave as thick a layer of fat on the skin as possible.

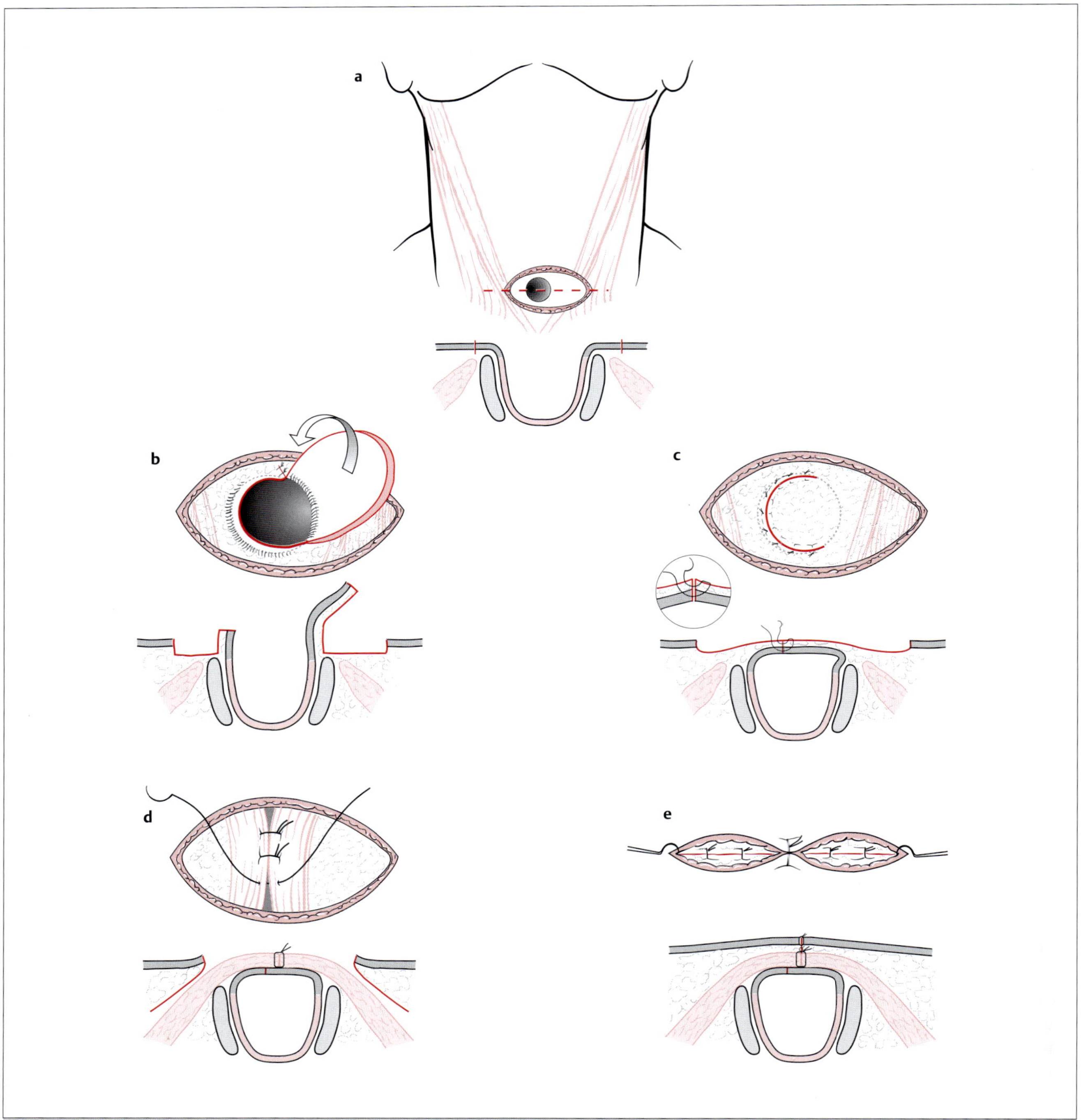

Fig. 5.50a–e Plastic-reconstructive closure of an epithelialized tracheostoma (frontal view with corresponding cross-section).

a Elliptical asymmetrical incision of the skin around the tracheostoma.

b Formation of a turnover flap which is hinged on the skin margin of the contralateral side. This brings the suture to lie laterally at the lumen of the trachea.

c Insetting the turnover flap. Mattress suture of the subcutaneous tissue to bury the epithelium in the trachea.

d Mobilization of the medial margins of the sternocleidomastoid muscles on either side and approximation over the previous tracheostoma (for a deep tracheostoma).

e Appearance after skin suture. The suture line lies along the RSTL. Care should be taken to gain as thick a subdermis of the mobilized skin as possible to allow shifting between skin and trachea during swallowing.

6 Nasal Surgery

Preliminary Remarks

Surgical Anatomy

A basic distinction is made between the internal and the external nose. Common to both is the supporting structure of cartilage and bone, which is covered by skin (externally) and mucosa (internally). The supporting tissues are referred to as the bony and cartilaginous frameworks. The terminology for the position of individual parts is orientated according to the upright patient (**Fig. 6.1**), which requires a certain amount of thought during surgery. A flat muscle layer is embedded in the subcutaneous layer (**s**ubcutaneous **m**usculo**a**poneurotic **s**ystem = SMAS) which, together with the muscles of the nose, allows limited movements of the cartilaginous nasal segments as well as regulation of the width of the vestibule (see **Fig. 6.31b**). These muscles are largely spared during surgery if the soft tissues are elevated directly off the perichondrium of the upper lateral cartilages (degloving of the dorsum of the nose). On the inside of the nose, the lumen is adjusted by the erectile tissue of the mucosa. This tissue is found not only in the region of the nasal turbinates (particularly the inferior turbinate), but also in the middle part of the nasal septum (the so-called septal turbinate or intumescentia septi).

The nasal frameworks are shown in detail in **Figs. 6.1** and **6.2** and some special aspects are also mentioned here for a better understanding of operative techniques. The basic structure of the framework consists of the bony nasal pyramid (nasal bones and the frontal process of the maxilla), into which is inserted a cartilaginous pyramid made up of the nasal septum (cartilaginous septum, quadrilateral cartilage) and the upper lateral cartilages (triangular cartilages). The upper lateral cartilages and the septal cartilage form a single cartilaginous unit (the septodorsal cartilage) and are therefore not joined by cartilaginous sutures (**Figs. 6.1c** and **6.2b**). Their positional relationship to each other is determined by internal cartilaginous forces, which may be disrupted by cartilage-splitting incisions, e.g., between the upper lateral cartilages and the septal cartilage ("division of the upper lateral cartilages").

The cartilaginous and bony frameworks are held together at three surgically relevant sites. First, the nasal bones overlap the upper lateral cartilages by a few millimeters. The integrity of this unit, consisting of nasal bones and upper lateral cartilages (Cottle's "keystone" or K-area, **Fig. 6.1d** [3]), is particularly important for correction of the deviated nose, and it is separated when reducing a prominent nasal hump, for example. A further junction is the suture line between the perpendicular plate of

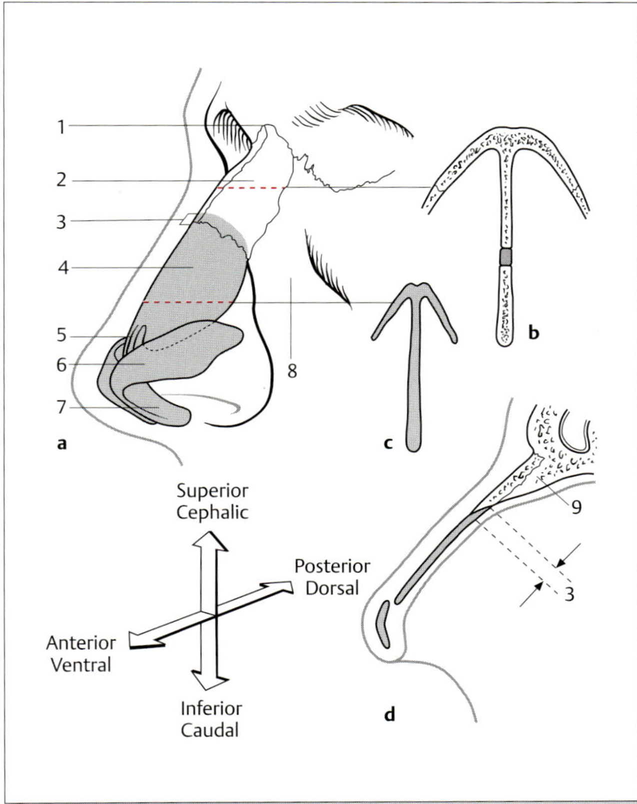

Fig. 6.1a–d Infrastructure of the nose.
a Architecture of the cartilaginous and bony pyramids.
b Frontal section through the bony dorsum of the nose ("bony vault").
c Frontal section through the cartilaginous dorsum of the nose ("pointed arch").
d Sagittal section through the keystone area ("K-area").
1 root of the nose (nasion, intersection between the internasal suture line and the nasofrontal suture line)
2 nasal bone
3 keystone area ("K-area")
4 upper lateral cartilage (triangular cartilage)
5 septum (anterior–inferior corner), not covered by upper lateral cartilages (Converse's weak triangle)
6 lower lateral cartilage: lateral crus
7 lower lateral cartilage: medial crus
8 maxilla: frontal process
9 frontal bone: nasal spine (together with the nasal bones, forms a solid bony block at the root of the nose)

the ethmoid and the cartilaginous septum (chondroethmoid suture), which is embedded with a sphenoid process between this suture line and the vomer (**Fig. 6.2b** [4]). A so-called "ascending septal ridge" can form at this interface. During septoplasty, e.g., for resection of this type of ridge, this attachment is separated by means of a complete vertical chondrotomy. The third anchorage point involves the septal cartilage and the premaxilla. The premaxilla is a distinct and separate bone (the os incisivum) which is inserted anterior to and between the maxillary bones (**Fig. 6.2a** [9]). Within the groove of the nasal floor, bordered on either side by bony extensions (premaxillary wings) and anteriorly by the anterior nasal spine, the septal cartilage rests in a fibrous sling that allows slight articulated movements. The premaxillary wings can appear asymmetrical and laterally protruding, thus causing septal deviations in the vestibular area, which can have an effect on breathing (the so-called basal crest). A horizontal chondrotomy during septoplasty will free this connection. *At least two* of the above-mentioned connections are essential to ensure sufficient stability of the cartilaginous pyramid and must either be preserved intraoperatively or reconstructed.

The nasal base is made up of the nasal tip, columella, and nasal alae. Its foundation is the paired lower lateral cartilages (**Fig. 6.2c**), which consist of a medial and lateral crus. The middle part diverges and is known as the intermediate crus. The degree of divergence determines, among other things, the width of the nasal tip. The nasal base is highly mobile with respect to the adjacent structures. The medial crus forms the cartilaginous base of the membranous septum, which can be moved in all directions against the relatively static caudal septal margin. The crura of the lower lateral cartilages are hinged to the adjacent upper lateral cartilages (**Fig. 6.3**), whose caudal margin is often curled outward for better stability ("returning" or "scrolling" of the upper lateral cartilages).

The following details of the bony pyramid are of particular interest from a surgical point of view. A strong crest is relevant during osteotomies at the level of the nasal radix (lacrimal crest), behind which the lacrimal sac is found and into which the medial canthal tendon inserts. It is at this level that lateral osteotomies usually end, with the thickness of the bone protecting the canthal tendon and lacrimal sac from injury. The nasal radix, or root of the nose, also lies at the level of the medial canthus and defines the level of transverse osteotomies. In complete mobilization of the nasal radix, which is necessary for a markedly crooked nose, a solid block of bone, made up of the nasal spine of the frontal bone and the overlying nasal bones, needs to be divided (**Fig. 6.1d**). This osteotomy line usually lies caudal to the nasofrontal suture line.

The internal nose starts with the vestibule (**Fig. 6.3**). This is defined anteriorly by the margin of the nostril and posteriorly by the nasal valve region. The vestibule consists medially of the membranous septum and laterally of the nasal alae, which are stabilized to only a small extent by the crura of the lower lateral cartilages. Large areas, reaching as far back as the bony piriform aperture, are free of cartilage and thus relatively unstable (see Correction of Alar Collapse, **Fig. 6.62**). The narrowest point of the nasal passage is the valve region (internal valves) at the junction of the vestibule and the nasal cavity. It includes the nasal valve proper, which is the space between the most caudal margin of the upper lateral cartilage laterally and the nasal septum medially. The width of this space, characterized by the nasal valve angle, which under normal circumstances is about 15°, is variable and depends on the activity of the nasal muscles—hence the use of the dynamic term "valve." The head of the lower turbinate is also situated at the level of the nasal valve and contributes to regulating its width. Given the narrowness of this cross-section (**Fig. 6.3a**), even small irregularities of the nasal septum can result in considerable obstruction of nasal breathing (nasal valve stenosis—not to be confused with vestibular stenosis). Certain malformations of the external nose are typically associated with narrowing (tension nose, **Fig. 6.3d**) or pathological dilation (saddle-nose deformity, **Fig. 6.3e**). Cephalad to the nasal valve region the nasal cavity widens, with the cartilaginous roof appearing pointed and the bony roof taking on a vaultlike form (**Fig. 6.1b, c**).

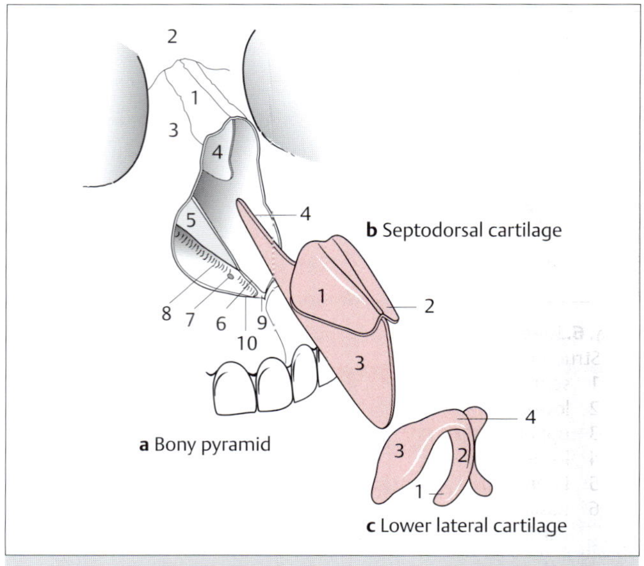

Fig. 6.2a–c The three basic units of the infrastructure.
a Bony pyramid.
1 nasal bone
2 frontal bone
3 maxilla: frontal process
4 perpendicular plate
5 vomer
6 premaxilla: body and wing
7 incisive canal: nasal foramen
8 maxilla: palatine process
9 premaxilla: anterior nasal spine
10 piriform crest
b Septodorsal cartilage. The septodorsal cartilage "inserts" into the bony pyramid.
1 upper lateral cartilage
2 "returning": the caudal border of the upper lateral cartilage scrolls upward
3 septal cartilage: quadrilateral plate
4 septal cartilage: sphenoid process
c Lower lateral cartilage.
1 medial crus
2 intermediate crus
3 lateral crus
4 dome

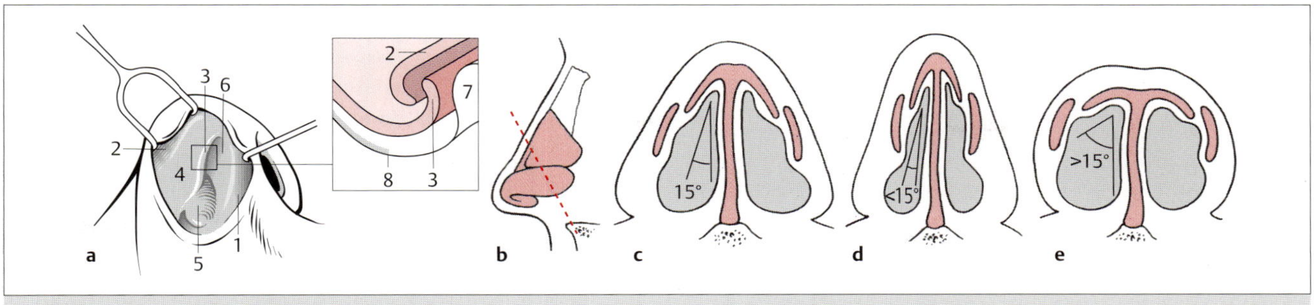

Fig. 6.3a–e Nasal vestibule and nasal valve.
a Structure of the nasal vestibule.
1 septal cartilage: caudal margin
2 lower lateral cartilage: lateral crus
3 upper lateral cartilage: caudal margin (returning)
4 lower lateral cartilage: protrusion of the lateral crus
5 inferior turbinate: head
6 nasal valve: angle between the upper lateral and the septal cartilage
Enlarged inset (scroll area):
7 "cul-de-sac" between the caudal margin of the upper lateral cartilage and the undersurface of the lower lateral cartilage
8 transition between skin and mucosa (dark area)
b Plane of section of c–e.
c Normal nasal valve angle (ca. 15°).
d Tension nose: excess growth of the septum produces a high nasal dorsum with reduction of the nasal valve angle and functional valve stenosis.
e Saddle nose: depressed nasal dorsum with a wide nasal valve angle ("ballooning phenomenon").

The nasal septum divides the nasal cavity into two parts. It consists of the septal cartilage (quadrangular cartilage), which is in fact a "septodorsal cartilage," and two bony parts (see also **Fig. 6.15**). The perpendicular plate of the ethmoid bone is a thin bony lamella; only at its junction with the septal cartilage is it thick enough to contain marrow. Any division made in this region should be done with an instrument and not by fracturing, which could result in dislocation of the adjacent cribriform plate of the skull base. The vomer, in contrast, is a very thick bone, which rises steeply up to the anterior wall of the sphenoid sinus. To mobilize it, the vomer should always be osteotomized or divided with nasal bone scissors. Small parts of the maxillary bone and palatine bone form the basis on which the vomer rests (**Fig. 6.2a**). The septal mucosa is firmly attached to the suture lines between the cartilaginous and bony parts of the septum, where it must be detached by sharp dissection. The attachment between premaxilla and septal cartilage in the region of the anterior nasal spine and the premaxillary wings is particularly strong.

The vascular supply of the anterior parts of the nose originates from the internal carotid artery (ophthalmic artery → anterior ethmoid artery), that of the posterior parts from the external carotid artery (maxillary artery → sphenopalatine artery) (**Fig. 6.4**). Tributaries from both systems unite in the caudal septal mucosa (Kiesselbach's plexus), which is a favored site for anterior nose bleeds. More serious nasal hemorrhage from the posterior nasal parts usually originates from the sphenopalatine artery, near its exit from the sphenopalatine (pterygopalatine) foramen. The course of the sensate nasopalatine nerve (incisive nerve) is important during septoplasty. After exiting from the sphenopalatine foramen, the nerve takes an anterior course in the septal mucosa and exits on either side through foramina in the nasal floor, ca. 1.5 cm dorsal to the piriform crest (lower osseous margin of the piriform aperture), in two bony canals toward the palatine side, which then unite to form the incisive canal. There the nerves innervate the mucosa behind the incisor teeth. When the septal mucosa is dissected in the vertical plane, the nerve can normally be protected. If the floor of the nose is also tunnelled, however, and septal tunnel and nasal floor tunnel are connected in the anterior part (the so-called maxillary–premaxillary approach; see Septoplasty, p. 57), then the nerve needs to be divided at its entrance into the bony canal. Without this division, connection of the vertical septal tunnel with the horizontal nasal floor tunnel will not be achieved. This may result in sensory disturbances of the mucosa behind the incisor teeth, which patients often perceive as "blisters." Usually, however, this type of sensory disturbance is no longer noticed after a few weeks.

Respiratory Function

The most important functions of the nasal airways are *conditioning* of the inspired air (humidification, warming, filtration) and *olfaction*. The most important organ for this processing of inspired air is the *respiratory mucosa*. The nasal turbinates provide a large contact area between inspired air and mucosa, and control the width of the airways by their erectile tissue. Larger particles (>10 µm diameter) are retained in the nasal mucosa; within a few minutes they are conveyed by mucociliary transport into the nasopharynx, from where they are swallowed. Humidification is accomplished by mucosal glands, which are primarily concentrated in the region between the internal valves and the heads of the turbinates. It is mainly there that the inspired air is humidified, although moisture is also regained during expiration.

Conditioning of inspired air and olfaction are closely associated with the structure of the nasal airways. Essentially, three segments can be distinguished (**Fig. 6.5**). The air flows from below into the nasal vestibule and is greatly accelerated through the bottleneck of the nasal valve area. This creates a negative pressure during inspiration, which can subsequently lead to

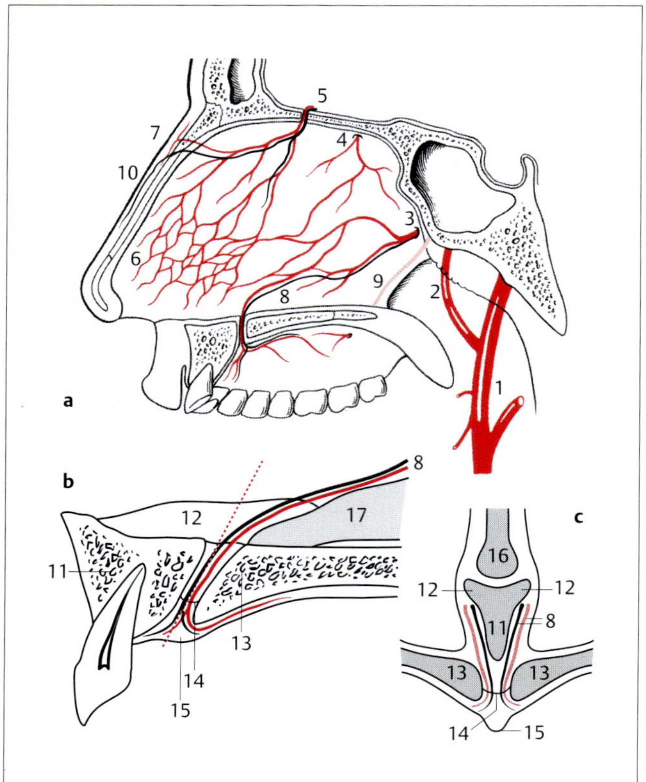

Fig. 6.4a–c Nerves and vessels of the nasal septum and the premaxilla. Arteries red, nerves black.

a Sagittal section through the septum.

b Sagittal section through the premaxilla (dotted line: plane of section of **c**).

c Frontal section through the premaxilla.

1 external carotid artery
2 maxillary artery
3 sphenopalatine foramen, sphenopalatine artery and nasopalatine nerve
4 posterior ethmoid artery
5 anterior ethmoid artery and nerve
6 Little area (Kiesselbach's plexus)
7 dorsal nasal artery
8 nasopalatine artery and nerve
9 descending palatine artery (light red)
10 external nasal artery
11 premaxilla with anterior nasal spine
12 premaxillary wing
13 maxillary bone: palatine process
14 incisive canal
15 incisive papilla
16 septal cartilage
17 vomer

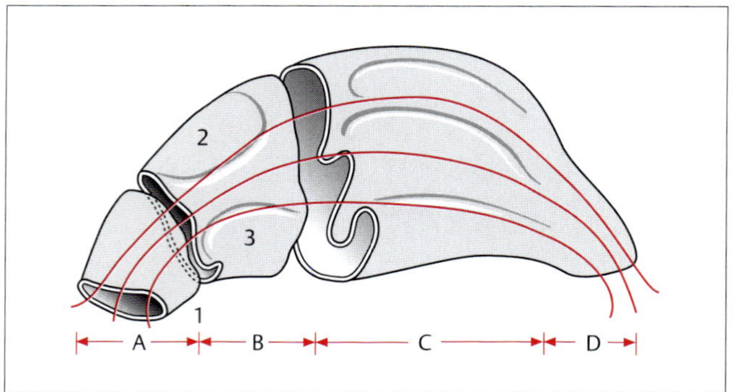

Fig. 6.5 Functional sections of the nasal cavity.

A Nasal vestibule: inflow section with "diffusor" (nasal valve)
B Turbinate area: air conditioning area
C Main nasal cavity: air conditioning area
D Choana: outflow section with "manifold" (nasopharynx)
1 Internal nasal valve area
2 Upper lateral cartilage
3 Head of inferior turbinate

"alar collapse" in the presence of insufficient stability or malformation of the nasal alae. The nasal airways widen considerably behind the nasal valve and the airflow now adopts a more horizontal course. During inspiration, the nasal valve acts like a nozzle (diffuser) ensuring that the air is distributed throughout all parts of the nasal cavity and thus comes into close contact with the mucosa. The inspiratory resistance created by the nasal valve is therefore an important physiological prerequisite for the conditioning of the inspired air. Surgical widening of the nasal valve to make it wider than normal does indeed lower airway resistance, but at the expense of warming and humidification, which can lead to desiccation of the mucous membranes not only of the nose and pharynx, but also of the larynx and trachea. Long-term effects on the bronchial system can be expected. In the region of the turbinates and the nasopharynx the air flow is accelerated and once again diverted by 90°. On its way from the nasal vestibule to the pharynx the air thus follows a semicircular path, turning through 180° (**Fig. 6.5**).

During expiration the air contacts particularly the cranial parts of the nasal cavity, where the olfactory mucosa is found, both on the septum as well as on the medial surfaces of the middle and superior turbinates. In this way, odors pass from the oral cavity to the olfactory organ ("gustatory olfaction"). Small drops of water are deposited in the region of the head of the turbinates and are then available again to humidify the inspiratory air. The oxygen-deficient air is accelerated in the nasal valve area and so transported away from the nasal vestibule. This prevents the "used" air from being drawn in again with the next intake of breath.

For these physiological reasons, two basic principles may be deduced, which are important for the *functional* surgery of the nose:

- A certain amount of respiratory resistance is essential; the nasal airways must not be too wide.
- The mucosal organ must be preserved. Extensive destruction of the mucosal surface compromises warming and humidification, as well as mucociliary transport.

Measuring Respiratory Function

There are no routine procedures available to measure the conditioning of inspired air—warming, humidification, and particle filtration. (Active, anterior) *rhinomanometry* is an established procedure for measuring the respiratory function of the nose, which is merely the prerequisite for these basic functions. It quantifies nasal airway patency. On one side of the nose respiratory volume is measured during inspiration and expiration, and on the other side the pressure difference required to move the air between the atmosphere and the pharyngeal cavity is measured. The values are valid only with an intact nasal septum; in the presence of a septal perforation they are distorted. Generally speaking, in addition to recording the values on a chart, volume flow as a measure of nasal breathing is given at a fixed pressure difference of 150 Pa. It is subject to considerable variation, but values between 300 and 500 mL/s are generally considered normal. In the presence of an obstruction to nasal breathing, a comparison of the measured values before and after decongestion of the nasal mucosa can provide information as to whether the problem is structural (e.g., septal deviation), mucosal (turbinate hypertrophy), or a combination of the two.

As a rule, rhinomanometry can only provide an overall statement about the function of one side of the nose, not a more exact spatial indication of the location of a functional impairment. A more detailed assessment of the shape of the graph makes this possible to some extent, but is only rarely undertaken in practice. The results obtained by measuring pressure gradient and volumes are very variable, so they are usually only regarded as supplementary to the information already found by inspection. Rhinomanometry is nevertheless recommended before operations on the internal and external nose, to provide pre- and postoperative comparison.

Using the echo sonographic technique, acoustic *rhinometry* measures the cross-section of the nasal cavity in relation to the distance from the nasal vestibule. It is a static procedure, which allows only conditional conclusions to be drawn on dynamic inspiration and expiration. The precision of the cross-section measurement decreases with the distance from the nasal vestibule, and assessment of nasal vestibule and nasal valve area is significantly limited by the need for a tight-fitting nasal adapter.

Olfaction should be determined preoperatively with the aid of a screening test (subjective, various odor qualities), mainly for medicolegal reasons. Disturbances of smell may well arise after surgery, e.g., as a result of scar formation or of infection or toxicity, but they may have been already present before surgery. Although they are only noticed later by the patient.

Instruments Required for Septoplasty/ Rhinoplasty

A multitude of instruments are available for septoplasty and rhinoplasty and are often offered in different variations, depending on individual experience. The selection shown in **Fig. 6.6** has been chosen largely on the basic principle that it is not necessary to have a special instrument for each and every operative step. On the contrary, as few instruments as possible should be used for as many functions as possible. Novices in functional and aesthetic surgery of the nose can familiarize themselves with the instruments presented here and, as they gain experience, may decide to dispense with some instruments or replace them with variations more suitable to their needs.

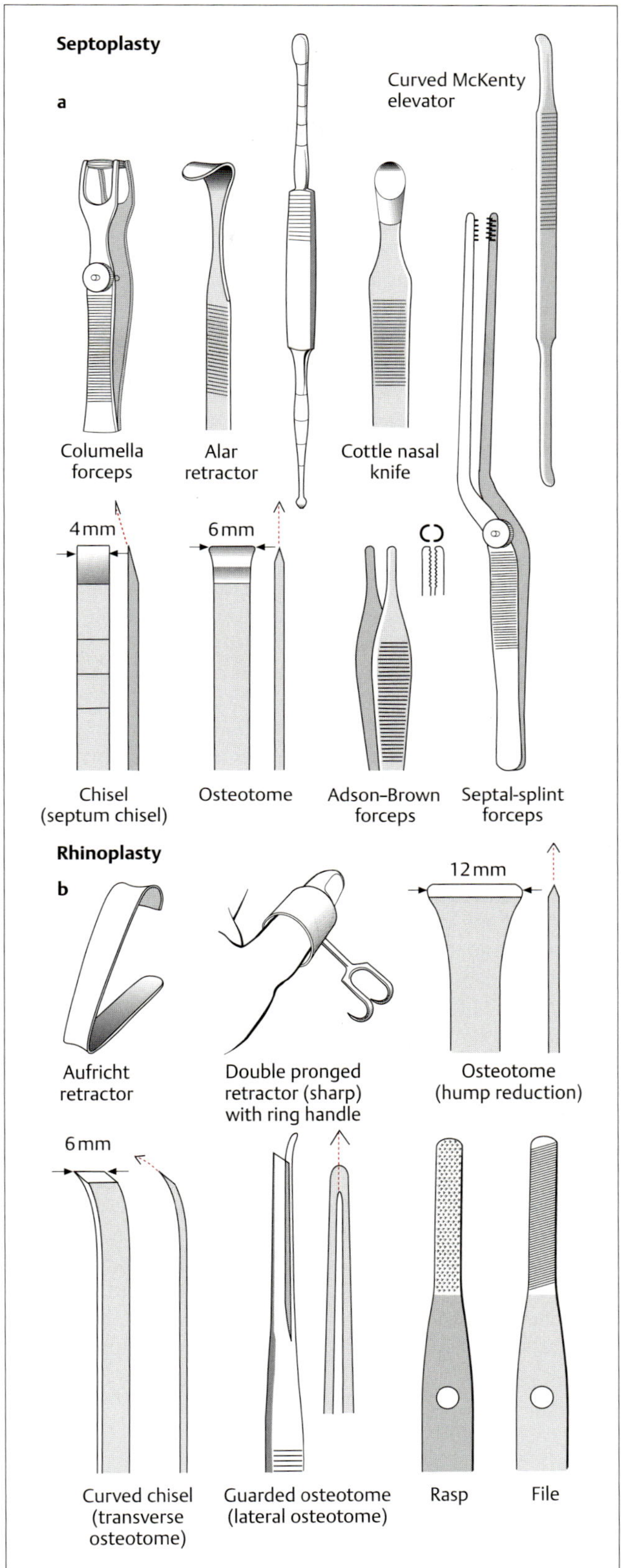

Fig. 6.6a, b Instruments (selection).
a Septoplasty
b Rhinoplasty

One general point is that when buying “nose instruments” it is important to ensure that they have large enough handles, even though very small tips are needed for the fine and intricate work involved. This applies especially to needle holders and scissors.

Septoplasty Instruments

The double elevator has a blunt and a sharp end. The blunt end is for subperichondrial dissection of septal mucosa (“over cartilage”), the sharp end for subperiosteal dissection (“over bone”). With more significant hemorrhage and subsequently unclear conditions, the suction elevator may also be used, with the suction opening pointing to the cartilage or bone.

The Cottle nasal knife is used to divide cartilage (chondrotomy), as well as for detaching fibrous strands, particularly in the area around the premaxilla. This bone contact soon makes the knife blunt, and it should be sharpened before any subsequent work on cartilage.

The McKenty curved elevator is used to create the inferior septal tunnel and should be only slightly bent to avoid placing the septal mucosa under too much tension.

It is important to distinguish between a chisel and an osteotome. The chisel has an oblique cutting surface, which allows the instrument to be driven into the bone away from the cutting surface (see arrows in **Fig. 6.6**). This is particularly required when there is a need to progress from thin bone into more solid bone. An osteotome, with two cutting surfaces, usually glides straight ahead and would at this point tend to glide away from the more solid bone. In septum surgery, therefore, a chisel is more helpful when making an osteotomy of the vomer near the more solid bone of the nasal floor.

An all-round forceps for septum surgery is the Adson–Brown forceps (or “plastic surgery forceps”), which has a row of teeth on either side of the forceps jaw (in this way acting like a multiple surgical forceps), allowing a gentle but stable grasp of soft tissues or cartilage.

Rhinoplasty Instruments

Good visualization is essential for work on the nasal dorsum. So-called “Aufricht retractors” (named after an American rhinosurgeon) should therefore be wide enough. Sharp double-pronged retractors for incisions and dissections in the nasal vestibule can be comfortably held with the aid of a thumb ring, freeing the surgeon’s fingers for use as a counter-support.

Osteotomes for nasal hump reduction should be as wide as possible, so that the bony part of the hump can be mobilized in one piece and thus avoiding multiple attempts, with the subsequent risk of producing unequal cutting levels. The corners of the blade should be rounded, to avoid inadvertently perforating the skin as it is elevated by the osteotome. It should be possible to hold the osteotome horizontally steady so it does not tilt laterally during osteotomy. This requires a stable handle.

Lateral and transverse osteotomies can be performed with either narrow chisels or osteotomes (e.g., 3 mm) directly through the skin via stab incisions; the usual practice, however, is via the nasal vestibule. The so-called “guarded osteotome” is effective for lateral osteotomies, especially for thicker bone, as it can be easily hooked into the piriform aperture while allowing stable guidance and control with the aid of the guard, which glides along the outside of the bony pyramid. Variously curved guarded osteotomes are available for left and right lateral osteotomies, although a straight osteotome is usually quite adequate. A transverse osteotomy can also be performed via the nasal vestibule with a chisel that is curved at the end (“transverse chisel”).

If the cartilaginous nasal septum is “too high” at the nasal dorsum after hump reduction, it may be successively reduced to the correct level under direct vision using scissors with angled blades. Small teeth on the serrated cutting surfaces prevent the mobile cartilage from evading the scissors. If smaller irregularities still remain over the nasal dorsum after hump reduction, they may be smoothed down with a rasp or file. The difference between the two instruments lies in the fact that files remove bone during both the forward and the backward movement, while rasps normally only remove bone with the backward movement. Because files only remove a small amount of bone with each movement, it is usually recommended to use a rasp as the main instrument for smoothing out irregularities. When using these instruments, it should be borne in mind that both types can work only on bone and not cartilage. Sharp ridges are often found at the transition between cartilaginous and bony dorsum, due to bulges of the upper lateral cartilages, and these can only be removed with the aid of a scalpel.

Depending on the frequency of their use, sharp instruments become blunt. They must therefore be sharpened regularly (scissors, chisel, osteotome) or exchanged (rasp). It is the sharpness of the osteotome in particular that determines the quality of osteotomies. With a sharpening stone available on the instrument table, osteotomes can be sharpened by the surgeon immediately before use.

Management of Fresh Nasal Injuries

Soft-Tissue Injuries

Surgical Principle

Soft-tissue injuries must be managed using atraumatic technique. With multilayered injuries, management proceeds from the inside out, especially with perforating injuries. With avulsions (e.g., secondary to dog bites) replantation has a prospect of success only with superficial injuries.

Indications

Gaping cutaneous wounds, perforations, defects.

Specific Points Regarding Informed Consent

The patient needs to be informed about tissue transplantation, the possibility of staged procedures, later fine adjustments, and potential functional and aesthetic impairment, especially with regard to more complex procedures to manage defects.

Operative Planning

Treatment should be initiated as soon as possible. Immediate reconstruction is preferable for defects, because healing by secondary intention makes later reconstruction more difficult due to extensive scar areas and distortions. With disrupted tissues, even small viable skin bridges are often enough to ensure adequate perfusion of injured areas. They should be carefully preserved.

Special Instruments

Atraumatic needle–suture combinations are required to achieve good aesthetic results on the face. Monofilament sutures should be used for repair of the skin. Lacerations can be adequately treated with tissue glue instead of sutures, especially in children. Occlusive dressings promote wound healing, especially with abrasions.

Anesthesia

General anesthesia may be required, depending on the scale of the injury and time needed for repair. In principle, however, the use of a local anesthetic is possible by infiltrating the injured area in a fan-shaped pattern.

Surgical Technique

Perforating injuries are closed in layers from the inside out (**Fig. 6.7**). Wound edges should be slightly everted to avoid the subsequent formation of retracted scars. Longer linear scars running perpendicular to the RSTL are converted into zigzag lines by creating small Z-plasties (W-plasty), which then come to lie partially in the RSTL and are thus cosmetically less conspicuous (see Chapter 5). In the nasal vestibule, semicircular shear injuries can occur at the piriform aperture, with involvement of the head of the turbinate. In these cases, the wound margins should be exactly re-approximated to preclude the development of a scar contracture with a pinhole stenosis of the vestibule.

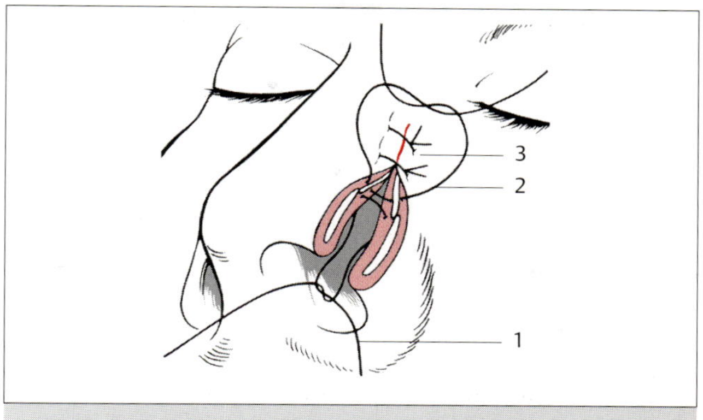

Fig. 6.7 Full-thickness laceration of the complete ala. Closure in layers from the inside out: suture repair of
1 vestibular skin and mucosa
2 cartilage
3 external skin

Avulsions can arise after dog bites, for example; often the victims are children. The missing piece of tissue is often lost or rendered unusable for replantation by severe crushing. A full-thickness skin graft is an option for defects involving only skin. The retroauricular skin is a suitable donor site. With chondrocutaneous defects of up to 1 cm in size, a free chondrocutaneous graft from the auricle is an option (see Chapter 5). Free grafts should be immobilized for 10 days by an external dressing and possibly supported from within the nose by suitable packing. Antibiotic cover is recommended, particularly when nasal packs are used.

If the skin has been soiled by ingrained dirt (a so-called "dirt tattoo") during an accidental injury (e.g., a cycling accident), then the particles must be scrubbed out intraoperatively with a sterile hand-washing brush. This is best done during the initial treatment; later attempts at cleaning the skin are usually much less effective.

> **! Risks and Complications**
> If, despite all due care and attention, unfavorable scar formation or even the distortion of adjacent structures due to the scars has occurred, then at least 6 months should elapse before revision surgery is attempted. Only then will sufficiently stable scar conditions have developed.

Foreign Bodies

Foreign bodies of every description are inserted into the nose, especially by small children, but also by psychotic patients. Unilateral, intractable purulent discharge from the nose should always prompt the search for a foreign body.

A round foreign body is removed by placing the end of a right-angle hook behind the object and pulling it forward (**Fig. 6.8**).

6

If the foreign body is in a child's nasal vestibule, its immediate removal may be attempted. If this is unsuccessful, however, further attempts should not be made, but removal should be undertaken under general anesthesia. This is also advisable for all foreign bodies in the nasal cavity, as they could slip down into the pharynx and block the bronchial airways.

Foreign bodies which have remained in the nasal cavity for a longer period of time can become encrusted and form a so-called *rhinolith* (preferentially in the inferior nasal meatus). Usually this can only be extracted after mobilization with a chisel.

Fractures of the Bony Nasal Pyramid

Typical fracture patterns occur, depending on the direction and strength of the force applied (**Fig. 6.9**):

- Lateral impact injury (**Fig. 6.9a, b**):
  - moderate force: lateral depression without involvement of the septum
  - severe force: bony, crooked nose with associated septal fracture.
- Frontal impact injury (**Fig. 6.9c, d**):
  - moderate force: dorsal nasal depression (saddle-nose deformity)
  - severe force: saddle-nose deformity with impacted fracture of the nasal septum.

The diagnostic examination includes inspection and palpation, ensuring that the nasal septum is examined for septal hematoma or septal fracture. With major trauma, associated injuries of adjacent organs should also be assessed (anterior skull base, frontal sinus, orbital walls, zygoma, maxilla). Imaging is particularly appropriate in these cases (CT for major injury). Assessment of slight displacements of the nasal pyramid may be rendered difficult by soft-tissue swelling. In such cases it is advisable to repeat the examination a few days later, after the edema has resolved.

Fresh fractures should be treated within 8 days of the injury.

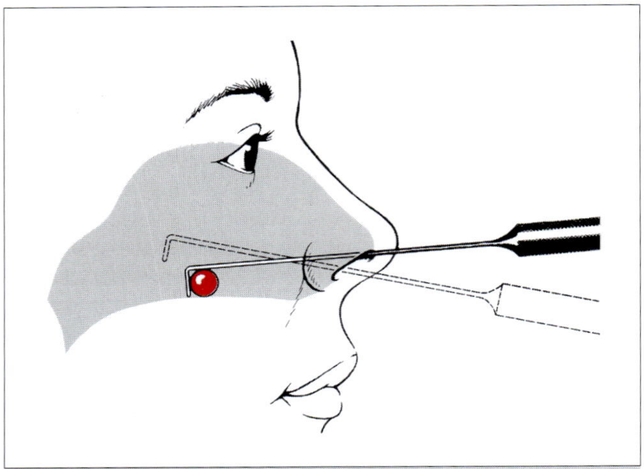

Fig. 6.8 Removal of a round foreign body from the nasal cavity. The blunt 90° hook is placed behind the foreign body.

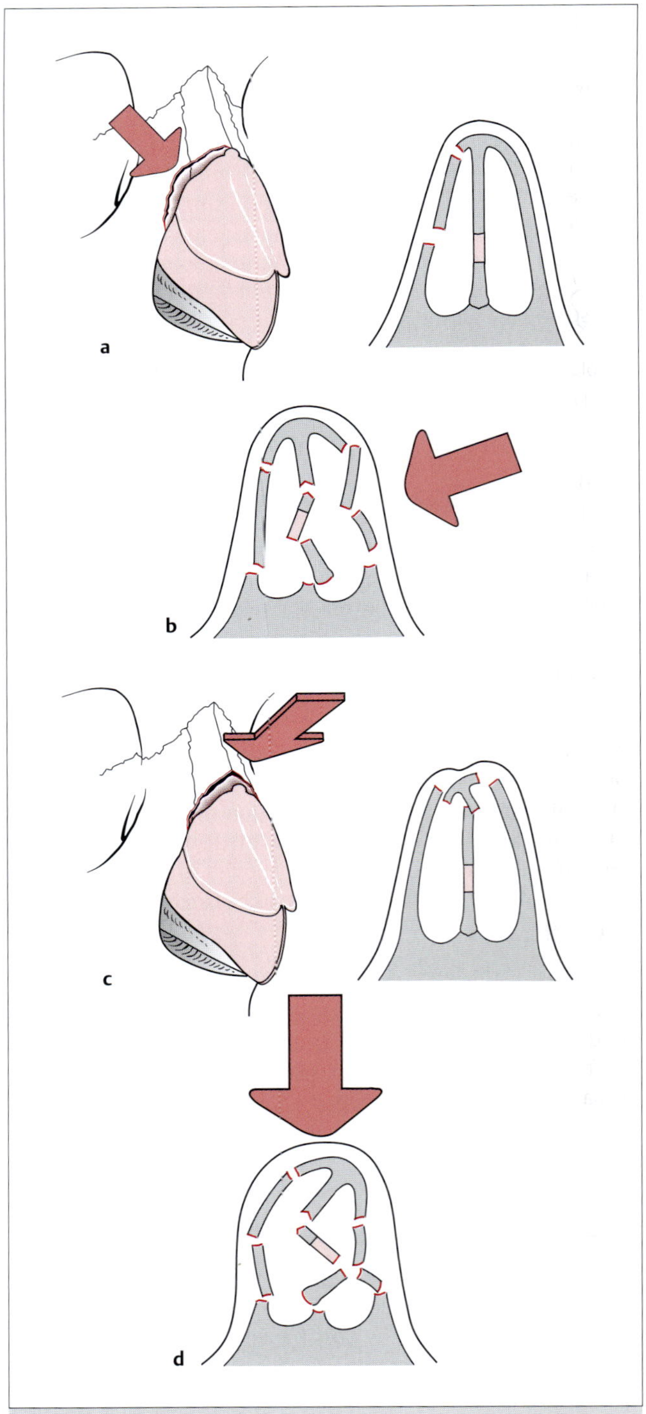

Fig. 6.9a–d Fractures of the nasal pyramid: injury mechanisms.
a Lateral impact injury (moderate force): lateral impression without lateral displacement of the pyramid; septum intact → endonasal reduction.
b Lateral impact injury (severe force): crooked nose with fracture of the septum → endonasal and external reduction of septum and pyramid; septoplasty may be necessary.
c Frontal impact injury (moderate force): dorsal nasal depression (localized saddle-nose deformity) → endonasal reduction.
d Frontal impact injury (severe force): saddle-nose deformity with impacted fracture of the septum → endonasal reduction and septoplasty.

Reduction of Fractures

Surgical Principle

The management of fractures of the nasal septum should adhere to the principles of septoplasty (see below, p. 57 ff). Dislocated bony walls of the pyramid are reduced (**Fig. 6.10**). Here the following principles apply:

> Depressions can only be reduced from an endonasal approach. Only lateral deviation of the nasal dorsum can be corrected by external pressure.
> Isolated depressions of the lateral nasal wall may give the misleading impression of a deviation of the nasal dorsum.

Indications

Fresh fractures (up to 8 days old) associated with cosmetically and/or functionally relevant sequelae. Septal fractures with mucosal injury or septal hematomas require immediate treatment, otherwise a wait of up to 8 days is possible (edema reduction).

Contraindications

Fractures older than 2–3 weeks. In this case it is better to wait 6–12 months and then correct the pyramid by means of a rhinoplasty after performing osteotomies. Fresh injuries may be superimposed on old fractures, rendering reduction impossible. The patient should therefore always be asked whether the nose was already "crooked" before the presenting injury.

Anesthesia

In a fresh lateral impact injury, deviation of the nasal dorsum without significant depression can be manually reduced to the midline without anesthetic. Depressions secondary to a lateral or frontal impact injury are best reduced from an endonasal approach under general anesthesia.

Surgical Technique

For endonasal reduction, a blunt instrument is introduced (e.g., the blunt end of a Cottle elevator), either to lift the nasal dorsum or to displace the lateral nasal wall outward (**Fig. 6.10**). If the cartilage fragments do not interlock by themselves, then they will need endonasal support in the form of packing for 8–10 days. In these cases, antibiotic prophylaxis is recommended. If the cartilage fragments have interlocked in the wrong position and disimpaction is difficult, they will need instrumental mobilization first. This is best achieved with a disimpaction forceps, which is introduced with one of its jaws into the nose to mobilize the lateral nasal pyramid wall with slight rotary movements.

Postoperative Care

After reduction an external splint is required, not so much for stabilization as for protection and to avoid any significant postoperative swelling. It is applied in the same manner as for elective septo-rhinoplasty (**Fig. 6.11**). The nasal dorsum is covered with a dressing consisting of overlapping strips of adhesive tape. The tissue in the supratip region has a tendency to swell considerably, and a swelling with the subsequent formation of a "polly beak" deformity (see **Fig. 6.42**) may develop if a hematoma appears. To counteract the development of swelling there, a strip of tape should be applied firmly over the supratip. The actual splinting can be achieved with a thermoplastic splint, or with plaster of Paris or other material. Care should be taken to ensure that no sharp edges penetrate the skin of the medial canthal region and that the eyelids can open and close without hindrance. A grid-patterned splint has the advantage that the vertical components of the grid are helpful for orientation and assist in bringing the nasal dorsum back into its midline position. The splint is secured with further strips of tape, similar to those laid on initially.

6

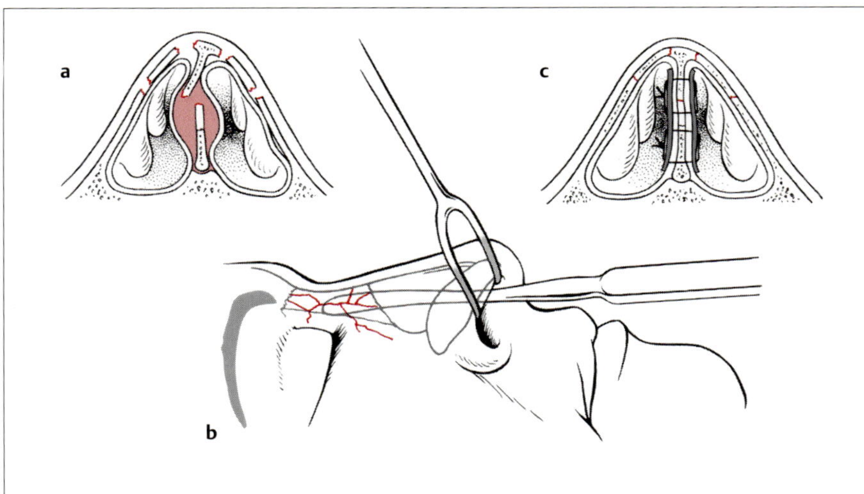

Fig. 6.10a–c Nasal pyramid reduction and septal revision.
- **a** Frontal impact injury with fractures of the pyramid and septum.
- **b** Reduction of the nasal dorsum using an elevator after management of the septal fracture.
- **c** Appearance after reduction and fixation of the septum with septal splints.

Septal Fracture / Septal Hematoma / Septal Abscess

Septal fractures that affect breathing require mobilization and correction of the nasal septum, in addition to reduction of the external bony pyramid (**Fig. 6.10**). The technique does not in principle differ from that used for septoplasty (see below, p. 57 ff). Bleeding occurs if the perichondrium is stripped from the underlying cartilage, resulting in the formation of a septal hematoma (**Fig. 6.10a**). Without treatment, the hematoma leads within a few days to absorption of the cartilage, which is dependent upon the perichondrium for its blood supply by diffusion. The result is the complete loss of the supporting function of the cartilaginous septum, with the development of a cartilaginous saddle-nose deformity. A septal hematoma can also develop relatively quickly into a septal abscess, which then leads to the destruction of the cartilage within a matter of hours. Apart from fever caused by infection, the presenting signs are complete blockage of nasal breathing with erythema and swelling of the skin in the region of the dorsum, columella, and nasal tip. Even light pressure on the nasal tip is painful. Such septal hematomas and abscesses can also develop after minor injuries (particularly in children), or even without any apparent external cause. The results of culture swabs taken from abscess fluid often return as sterile; occasionally staphylococcus or streptococcus is isolated. Antibiotic treatment is indicated in addition to surgery.

6

Surgery for Septal Hematoma/Abscess

Surgical Principle

After incision and drainage of the hematoma or abscess, any cartilage necrosis will require debridement and immediate reconstruction. Prevention of recurrence is essential, e.g., by the use of septal splints.

Specific Points Regarding Informed Consent

Children can still develop disturbances of growth in the course of time, despite appropriate management (see **Fig. 6.28**). Parents should be informed that definitive surgical treatment of residual deformities may possibly still be required after growth is complete. In cases requiring immediate reconstruction of the nasal septum, mention should be made of the possible need to harvest cartilage from the auricle or the use of foreign cartilage.

Special Instruments and Implants

After incision and drainage of the hematoma and abscess, intraseptal granulations should be curetted and the operative site irrigated with an antibiotic solution.

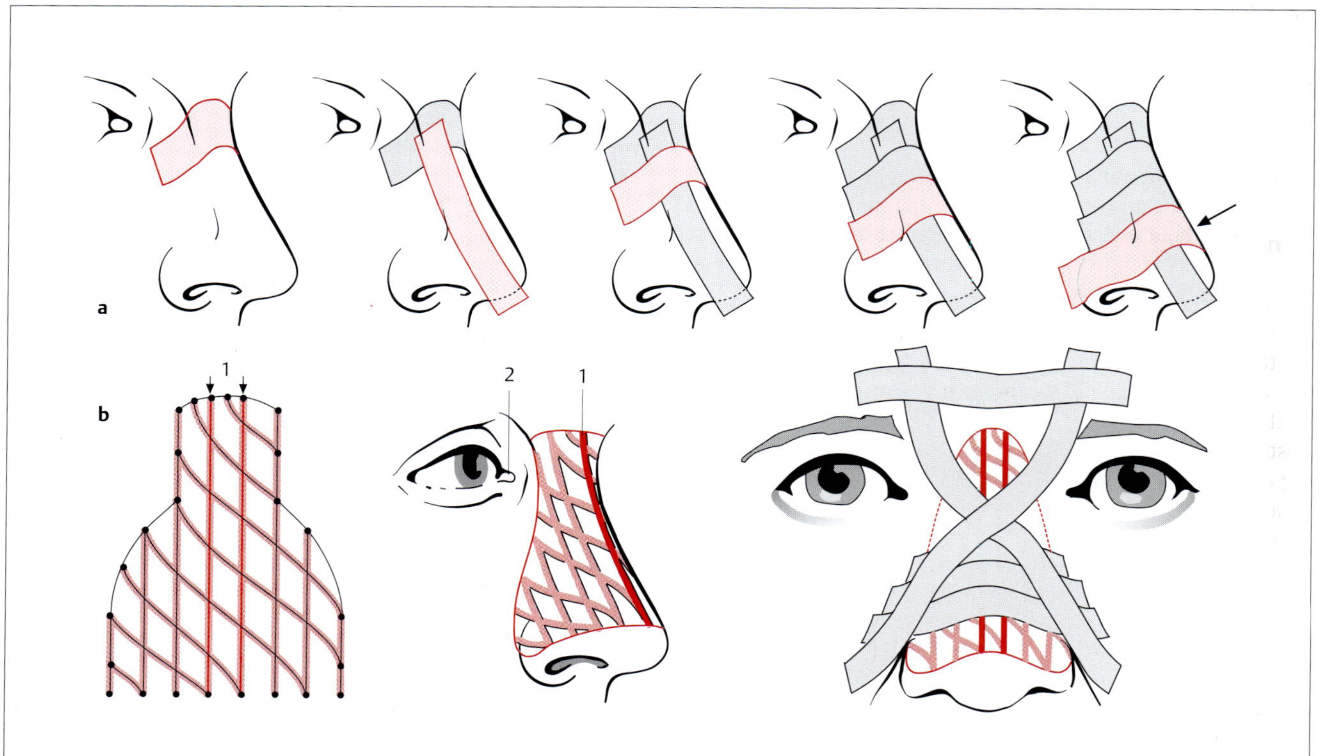

Fig. 6.11a, b Nasal dressing and splinting.
a Nasal dressing consisting of overlapping strips of adhesive tape. A "suspension" around the tip of the nose takes the tension off the endonasal sutures. Swelling of the supratip region must be avoided by firmly applying a strip of tape (arrow).
b Splinting and fixation: a splint constructed from grid-patterned thermoplastic material is trimmed to form so that the grid is orientated exactly vertically over the dorsum of the nose (1). This helps in bringing the mobile nasal dorsum exactly into its midline position. The splint must spare the medial canthal regions (2).

Anesthesia

General anesthesia is advisable.

Surgical Technique

The region of the hematoma/abscess is exposed via a hemitransfixion incision (see Septoplasty, p. 57ff) and a tunnel is developed beneath the mucosa until healthy cartilage or bone is reached. Soft, unstable nasal septal cartilage is removed and a culture swab of the abscess fluid is taken. After irrigating the cavity several times, the perichondrium and the periosteum are freed of granulations with a curette. These measures may need to include the undersurface of the upper lateral cartilages as well as the region around the membranous septum. After several rinses with an antibiotic solution, the perichondrial surfaces should be smooth on all sides.

If the caudal septal cartilage has been destroyed, immediate reconstruction is advisable, even in the presence of a septal abscess, to prevent contraction of the soft tissues. Options for autologous supporting material include either bony parts of the vomer and perpendicular plate or autologous conchal cartilage from the auricle. If it is available, solvent-dehydrated irradiated human costal cartilage is very suitable and can be rehydrated in an antibiotic solution.

Even if these grafts and implants only act as temporary spacers, they not only prevent soft-tissue contracture, but also considerably facilitate any later definitive treatment.

Prophylaxis against renewed intraseptal fluid collection can be achieved either by trans-septal absorbable mattress sutures or by sutured-in septal splints (**Fig. 6.10c**; see also **Fig. 6.18**). Unlike sutures, intranasal septal splints have the advantage of providing compression over a larger surface area. They should remain in situ for approximately 1 week.

Postoperative Care

The packs should remain for 3 days and the septal splints for up to 1 week under antibiotic protection. Otherwise postoperative care does not differ from that for septoplasty.

Alternatives

Localized unilateral septal hematomas (but not abscesses) may also be aspirated with a needle and then packed. If they are not too large, they may be left for spontaneous absorption, given that any aspiration is associated with the possibility of bacterial spread and secondary infection. A unilateral hematoma does not carry the risk of cartilage necrosis because nutrition of the cartilage is guaranteed by the perichondrium of the contralateral side. Hematomas situated over bony regions of the septum are less at risk because the bone does not receive its nutrition by diffusion, but via blood vessels.

6

Surgery of the Nasal Septum

Functions of the Nasal Septum

The cartilaginous nasal septum is the central supporting structure for the cartilaginous nose and the enveloping soft tissues. Septal deviations have functional consequences especially in the areas of natural narrowings, i.e., the nasal vestibule and at the level of the nasal valve area. Deviations situated more posteriorly (e.g., vomerine spur) can also represent a breathing obstruction, although they tend to be less serious than anterior deformities. Deviations of the cartilaginous septum are therefore of particular functional importance and must be corrected by mobilization, reduction, resection, and, if necessary, reconstruction. Consideration must be given to the supporting function of the caudal nasal septum, which needs to be reconstructed by septoplasty or preserved during straightening procedures. As **Fig. 6.12** clearly shows, it is not merely a problem involving the internal nose; loss of the supporting function of the nasal septum also has manifold consequences which also affect the external form of the nose. The left column in **Fig. 6.12** shows the normal situation, with cross-sections parallel to the columella at the level of the lower lateral cartilages (1) and the nasal valve (2), as well as a cross-section through the columellar base and the alae of the nose (3). By comparison, the right column shows the effects resulting from destruction of the septal cartilage, with subsequent reduction in the height of the caudal septal margin. The lower lateral cartilage domes usually have an acute-angled form as seen from the basal view, with the fibrous tissue between the domes riding on the anterior septal margin, thus determining the height of the nasal tip (the nasal tip projection is the distance between the nasal tips as seen from the vertical facial plane—see **Figs. 6.39** and **6.40**). Cartilage and soft tissues are thus under tension. The nostrils are oval and the columellar base is only slightly wider, due to the diverging medial crura of the lower lateral cartilages. The intact septodorsal cartilage has a nasal valve angle of approximately 15°. In the transverse section through the columellar base, the latter lies caudal to the alar rims, the membranous septum is elongated and the cross-sections of the medial crura of the lower lateral cartilages are close together. This creates a space between the membranous septum and the alar rim, which is large enough to prevent the nostrils from being sucked in toward the membranous septum during inspiration.

The alterations encountered when the septum height is reduced are correspondingly complex in nature. The nasal basal view now demonstrates a reduction in nasal tip projection. The fibrous tissue between the lower lateral cartilages is no longer held under tension by the nasal septum; the domes flatten off and diverge. The result is a wide nasal tip, which is amorphous

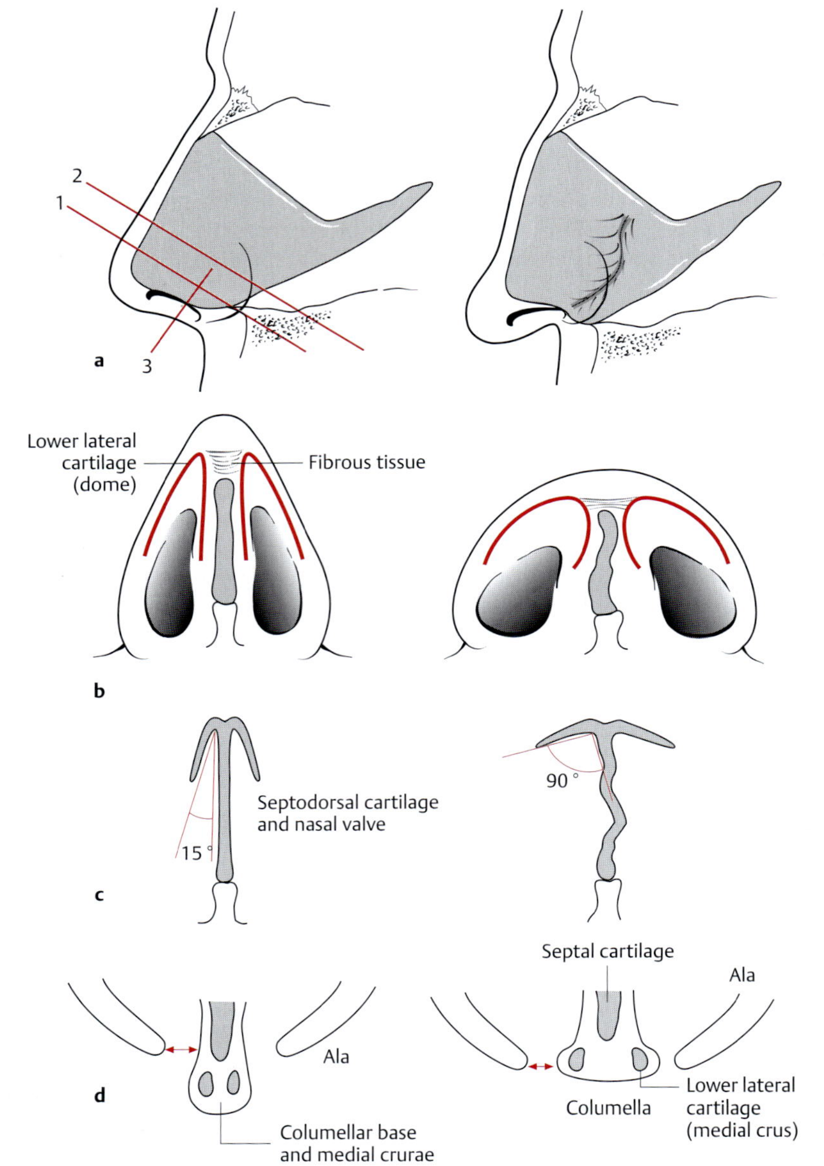

Fig. 6.12a–d The role of the nasal septum as the central supporting structure for the nasal tip, nasal dorsum, and nasal base. Left column: normal situation. Right column: sequelae after loss of the supporting function of the septal cartilage.

- **a** Lateral view indicating the section planes 1–3.
- **b** Section through the nasal tip (1): the domes are supported over the upper septal margin and held under tension by fibrous tissue. This gives the domes an acute angle, making the tip of the nose slender (left). Loss of height of the caudal edge of the septum "relaxes" the cartilage, making the domes and the tip as well as the nostrils "round." Nasal tip projection is reduced and the columella becomes wide and short. The distance between the alae is increased (right).
- **c** The angle of the nasal valve is widened (ballooning phenomenon).
- **d** The columellar base is held in a caudal direction by the septum and placed under tension. This makes it narrow. The medial crurae of the lower lateral cartilages are close together and their distance from the nostrils is wide (double arrow left). If the caudal edge of the septum is displaced posteriorly, the columellar base retracts and becomes wider. The vestibule is then narrower (double arrow right).

or undefined because of the loss of the domes. The loss of height results in excessive soft tissue, which widens, so the distance between the two nostrils is greater and the normally oval nostrils adopt a more rounded form. Reduction of the cartilaginous nasal dorsum causes the nasal valve angle to increase up to 90° (a situation known as the "ballooning phenomenon"). This results in a deflection of the principle air flow toward the floor of the nose, which is associated with an overloading and desiccation of the mucous membranes. The transverse section through the columella now shows the columella to be lying at the same level as the alar rims (retracted or "hidden" columella) and at the same time widened as a result of the loss of tension (the cross-sections of the medial crura of the lower lateral cartilages are farther apart). The now reduced distance between nostrils and columella results in vestibular stenosis, with the risk of total collapse from negative pressure during inspiration.

This list of the dynamic processes that result from the loss of the supporting function of the cartilaginous nasal septum shows that three aspects in particular must be borne in mind during surgery of the nasal septum:

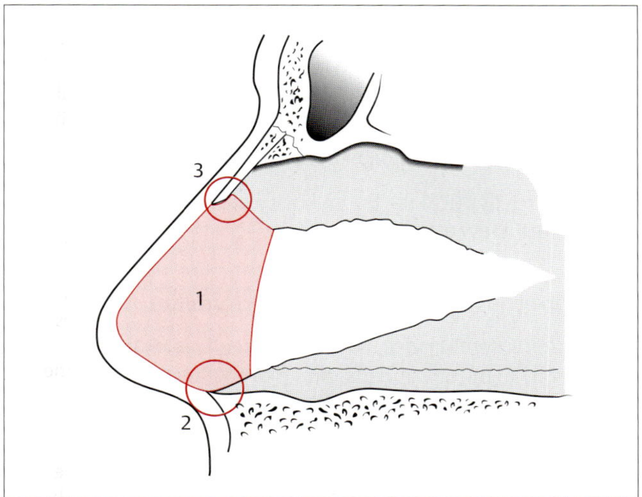

Fig. 6.13 The objectives of septoplasty/septal reconstruction. Preservation or reconstruction of the cartilaginous support by:
1 adequate size, form and stability
2 preservation or reconstruction of the connection with the premaxilla
3 adequate fixation by (partial) preservation of the suture line to the perpendicular plate or by suturing the upper lateral cartilages and septum at the level of the keystone area

- The caudal third of the nose, including the nasal base, represents a complex system under tension. This tension is produced by the size, form, and position of the septal cartilage.
- Straightening of a caudal septal deviation must not be achieved at the cost of the supportive function, otherwise the changes mentioned above may develop in more or less pronounced form.
- If deformities have developed as a result of the loss of the supportive function, then they should not, if at all possible, be corrected by surgery of individual issues (e. g., nasal tip correction or cartilage grafting for the depressed nasal dorsum), but rather an attempt should be made to correct the underlying pathology: restoration of stability, size, and position of the caudal nasal septum (**Fig. 6.13**).

Surgery of the nasal septum usually involves mobilization of the cartilaginous septum. It is therefore essential to have knowledge of the natural fixation points, which need to be either preserved or reconstructed after separation (**Fig. 6.13** [2, 3]):

- *preservation* of the connection with the perpendicular plate and/or the premaxilla, or
- *fixation* to the upper lateral cartilages at the junction with the nasal bone and at the anterior nasal spine.

Septoplasty

Surgical Principle

The literature often describes submucous resection of the septum (Killian) and septoplasty (Cottle) as if they were basically equivalent. These two operative techniques are, however, different in principle.

During *submucous resection of the septum* the central cartilaginous and osseous components of the nasal septum are removed, while preserving a sufficiently large cartilaginous frame at the nasal dorsum and columella. If the stability of this frame becomes inadequate after extensive resection, a typical deformity will result, as shown in **Fig. 6.12**. Because it is important not to disrupt the unit of mucosa and cartilaginous frame, the incision through the mucosa to gain access to the area of resection lies immediately at the anterior border of the intended cartilaginous window. This approach therefore does not allow the exposure of deviations of the cartilaginous frame. Submucous resection of the septum thus corrects mainly septal ridges at the junction between septal cartilage, vomer, and perpendicular plate, or corrects a vomerine spur. It has already been pointed out that obstruction of nasal breathing due to this deformity is often only moderate.

In contrast, the principle of *septoplasty* not only permits correction of the central parts of the septum, but also allows surgery of the *cartilaginous framework*. Cottle's standardized approach (maxillary–premaxillary approach) enables the complete exposure of the infrastructure of the nasal septum. Because deviations of the cartilaginous framework lie at the narrow parts of the nasal airways, they are of considerably greater functional importance than deviations of the central septum. Although the procedure has undergone changes over the years, certain basic operative steps still apply:

1. Incision (right hemitransfixion).
2. Approach: subperichondrial and subperiosteal septal tunnels.
3. Mobilization (chondrotomies, osteotomies).
4. Resections (cartilage and/or bone).
5. Reconstruction/replacement.
6. Fixation (suture, septal splints).

Only knowledge and use of an approach which provides access to *all* parts of the septum will allow its correction, and this is therefore recommended as the basic technique. Depending on the presenting pathology, an adapted modification is then possible. Cottle's technique is to proceed along the floor of the nose from bilateral tunnels, which are developed beginning at the piriform aperture in a dorsal direction (maxillary approach). These nasal floor tunnels are connected to superior septal tunnels, proceeding from the caudal septum and the premaxilla (premaxillar approach). Connecting the septal tunnels to the nasal floor tunnels, however, necessitates division of the nasopalatine nerve at the incisive canal (**Fig. 6.4**), which is why the maxillar–premaxillar approach is mainly recommended only for special indications (protruding basal crest of the nasal septum, difficult revision surgery, closure of septal perforations).

Otherwise, tunnelling of the septum should only be performed in a vertical plane, sparing the horizontal nasal floor.

Indications

- Obstruction of nasal breathing secondary to dislocation of the caudal margin of the septum, deviations of the cartilaginous nasal dorsum or the caudal septal margin, septal basal crest (caudal septum and premaxilla), ascending septal ridge and vomerine spur (septal cartilage, vomer, perpendicular plate), deviated perpendicular plate.
- Septal fractures or their sequelae (in particular vertical fractures at the level of the nasal valve, transverse fracture), vestibular stenoses associated with a crooked or tension nose.
- Septal reconstruction for saddle-nose deformity.
- For improved access during surgery of the paranasal sinuses, for posterior epistaxis, as an approach for choanal atresia, and for access to the hypophysis.

Contraindications

- Acute rhinitis.
- Severe general disorders, especially coagulopathies.
- High-grade atrophy of the septal mucosa (e.g., after multiple previous operations).

Specific Points Regarding Informed Consent

- Alterations of the form of the external nose.
- Olfactory dysfunction.
- Septal perforation.
- Possibility of harvesting a graft (auricle, rib).

Operative Planning

It is to be expected that any cartilage material still available from earlier injuries or operations will be insufficient to restore an adequate supporting function of the cartilaginous nose. The so-called "cotton bud test" can assist in providing an estimate: the nasal septum is palpated with a cotton bud to identify any areas that are still stable or free of cartilage. The possible harvesting of a graft should be provisionally included in the informed consent, to avoid resorting to compromises when faced with a lack of cartilage during the operation. In difficult cases, especially with re-explorations, it may be useful to include subsequent revision surgery to remove residual deformities in the operation plan.

Special Instruments and Implants

A selection of instruments for septoplasty is shown in **Fig. 6.6a**.

Anesthesia

Septoplasty is usually performed under general anesthesia. Only in selected cases of isolated operations in the vestibular area (e.g., isolated dislocation of the caudal septal margin—very rare) can local anesthesia be sufficient.

Surgical Technique

The operation is divided into the following steps:

(a) Preparation, Incision, Approach

- These are identical for the majority of septal deformities, with just a few exceptions.

(b) Correction of Various Septum Deformities

- Ascending septal ridge, basal crest (see **Figs. 6.19** and **6.20**).
- Dislocation of the caudal septal margin (see **Fig. 6.21**).
- Deviation of the septal cartilage:
  - caudal septal margin (see **Fig. 6.22**).
  - superior septal margin (see **Fig. 6.23**).

(c) Defects or Insufficiency of the Caudal Septum

- Partial septal reconstruction
- Total septal reconstruction (septal replacement) (see **Figs. 6.25, 6.26, 6.27**)

(d) Replacement, Fixation, Packing

These measures, on the other hand, are usually performed in a uniform manner.

Because of the mainly uniform approach, independent of the presenting pathology, points (a) and (d) will be discussed together (**Figs. 6.14, 6.15, 6.16, 6.17,** and **6.18**).

Preparation. The head is positioned slightly elevated (chin in the direction of the chest) to allow visualization of both the nasal floor and the superior parts of the septum, without the surgeon having to adopt extreme head positions. The operative site is prepared before sterile draping: decongestion of the mucous membranes (e.g., by inserting strips of sponge soaked in xylometazoline), possibly cleansing the nasal vestibule with alcohol (where staphylococci are found in about half of all patients), infiltration of the membranous septum (for practical reasons a ready-prepared combination of local anesthetic and epinephrine 1:200 000 has proved useful). Extensive infiltration of the septal mucosa to facilitate later tunnelling (so-called "hydraulic dissection") is not generally recommended, as this usually inflates only the mucosa and does not separate the perichondrium from the cartilage, in addition to the complications that have been described (blinding). Disinfection of the face is an option, but not absolutely necessary. Antibiotic prophylaxis (e.g., for re-explorations using grafts, potentially infected adjacent regions) should be administered in the form of perioperative prophylaxis. A right-handed surgeon stands to the right of the patient.

Incision: right hemitransfixion (**Fig. 6.14**). For the right-handed surgeon, the right nasal vestibule is more easily visualized than the left, which is why the incision is always performed on the right, even if the caudal septal margin is dislocated to the left. The caudal septal margin is exposed using a columella forceps and an alar retractor: the clamp grasps only the mobile membranous septum. The skin covering the cartilaginous margin is placed in tension by moving the clamp to the left and pos-

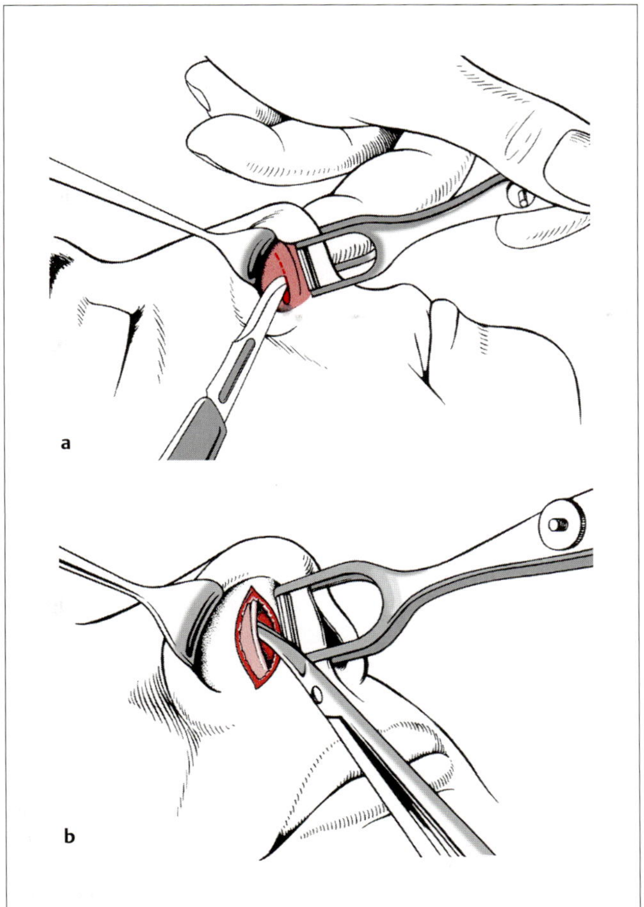

Fig. 6.14a, b Incision.
a Right hemitransfixion.
b Identification of the caudal septal margin and the subperichondrial plane of dissection (approach to the left anterior tunnel).

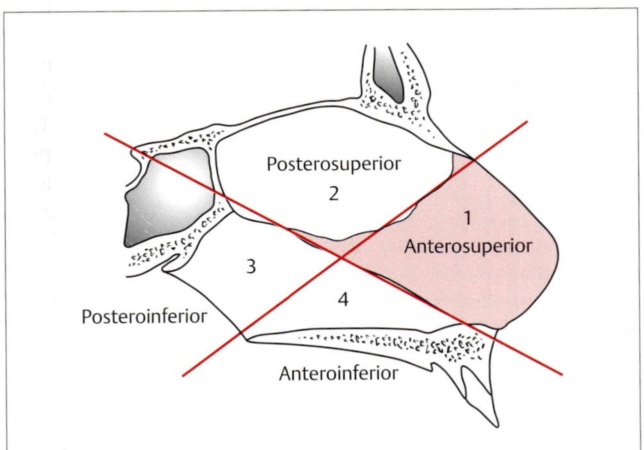

Fig. 6.15 Position of the four septal tunnels (unilateral) over the:
1 quadrangular plate
2 perpendicular plate
3 vomer
4 vomer and premaxilla

teriorly. The alar retractor (assistant) exposes the attachment of the upper lateral cartilage and at the same time protects the ala from an inadvertent laceration. The middle finger of the surgeon's right hand can displace to the right a septum which has dislocated to the left and stabilizes the septal cartilage for the incision.

The hemitransfixion (Latin: hemi = half, transfigere = to pierce through) incision is made, using a No. 15 scalpel blade, in the skin (not in the mucosa) about 2 mm *behind* the cartilage edge, from the anterior nasal spine to just before the attachment of the upper lateral cartilage (the anterior–inferior septal corner). The incision proceeds in a posterior-to-anterior direction to avoid blood dripping down and obstructing the view. Incision of the cartilage should be avoided.

Note: A transfixion (see **Fig. 6.32a**) differs from a hemitransfixion in that it not only transects the entire membranous septum through to the opposite side, but also lies caudal to the septal end. It enables the membranous septum to be completely separated from the nasal septum, together with the columella and the medial crura of the lower lateral cartilages.

Approach: septal tunnels (**Figs. 6.15** and **6.16**). The cartilaginous framework is exposed by subperichondrial septal tunnels and the bony framework by subperiosteal septal tunnels.

It is generally recommended, whenever possible, to leave the cartilage attached on one side to the septal mucosa, as this reduces the risk of a too generous mobilization and dislocation. With a unilateral anterior deviation, one would create an anterior tunnel only on that side. The left tunnel is routinely created first when dealing with an ascending septal ridge on the left side.

Finding the *correct plane* for the dissection is essential. The fibrous strands are separated from the caudal septal margin with a pointed instrument (e.g., closed small pointed scissors, **Fig. 6.14b**). At times they will require transection. The correct plane can often only be identified 2–3 mm behind the cartilage edge. After elevating the perichondrium, the cartilage shines through with a bluish tinge. The "incorrect plane" is recognized by its reddish color and pinpoint bleeding. In this case, the remaining perichondrial layer must once again be separated from the cartilage with a pointed instrument. Once the subperichondrial layer has *definitely* been reached, tunnelling beneath the quadrangular plate to its junctions with the perpendicular plate (chondroethmoid suture) and the vomer (chondrovomerine suture) is usually achieved without difficulty using the blunt end of a Cottle elevator, provided no significant deviations are encountered which place the mucosa under tension, or old cartilage fractures to which the mucosa is attached by scar tissue. At these points, further sharp dissection must be undertaken. In this manner, a left anterosuperior tunnel is created.

The mucosa is elevated off the junction with the perpendicular plate using the sharp end of the Cottle elevator and a posterosuperior tunnel is dissected, ensuring constant contact of the instrument with bone as far as the junction between the perpendicular plact and the vomer (or the sphenoid process of the septal cartilage). On completion of these steps, a left anterosuperior and a left posterosuperior septal tunnel will have been created.

6

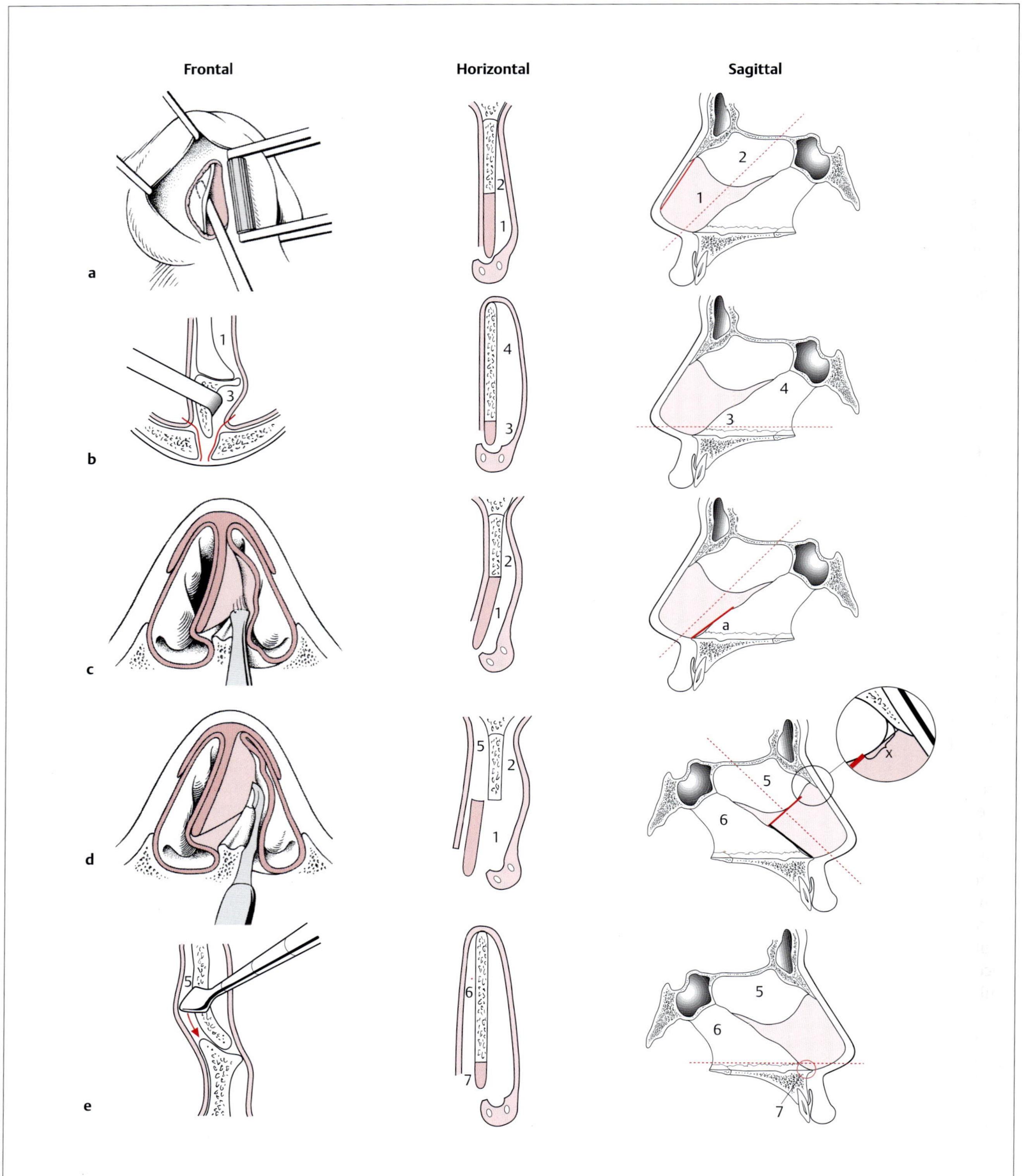

Fig. 6.16a–e Septoplasty: standard approach to the infrastructure. Presentation of the individual steps in the frontal, horizontal, and sagittal planes; the horizontal section plane is marked in each case in the right column.

a Superior tunnel left anterior (1) and posterior (2).

b Inferior tunnel left anterior (3) and posterior (4).

c Horizontal chondrotomy at the cartilaginous base of the septum.

d Vertical chondrotomy at the osseocartilaginous junction, sparing the region immediately below the nasal bones (x) and the right posterosuperior (5) and inferior (6) tunnels.

e Anteroinferior tunnel on the right. The posteroinferior tunnel may be opened from above by sharp division of the fibers at the bony suture (the so-called “posterior approach”) to allow the anterior section to be exposed from here (7).

> Tunnelling over cartilage is done with blunt instruments to avoid injury to the cartilage, whereas sharp instruments are used over bone.

The left inferior tunnels may be created relatively simply in a posterior-to-anterior direction via the superior tunnel, provided there is no relevant septal deviation. For this purpose, the mucosa is elevated in the posterior septal segment at the junction between perpendicular plate and vomer, using the sharp end of the elevator, and the tunnel is then exposed from above down to the nasal floor (the so-called posterior approach to the inferior tunnel). With contact between the instrument and the bone of the nasal floor, this posteroinferior tunnel may then be easily enlarged in a posterior-to-anterior direction as far as the level of the premaxillary wing and the anterior nasal spine. Dissecting in the vertical plane in this region avoids injuring the nasopalatine nerve. At the end of this stage, a complete left-sided tunnel of the nasal septum will have been developed (**Fig. 6.16b**).

With a protruding ascending septal ridge or a basal crest, this posterior approach to the inferior tunnel is not possible. Instead, the mucosa must be elevated from the undersurface of the ridge or crest from an anterior direction. For this purpose, the strong fibrous strands are first separated from the bone at the piriform aperture, exposing the transition from premaxilla (septum) to nasal floor at the piriform crest. This then allows a curved elevator (e.g., a McKenty elevator) to be inserted, with bone contact, to separate the mucosa subperiosteally from the premaxillary wings and from the undersurface of an ascending septal ridge (**Fig. 6.16b**). In this case the mucosa is not elevated off the protruding parts of the ridge until it has been mobilized by osteotomy, thus taking the tension off the mucosa which is often very thin at this point. In the case of ridges and crests, therefore, the superior and inferior tunnels are not initially connected.

To develop the right posterior tunnel, the septal cartilage must be mobilized and displaced to the right. For this purpose, a *horizontal chondrotomy* is made first (**Fig. 6.16c**). A sharp instrument (e.g., Cottle knife, No. 15 scalpel blade) is used to transect the cartilage at its attachment to the premaxilla and vomer to about the middle of the septum (the beginning of the sphenoid process of the cartilage). Then the attachment to the perpendicular plate is *subtotally* released by a *vertical chondrotomy* (**Fig. 6.16d**). Immediately before the osseocartilaginous junction, the cartilage is incised (e.g., with a Cottle elevator) and the incision extended in a caudal-to-cranial direction. Whenever possible, at least 5 mm of the suture line should be preserved to avoid rotation of the septum after any bilateral elevation of the mucosa and chondrotomies (see **Fig. 6.29**). If, however, there are significant septal deviations beneath the nasal dorsum, then the vertical chondrotomy must be extended until bony contact with the nasal bones is obtained, to be directly repaired at a later time (see below).

Access is gained via the chondrotomies to the right side, in the correct plane directly beneath the periosteum, after displacing the mobilized cartilage to create the right posterior tunnels (superior and inferior) (**Fig. 6.16c**). The posteroinferior tunnel may be extended into an anteroinferior tunnel via the posterior approach. At the end of this step, the septal cartilage is still partially attached to the perpendicular plate, to the nasal bones via the upper lateral cartilages, and to the septal mucosa of the right side. It may now be swung to the side like a swinging door, allowing complete visualization of the remaining septal parts, from the nasal floor to the dorsum and from the premaxilla to the choanae.

Replacement. After correction of the nasal septum pathology is complete (see below), it is necessary to initiate replacement and fixation of the mobilized nasal septum, followed by packing of the nasal cavity to achieve hematoma prophylaxis and stabilization (**Fig. 6.17**). At the end of the operation, as few areas of the septum as possible should remain free of cartilage and bone. Any supporting tissue which is not required for reconstruction should be replaced after straightening with the cartilage and bone crusher. The nasal cavity should first be packed, at least temporarily (e.g., with foam packs), to avoid dislocation of the fragments. The packs press both mucosal layers lightly together, while replacement is being accomplished in a posterior-to-anterior direction.

Fixation. Before suture repair of the hemitransfixion, fixation of the cartilaginous septum must be checked. For this purpose, the caudal septal margin is grasped with an Adson–Brown forceps and moved. If it can be pushed into the nose, then it will definitely need suture fixation to the anterior nasal spine (**Fig. 6.17**). Mobility of the septal cartilage is to be anticipated, particularly when the septum has been tunnelled on both sides and the posterior chondrotomy extends as far as the undersurface of the nasal bones. In this case, the cartilaginous nasal septum is "hanging on" only by the upper lateral cartilages, and soft-tissue pressure will lead to inward rotation of the cartilaginous nasal septum (see **Fig. 6.29**).

Packing or other stabilization measures. Stabilization and prophylaxis of a septal hematoma may be accomplished by nasal packs, septal splints, or trans-septal mattress sutures. Depending on the complexity of the operation and the extent of mobi-

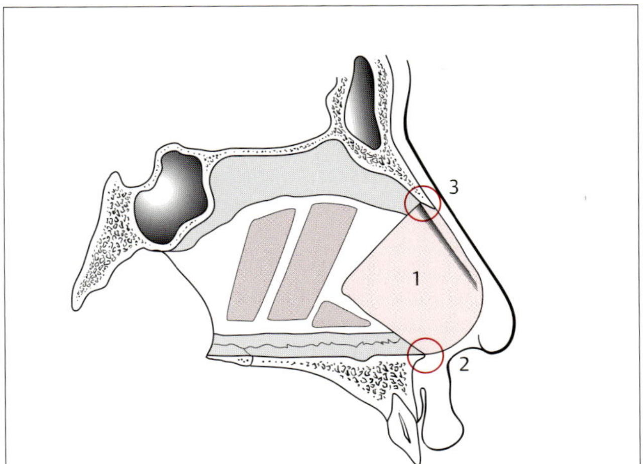

Fig. 6.17 Replacement and fixation.
Straightened pieces of cartilage and bone are used to fill the "empty mucosal pockets" and to support the mobilized septal cartilage from below. The caudal septum must be of adequate size (1) and secured (2 and 3) before the hemitransfixion can be repaired.

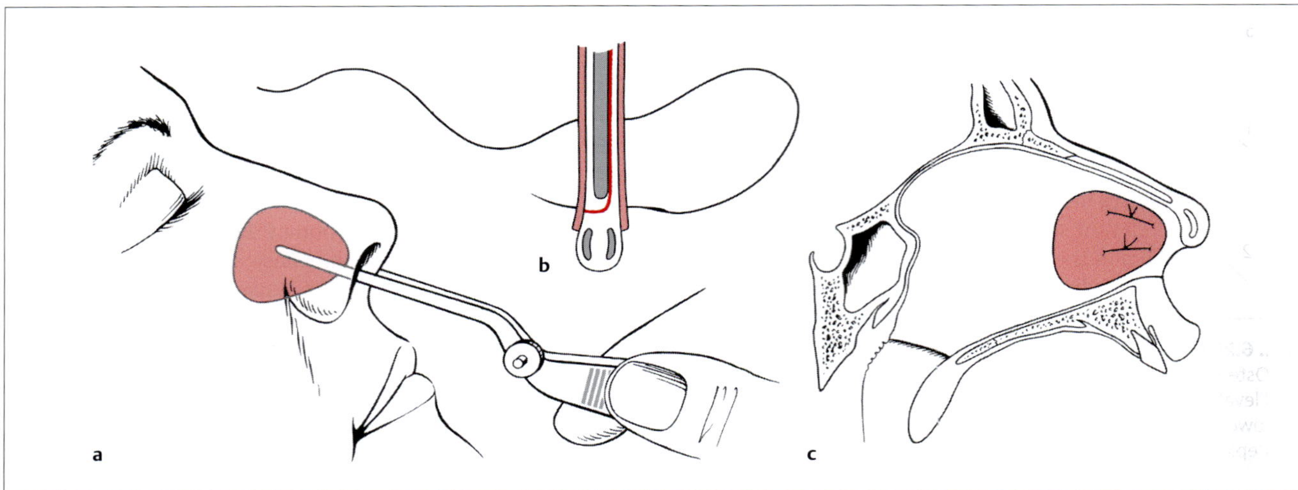

Fig. 6.18a–c Fixation of the septum with septal splints.
a The fashioned septal splints are fitted and secured using a septal-splint clamp.
b Horizontal section demonstrating the absorbable mattress suture.
c The septal splints secured by two mattress sutures.

lization, a combination of these methods is recommended, with nasal packs nearly always being beneficial. Prophylaxis against hematoma formation over the cartilage is imperative (see p. 54). Trans-septal continuous mattress sutures using absorbable suture material are well suited for stabilization and hematoma prophylaxis in the cartilaginous region and near bone-free septum regions. They should not be placed too closely together, however, nor tied too tightly, in order avoid mucosal necrosis. A combination with nasal packing is recommended, at least for one night. The same applies for septal splints (**Fig. 6.18**), which are positioned with the aid of a septal-splint clamp and secured with two or more trans-septal mattress sutures. These should be absorbable sutures because small pieces of residual suture material tend to remain within the septum on removal. Septal splints compress the mucosa over a wider area than sutures alone and thus have less tendency to produce mucosal necrosis, provided the mattress sutures are not pulled too tightly. Care should be taken to ensure that the splints reach as far as the columellar margin, but do not cut into the upper nostril rim. Injury to the soft triangle there (see **Fig. 6.33a**) can result in an irreparable deformity from scar contracture. The septal splints are removed after 3–6 days, depending on the complexity of the reconstruction.

Nasal packs, inserted together with mattress sutures or septal splints, may be removed on the first postoperative day. A wide variety of materials are used for packing. Basically, they should exert a sufficient amount of pressure on the septal mucosa across as wide an area as possible, safeguard the mucosal surface, be easily removed, and provide safety against slipping down the nasopharynx. The use of several unsecured packs should be avoided, given that parts may be easily overlooked during removal and thus left behind.

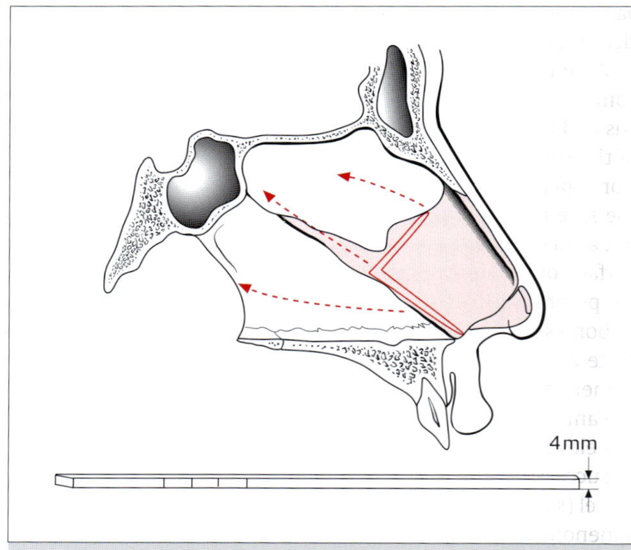

Fig. 6.19 Osteotomy of an ascending septal ridge and mobilization of the perpendicular plate.
Three osteotomies are made using the 4-mm chisel and residual bony bridges are fractured or, with thick bone, selectively osteotomized.

Correction of Individual Septal Deformities or Defects

Resection of an ascending septal ridge/basal crest (**Figs. 6.19** and **6.20**). Ridges and crests are formed of septal cartilage in their cranial part and of bone on their undersurface. Basal crests can significantly narrow the piriform aperture. They are composed of the bony premaxillary ala covered by the septal cartilage, which usually deviates to the ipsilateral side. They are exposed via superior and inferior tunnels, initially leaving the mucosal attachment untouched over its lateral prominent part. Cartilage and bone are removed tangentially, using a sufficient-

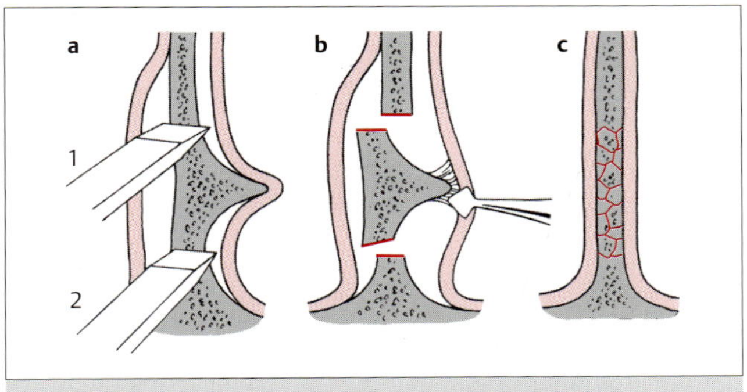

Fig. 6.20a–c Resection of a vomerine spur.
a Osteotomies, first above (1), then below (2) the spur.
b Elevation of the mucoperiostium from the tip of the spur, followed by extraction.
c Replacement after straightening with a crusher.

ly wide chisel or osteotome, and thus mobilized. This relaxes the mucosa, allowing the basal crest to be dissected out. Hemorrhage from the wound surface of the bone is controlled by compression. Because this bleeding can impair visibility when working on the posterior parts of the septum, removal of the basal crest is delayed until all parts of the septum have been clearly exposed.

Ascending septal ridges follow the cranial margin of the vomer. Their undersurface consists of the bony vomerine sulcus and their cartilaginous part mainly of the sphenoid process of the septal cartilage (**Fig. 6.19**). Here too anterior and posterior septal tunnels are required, bearing in mind again that, on the side of the ridge, the superior and inferior tunnels should not at first be connected at the ridge margin. The posterior cut surface of the vertical chondrotomy in fact serves as the starting point for the osteotomies, preferably using the 4-mm chisel or bone scissors. At first, the thinner bone of the perpendicular plate is osteotomized above the ridge, followed by the thicker vomer below. In the dorsal region, the thin bony lamella toward the anterior wall of the sphenoid cavity is easily fractured with the elevator, allowing the ridge to be mobilized. If fracturing is unsuccessful because of dense bone, then a curved transverse chisel (see **Fig. 6.6b**) is placed in front of the anterior wall of the sphenoid cavity against the septum bone, which is perforated with a few blows and then mobilized. The ridge can then be displaced to the contralateral side, thus relaxing the still-attached mucosa. Superior and inferior tunnels are then connected over the margin of the ridge using an elevator and the mobilized osseocartilaginous fragment is removed (**Fig. 6.20b**). With ascending septal ridges the perpendicular plate of the ipsilateral side is often slanted, so it is mobilized by osteotomy below the nasal dorsum. The bone of the perpendicular plate is very thick only in the region of the bony nasal pyramid and becomes paper-thin beneath the skull base. Once the thicker bone has been divided, the lamina can usually be fractured off the skull base with mild pressure of the elevator and then extracted.

Dislocation of the caudal septal margin (**Fig. 6.21**). An isolated dislocation of the caudal septal margin into a nostril is extremely rare. Usually the underlying cause is an osseocartilaginous crooked nose, which must be corrected accordingly (see Crooked Nose, p. 87). With an incomplete vertical cartilaginous fracture, however, it may be that only the caudal cartilaginous nasal septum has come out of the premaxillary groove on one side. Often the cartilage of the nasal septum is even found on the floor of the nose.

The caudal septum is exposed via a right hemitransfixion incision. Usually both anterosuperior tunnels need to be created because the septum has deviated to one side where it is

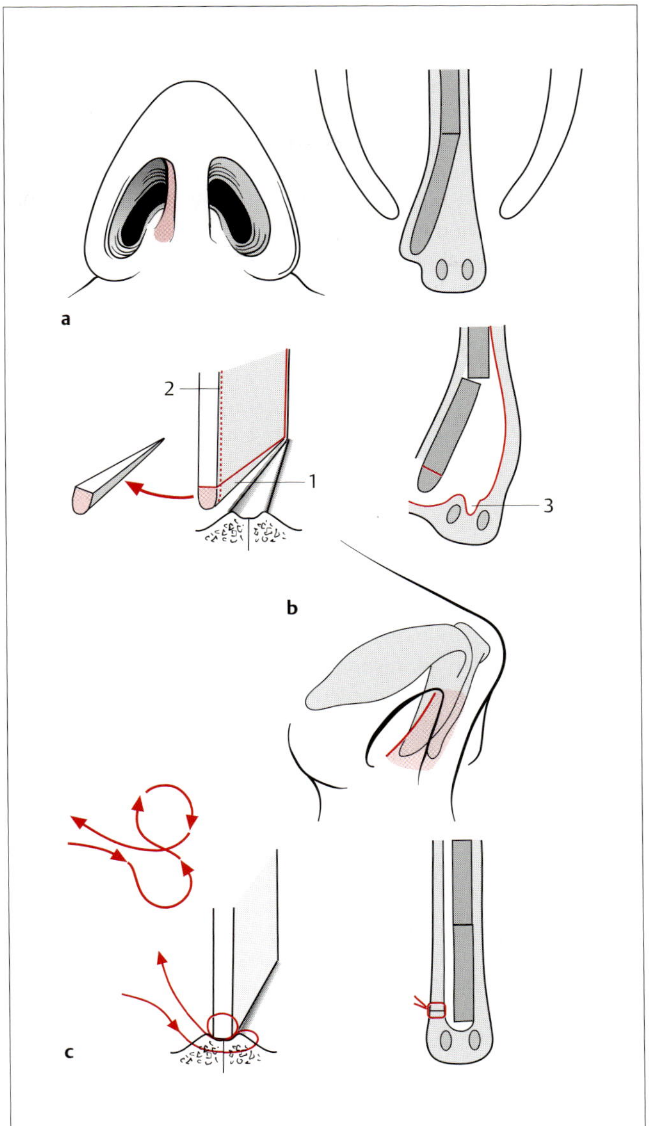

Fig. 6.21a–c Displacement (dislocation) of the caudal septal margin and cartilaginous crooked nose with an otherwise straight nasal dorsum (basal view and horizontal section).
a Lateral displacement of the caudal septal margin in the presence of a vertical cartilaginous fracture, stenosis of the right vestibule.
b Shortening of the septum at the base (septum table) (1) and if necessary at the caudal margin (2). Vertical chondrotomy of the cartilage fracture resulting in a "swinging door." Columellar pocket (3) from the nasal spine to the upper margin of the nostril (shaded area in the lateral view).
c Repositioning of the septum and fixation to the periosteum of the nasal spine with a figure-of eight suture.

fixed in this position by the septal mucosa. This is followed by horizontal and vertical chondrotomies. The horizontal chondrotomy should simultaneously shorten the septum, which is relatively too high, sufficiently to allow it to be settled in a midline position without leaving too large a gap to the premaxilla. The vertical chondrotomy lies in the region of a (usually present) cartilaginous fracture line. The septum mobilized in this way is still attached to the upper lateral cartilages. Positioning of the caudal septal margin is facilitated by creating a columellar pocket, which should extend from the anterior nasal spine to the upper margin of the nostril (not to the tip of the nose). This pocket should not be dissected too deeply, especially in the lower area, otherwise a retracted and widened columella could result. Shortening of the caudal septal margin if it seems "too long" should also be considered. The caudal septum normally projects beyond the nasal spine by 1–2 mm (with a normal-sized nasal spine). Even shortening it to the level of the nasal spine will result in retraction of the columella, especially if a columellar pocket has been created. The caudal septal margin should therefore only be resected, with care, if it projects beyond the spine by more than 1–2 mm.

Fixation of the mobilized caudal septum to the nasal spine is accomplished with an absorbable or nonabsorbable figure-of-eight suture to ensure it is securely anchored over the middle of the nasal spine. In the region of the nasal spine, the suture is placed through the abundant fibrous tissue found there. In order to place such an anchoring stitch it is therefore necessary to avoid laying the bone completely bare when exposing the nasal spine with an elevator (e.g., Cottle knife).

Deviations of the septal cartilage: caudal margin (**Fig. 6.22**). If the septum is placed under excessive tension by pressure from above, it dislocates out of the premaxillary groove (basal crest) and buckles. Release of septal tension can be accomplished by resection of "excess" cartilage at the premaxilla, if necessary together with part of the premaxillary ala (**Fig. 6.22b**). Unlike the tangential resection of a basal crest, here a complete strip of cartilaginous septum must be resected. Tension in the cartilage is only completely released, however, if the septum is tunnelled on both sides; otherwise the mucosa on the concave side, which is relatively short, keeps the septum bent like a bow. If the cartilage can be straightened up by these measures alone, then no further surgery to the cartilage is necessary.

However, despite maximal release of tension, the cartilage usually remains deviated because its growth has been disrupted. In this case, either the entire cartilaginous septum can be removed and a complete septum replacement (see below) performed, or other measures are available.

Often, superficial cross-hatching of the cartilage on one side is recommended. This exploits the tension forces within the cartilage: if they are neutralized on the scored side, the contraction forces on the contralateral side prevail and the cartilage arches away from the scored side (the scored surface becomes convex). This effect was examined in detail by Gibson and Davis and may be useful, e.g., for correction of the auricle (see Chapter 15), but it has significant disadvantages for the nasal septum:

- It is not known how many and how deep incisions should be made on the concave side of the septal cartilage to straighten an existing deviation exactly.

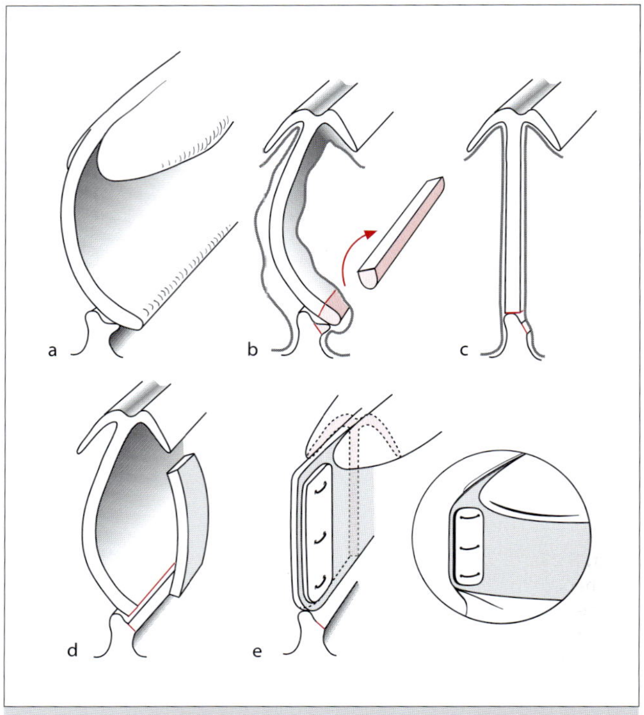

Fig. 6.22a–e Bending of the caudal septum.
a Extensively bent cartilage with basal crest.
b Relaxation of the cartilage by bilateral tunnelling and shortening at the base.
c Straightening and refixation.
d Residual bowing despite relaxation of the cartilage: prepared cartilaginous strut, bent in the contralateral direction.
e Straightening achieved with strut, sparing out the nasal valve.

- Cartilage scoring weakens stability, so that its supportive function may be compromised in the long term.
- It is a dynamic process, the final state of which cannot be exactly predicted.

Nevertheless, superficial scoring may be useful when combined with cartilage reinforcement. For this purpose, a thin, straight or slightly curved strip of cartilage is harvested from the posterior septum and sewn onto the caudal nasal septum. If it is curved, then its concave surface should come to lie on the concave side of the septum (**Fig. 6.22d**). The two cartilages are joined together with several absorbable mattress sutures. The cartilaginous frame straightens and reinforces the caudal septal margin. It must lie caudal to the attachment of the upper lateral cartilage, to avoid narrowing the nasal valve. A "nasal spine suture" is recommended.

Deviations of the septal cartilage: cartilaginous nasal dorsum (**Fig. 6.23**). A C-shaped or reverse C-shaped deviation of the nasal dorsum rarely presents as an isolated finding. It is commonly a component of an osseocartilaginous crooked nose. In this case, the bony pyramid, in addition to the cartilaginous part, must be straightened by osteotomies (see Crooked Nose, p. 87).

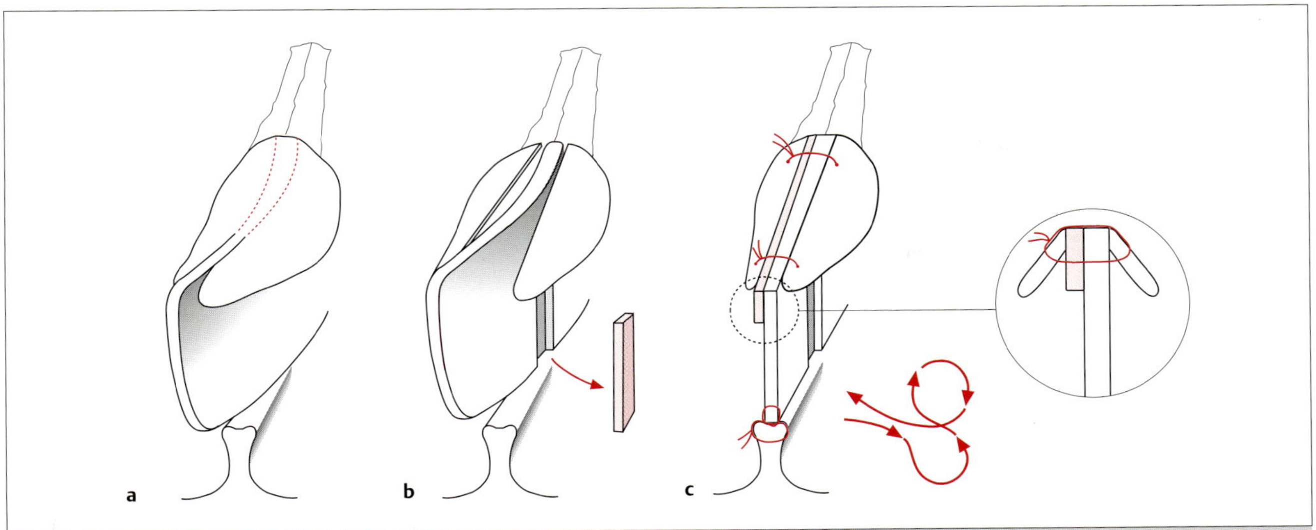

Fig. 6.23a–c Bending of the superior septal margin (cartilaginous C-shaped crooked nose).
a Reverse C-shaped curve of the nasal dorsum (in the presence of a vertical cartilaginous fracture at the junction with the perpendicular plate).
b Partial resection of the fracture area and detachment of the septum at the base and at the upper lateral cartilages.
c Spreader graft has been inserted on the right and the upper lateral cartilages and septum have been reattached to the nasal spine.

Dislocation of the caudal septum in the same direction as the deviation of the nasal dorsum is an almost regular feature. The cartilaginous septum must be mobilized accordingly via bilateral tunnels and chondrotomies, leaving it still attached only to the upper lateral cartilages and the K-region. Since in this case the nasal dorsum is also involved, it will need to be exposed by degloving. The appropriate techniques are shown and described in **Figs. 6.32** and **6.33**. At this point, only the operations involving the framework itself are discussed, because it belongs in the section related to nasal septum deviations.

Although in this situation too, the "relatively short" upper lateral cartilage on the concave side contributes to the deviation of the nasal septum, its separation from the septum will not normally correct the bowing entirely. Maximal release of the superior septal margin is achieved by separating both upper lateral cartilages. For this purpose, an Aufricht retractor is inserted under the nasal dorsum and then the upper lateral cartilages are separated from the septum with a No. 15 blade via the superior tunnel, beginning on the undersurface of the nasal bones and extending to the nasal valve. After bilateral division, the septal cartilage remains connected only by its superior attachments to the perpendicular plate, where it must therefore be protected. As in the procedure for a deviation of the nasal septum, the cartilaginous deviation is corrected by suturing on a (or bilateral) strip(s) of cartilage (a so-called "spreader graft"). This extends from the nasal bones to the anterior inferior corner of the septum, with a height of 3–4 mm. Fixation is achieved with absorbable sutures, placed in the following manner: right upper lateral cartilage—spreader graft—septal cartilage—spreader graft, (if bilateral)—left upper lateral cartilage. This suture brings each cartilage included in the stitch to the same level, with no edges becoming visible afterward. Fixation of the spreader graft is difficult, which is why the more easily placed caudal suture is best inserted first. Once the cartilage has been secured at one point, the remaining one or two sutures are more easily placed. Here too, a nasal spine suture is recommended because of the mobilization of the septum over the premaxilla.

Defects of the caudal septum: partial septal reconstruction (**Fig. 6.24**). Even with extensive deformities or defects of the caudal septum, there is often a strip of cartilage still present beneath the nasal dorsum. This can form the base for a reconstruction. The advantage lies in the fact that this strip of cartilage forms a pivot point with its attachment to the K-region, thus already providing two essential fixation points for the nasal septum. The aim of partial septal reconstruction is then "merely" to stably fill the gap between this residual cartilage and the premaxilla. Autologous cartilage serves as a graft, taken either from residual septum, the auricle (**Figs. 6.26** and **6.27**), or even a rib (see **Fig. 6.52**). The sufficiently long, or even too long, cartilaginous graft is first secured to the residual septum with two absorbable mattress sutures. One of these is brought out as a guide suture through the columella in the midline at the level of the upper nostril rim (**Fig. 6.24b**). Traction on this suture allows the nasal tip and dorsum to be brought to the correct level. A further absorbable traction suture is then inserted at the inferior end of the cartilaginous graft and also brought out through the columellar skin in the region of greatest retraction of the columellar base. Traction on this suture allows the correct position of the cartilaginous graft to be determined with respect to the premaxilla. The correct position is achieved when the columella projects about 2 mm beyond the alae, when viewed from the side, and the angle between upper lip and columella is 95° or more. Traction on suture 1 (nasal dorsum—nasal tip projection) and traction on suture 2 (position of the caudal columella) define the correct position in which the cartilaginous graft should be secured to the premaxilla. This position must be

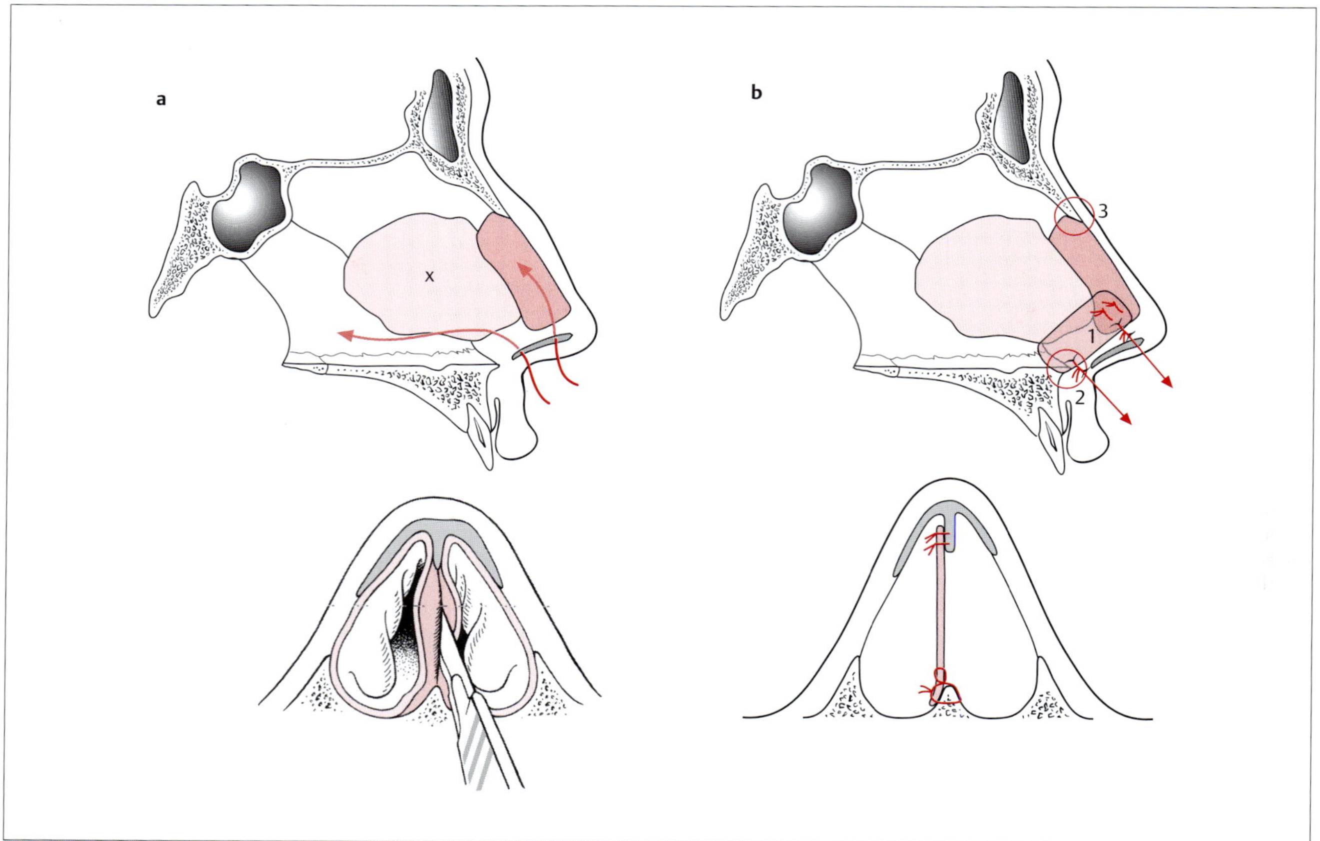

Fig. 6.24a, b Partial reconstruction of the caudal septum.
a Residual cartilage is placed beneath the nasal dorsum. Elevation of the septal mucosa from above and below the cartilage-free area (x). The mucosal layers of this area must be separated from each other by sharp dissection. The approach is via a hemitransfixion incision above and below the cartilage defect (arrows).
b Interposition of cartilage graft (1), which is secured by overlapping it over the residual septum, allowing the dorsum to be elevated with the aid of guide sutures (arrows) with the keystone area (3) as the pivot point. The graft is secured to the nasal spine (2).

maintained by an assistant who holds the sutures in place until secure stabilization and fixation have been achieved.

Even though the cartilaginous graft should ideally sit *on* nasal spine and premaxillary groove, a more stable anchorage is achieved in practice if the graft sits in a paramedian position next to the nasal spine, which it overlaps. Because of the increased load, nonabsorbable suture material is recommended here for the nasal spine suture. Additional stabilization is achieved by suturing in septal splints; the traction sutures should then be cut short, flush to the columellar skin, only after fixation of the septal splints with mattress sutures. The splints should remain in place for 5–6 days or even longer.

Defects of the caudal septum: total septal replacement (**Fig. 6.25**). For total septal replacement a stable, a roughly triangular plate of cartilage is required. Depending on the initial situation, the minimum length is about 2 cm for the nasal dorsum and 2.5 cm for the caudal septal margin. In principle, grafts should be harvested as large as possible, to be subsequently reduced to the correct size in situ.

Although a single piece of cartilage is the best option, one can manage with combined cartilaginous grafts (**Fig. 6.27**). Sufficiently large cartilaginous parts from the auricle can only be harvested from the concha. For this purpose, either a retroauricular or a preauricular approach is suitable (**Fig. 6.26**). The incision for a preauricular approach should run in the vertical part of the concha and preferably divide both skin and cartilage together. After the skin has been elevated from the anterior surface, as large a piece as possible is removed, encompassing both cavum and cymba and divided by the helical crus. Without any further measures, however, conchal cartilage is not entirely suitable for septal reconstruction, being too soft and concave. The cut helical crus also renders its surface uneven. Furthermore, it is not possible to shave off this cartilaginous edge because it would leave a defect in the cartilage, which is very thin at this point. These disadvantages can be partially counterbalanced by using double-layer grafts (**Fig. 6.27d**).

Unlike partial septal reconstruction, total reconstruction needs to recreate two fixation points: the K-region and the premaxilla. Exposure of the nasal dorsum is required to place the necessary suture at the K-region, as shown in **Figs. 6.32** and **6.33**. First, the cartilage graft is inserted between the layers of the septal mucosa and the detached upper lateral cartilages so

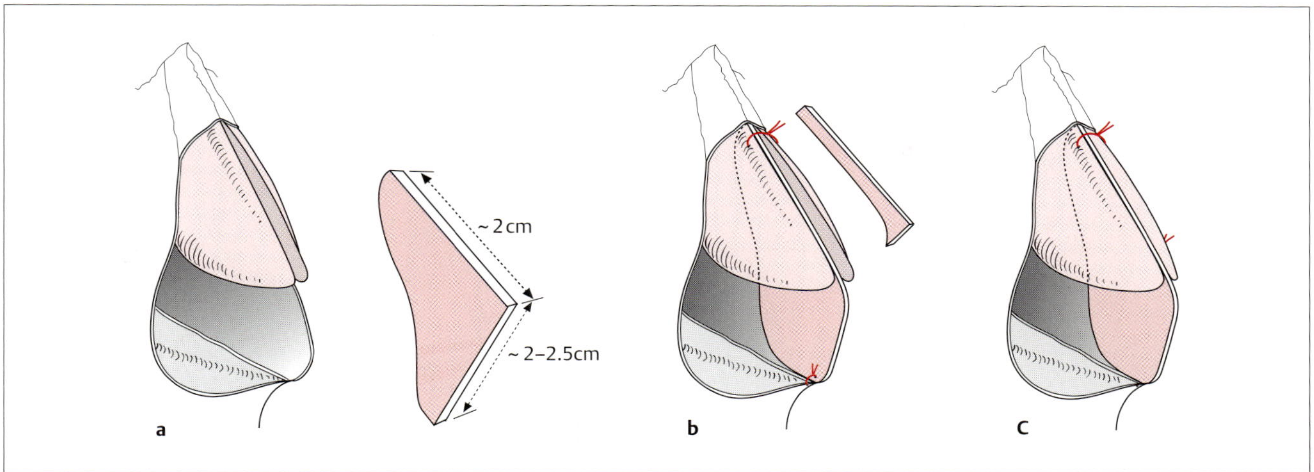

Fig. 6.25a–c Total replacement of the caudal septum.
a Initial situation and pre-prepared cartilage graft.
b Fitting the graft and resection of superfluous cartilage. Fixation to the keystone area and nasal spine.
c Final appearance after re-fixation of the upper lateral cartilages to reconstruct the nasal valve.

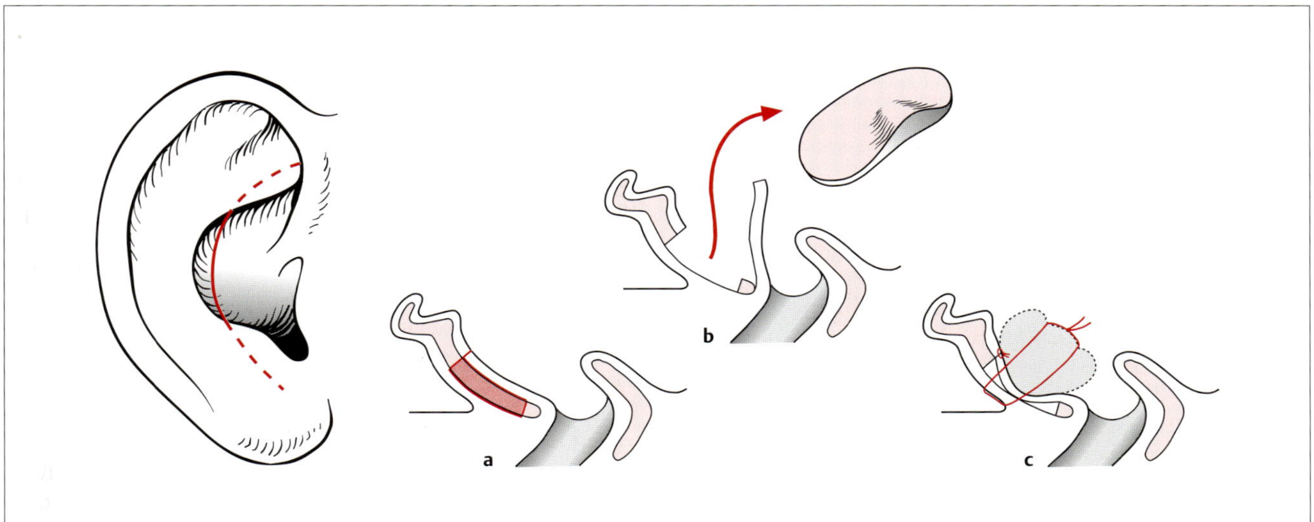

Fig. 6.26a–c Harvesting the cartilage graft from the auricular concha (anterior approach).
a Incision through skin and cartilage of the anterior surface, extending from the antihelical crus to the antitragus. Elevation of the skin from the anterior and posterior surfaces.
b The cartilage is removed, leaving a residual strip at the entrance to the auditory canal.
c Wound closure with a tie-over gauze to prevent hematoma formation.

that it has contact with the nasal bones, where it is secured with an absorbable suture passing through all layers: left upper lateral cartilage—septal graft—right upper lateral cartilage (**Fig. 6.25b**). This creates the necessary pivot point for the exact positioning of the cartilaginous graft. As with partial septal replacement, positioning of the graft to the nasal spine via an endonasal approach is now undertaken using two traction sutures. Using the open approach is technically easier, for the suture of the K-region in particular. Once the cartilaginous graft has been firmly anchored to both fixation points, any excess cartilage in the dorsum area is excised. If there was a significant preoperative saddle-nose deformity, the caudal parts of the upper lateral cartilages will now still be too low (ballooning of the nasal valve). In these cases, the upper lateral cartilages are raised to the level of the upper septal margin (see **Fig. 6.25c**), where they are secured by suturing (reduction of the nasal valve angle).

Even with total reconstruction, temporary stabilization with septal splints may be useful following an endonasal approach.

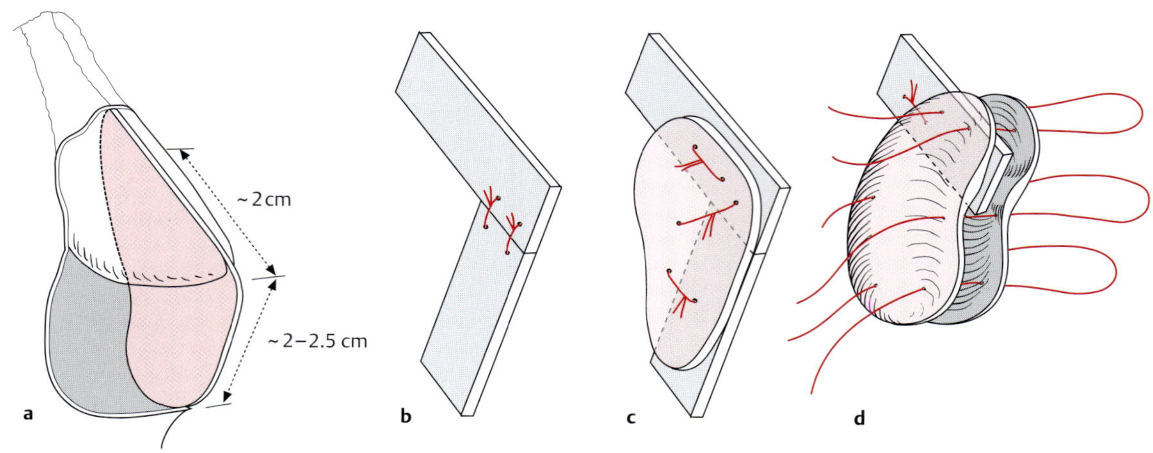

Fig. 6.27a–d Alternative options for reconstructing the caudal septum.
a Required graft size (average values).
b Assembled graft, made up of two pieces of septal cartilage.
c Auricular cartilage is sutured on to provide additional support.
d Assembled graft, made up of residual septum and both conchal cartilages (concave surfaces are correspondingly sewn together).

Rules, Tips, and Tricks

It can be difficult to find the correct subperichondrial plane during septoplasty. Novices in particular should bear in mind that if you think you are in the correct plane, then you will find the *really* correct plane a little deeper. If in doubt, check again with a sharp instrument 5 or 10 mm away from the caudal septal margin, to see whether another layer can be elevated. In contrast, when tunnelling to the contralateral side via a chondrotomy, the correct plane is almost always found automatically.

The decisive point during septoplasty is good visualization in the septal tunnels. The spaces between the planes can fill with blood very quickly, making any further dissection under vision possible only with the aid of a suction elevator. Reasons for more significant hemorrhage with hindered visualization may arise from, among other things, dissection in the incorrect plane (always check the plane) or chiselling at the premaxilla before creating the posterior tunnels. It is therefore advisable first to create the tunnels unilaterally right back so that more blood can collect in the deepened plane and so allow dissection under direct vision in the anterior septal areas, at least for a certain amount of time. “Blind dissection” is only wise provided the instrument has good bone contact.

In scar areas secondary to previous surgery or trauma, dissection in cartilage regions must also be sharp, otherwise mucosal defects can easily develop (*scar tissue = sharp dissection*).

Mucosal tears over a sharp-edged septal ridge are often unavoidable, yet also unproblematic, if:

- they are exclusively *unilateral*
- only a mucosal tear and not a mucosal defect is present.

Removal of a septal ridge will result in excess mucosa, which allows a tension-free re-approximation of the wound edges (even without sutures).

There is a significant risk of septal perforation developing from tears on corresponding sides. In this case the following steps should be taken:

- Place a mucosal adaptation stitch on either side, preferably as a mattress suture to evert the wound edges (see **Fig. 6.30**).
- Use autologous cartilage or bone or even fascia as an interposition. Both mucosal layers must be securely separated from each other. In this situation the intraseptal application of fibrin glue may be helpful.

In all these cases, nasal packs should be left for several days under antibiotic protection to allow the wound surfaces to adhere.

A vomerine spur should only be removed after complete elevation of the mucosa; otherwise a long mucosal tear will develop. Neither should the spur be fractured by leverage, as this may lead to abnormal fractures (fracture lines as far as the carotid canal with fatal hemorrhage have been reported). If required, a transverse curved chisel may be used on the anterior wall of the sphenoid sinus.

Trans-septal mattress sutures should be placed consecutively and at sufficient intervals for fixation and prevention of hematomas; otherwise there is an imminent risk of mucosal necrosis. Should unilateral mucosal defects up to the size of a fingernail develop (sometimes also as a result of a gaping hemitransfixion incision), then there is still the possibility of achieving healing by secondary intention without revision surgery. In this case, any foreign material in the depths of the wound (nonabsorbable suture) should be removed and the wound surface "sealed" several times a day with an antibiotic ointment. Healing may require 2–3 weeks, and only then should a decision be made about any possible further operative measures.

For operations on the *nose of a child*, disturbances of growth should be anticipated. The indication for septoplasty in children and adolescents under the age of 16 years should therefore be considered most carefully. Children often tolerate even the complete blockage of *one* side of the nose well. Septoplasty may, however, be indicated for bilateral deviations associated with severe obstruction of nasal breathing and for secondary complications (e.g., sinusitis, otitis media). Surgery should be performed with maximal protection of the cartilage, paying particular attention to the suture lines (**Fig. 6.28**). Because in children, depending on age, the nasal septum and the external nose consist mainly of cartilage, the chondroethmoid suture (between cartilage and perpendicular plate) lies close to the skull base and the chondrovomerine suture close to the floor of the nose. Injuries to the cranial suture typically result in a saddle-nose deformity, and injuries to the inferior suture lead to hypoplasia of the cartilaginous nose with growth disturbances of the premaxilla (maxillonasal dysplasia, Binder syndrome). The typical characteristics of this after completion of growth are the bony pseudohump with hypoplasia of the cartilaginous nose resulting in an amorphous and round nasal tip and round nostrils, as well as a deep retraction of the columellar base with a nasolabial angle less than 90°. Premaxilla and maxilla are hypoplastic, and microgenia with malocclusion may be present. If septoplasty had been done previously, this was usually for trauma. It is then not possible to say whether the disturbance of growth was caused by the operation or the previous injury. It is essential during septoplasty to preserve the above-mentioned structures whenever possible. Incomplete fracture lines are divided and any untidy cartilaginous parts sparingly resected.

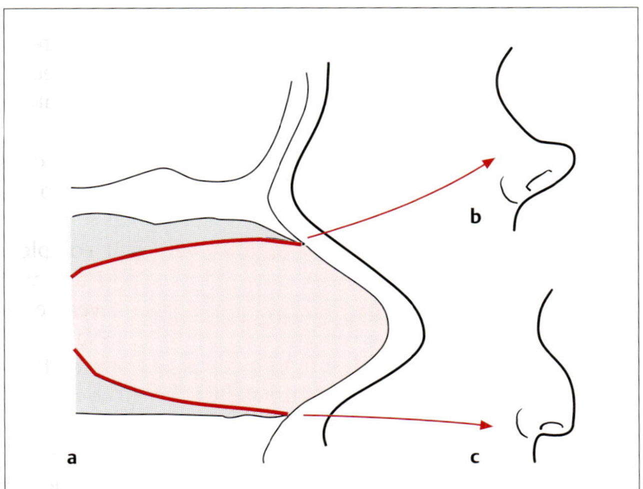

Fig. 6.28a–c Growth zones and disturbances of growth.
a Growth zones at the junctions of cartilage to the vomer and to the perpendicular plate.
b Saddle-nose deformity resulting from disturbance of the superior growth zone.
c Hypoplasia of the cartilaginous nose resulting from disturbance of the inferior growth zone.

Cartilage-free areas should be filled with the removed pieces of cartilage, leaving as few gaps as possible.

! Risks and Complications

A significant risk associated with septoplasty is dislocation of the cartilaginous septum as a result of the necessary mobilization. This can be expected especially when complete bilateral septal tunnels have been created and, after completion of the horizontal chondrotomy, the vertical chondrotomy has been extended beneath the nasal bones. The septal cartilage is then attached to the nasal bones only by the upper lateral cartilages, resulting in a pivot point at the K-region (**Fig. 6.29**). Pressure from the soft-tissue envelope leads to an internal rotation of the nasal septal cartilage around this pivot point. The complex sequelae are depicted in detail in **Fig. 6.12**. It is worth pointing out again here that they are not brought about by cartilage resection, but merely by mobilization. Rotation of the cartilage can be recognized from within the septal tunnels by an overlapping of the incision margins of the vertical chondrotomy (**Fig. 6.29a**).

A cartilaginous saddle-nose deformity, either discreet or more pronounced, is often regarded as the typical result of a too-extensive submucous septum resection. It can, however, also develop from a septoplasty without resection. This stigma is avoidable. After septoplasty, the surgeon should make it a rule to assess the mobility of the caudal septum with forceps before suture repair of the hemitransfixion. If it is possible to rotate the cartilage into the nose, then it is too mobile and must be secured. A traction suture in the lower part of the caudal septal margin is used to bring it into the correct position and fix it with a nasal spine suture (**Fig. 6.29**).

Postoperative Care

After endonasal operations, some degree of crusting should be expected after removal of the nasal packs. Adherent fibrin deposits may develop in predisposed individuals. If packs are left longer these effects are usually less, although patients usually find the complete obstruction of the nasal airways by packs to be significantly more unpleasant than nasal breathing that is restricted, but in principle still possible, after removal of the packs. Removal of crusts and slough should not be forced, because this encourages their renewed development. Moreover, it is essential to soften the crusts by applying ointment until they either fall off on their own during nasal irrigation or can easily be removed with suction. Patients themselves can perform the main part of nasal care: irrigating the nose with saline several times a day and then blowing the nose free of the solution with moderate force, after waiting a short while to allow its endonasal effect. This is followed by the application of a nasal oil. Daily inhalations are also recommended. Decongestant nose drops should be used after surgery only in exceptional cases.

Note that it is not recommended to use nasal oils or ointments for more than 1–2 weeks, because they adhere to the cilia of the respiratory mucosa and the subsequent disruption of the mucociliary transport system may result in even more severe crusting.

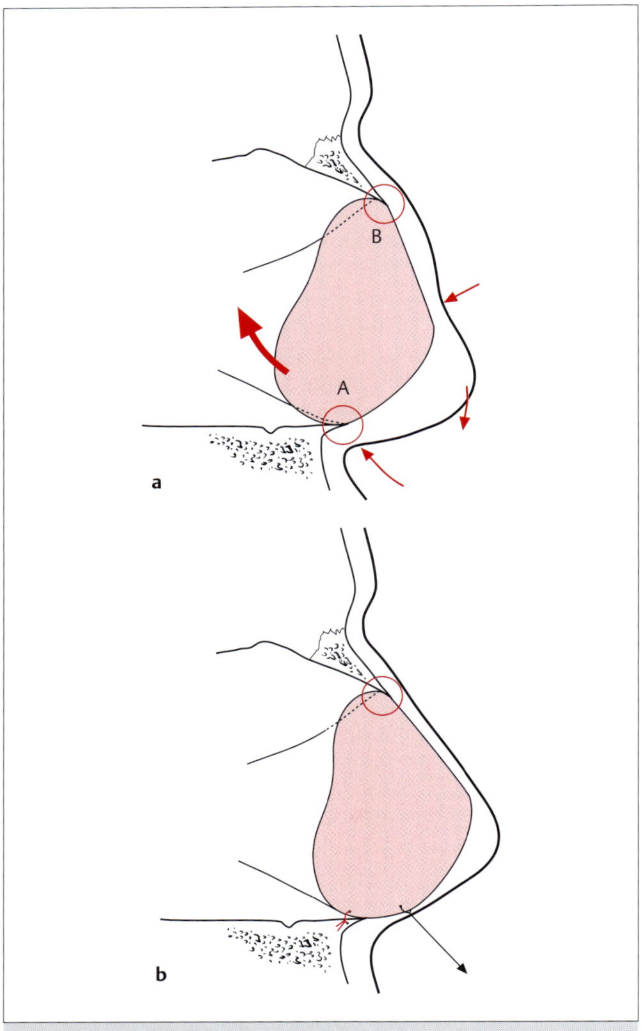

Fig. 6.29a, b Cartilaginous saddle-nose deformity resulting from rotation of the septum.
a After mobilization (septal tunnel, chrondrotomies, and detachment from the premaxilla [A]), the septum rotates around the pivot point at the keystone area (B) "into the nose" (thick arrow) as a result of soft-tissue pressure. The soft tissues follow in the direction of the thin arrows.
b Correction is achieved by reduction using a guide suture placed through the caudal septal margin which is secured to the nasal spine.

Septal Perforation

Surgical Principle

Bilateral closure of the perforation using local mucosal transposition flaps and cartilage interposition.

Indications

Only perforations that cause relevant symptoms should undergo surgical closure. These are predominantly perforations of the anterior nasal septum. Typical presenting symptoms are:

- Obstruction of nasal breathing (increased resistance by turbulence).
- Nasal bleeding and crusting (particularly at the posterior margin of the perforation).
- Frontal headache (pain resulting from inflammation of the posterior margin of the perforation).
- Whistling sound on inspiration (small perforation).

When the cause of the perforation is known, the prospects of a successful closure are more favorable in the long run because, with an unknown cause, the causative agent may still persist after surgery. The most common causes include:

- Previous surgery of the nasal septum or repeated treatment for epistaxis.
- Deviation of the anterior nasal septum associated with anterior rhinitis sicca, crusting, and subsequent digital manipulations.
- Long-term use of a cortisone nasal spray.
- Systemic diseases (Wegener disease) or cocaine abuse.

Contraindications

- *Location*: Perforations of the middle and posterior parts of the septum are usually protected by the turbinates, and they are located in sufficiently moist surroundings. Even if they are large, they do not necessarily cause any significant problems. Provided there are no relevant symptoms, operative closure of a perforation is not required merely because it is present.
- *Dimension*: A sufficient amount of mucosa must be available in the vicinity for good prospects of closure. Unfavorable size and location of the perforation may present a contraindication for closure.
- *State of the mucosa*: Dry and crusted mucous membranes must be treated beforehand (ointment, saline irrigation, inhalations). If problems with wound healing are anticipated, then the indication to operate should be considered with great caution (diabetes, smoker, mucosal atrophy secondary to cortisone use). If there is a history of earlier cocaine use, abstinence must be guaranteed. If the mucous membranes are atrophic and thin on inspection and, in particular, if they are no longer separated by cartilage and bone, then surgery may be impossible, given that it presumes separation of both layers of the septal mucosa.

Specific Points Regarding Informed Consent

Permanent and complete closure of a septal perforation cannot be guaranteed. However, often patients benefit even from a partial closure, resulting in epithelialization and protection of the posterior margin of the perforation. Usually auricular cartilage is required as a cartilage interposition graft. Any existing external pathological changes (e.g., cartilaginous saddling, columellar retraction) should be corrected in a follow-up operation. The same applies for residual deviations of the septum, especially in the area of the nasal valve and the region beneath the nasal dorsum, where cartilage removal is not possible. This would lead to a septal defect after transposition of the mucosa. Because complete tunnels in the nasal floor need to be created, the inevitable division of the nasopalatine nerve may lead to sensory disturbances behind the incisors. Injury to the opening of the nasolacrimal canal is theoretically possible when elevating an inferior transposition flap.

Operative Planning

The availability of mucosa between the superior margin of the perforation and nasal dorsum is imperative for the success of the operation. Its width should be at least as large as the height of the perforation. The perforation is generally longitudinally oval, i.e., its height is less than its width. The horizontal diameter is not usually the limiting factor for the successful closure. A check should be made for cartilage-free areas ("cotton bud test," see p. 58) with regard to the ability to separate the mucosal layers in this region.

Surgical Technique (Schultz–Coulon) (Fig. 6.30)

Usually an endonasal approach is adequate. In difficult cases, however, an external approach via a transcolumellar incision may be useful because it allows more exact work between the mucosal layers in the midline. Furthermore, visualization of the perforation from above is clearly better after separation of the upper lateral cartilages.

Closure of the perforation is achieved by up to four transposition flaps (Schultz–Coulon). Because these remain pedicled posteriorly and anteriorly, they are referred to as bipedicled, or bridge, flaps. The decisive flaps are the two superior bipedicled flaps that cover the largest part of the perforation. They may even be adequate on their own for smaller perforations (up to 10 mm diameter). Inferior bipedicled flaps will also need to be developed for larger perforations, although they have less mobility and thus only cover the lower part of the perforation. Their task is essentially to allow a tension-free suture.

At first, the layers of septal mucosa must be elevated from residual cartilage and bone according to the rules of septoplasty. Even in regions free of cartilage and bone, elevation of the mucosal layers is usually easily accomplished using blunt instruments, provided perichondrium and periosteum are well preserved after any previous surgery. Should these be absent in places, however, then sharp dissection with a scalpel is required, elevating the layers millimeter by millimeter (see **Fig. 6.24a**). Dissection of the superior tunnel continues at first as far as the superior margin of the perforation, taking care not to divide the perforation margin. This avoids any uncontrolled tear of the perforation margin when inserting the nasal speculum. The piriform aperture is completely exposed for the inferior tunnel and the nasal floor tunnel, where tunnelling proceeds with bone contact in a subperiosteal plane as far as the insertion of the inferior turbinate. Only now is the perforation margin gradually opened up from above with the scalpel and the mucous membranes completely elevated in the remaining regions of the perforation. Superior and inferior tunnels extend posteriorly until shortly before the posterior margin of the vomer.

Using a No. 15 scalpel blade, incision of the septal mucosa for the superior bipedicled flap begins posteromedially and above the inferior margin of the middle turbinate. It assumes a curved course in an anterior direction, initially with bone contact (perpendicular plate), and lies as close to the nasal bridge as possible. It ends at the septum, shortly behind the insertion of the upper lateral cartilage. Bleeding from branches of the anterior ethmoid artery is controlled by bipolar coagulation to avoid obstruction of view. If necessary, the incision is extended posteriorly and caudally with angulated scissors. It should now be possible to transpose the bipedicled flap in an inferior direction. If it is possible to approximate the flap to the inferior margin of the perforation without tension, creation of an inferior bipedicled flap may be dispensed with. Otherwise, the mucosa of the inferior nasal meatus is incised with the scalpel in a posterior-to-anterior direction after medial fracturing of the inferior turbinate. This may prove difficult, especially in the anterior parts, because of the formation of niches in the area of the lacrimal duct. Using a sharp elevator, the final adhesions to the bone are then released and the inferior bipedicled flap is transposed medially.

Bilateral flaps are always necessary to completely epithelialize the perforation. Transposition of the superior bipedicled flap exposes the infrastructure of the nasal septum beneath the nasal dorsum. It must therefore be preserved as a whole, as otherwise a perforation would develop at this point. For this reason no major corrections with resections can be made at this stage, even with relevant septal deviations, but only replacements following osteotomies.

The former margins of the perforation are now sutured in a posterior-to-anterior direction. Mattress sutures are most suitable, even though they are technically difficult, because they evert the wound edges and so wound surface comes to lie on wound surface (**Fig. 6.30c**). Before closure of the hemitransfixion or of the transcolumellar incision, cartilage is interposed in the former perforation area. Conchal cartilage from the auricle is most suitable and may be crushed or scored to straighten it.

Rules, Tips, and Tricks

Dealing with Intra-operative Problems

The following rules apply for the successful closure of a septal perforation:

- Suturing must be accomplished without tension. The suture technique is also important (mattress suture).
- Elevate *large* flaps, even for *small* perforations. Settling for small measures will inevitably result in recurrence.
- Sutures do not hold in mucosa, but rather in perichondrium or periosteum, which will therefore need maximal protection. Sutures inserted through the mucosa must not exit through the raw surface of the wound margin, but should also include periosteum/perichondrium.
- If the mucosa is relatively thin in areas free of infrastructure, its elevation may be very difficult. It can be facilitated by hydrodissection using local anesthetic and a long, thin needle.

! Risks and Complications

Postoperative hemorrhage usually originates from the superior incision margin of the bipedicled flaps, where branches of the anterior ethmoid artery and the highly vascular erectile tissue of the septal turbinate are located. Since "blind" packing puts the stability of the sutures at risk, hemostasis is best achieved with bipolar coagulation.

Postoperative Care

As far as possible, suction should be dispensed with for 2–3 weeks to avoid tearing open the mucosa. Saline irrigations, nasal oil, and inhalations should suffice.

Alternatives

There is really no effective alternative to the closure of a septal perforation using local mucosal transposition flaps (rotation flap, bipedicled flap) as indicated here. This applies particularly to mere interposition, using fascia for example, as well as to the transposition of skin (e.g., concha–vestibular flap). The use of silicone obdurators is not proven (foreign body, crusting, large volume).

With a sufficiently wide posterior pedicle, the bipedicled flap using septal mucosa can be converted into a rotation flap by dividing the anterior pedicle. This facilitates its transposition and prevents the troublesome development of puckering.

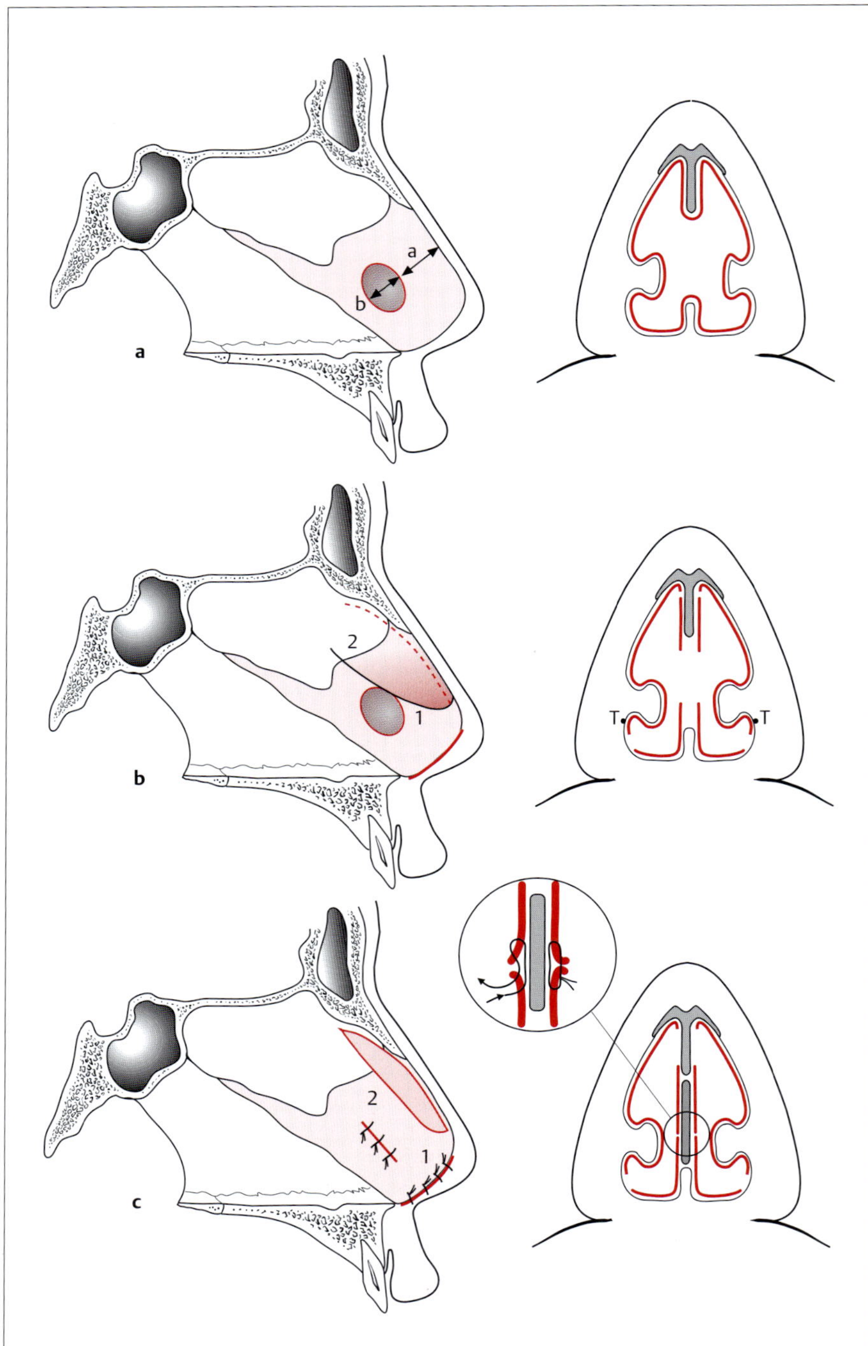

Fig. 6.30a–c Closure of a septal perforation using bipedicled flaps of the nasal mucosa (Scgultz–Coulon) (sagittal and basal views).

- **a** Preoperative assessment of the available mucosa: distance a should be larger than the vertical diameter of the perforation (b).
- **b** Tunnelling and separation of the perforation via a hemitransfixion incision. The superior bipedicled flap, with its anterior (1) and posterior (2) pedicle, is formed by incising the mucosa along the nasal dorsum. This incision ends behind the nasal valve. The basal view shows how the inferior bipedicled flaps have been elevated by an incision in the lower nasal meatus, sparing the opening of the lacrimal duct (T), and have already been transposed.
- **c** The superior and inferior flaps are inset with mattress sutures, with interposed cartilage. An osseocartilaginous area beneath the nasal dorsum is left to heal by secondary epithelialization.

Surgery of the External Nose (Rhinoplasty)

Preliminary Remarks

Surgery of the external nasal pyramid is undertaken for aesthetic reasons (e.g., a prominent hump) or for combined functional and aesthetic reasons (e.g., tension nose, crooked nose, saddle-nose deformity). The term "aesthetic surgery" relates to the normalization of an external deformity, while "cosmetic surgery" addresses the improvement of an otherwise normal form. In general, however, a clear line is not drawn between these two terms.

The form and function of the nose must be considered as a single entity. A deformity is usually associated with a disturbance of function. "Functional and aesthetic surgery of the nose," therefore, has the aim of reconstructing this entity. Earlier in this chapter, reference has already been made to the significance of the nasal septum (see **Fig. 6.12**). Functional and aesthetic surgery of the nose usually involves a combined operation on the nasal septum and the external nose (septo-rhinoplasty). Although they are discussed separately in this surgical textbook, they are generally operated on in one session, with the operation typically proceeding along the following steps:

- Septoplasty part 1: incision, approach, mobilization and resection, temporary nasal pack.
- Rhinoplasty with incision, approach, correction.
- Septoplasty part 2: replacement, reconstruction, fixation, suture repair of the incisions.
- Definitive nasal pack, external dressing, splint.

Although the two operative components are usually, and wisely, performed together, there is also a major problem in septorhinoplasty: Unlike an operation purely on the external nose (rhinoplasty), which is performed around an unaffected septum as the central support, the simultaneous correction of the nasal septum, together with the mobilization and reconstruction involved, results in dynamic healing processes that over the course of weeks and months may be associated with changes of the position of the septum, recognizable by changes in its outer form. The late results of the external form may therefore differ considerably from the immediate postoperative outcome, making any reliable prognosis difficult. Revision surgery may therefore be necessary and is sometimes unavoidable, despite the most careful of surgical techniques. Patients should be made particularly aware of these special circumstances when the informed consent is discussed, and the potential need for later refinements, which should not be performed until a year after the initial operation, should be specifically mentioned.

Given that septo-rhinoplasty serves the reconstruction of both form and function, purely aesthetic or cosmetic operations should not be undertaken at the expense of function. Such operations often involve resections of the cartilaginous infrastructure of the external nose to achieve reductions or narrowings, and this can easily result in a loss of the supportive function, even after a period of years. Surgery in these cases becomes a trade-off between improvement of the external form and disturbance of function.

Basic Techniques

Incisions and Approaches to the Nasal Dorsum

Endonasal Approaches

Surgical Principle

The endonasal *incision* is always made in the skin of the vestibule, not in the mucosa. *Access* to the nasal dorsum is achieved by elevation of the soft-tissue envelope (**Fig. 6.31b**) *over* the perichondrium and *beneath* the periosteum (so-called degloving or décollement).

Indications

Operations to the nasal dorsum, such as osteotomies or nasal hump reduction.

Contraindications

Necrosis may develop with very atrophic skin due to severe scarring secondary to trauma or multiple previous operations.

Specific Points Regarding Informed Consent

Irregularities after surgery of the nasal dorsum are not always avoidable, especially with very thin nasal skin. Refinements may be necessary, but should not be undertaken earlier than 6 months after the initial operation. Skin atrophy (particularly after revision surgery) may result in erythema and teleangiectasia of the skin of the nasal dorsum (rubeosis). Sensory disturbances of the skin, in rare cases even chronic pain, may result from the (unavoidable) division of nerves (**Fig. 6.31a**).

Operative Planning

The choice of endonasal incisions depends, among other things, on whether simultaneous operations on the lower lateral cartilages are intended. Reduction of volume in the region of the lateral crus will require a transcartilaginous incision rather than an intercartilaginous approach (see **Fig. 6.59**). An external approach (see below) is recommended for more complex surgery of the nasal tip.

Special Instruments (see also Fig. 6.6)

A scalpel with a No. 15 blade is suitable for the incisions. A sharp, double-pronged retractor (e.g., a ring retractor) is used to expose the nasal vestibule. Degloving is achieved either with a scalpel or with slightly angulated pointed scissors to expose the perichondrium in the correct plane. A slightly curved (McKenty) elevator is used for subperiosteal tunnelling in the K-area. A sufficiently wide Aufricht retractor will allow direct vision of the cartilage and bone of the nasal dorsum.

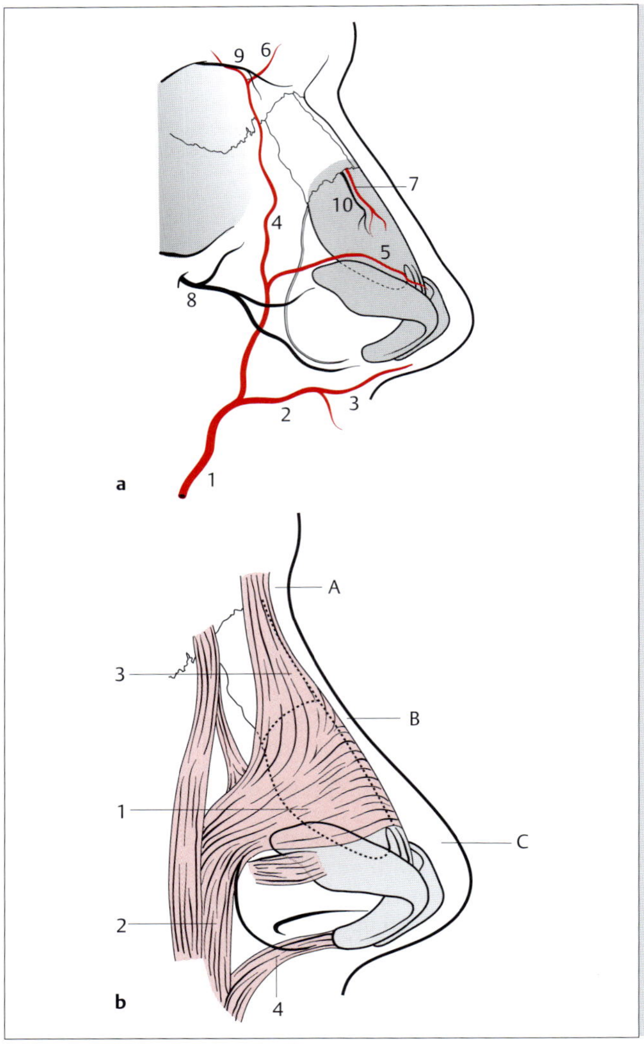

Fig. 6.31a, b Soft tissues, vessels, and nerves of the external nose.
a Neural and vascular supply.
Arteries (red):
1 facial artery (from the external carotid artery)
2 superior labial artery
3 terminal branch between the medial crura of the lower lateral cartilages
4 angular artery
5 superior alar artery (between the upper and lower lateral cartilages)
6 supratrochlear artery (from the internal carotid artery)
7 anterior ethmoid artery (from the internal carotid artery); exit point between the nasal bone and the upper lateral cartilage
Nerves (black):
8 infraorbital artery
9 supra- and infratrochlear nerves
10 external branch of the anterior ethmoid nerve
b Thickness of the skin and superficial musculoaponeurotic system (SMAS). Various thicknesses of the skin (arrows): thick at the root of the nose (A) and supratip region (C), thin over the keystone area (B).
External nasal muscles:
1 *Name:* pars transversa; *origin:* maxilla; *attachment:* nasal dorsum
2 *Name:* pars alaris; *origin:* incisive fossa; *attachment:* skin, nasal alae
3 *Name:* procerus muscle; *origin:* division from frontal muscle; *attachment:* periosteum, nasal dorsum
4 *Name:* depressor septi muscle; *origin:* incisive fossa; *attachment:* medial crus

Surgical Technique (Fig. 6.32)

Incisions made exclusively on one side (hemitransfixion and intercartilaginous incision) are sufficient for minor operations on the nasal dorsum (e.g., for smoothing out irregularities). Better visualization is achieved, however, by extensive separation of the lower lateral cartilages from the rest of the pyramid. For this purpose a transfixion incision is made to divide the skin of the membranous septum *anterior* to the caudal septal margin, reaching from the level of the upper lateral cartilages to about the level of the anterior nasal spine. Bilateral intercartilaginous incisions are made between the cephalic margin of the lower lateral cartilages and the caudal margin of the upper lateral cartilages, at the lowest point of the cutaneous indentation between both cartilages (the so-called cul-de-sac: see **Fig. 6.3a**) and should preferably meet the transfixion incision at right angles, because at the end of the operation the connecting point of these two incisions must be identified precisely and re-approximated exactly. Such incisions, with an almost semicircular course, otherwise tend to heal with a circular contraction and subsequent deformation of the nasal valve after improper, or even omitted, suture repair.

The upper lateral cartilages are identified with spreading movements of the tips of pointed scissors over the anterior–inferior corner to expose the perichondrium in the region of the nasal dorsum. The soft-tissue envelope can now be elevated in this plane under direct vision, with the SMAS lying immediately over the Aufricht retractor. Once the K-area has been reached (which is best confirmed by palpation), the periosteum is then incised transversely at this point and elevated with the curved elevator as far as the nasal root. Subperiosteal dissection at the nasal root is used to elevate the procerus muscle from the bone. This considerably facilitates extraction of a mobilized osseocartilaginous nasal hump because the muscle fibers have already been detached.

Lateral undermining of the nasal dorsum should only be performed as far as the reduction of a nasal hump, for example, requires.

Rules, Tips, and Tricks

If the volume of the of the lower lateral cartilages is intended to be reduced by trimming off a cephalic strip of cartilage, then a

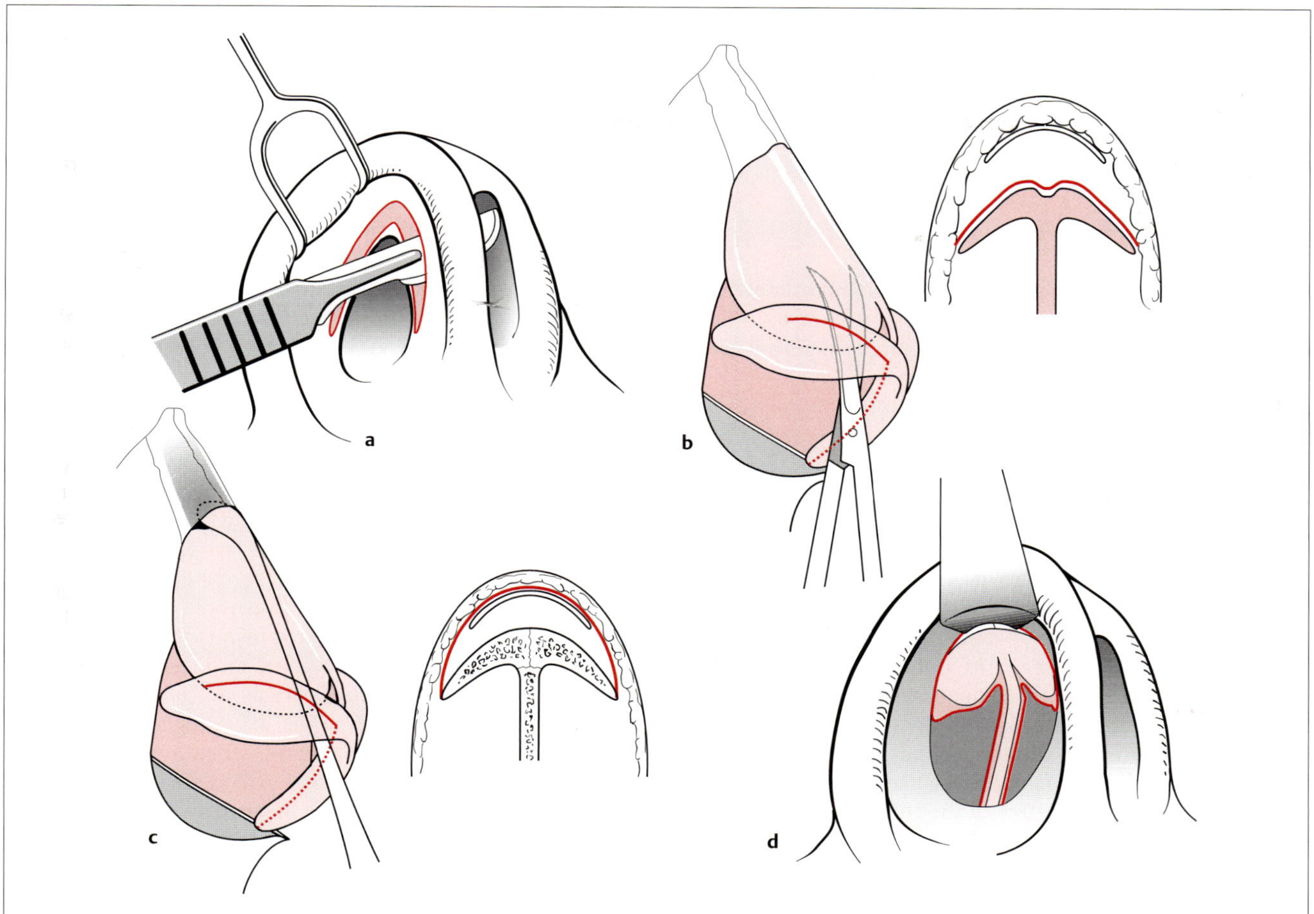

Fig. 6.32a–d Endonasal approach to the nasal dorsum.

a Intercartilaginous incisions (between upper and lower lateral cartilages) on either side and transfixion (in the membranous septum between the lower lateral cartilages and the caudal edge of the septum).

b Elevation of the skin over the nasal dorsum (degloving) close to the perichondrium (red) using angulated pointed scissors; the transverse section shows the skin held up with an Aufricht retractor.

c On reaching the keystone area, the plane of dissection changes from the epiperichondrial to the subperiosteal; the periosteum (red) has been released together with the skin by a McKenty elevator and raised.

d Exposure of the nasal dorsum with the Aufricht retractor; the procerus muscle has also been elevated together with the periosteum and the bony root of the nose has been exposed.

transcartilaginous incision should be selected instead of an intercartilaginous incision (see **Fig. 6.59**). Direct undermining of the nasal skin with a scalpel (No. 15 blade) without direct vision is also possible, although the plane of dissection does not then usually lie immediately over the perichondrium, but rather more superficially. With significantly "retroussé" upper lateral cartilages, it may be difficult to identify the caudal lateral area of the upper lateral cartilages in the correct plane. In this case it is best to identify the junction between the cephalic margin of the lower lateral cartilage and the caudal margin of the upper lateral cartilage, followed by the conservative excision of the raised free edge of the upper lateral cartilage. The cut edge of the cartilage may then be deflected toward the nasal cavity and the perichondrial plane can subsequently be identified.

External Approach

Surgical Principle

The skin is elevated off the columella, nasal tip, and nasal dorsum after making an incision at the columella and extending it in an endonasal direction along the caudal margin of the lower lateral cartilage. This allows corrections under direct vision, which is a particular advantage when preserving or restoring symmetry.

Indications

Simultaneous operations on the nasal tip and pyramid, especially for more complex deformities and revision surgery. There is also good visualization of the nasal septum, which is advantageous when undertaking technically more demanding reconstructions with grafts and closing a septal perforation.

Contraindications

Severely scarred columella with the risk of skin necrosis. Increase of nasal tip projection in case of a short columella due to the associated risk of wound breakdown from suturing under tension.

Specific Points Regarding Informed Consent

Information regarding the possibility of wound breakdown and visible scar formation. Long-lasting (≥1 year) sensory disturbances in the area of the columella and more significant swelling, particularly of the supratip region.

Surgical Technique (Figs. 6.33 and 6.34)

The columellar incision should be barely visible later, if the orginal incision and suture technique have been sufficiently precise.

An incision in the form of an inverted V has proved useful for the columellar incision (**Fig. 6.33**). The tip of the inverted V is at the level of the narrowest part of the columella (usually the junction between the lower third and the upper two thirds). The lateral points are over the wider basal part of the columella, slightly medial to the junction with the membranous septum. The inverted V formed in this manner has the advantage of being relatively wide at its base, with the lateral corner points still situated in the anterior surface of the columella. This makes it easier to avoid creating a step-off at the junction with the horizontal incisions at the membranous septum. Any irregularity in this area gives the optical impression of a permanent "dewdrop." The V-shaped incision is best made with a No. 11 scalpel blade, as this allows the exact creation of the sharp angle. Injury to the medial crus of the lower lateral cartilage need not be feared with this incision, because only fibrous tissue and possibly a minor blood vessel are to be found beneath the skin here (**Fig. 6.31a**). The vessel may bleed most annoyingly, however, and interfere with further surgery, in which case it should be cauterized with fine bipolar diathermy forceps.

The further incisions are done with a No. 15 scalpel blade. The transverse incision of the skin over the medial crura of the lower lateral cartilages, with its connection to the incision already made, must be done very carefully because the cartilage lies immediately beneath the skin and is often very thin. There is no protective subcutaneous layer of fatty tissue at this point. The further incision is endonasal, running initially at right angles toward the nasal tip, and is also superficial because of the thin skin coverage. In the region of the domes of the lower lateral cartilages, the so-called soft triangle ("facet area") should be protected. The soft triangle is a cartilage-free area of skin at the anterior margin of the nostril. Here, the endonasal incision must directly follow the caudal margin of the lower lateral cartilage. If the incision comes to lie too near to the nostril margin on the inside, the latter may become distorted by the scars—aesthetically an extremely undesirable outcome, which is almost impossible to repair. The incision ends about 5–10 mm lateral to the dome. In special cases, when a more extensive exposure is required, it may also be extended further.

Elevation of the thin skin from the medial crura of the lower lateral cartilages is problematic. Undermining the skin over the cartilage with fine pointed scissors is the best method of protecting the cartilage. The small bridge of tissue that sub-

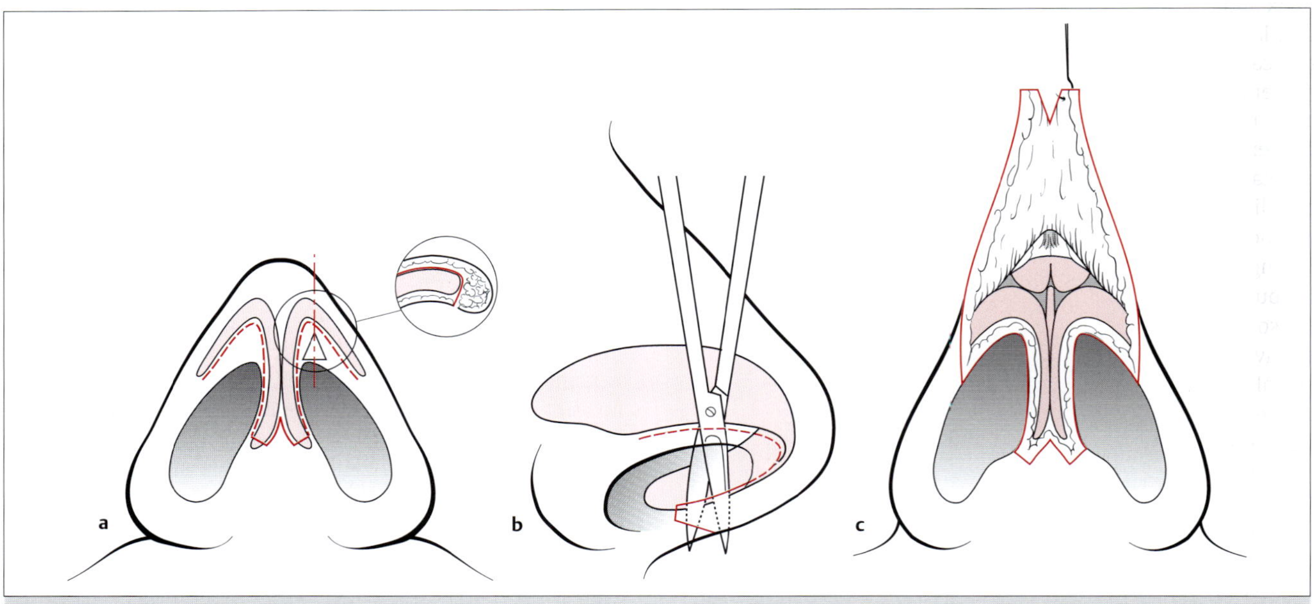

Fig. 6.33a–c External approach to the nasal dorsum and nasal base.
a Angulated columellar incision (continuous line) and marginal incision (dotted line because it is hidden). Protection of the "soft triangle" (inset with cross-section): the cutaneous fold along the upper margin of the nostril must be especially protected during the incision.
b Detachment of the columellar skin off the lower lateral cartilages with pointed scissors.
c Exposure of the lower lateral cartilages and the nasal dorsum after degloving.

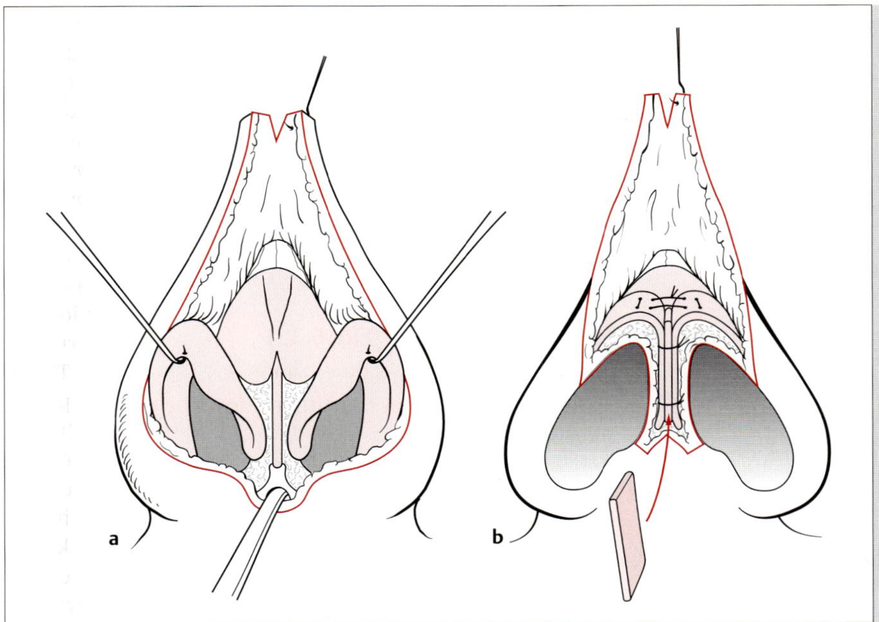

Fig. 6.34a, b External approach to the septum with subsequent reconstruction.
a Separation of the medial crura and domes of the lower lateral cartilages.
b Stabilization of the nasal tip with a columellar strut after an external approach. Interdomal suture.

sequently remains at the caudal incision margin may then be easily divided with a cut of the scissors. Once the cartilage has been exposed, further detachment of the columellar skin is usually unproblematic and best done with small angled scissors. Dissection of the dome region may still be critical, but should not usually pose any major difficulties if the caudal margin of the lower lateral cartilage is followed consistently and scissors are used to divide the skin of the vestibulum. While these steps are undertaken, the columella should be held with a sharp skin hook and not with forceps. After the domes of the lower lateral cartilages are exposed (while preserving the perichondrium), the cartilaginous nasal dorsum is identified using spreading movements of the scissors. The nasal dorsum is further exposed as in the endonasal approach. When doing so, any dissection that extends too far laterally between the lower and upper lateral cartilages should be avoided, as visibility may be lost due to bleeding from an artery that runs in this area (**Fig. 6.31a**).

The external approach also allows the opportunity of exposing the septum to view (**Fig. 6.34**). For this purpose, the fibrous tissue between the medial crura is first divided with scissors until access is gained in front of the nasal spine via the avascular gliding plane to the muscles of the upper lip (the so-called "magic plane"). After dividing the fibrous anchorage of the domes of both lower lateral cartilages, the latter can be displaced laterally with single hooks to allow the caudal septal margin and the upper lateral cartilages to be dissected free. If the upper lateral cartilages are also separated, this will allow free visualization of the entire nasal septum, not only from a caudal direction but also from above.

Because separation of the medial crura from the septum and division of the fibrous tissue between the domes mean that essential suspension points of the lower lateral cartilages are lost (see **Fig. 6.54**), it is recommended to stabilize the nasal tip before suture repair of the columella with a cartilaginous strut, which is inserted between the medial crura of the lower lateral cartilages (**Fig. 6.34b**). The lower lateral cartilages are also additionally stabilized with an "interdomal suture" to avoid later separation. Exposure of the medial crura of the lower lateral cartilages allows the required sutures (usually absorbable 4/0 material) to be placed directly through the cartilage so they do not need to be inserted through the skin of the membranous septum.

Skin closure begins at the tip of the inverted V with a monofilament 5/0 suture. All five corner points must be exactly reapproximated without any step-off, after which intermediate sutures are placed in between each stitch. The lateral area needs only one suture placed roughly in the middle of the columella and a further (absorbable) suture to repair the marginal incision of the lower lateral cartilage.

Rules, Tips, and Tricks

A columellar incision is practically invisible later on, provided the incisions are correctly made and the suture repair is precise. A fine white incision line will be visible only if the skin is closed under tension. Correct placement of the approximating stitch in the lateral area of the incision on the inner surface of the alae is also important: a step-off can be avoided if the vestibular skin on the undersurface of the lower lateral cartilage is taken only with a superficial bite (without transfixing the cartilage), while the needle is inserted deeply into the wound margin of the nostril. The lower lateral cartilage thus "disappears" behind the caudal incision margin.

A further consideration is the tangential displacement of the wound edges at the lateral incision margin, where a skin fold can develop on the undersurface of the lower lateral cartilage. The tangential displacement must be compensated for by the lateral suture, by placing the stitch of the lower lateral cartilage obliquely in the direction of the nasal tip through the incision margin adjacent to the nostril.

! Risks and Complications

The most feared risk is a visible columella scar, and the worst complication is necrosis of the columella.

Retracted columella scars are very difficult to revise. They can be avoided by using an everting suture technique and ensuring a stable cartilaginous support, which is usually absent in the soft-tissue region between the medial crura of the lower lateral cartilages. Although the columellar skin is relatively thick there, it can nevertheless still retract, especially if the fibrous tissue between the medial crura has been excised. The insertion of a cartilaginous frame between the medial crura, which ends exactly in line with the caudal margin of the lower lateral cartilage, is the best guarantee for healing without retraction. Necrosis of the columella can be expected especially in the presence of severe scar formation as well as with wound breakdown (diabetics, smokers) and significant wound tension. Here the indication for an open approach should be most carefully considered and, if in doubt, an endonasal access chosen. Once necrosis of the columella has occurred, it usually requires a technically demanding staged procedure, in most cases with the use of a forehead flap (see Chapter 5).

Postoperative Care

Crust formation at the columellar incision is dissolved with ointment, and the sutures are removed on about the seventh postoperative day. Sunblock can be used in the scar area for approximately 6 months to avoid pigmentation of the scar.

Osteotomies

Surgical Principle

Osteotomies serve to remove parts of the bony pyramid (hump) or to mobilize them in order to displace them.

Indications

Hump reduction with mobilization of the lateral walls to close the subsequent "open roof." Mobilization of the pyramid of a crooked or wide nose.

Contraindications

Osteotomy of mobile bony areas.

Specific Points Regarding Informed Consent

Step-offs (palpable or visible), particularly in the region of the nasal dorsum. Excessive callus formation (extremely rare).

Operative Planning

See Surgical Technique.

Special Instruments

There are numerous osteotomes (bevel on both sides, for a straight osteotomy line) and chisels (bevel on one side only, for a curved osteotomy line), which differ mainly in their type of handle and their width. A well-established set of tools is listed in the section on instruments above (**Fig. 6.6b**).

Surgical Technique

Osteotomies at a Glance (Fig. 6.35)

Standard osteotomies include:

- Paramedian osteotomy (on either side of the internasal suture line).
- Lateral osteotomy (in the frontal process of the maxilla).
- Transverse osteotomy (horizontal osteotomy at the level of the medial canthus, through the frontal process of the maxilla and the nasal bones, *not* through the suture lines to the frontal bone, which lie more cranially).

This is also the order in which the osteotomies are usually made.

In special cases, *supplementary osteotomies* are useful:

- Intermediate osteotomy (between paramedian and lateral osteotomy) for curved and severely deviated bony lateral wall.
- Wedge resection after an additional osteotomy above the lateral osteotomy for resection of a bony wedge to compensate for asymmetrical pyramid walls, e.g., for a growth-related crooked nose.

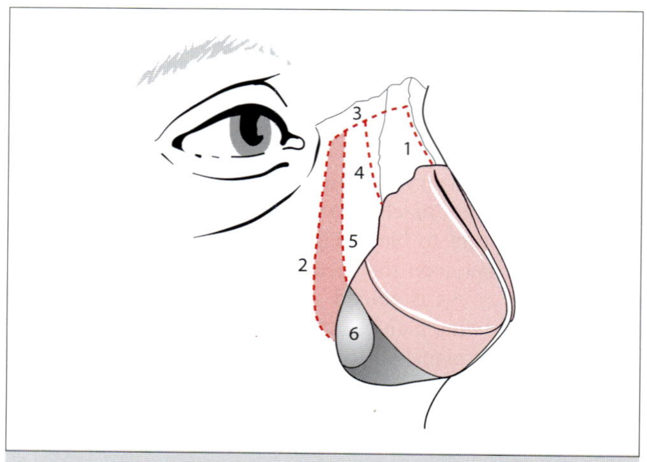

Fig. 6.35 Overview of osteotomies.
Standard osteotomies:
1 paramedian osteotomy (lateral to the internasal suture line)
2 lateral osteotomy (extends to the level of the medial canthus, protects the inferior turbinate [6])
3 transverse osteotomy (is situated at the level of the medial canthus)
Supplementary osteotomies:
4 intermediate osteotomy (between paramedian and lateral osteotomies)
5 wedge resection

Only after completion of at least the three basic osteotomies should it be possible to move the pyramid freely. If a complete transverse osteotomy is dispensed with, e.g., to treat a crooked nose, and the pyramid is just pushed into the midline against resistance, the final outcome is often unsatisfactory because the straight position is merely simulated by the soft-tissue swelling caused by the surgery.

Paramedian Osteotomy (Fig. 6.36)

A paramedian osteotomy is usually made via an extramucosal approach, i.e., without division of the endonasal mucous membrane on the undersurface of the nasal bones. For this purpose, the mucosa at this point is easily elevated from a trans-septal access with the aid of an elevator. If a septoplasty has been done beforehand, then the osteotome may also be inserted from a trans-septal approach. If no septal tunnels have been created, then the osteotome can still also be placed on the piriform aperture in a direct paramedian position via the intercartilaginous incisions. In this case the endonasal mucosa is not elevated and the osteotomy is made from a transmucosal approach, which does not usually present any problems with regard to healing (rarely: subcutaneous mucosal cysts).

Using a 6-mm wide osteotome for preference, the osteotomy is continued as far as the level of the medial canthus, from where it may deviate slightly in a lateral direction to facilitate the connection with the later transverse osteotomy, especially if it is made to close an "open roof."

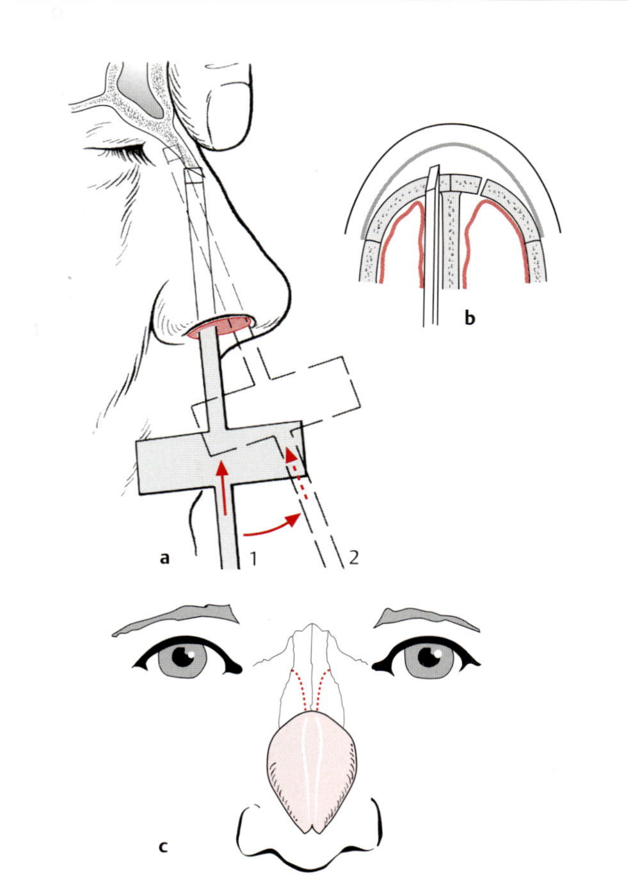

Fig. 6.36a–c Paramedian osteotomy.
a Trans-septal insertion of the osteotome under digital guidance: commence in position 1 until the instrument is palpable beneath the skin; continue in position 2, parallel to the dorsum of the nose.
b Frontal view: the mucosa is protected by an extramucosal trans-septal approach.
c The osteotomies diverge slightly in a lateral direction and end at the level of the medial canthus.

Lateral Osteotomy (Fig. 6.37)

The planned course of a lateral osteotomy may first be marked out on the skin with a pen. This line is based on the "nasal baseline" between the medial canthus and the alar–facial groove. The osteotomy begins just above this line at the piriform aperture, from where it is directed toward the line and runs 1–2 mm above and parallel to it before reaching the level of the medial canthus.

For the endonasal version, a vertical lateral vestibular incision is made in the skin at the level of the head of the inferior turbinate, and the bony margin of the piriform aperture is identified. A subperiosteal tunnel is created on the lateral surface along the planned osteotomy line, using a sharp elevator (e.g., the sharp end of a Cottle elevator). At the level of the canthus, the subperiosteal tunnel is extended with the elevator in the direction of the nasal root for the subsequent transverse osteotomy.

The osteotomy can be well controlled with the aid of a guided osteotome. On the one hand, the guide is easily palpable from the outside through the skin, while on the other hand it prevents the instrument from slipping into the nasal cavity. The guide can be easily engaged at the piriform aperture, about 5 mm above the nasal baseline. At the beginning of the osteotomy, the handle must be directed medially and superiorly because of the curvature of the aperture. Because the osteotomy line must follow this curved surface, the handle will follow a quarter-circle movement, proceeding from medial–superior to lateral–inferior. At the start of the osteotomy the bone is very thick (dull pitch, more effort); about halfway it becomes thinner (high pitch; use less force to avoid splitting the bone) and then somewhat thicker again at the level of the medial canthus. Because the lateral guide moves ahead of the actual blade, the guide must be palpable cranial to the medial canthus at the end of the osteotomy. If the osteotomy pitch becomes clearly duller, then the osteotome has already reached the thick frontal bone at the frontomaxillary suture. The lateral osteotomy usually ends a few millimeters caudal to this suture line.

Transverse Osteotomy (Fig. 6.38)

Here a curved chisel is used, which is introduced via the lateral vestibular incision. First the lower point of the chisel is positioned at the end of the lateral osteotomy line and advanced into the bone with light taps of the hammer to allow it to catch. Only then is the chisel handle moved as far laterally as possible

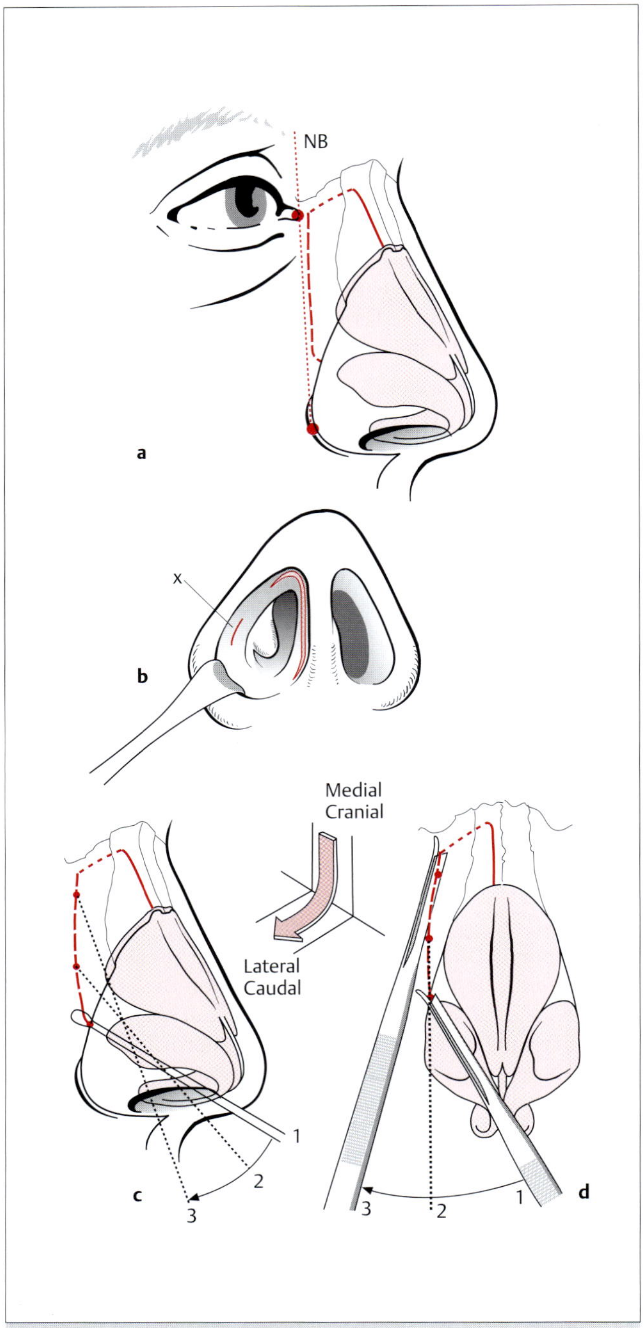

Fig. 6.37a–d Lateral osteotomy.

a Position of osteotomy at the nasal baseline (NB) (alar-facial groove to medial canthus), starting slightly higher to protect the head of the turbinate.

b Lateral vestibular incision (x) in the vestibular skin at the level of the head of the inferior turbinate (in addition to the hemitransfixion and intercartilaginous incision).

c Osteotomy using the guarded osteotome. The handle is moved in the sagittal plane from above (position 1) downward (positions 2 and 3). The position of the planned transverse osteotomy is depicted as a dotted line.

d In the frontal plane, the handle is moved from medial (position 1) to lateral (positions 2 and 3). Taking both movements together, the handle roughly follows a quarter circle, from medial–cranial to lateral–caudal.

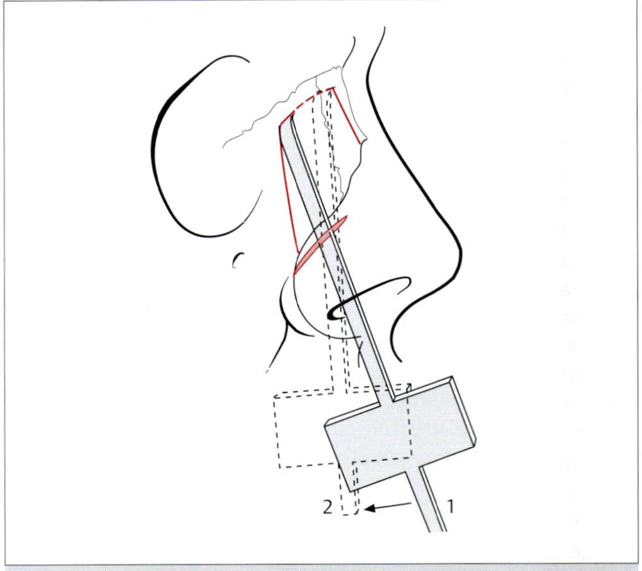

Fig. 6.38 Transverse osteotomy.
The curved chisel is inserted via a lateral vestibular incision and positioned at the cranial end (medial canthus) of the lateral osteotomy (position 1). From there a fracture line is gradually created in the direction of the nasal root (position 2).

to cut the bone to the whole width of the chisel. Then the chisel is advanced in the direction of the nasal root and the transverse osteotomy completed on one side. Because the bone is very thick, particularly in the region of the nasal root (the block of bone made up of the nasal spine of the frontal bone and the nasal bones, see **Fig. 6.1d**), an attempt should not be made there to chisel it through completely from one side, but rather complete mobilization should only be attempted after the transverse osteotomy of the contralateral side has been accomplished. Otherwise there is a danger of splitting the bone in the region of the nasal root.

In principle, lateral and transversal osteotomies can also be directly made percutaneously instead of endonasally and this has indeed proved effective, especially for transverse osteotomies. With thick bones, an endonasal transverse osteotomy has an unfavorable force vector, often making very hard taps with the hammer necessary. The very thick nasal spine of the frontal bone, which lies beneath the nasal bones, can be chiselled through with the aid of a 3- or 4-mm wide osteotome via a stab incision at the nasal root and the osteotomy then extended on either side toward the medial canthus. The periosteum is divided directly with the sharp osteotome and not elevated beforehand. Special attention should be paid to the direction of the osteotomy (recognizable by the position of the osteotome handle). The direction runs perpendicular to the surface of the bone and not in the direction of the skull base.

In principle, a lateral osteotomy can also be performed percutaneously via a stab incision, made roughly in the middle of the osteotomy line, also dividing the periosteum with the sharp 3- or 4-mm wide osteotome. The skin is easily retracted over the whole length of the osteotomy using the osteotome inserted through the stab incision.

Rules, Tips, and Tricks

Dealing with Intra-Operative Problems

As with all endonasal incisions, it is recommended to infiltrate the corresponding vestibular skin with local anesthetic and epinephrine before the start of the operation. This considerably reduces bleeding from the wound margins. Only the incision line is infiltrated and not the whole region around the subsequent osteotomy.

A clean osteotomy presupposes sharp instruments. This is best guaranteed if the osteotomes and chisels are sharpened at the operating table with a sharpening stone. With very thick bone, it may even be advisable to sharpen the instrument anew for each side.

Osteotome and chisel are advanced with double taps of the hammer. A light "testing tap" (to test the firm positioning of the instrument) is followed by a harder "working tap," which makes the actual cut in the bone. This avoids any inadvertent slipping of the instrument and perforation of the skin.

Osteotomies can raise the blood pressure of the surgeon, and also that of the patient. The anesthethist should be notified in good time that osteotomies are about to be made, so that they can react accordingly. Reduction of intra-operative bleeding considerably reduces postoperative swelling and hematoma formation. This can also be assisted by compression of the soft tissues for 1–2 minutes after every osteotomy.

If it is not possible to move the pyramid freely to the left and right between two fingers, then mobilization should not be forced, as this will result in irregular fracture lines. The region of resistance should rather be "re-osteotomized," possibly even percutaneously, if it is in the nasal root area.

If an intermediate or supplementary osteotomy is required for a wedge resection, then this is done *after* the paramedian osteotomy and *before* the lateral osteotomy. Osteotomy of a mobile area of bone is not possible.

Small protruding ridges of bone, particularly at the nasal root after a transverse osteotomy, should undergo additional osteotomy, as they are usually clearly visible after the swelling has resolved. For this purpose, a percutaneous osteotomy is also very helpful.

! Risks and Complications

Lateral osteotomies that are extended too high often result in visible and palpable step-offs. This can often be corrected intra-operatively by "re-osteotomizing" a little lower (possibly percutaneously). In the further postoperative course small fragments of bone may result in the formation of sequestra, which lead to swelling and erythema of the skin, especially in the region of the medial canthus. In such situations, the sequestrum is best removed via a stab incision.

A transmucosal osteotomy can displace the mucosa beneath the skin and may lead to the formation of a subcutaneous cyst. In this case, the cyst must be completely removed and the connection with the inside of the nose closed. This requires optimal visualization, which is best achieved only via an open approach (see **Fig. 6.63**). Alternatively, a direct skin incision over the cyst, taking the RSTL into consideration (see Chapter 5), is also a conceivable option, although it usually leaves a visible scar.

Measuring Points, Lines, and Angles

In describing and planning operations on the nose, there are several measuring points on the soft tissues of the face that allow proportions and angles to be determined (**Fig. 6.39**). They play an important role above all in the analysis of the profiles of the nose and face.

These points are based on the frontal plane of the face through the nasion (nasal root), subnasale (junction of the columella with the upper lip), and pogonion (the most anterior point of the chin). Normally these three measuring points lie in one line. Together with the line through the root of the nose and the nasal tip, the frontal plane of the face forms the nasofrontal angle, which is a measurement of the projection of the nasal tip (distance of the nasal tip from the facial plane—see **Fig. 6.53c**). The nasofrontal angle also reflects the indentation of the nasal root below the glabella. Another important angle is the nasolabial angle, between columella and upper lip. This should be between 95° and 110°.

Only a few lines and points are relevant in assessing the form of the nose from an aesthetic point of view (**Fig. 6.39b**). They are mainly produced by light reflections on the skin of the nose. The brow–tip aesthetic line takes a curvilinear course from the eyebrows on either side of the junction between nasal dorsum and nasal wall and ends at the level of the supratip region. Minor irregularities of this line are suggestive of a "crooked" nose. The domes of the lower lateral cartilages produce two small light reflections on the tip of the nose, which become all the more conspicuous the more marked the nasal tip is. The distance between the two reflections is responsible for the impression of a wide or a narrow nose. The lines connecting the alar–facial groove and the columella take an oblique course and meet in the form of a V at the columella. The columella is therefore caudal to the nasal alae and is normally visible when looked at in profile. If, however, the columella is retracted ("hidden columella"), e. g., as a result of a loss of the septal cartilage, then the nasolabial angle is also decreased (<90°).

Plans for correcting the profile of the nose must start from the nasal tip projection (**Fig. 6.40**). With a normal nasofacial angle of ca. 36°, the nasal base demonstrates oval nostrils with an oblique axis (**Fig. 6.40a**). With a prominent hump deformity, the nasal base and nasal tip projection are normal. The excess of cartilage and bone to be removed thus lies above the line connecting nasal root and nasal tip (**Fig. 6.40b**). A ptotic nasal tip with a reduced nasofacial angle can, on the other hand, simulate a prominent hump deformity (so-called pseudohump). Reducing the hump without raising the nasal tip projection would result in the formation of a saddle nose. A reduced nasal tip projection is recognizable at the nasal base by transverse-oval or rounded nostrils with a rounded tip and increase of the distance between the alae. The columella is shortened (**Fig. 6.40c**).

An over-projection of the nasal tip can resemble a prominent hump nose in profile (**Fig. 6.60d**). The anatomical situation is completely different here, however, and usually also results in obstruction of nasal breathing. Excess growth of the cartilaginous nasal septum reduces the nasal valve angle (between the upper lateral cartilages and septum), resulting in a nasal valve stenosis (**Fig. 6.3d**). The nasal vestibule, situated caudal to the nasal valve, is narrow. This is partially caused by the slit-like

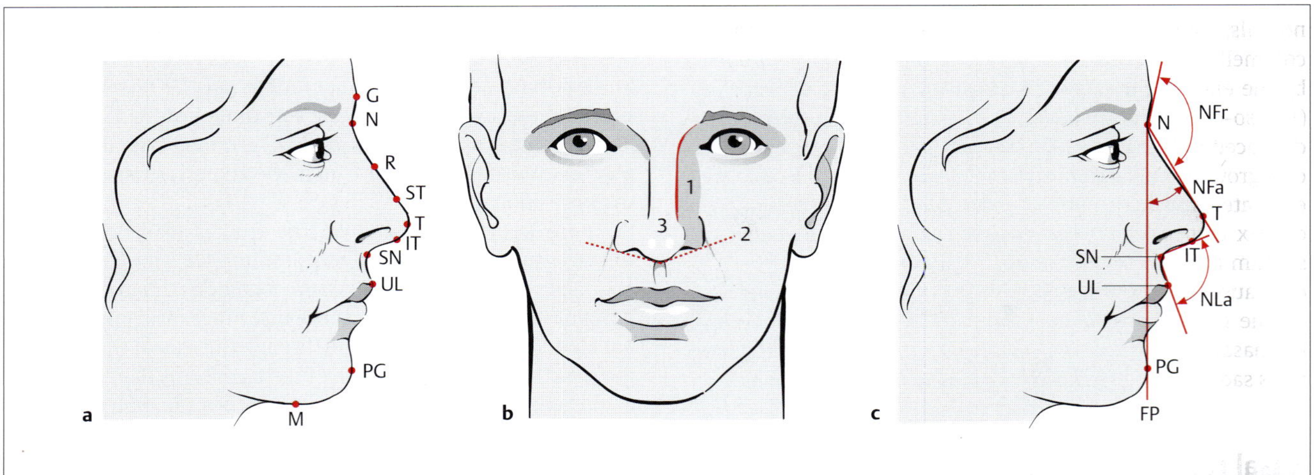

Fig. 6.39a–c Measuring points, lines, and angles.

a Soft-tissue measuring points.

- G glabella
- N nasion (nasal radix)
- R rhinion (osseocartilaginous junction, corresponding to the K-area)
- ST suptratip region
- T nasal tip (corresponding to the domes of the lower lateral cartilages)
- IT infratip region (between the tip and the upper nostril rim)
- SN subnasale (junction of the columella with the upper lip)
- UL upper lip (vermilion border)
- PG pogonion (anterior chin)
- M menton (inferior chin)

b Lines.

1. brow–tip aesthetic line: this line should run without interruption in a curve from the eyebrow to the tip of the nose, and divides the light reflections of the nasal dorsum from the shadow of the nasal wall
2. the lines connecting the alar–facial groove and the columella take a V-shaped course; a horizontal course is characteristic of a retracted columella
3. light reflections, produced by the domes of the lower lateral cartilages (they define the width and form of the nasal tip)

c Facial angles.

- FP facial plane (through the nasal radix N and tip of the chin PG)
- NFr nasofrontal angle
- NFa nasofacial angle (between NT and FP); it is ca. 36° and is a possible measurement for the nasal tip projection
- NLa nasolabial angle (between SN–IT and SN–UL); it is between 95° and 110°

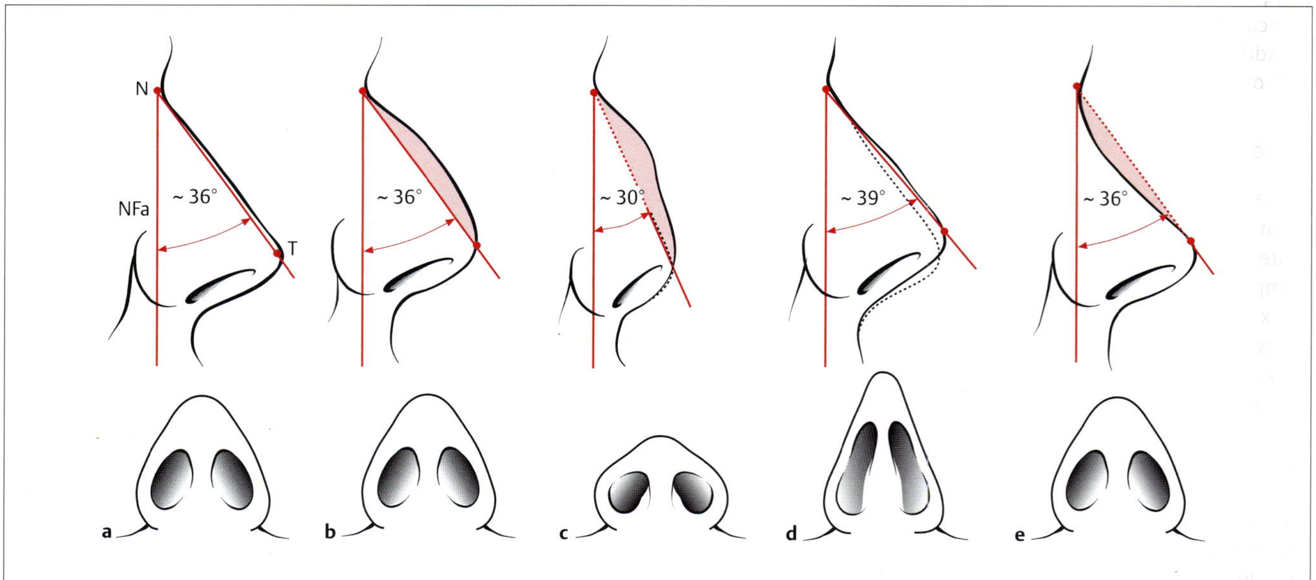

Fig. 6.40a–e Nasal tip projection and profile correction.

a Normal profile: nasal tip projection and nasal base are normal.

b Hump nose: projection and base are normal.

c Pseudohump: projection reduced, base wide, columella short, nostrils rounded.

d Tension nose: projection too high, base narrow, columella wide, slitlike nostrils.

e Bony saddle: projection normal, base normal.

nostrils, which are constricted even further medially by a wide columella base. The widening of the columella is produced by the ends of the medial crura of the lower lateral cartilages (the so-called "footplates"), which are directed outward and displaced in the direction of the nasal tip as a result of the excess growth. The tension causes the nasal ala to take on a more elongated appearance rather than the usual outwardly slightly convex course. The distance between the alae and the nasal septum is shortened. The negative pressure during inspiration can cause collapse of the alae.

The saddle nose is the opposite of the hump nose, although the nasal dorsum alone is only rarely involved (osseocartilaginous saddle nose, **Fig. 6.40e**).

Nasal Hump Deformity

Surgical Principle

Reduction of the osseocartilaginous nasal hump and closure of the "open roof" using osteotomies.

Indications

Excess projection of the nasal dorsum *after* determining the desired nasal-tip projection.

Contraindications

Pseudohump.

Specific Points Regarding Informed Consent

Irregularities of the nasal dorsum, particularly with thin skin associated with the possible need of fine adjustments, should be addressed after 6 months at the earliest. Erythema of the skin of the nasal dorsum (rubeosis).

Operative Planning

The extent of the reduction of the nasal dorsum must depend upon the nasal-tip projection. A ptotic nasal tip should be elevated by appropriate measures (see **Fig. 6.56**). Often a planned hump reduction is then no longer necessary, or only to a lesser extent. On the other hand, lowering of the nasal tip in the course of wound healing should be taken into account, making an additional reduction, particularly of the cartilaginous nasal dorsum, necessary to avoid creating a "polly beak" (**Fig. 6.42**).

Special Instruments

An adequately wide osteotome (≥12 mm) is required for a symmetrical hump reduction. The corners of the blade should be slightly rounded to avoid injury to the skin of the nasal dorsum (see **Fig. 6.6b**).

Surgical Technique (Fig. 6.41)

The dorsum of the nose is exposed by an endonasal or an external approach (see Basic Techniques, p. 73). If the septum has previously been corrected, then hump reduction should be done from an extramucosal approach, after elevating the mucosa from the undersurface. Otherwise, hump reduction is done in a transmucosal manner.

The exact positioning of the patient is important for a symmetrical reduction: the head must not be rotated to one side. Only in this way can the horizontal guidance of the instruments be correctly ensured.

First, an incision is made around the cartilaginous part of the nasal hump. For this purpose, a No. 11 scalpel blade may be used. For a right-handed surgeon, the blade first divides the upper lateral cartilages on the left side of the aperture, at the level of the intended new height. At this point, the knife is drawn through the cartilaginous nasal septum and the right upper lateral cartilage, keeping it exactly in the horizontal plane. An Aufricht retractor serves to protect the skin of the nose and as a counter-support. The scalpel is now drawn in a cephalic-to-caudal direction and the cartilaginous part of the nasal hump, made up of parts of the upper lateral cartilages and the nasal septum, is detached. It remains attached only to the nasal bones. Upper lateral cartilages and septum are usually still attached to the caudal resection margin. If in doubt, it is preferable to remove too little, as it is easy to resect more later using angled scissors, especially from the cut edge of the nasal septum. If too much is removed at the start, however, any subsequent replacement with cartilage grafts is difficult and the outcome unreliable.

The cartilaginous nasal hump can now be lifted like a lid and a wide osteotome inserted. It is placed against the bony aperture and must be held exactly horizontally. The correct course of the osteotomy (not too high and not too low) can best be assessed from the direction of the handle, looking at it from the side. As far as possible, removal of the hump is done in one blow, with the osteotomy usually already ending caudal to the nasion. With a very broad nasal dorsum and an insufficiently wide osteotome it may be necessary to do separate left and right osteotomies at the beginning. In principle, a chisel may also be used, especially if too superficial a hump reduction is feared in the presence of thick bone. In this case, the chisel is used first with the bevelled surface facing upward, until one half of the bony hump has been osteotomized. Then it is turned through 180° (bevelled surface downward) to complete the osteotomy. This technique avoids making too deep a reduction in the area of the nasal root.

Provided the periosteum together with the overlying procerus muscle has already been elevated, the osseocartilaginous hump is easily removed. If bridges of fibrous tissue are still attached, the hump must not be torn out using force. The fibrous bridges must be selectively divided with scissors or scalpel.

If the bony nasal root has a deep depression, reduction of the nasal hump usually ends below the level of the medial canthus. In this case, short supplementary paramedian osteotomies are usually required. They are directed slightly laterally as supplementary osteotomies using an osteotome or chisel (bevelled surface facing medially). The "open roof," which results after hump reduction and in the depths of which the raw edge of the

6

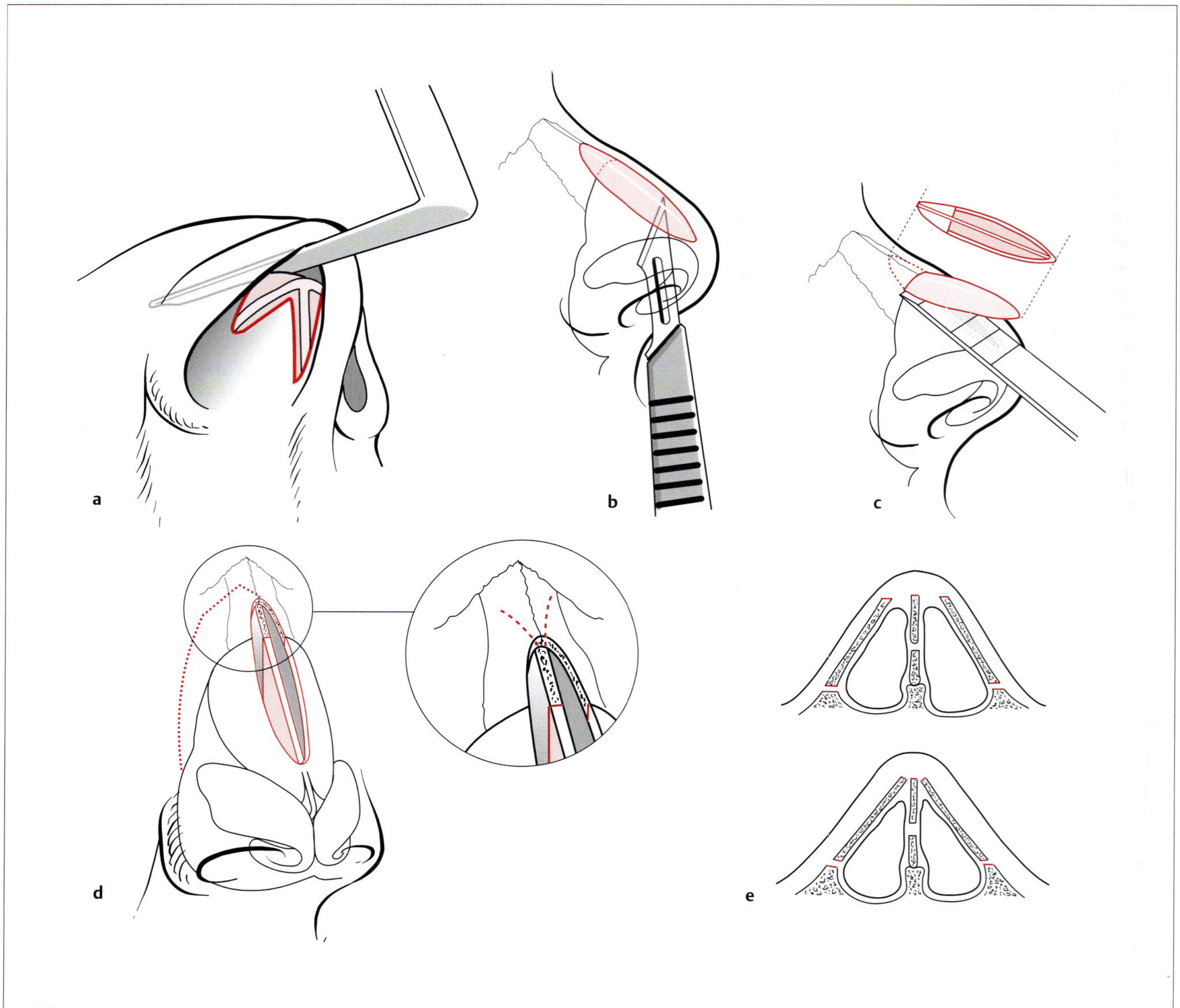

Fig. 6.41a–e Technique of nasal hump reduction.
a Exposure of the nasal dorsum with the Aufricht retractor.
b Circumferential incision around the cartilaginous part of the hump.
c Osteotomy of the bony part of the hump using the 12-mm wide osteotome. The resected part usually contains only a small bony part and a strip of septum on its undersurface.
d Completion with outwardly directed paramedian osteotomies, if necessary with bony resection of the nasal radix.
e Closure of the open roof after mobilization of the pyramids by lateral and transversal osteotomies.

cartilaginous nasal septum and possibly the adjacent perpendicular plate can be seen, must now be closed. This is all the easier if additional bone is chiselled away between the supplementary paramedian osteotomies or removed with a rongeur.

The dorsum of the nose should be assessed for any irregularities before mobilization of the bony pyramid. These are better palpated with a finger than recognized by eye. A moist finger is stroked lightly over the skin of the nasal dorsum to identify the site of any cartilaginous or bony ridges. Cartilaginous ridges are smoothed out with the scalpel or with angled (serrated) scissors. Care should be taken to ensure that the raw edge of the cartilaginous septum lies slightly below the level of the upper lateral cartilages. Attention should also be paid to adequately reducing the height of the septum, especially in the region of the nasal valve. If, after reduction of the hump, the upper lateral cartilages are still connected to the nasal septum at this point and further reduction is required, then they should be completely detached.

If the nasal dorsum now lies at the correct level and all raw edges have been smoothed out, then the open roof is closed by lateral and transverse osteotomies.

Rules, Tips, and Tricks

As a general rule, it is better to remove too little cartilage and bone than too much. Subsequent resection from cartilage and bone is always possible and one can gradually approach the desired final profile. Excessive reduction can only be evened out with a dorsal onlay graft, which may leave conspicuous irregularities. Uneven ridges in the cartilaginous region can only be smoothed out with sharp instruments. This often involves the junction between upper lateral cartilages and nasal bones. A rasp can only smooth out the bony part of these edges; cartilage does not lend itself to adjustments with a elevator.

Work on the nasal dorsum should be completed before mobilization of the bony pyramid, because mobile areas of bone can no longer be dealt with using a chisel and only with difficulty using a elevator. Furthermore, it should be borne in mind that, especially with a very wide "open roof," the dorsum can gain slightly in height after mobilization. This effect should be considered when undertaking hump reduction.

Risks and Complications

Three postoperative deformities in particular should be pointed out:

Polly Beak Deformity (Fig. 6.42)

If the nasal tip settles during the postoperative healing phase, then the domes may come to lie below the level of the cartilaginous nasal dorsum. The result is a distortion of the nasal profile, which resembles a parrot's (polly) beak. Noses with a deep nasal root, a high dorsum, and low nasal tip (the "risky nose") are predisposed to this frequent postoperative deformation. The nasal dorsal profile may appear pleasing at the end of the operation, but the nasal tip occasionally descends in the further postoperative course because of the loss of support of the lower lateral cartilages secondary to the approaches required to access the dorsum. The cartilaginous nasal dorsum then becomes relatively "too high." In some cases, excessive thickness of the subcutaneous soft tissue in the region of the supratip is responsible for the deformation (so-called "soft-tissue polly beak").

Because descent of the nasal tip by a few millimeters is almost routinely expected after rhinoplasty, the foreseeable final projection of the nasal tip should determine the degree of hump reduction. To prevent the creation of a polly beak, it is therefore recommended to reduce the cartilaginous dorsum by 2–3 mm more than the immediate postoperative result would require. If such a deformity has occurred, then revision surgery should be undertaken after 6 months at the earliest, although 1 year would be even better. Admittedly, elevation of the nasal tip is an alternative worth considering, but it may be easier to resect the cartilaginous and, if necessary, the bony dorsum by the required amount at a later session. An open roof with the subsequent need for renewed osteotomies does not usually occur, so revision is usually confined to the nasal dorsum.

Long Nose / Short Nose (Fig. 6.43)

If the nasolabial angle is still within normal limits (90–95°) before hump reduction, then the nose may appear optically "too long" after hump reduction. In this case nasal tip rotation together with a modest increase of the nasolabial angle may be appropriate (see **Fig. 6.57**).

However, it is not advisable to regularly combine a hump reduction with a nasal tip rotation (shortening of nasal length). If the nasolabial angle is already marginally increased preoperatively, then any further rotation would lead to an aestheti-

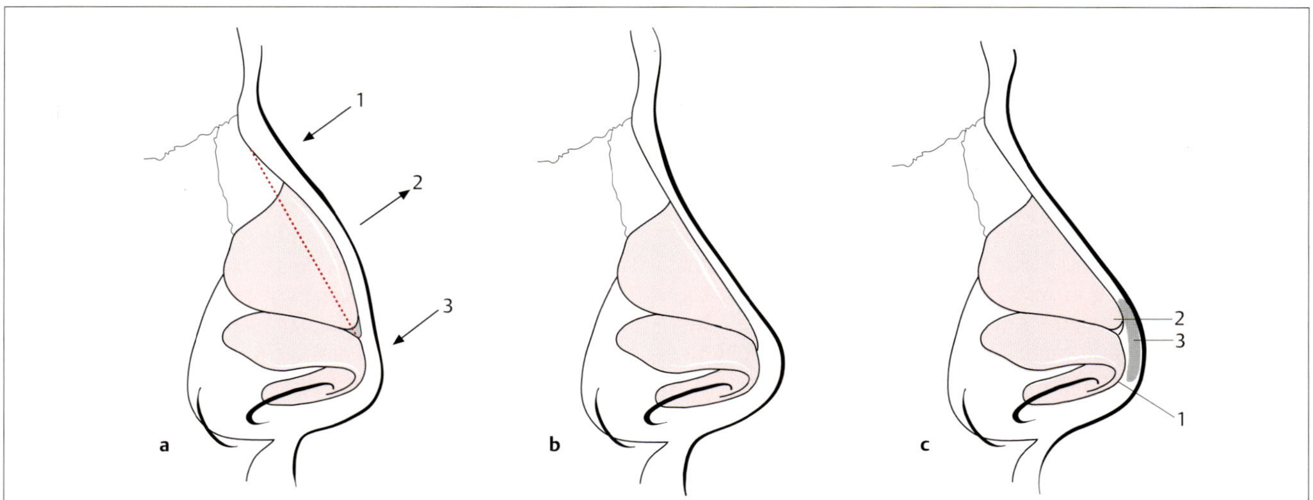

Fig. 6.42a–c Polly beak deformity.
a Risk factors.
1 deep nasal radix
2 high nasal dorsum
3 ptotic nasal tip (dotted line: planned hump reduction)
b Early result after hump reduction.
c Late result.
1 ptotic nasal tip
2 relatively prominent nasal dorsum
3 occasionally soft-tissue swelling in the supratip region ("soft-tissue polly beak")

6

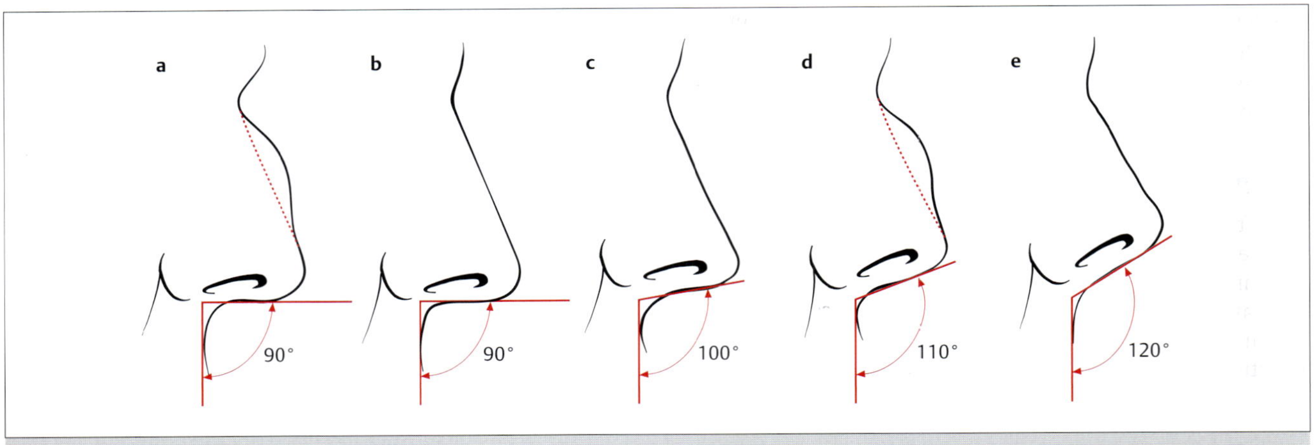

Fig. 6.43a–e Shortening of the nasal length by rotation of the tip.
a Acute nasolabial angle preoperatively (dotted line: planned hump reduction).
b After hump reduction, the nose is relatively "too long" (angle unchanged).
c Shortening of the length of the nasal dorsum by "tip rotation" (obtuse angle).
d Open nasolabial angle preoperatively.
e "Over-rotation" of the tip after hump reduction ("short nose").

cally most unfavorable short nose, where the nasal base plane is upright and the nostrils are clearly visible when seen from the front. Hump reduction of an already short nose is therefore risky, and all operative steps should be avoided which may lead to a further rotation of the tip and to shortening of the length of the nasal dorsum (columellar pocket, resection of the caudal septal margin, resections from the cephalic lower lateral cartilages or caudal upper lateral cartilages).

Open-Roof Deformity (Fig. 6.44)

If after hump reduction the open roof is not completely closed by osteotomies, a bony gap may result over the nasal dorsum. If the intranasal mucous membrane adheres to the overlying skin, neuralgiform pain may arise. In this case, skin and mucosa must be separated at a revision operation and the bony gap filled, e.g., with cartilage. Some cases will require renewed osteotomy after the scar tissue between the bone edges has been removed.

However, neuralgiform symptoms may also be the result of division of the external nasal nerve. Both nerves exit between the nasal bones and the upper lateral cartilages, running from the inside of the nose to the surface, and provide sensory capabilities to the dorsal nasal skin (see **Fig. 6.31a**). Their division during hump reduction may be unavoidable, even using the correct surgical technique. A resulting neuralgia, on the other hand, is very rare and cannot be rectified or improved by renewed surgery. Conservative management is required.

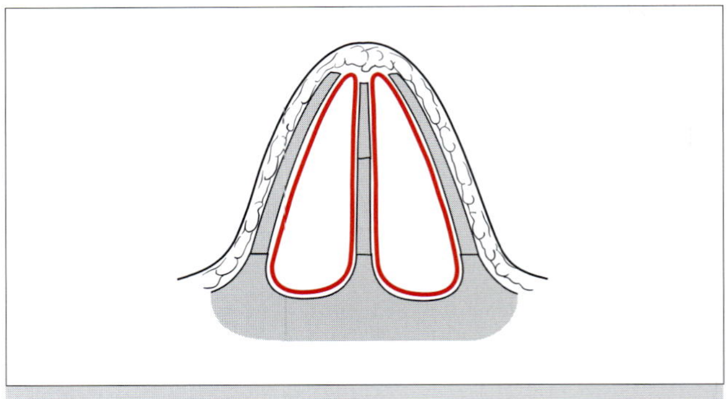

Fig. 6.44 Open roof deformity.
Bony defect of the nasal roof. Skin and mucosa are adherent to each other.

Further Risks and Complications

The postoperative formation of rough edges in the region of the nasal dorsum has already been mentioned. These appear especially with very thin nasal skin. In difficult cases it may be necessary, after removing more of the dorsum, to cover it with a finely formed and smoothed septal graft, ensuring in particular that the graft recreates the brow–tip aesthetic line. Artificial "thickening" of thin skin by inserting autogenous or allogenic fascia may be attempted, but due to absorption, this hardly ever results in a thick enough soft-tissue envelope.

When reducing a hump, the connection between septal cartilage, upper lateral cartilages, and nasal bones is separated. This may become risky, especially if the suture line between septal cartilage and perpendicular plate has also been completely divided. The nasal septal cartilage then loses an important point of suspension and may "slide" into the nasal cavity. This results in a visible step-off at the rhinion (K-area). If such a displacement of the nasal septal cartilage has already occurred immediately after hump reduction, it should be secured with an absorbable suture to the remnants of the upper lateral cartilages, which are still connected to the nasal bones.

During hump reduction, especially with a transmucosal approach, parts of the mucous membrane can become displaced beneath the skin over the dorsum and result in the development of subcutaneous cysts. This complication has already been referred to in the section on osteotomies above (p. 78).

Erythema of the skin over the dorsum, especially after revision operations for hump reduction, is unavoidable, even with correct operative technique. Later laser treatment of the visible vessels over several sessions may be beneficial.

Postoperative Care

A "soft-tissue polly beak" can develop secondary to a postoperative hematoma in the region of the nasal tip. It is therefore recommended to keep a firm plaster dressing in place for 14 days after surgery (see **Fig. 6.11a**). Any soft-tissue thickening that may develop can be treated with repeated subcutaneous injections of a crystalline steroid suspension.

Crooked Nose

Deviation of the nasal dorsum from the median-sagittal plane is referred to as a crooked, or twisted, nose. The dorsum may be either straight or curved in a C shape (**Fig. 6.45**). Crooked noses with C-shaped or reverse C-shaped deviations of the dorsum, particularly the cartilaginous part, have already been described. Here the bony pyramid is straightened by osteotomies and the deviation of the cartilaginous nasal dorsum is corrected, e.g., using spreader grafts.

The nasal bones form a unit with the septodorsal cartilage (**Fig. 6.45a**). If the nasal bones deviate to one side, then the upper lateral cartilages, and with them the nasal septum, must do so too (**Fig. 6.45b**). The impact on the nasal septum is as follows: the septum is attached to the nasal dorsum. If the dorsum deviates to one side, then the septal cartilage and the perpendicular plate are usually dislocated from their junction to premaxilla and vomer to the contralateral side (ascending crest). Cartilage and perpendicular plate are deviated in an oblique position, with the insertion of the plate to the undersurface of the nasal bones at an acute angle (need for osteotomy of the perpendicular plate at their junction to the nasal bones). As a result of this, there is almost always also a dislocation of the caudal septal margin to the side of the deviation of the bony nasal dorsum, which dictates the direction ("bone dominates cartilage"). However, the caudal septum need not necessarily be luxated from the premaxilla. It is just the deviation of the dorsum that forces the anterior inferior corner of the caudal end to deviate from the midline. In this case, correction of the nasal septum alone would only straighten the cartilaginous part of the nose, which might result on the one hand in a visible deviation in the K-area (a nasal dorsum that was seemingly straight before surgery suddenly appears twisted), or on the other hand in recurrent deviations of the nasal septum. With this deformity, it is the straightening of the pyramid that is decisive and which the attached cartilaginous structures follow.

Two situations must be differentiated here:

- Trauma in *adulthood*: The lateral nasal walls are of equal length and merely displaced (**Fig. 6.46**).

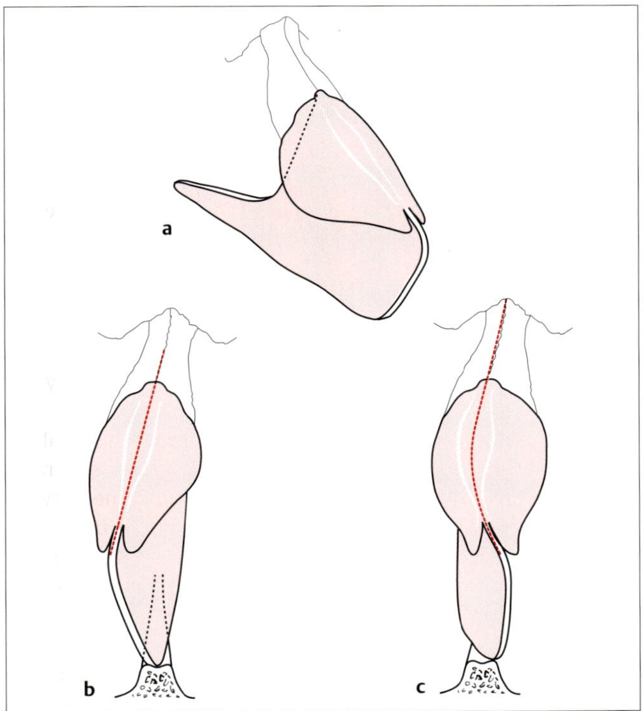

Fig. 6.45a–c Types of crooked nose.
a Functional unit made up of nasal bones and septodorsal cartilage.
b Crooked nose with a straight nasal dorsum in itself ("dislocation").
c Crooked nose with a convex nasal dorsum ("C form").

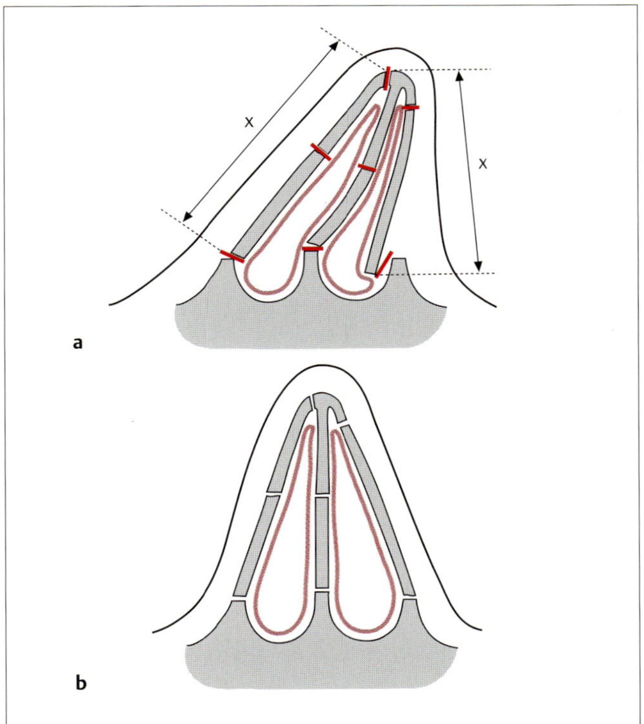

Fig. 6.46a, b Correction of a crooked nose after trauma in adulthood.
a Displacement of the fragments, but equal lateral heights (x).
b Reduction after osteotomies ("fibrotomies") of the previous fracture lines.

- Congenital crooked nose or trauma during *childhood*: The lateral nasal walls are asymmetrical as a result of disturbances of growth, and are of unequal length (**Fig. 6.47**).

Surgical Principle

Mobilization of the bony nasal pyramid by osteotomies. Mobilization of the nasal septum and, if necessary, correction of asymmetries of the lateral nasal walls by resection of the excess length.

Indications

Malalignment of the osseocartilaginous nasal dorsum. Usually the nasal valve is constricted on the contralateral side of the deviation as a result of the slant of the nasal septum.

Contraindications

A seemingly crooked nose secondary to a predominantly asymmetrical face where an optical alignment is not possible and alignment of the nose is the primary aim of the operation. Crooked nose simulated by a lateral depression (see **Fig. 6.9a**).

Specific Points Regarding Informed Consent

If there is an obvious facial asymmetry in addition to the crooked nose, then the patient must be informed that the nose may still appear crooked even after a correctly performed operation. Furthermore, crooked noses have a "memory effect," which can lead to recurrence despite the most careful technique. Subluxation of the caudal septal margin is very often merely the trademark of what is, for all intents and purposes, a crooked nose. Surgery of only the nasal septum may then result in a deviation of the axis of the nasal dorsum at the K-area and give the patient the impression of a newly developed crooked nose. On the other hand, if the patient wants just a septoplasty, then the possibility of this deformity should be pointed out.

Operative Planning

An detailed examination and operative planning should be conducted before surgery, given that soft-tissue swelling easily obscures any deformity on the operating table. The malalignment of the nasal dorsum is best recognized by viewing the nose from above (the surgeon stands behind the patient's head). For markedly crooked noses with asymmetries of the lateral nasal walls, resections to correct the malalignment should be planned preoperatively (see below).

Surgical Technique

If no extensive operative measures to the nasal tip are intended, correction of a crooked nose is done mainly via endonasal approaches. The incisions correspond to those used for hump reduction. Care must be taken to undermine the nasal dorsum adequately (degloving), because the mobilized osseocartilaginous infrastructure must be rotated beneath the soft-tissue envelope (see **Fig. 6.31b**) into the median plane.

Simple Lateral Displacement Secondary to Trauma in Adulthood (Fig. 6.46)

Here the nasal walls are in principle equal on either side and are merely displaced. The original fracture has also involved the nasal septum, which will first require mobilization by chondrotomies, leaving the mucous membrane on one side intact if possible. This creates a pivot point at the premaxilla, around which the nasal septum can be straightened up after division of any cartilaginous fracture lines with the nasal dorsum. In practical terms, therefore, the old fracture lines must be re-opened to straighten up the pyramid. This is achieved not by osteotomies but by "fibrotomies," because these fractures will usually have healed as fibrous unions. The osteotome follows the fracture lines almost automatically, given that it takes the path of least resistance. If this does not succeed, then standard paramedian, lateral, and transversal osteotomies should be used. Care should be taken to achieve complete mobilization, particularly in the region of the nasal root, because any elastic resistance will make a residual or recurrent deviation more likely.

A C-shaped deviation of the cartilaginous nasal dorsum may be corrected by using a spreader graft (see **Fig. 6.23**).

Asymmetrical Nasal Walls Secondary to Disturbances of Growth (Figs. 6.47 and 6.48)

In this case, the nasal walls of are differing lengths (i.e., there is a short side and a long side). Apart from mobilization, the

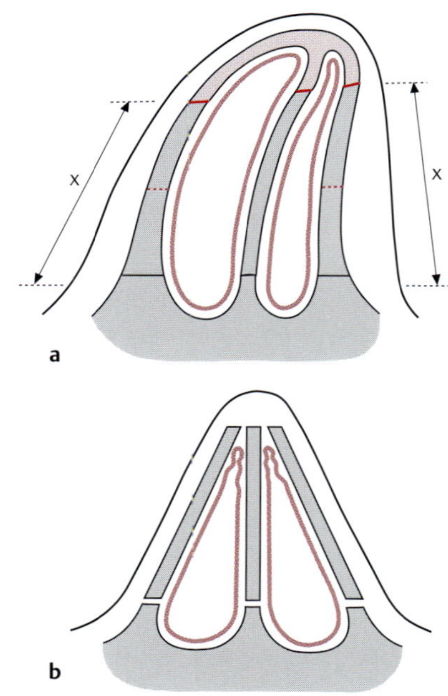

Fig. 6.47a, b Correction of a crooked nose due to disturbances of growth: asymmetrical hump reduction.
a Achievement of symmetry of height by "lowering" the "long" side to achieve equal heights (x) of the lateral nasal walls (intermediate osteotomies may also be required).
b Appearance after mobilization and reduction.

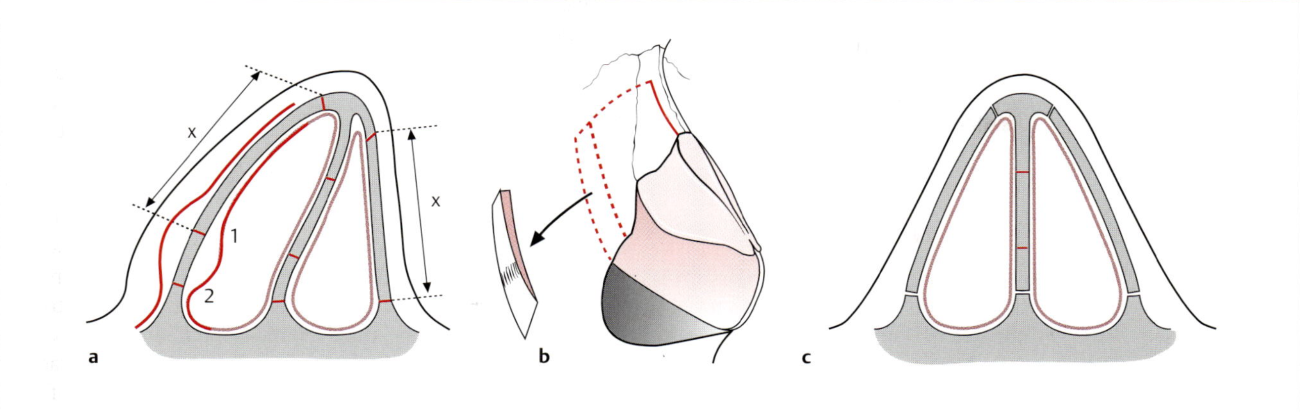

Fig. 6.48a–c Correction of a crooked nose due to disturbances of growth: achievement of symmetry by bony wedge resection.
a The positions of the various osteotomies is depicted. To achieve the same height of the lateral nasal walls, a wedge of bone is removed from the "long" side. For this purpose the medial periosteum must also be elevated and the anterior (1) osteotomy must be performed before the posterior (2) osteotomy.
b Resection of a wedge- or trapeze-shaped strip of bone.
c Appearance after reduction.

aim of the operation in marked cases is to achieve nasal walls of equal height by resection at a suitable site.

With a crooked nose resulting from disturbances of growth combined with a hump deformity, correction can be achieved by an asymmetrical hump reduction (**Fig. 6.47**). For this purpose, when chiselling the hump, the osteotomy cut is made slightly lower on the long side, leaving behind nasal walls of equal length when the hump is removed. The resulting open roof is closed by lateral and transverse osteotomies.

With a correct nasal profile, the bony resection can also be made at the base by means of a wedge resection (**Fig. 6.48**). For this purpose, paramedian osteotomies are made first, followed by a lateral osteotomy on the short side. On the long side, the bony base of the pyramid is tunnelled both laterally and medially in a subperiosteal plane up to the medial canthus. The bone of the pyramid is visualized between the blades of a narrow speculum. Then a strip of bone is mobilized by osteotomies, with the osteotomy nearest the nasal dorsum being cut first. Usually the osteotomies converge at the level of the medial canthus, allowing a wedge of bone to be extracted. After complete mobilization of the pyramid by transverse osteotomies, the infrastructure can be rotated in the midline. Here too, the septum must be mobilized first by chondrotomies and partial resection of the perpendicular plate.

Rules, Tips, and Tricks

The adequate release of the infrastructure from the tethering soft-tissue envelope (release of the asymmetrical muscular pull by the SMAS and the nasal muscles) as well as the complete mobilization of the bony pyramid are both imperative for bringing the crooked nose permanently back into midline. Division of the nasal root plays a special role here. The bony block consisting of the nasal bones and the nasal spine of the frontal bone makes it particularly pronounced. Chiselling through this bony block should be accomplished by a combined approach from both sides. It has proved useful to first initiate the transverse osteotomy from the "long" side and then to complete the separation with a transverse osteotomy from the "short" side. This allows the nasal dorsum to be brought into midline with the final blows of the chisel. If it is not possible to move the pyramid to either side between two fingers without resistance, then there is still a bridge of bone holding it back. If complete mobilization is not successful via an endonasal approach, the surgeon should not shy away from supplementing the transverse osteotomy via a percutaneous approach. In most cases an osteotomy of the perpendicular plate near the nasal bones has to be performed trans-septally from the side contralateral to the deviation of the dorsum. To avoid dislocation of the bone, the septal mucosa should stay attached on the other side.

! Risks and Complications

The possibility of a recurrent crooked nose is very much to the fore. The "memory effect" can be so pronounced that, even after optimal mobilization, a lateral deviation appears once again in the course of weeks or months. Any successful revision surgery is doubtful in these cases, and the indication should be made with due caution. Manual treatment of the nose by the patient (daily pressure against the tendency to deviate) over several weeks and months may be of help as long as the osteotomies have not yet consolidated (nasal manipulation). Defining the suitable pressure point and information for the patient are essential.
Wedge resection in one piece is often not possible. Bony fragments can easily be left behind at the medial canthus and should be removed if possible, as they tend to form sequestra.

Alternatives

Minor asymmetries of the nasal dorsum, which are usually the result of a concavity of one of the sidewalls, may also be "optically" corrected by a suitably tailored cartilaginous graft ("camouflaging"). Via an intercartilaginous incision, a precise pocket is created in the region of the concavity, through which a strip of septal cartilage is inserted. Sculpting of the graft may be facilitated by careful use of the cartilage crusher. The goal is to create symmetrical brow–tip lines.

Saddle-Nose Deformity

The term "saddle" refers to the position of the nasal dorsum. The purely cartilaginous saddle nose is a problem of the nasal septum and is treated by reconstruction of the septum (see **Figs. 6.24** and **6.25**). Only rarely is it an isolated indentation of the nasal dorsum in the presence of a normal nasal-tip projection. In this case a dorsal onlay graft may suffice (**Fig. 6.40e**). A marked saddle nose, on the other hand, is a complex deformity, which is not merely confined to the nasal dorsum, but also involves the nasal tip, nasal base, and columella–upper lip complex. In this case extensive reconstruction is necessary, requiring sufficiently large and stable cartilaginous grafts.

Surgical Principle

Reconstruction of the nasal dorsum alone using a graft or complex reconstruction of the nasal septum, dorsum, nasal base, and tip, possibly supplemented by reconstruction of the maxilla.

Indications

Deformity of the nasal dorsum or deformity of the nasal valve region associated with a complex deformity of the nose and possibly the mid face.

Contraindications

Elevation of the nasal dorsum is only possible with sufficient elasticity of the soft-tissue envelope. This may no longer be guaranteed in the presence of cutaneous scars and contracture secondary to previous surgery.

Specific Points Regarding Informed Consent

The absorption of cartilage grafts is a possibility, as is their dislocation or buckling. This may become conspicuous, particularly in the region of the dorsum. During the operation, it may also become necessary to harvest additional cartilage, e.g., from the auricle or even a rib. With respect to harvesting costal cartilage, it should be pointed out to the patient that, apart from the cutaneous scar, there is also the risk of breaching the pleura as well as the occurrence of postoperative intercostal neuralgia.

Operative Planning

A cartilage graft, inserted via an endonasal approach, is often sufficient for a simple indentation of the nasal dorsum. This presupposes a normal nasal base (**Fig. 6.49a**).

A complex saddle-nose deformity requires correction of all deformed details, which are analyzed preoperatively by an endonasal examination as well as from anterior, lateral, and basal views (**Fig. 6.50**):

- Broad nasal dorsum with irregular brow–tip aesthetic line.
- Possible skin creases covering the medial canthus ("epicanthic folds").
- Wide distance between the alar–facial grooves.
- Nasal dorsal depression.
- Ptotic, broad, or rounded nasal tip.
- Acute nasolabial angle (<90°).
- Short, retracted columella and long upper lip.
- Transverse-oval or round nostrils.
- Increased nasal-valve angle ("ballooning phenomenon").
- Possible hypoplasia of the maxilla and premaxilla, with or without malocclusion.

The presence of teeth deformities (e.g., cross-bite) should prompt orthodontic treatment before reconstruction of the saddle nose.

Special Instruments and Implants

Autogenous cartilage grafts may be harvested from the nasal septum, from the concha of the auricular cartilage, or from a rib. Orthotopic nasal septal cartilage is well suited as graft material in terms of form and stability, but its volume is not sufficient for extensive reconstructions. The elastic auricular cartilage has the disadvantage that straight grafts (septal reconstruction, dorsal onlay graft) can be constructed from it only to a limited extent because conchal cartilage is convex and also has a cartilage ridge originating from the extension of the helical crus (see **Fig. 6.26**). Cartilage scoring is only able to turn it into a flat graft to a limited degree. Costal cartilage provides sufficient cartilaginous material and lends itself well to sculpting. Harvesting it is more demanding, however, and grafts that have been formed by scoring can still warp during the further postoperative course.

Alloplastic implants (silicone, Gore-Tex, and others) have a tendency to become infected and to extrude. Their use should, whenever possible, be restricted to exceptional cases.

Surgical Technique

Correction of a Saddle-Nose Deformity Using a Dorsal Onlay Graft (Fig. 6.49)

A suitable cartilage graft may be harvested from the cartilaginous septum. Its undersurface must correspond exactly to the contour of the osseocartilaginous infrastructure. Cavities between graft and original nasal dorsum will lead to scar contracture and deformity of the graft. The surface of the graft should be flat and the lateral margins boat-shaped. The widest part should correspond to the K-area. Exact sculpting of the graft at the junction between nasal dorsum and lateral nasal wall produces the desired and distinctive brow–tip aesthetic line.

The graft must be inserted exactly in the midline. If only one intercartilaginous incision is made, the pocket formed by degloving will often follow an oblique course and the graft then does not come to lie completely straight once the soft-tissue swelling has receded. It is therefore recommended to make bilateral intercartilaginous incisions, which are then connected

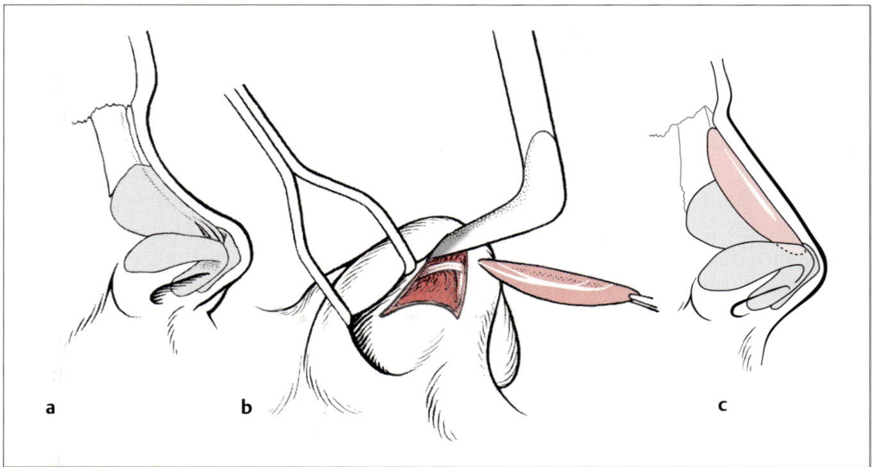

Fig. 6.49a–c Correction of a saddle-nose deformity using a dorsal onlay graft.
a Nasal dorsal depression with a normal position and shape of the nasal tip.
b Insertion of a cartilaginous graft (harvested from the septum, auricle, or elsewhere) via an extended intercartilaginous incision after degloving. The undersurface of the graft must correspond exactly to the supporting surface. It is boat-shaped (narrow at both ends, wider in the middle) and should recreate the brow–tip aesthetic line.
c Well-balanced profile line after positioning of the graft, which should come to lie beneath the lower lateral cartilages in the region of the nasal tip.

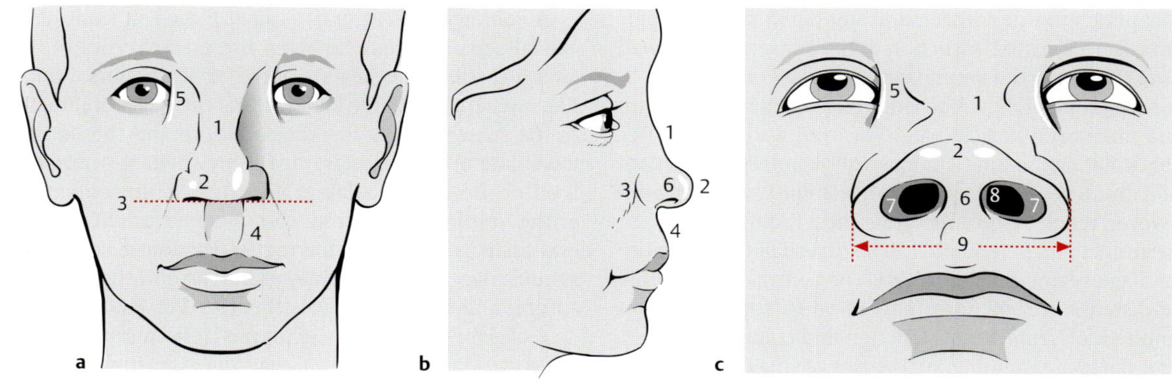

Fig. 6.50a–c Saddle-nose deformity: preoperative analysis.
a Frontal view.
b Profile view.
c Basal view.
1 irregular, broad dorsum with irregular brow-tip aesthetic line
2 irregular, widely separated light reflections over the domes (broad nasal tip)
3 retracted columella (columella and alar–facial grooves are on the same line)
4 “long” upper lip
5 epicanthic folds (the skin fold covers the medial canthus)
6 “short” columella
7 “round” nostrils
8 nasal valve 90° (ballooning)
9 wide nasal base

by an incomplete transfixion. This subsequently provides a wide access to the nasal dorsum and symmetrical degloving is facilitated by the lateral displacement of the lower lateral cartilages. The subperiosteal pocket over the bony nasal dorsum must lie exactly in the midline, otherwise the graft will deviate to the side at the nasal root.

Reconstruction of a Complex Saddle-Nose Deformity (Fig. 6.51)

Because there are numerous individual deformities (**Fig. 6.50**), it is wise to divide the operation into the following steps:

- Reconstruction of the nasal septum and, if necessary, the septal base (premaxillary grafts).
- Augmentation of the nasal dorsum using a graft.
- Reconstruction of the nasal base.

An open approach is best suited for providing good visualization when inserting and symmetrically securing the grafts. A costal cartilage graft is often necessary.

Technique of Harvesting and Sculpting a Costal Cartilage Graft (Fig. 6.52)

After infiltration anesthesia of the skin (for hemostasis), a skin incision about 6 cm long is made along the inferior margin of the pectoralis major muscle (or in the submammary fold of female patients), beginning paramedian to the sternum. Fascia and muscle are divided and the palpable rib (usually the sixth rib) is exposed together with its perichondrium. The costochondral junction is identified laterally (cartilage light yellow/bone dark gray). Next, the perichondrium is incised along the surface of the rib and in line with its course. The incision should just penetrate the surface of the cartilage to allow the full thickness of the perichondrium to be elevated. This longitudinal incision is supplemented by several vertical incisions, thus creating a series of three or four H-shaped perichondrial incisions. The perichondrium is elevated off the cartilage, together with the inserting muscle fibers, with the aid of an elevator (a Henke tonsil elevator is particularly suitable) and dissection is continued in a strictly subperichondrial plane on the surface of the rib, first from above and then from below. Ribs are significantly flatter in their lateral part than medially. Medial and lateral division of the cartilage is best performed with a V-shaped cartilage incision. The notch formed in this way is gradually deepened until only a thin attachment of cartilage remains at a deep level. There is occasionally a synchondrosis with the adjacent caudal rib, which is divided in the same manner. The remaining cartilaginous attachments are easily fractured with the elevator and the cartilage is elevated out of its perichondrial bed. It should measure at least 4–5 cm in length. Careful dissection will leave the medial perichondrium intact, and any significant postoperative pain is very unusual. A suction drain is inserted, followed by repair of the fascia and wound closure in layers.

If the parietal pleura is breached, it can be closed by suture repair and intercostal muscle patch (or even fibrin glue) after adequately inflating the lung. Drainage of the interpleural space is not usually necessary. Intraoperative injury to the pleura does, however, require a postoperative chest radiograph.

All the grafts that are required can be carved out of the entire costal cartilage segment (**Fig. 6.52d**). The central components are largely stable in their form and serve to supply straight grafts required for septal reconstruction and columellar struts. The lateral parts are suitable for the dorsal inlay graft and, if required, for premaxillary grafts.

Three-Step Saddle-nose Reconstruction (Fig. 6.51)

With hypoplasia of the maxilla, reconstruction of the nose begins with the insertion of premaxillary grafts, which form the basis for reconstruction of the septum. For this purpose, subperiosteal pockets are created at the lower margin of the piriform aperture, on either side of the anterior nasal spine, which is often only rudimentarily preformed, and extended beneath the alar–facial grooves. Two appropriately sculpted grafts are inserted into these pockets. They displace the soft tissues anteriorly and thus support correction of the retracted columella.

Reconstruction of the cartilaginous nasal septum corresponds to the procedure for total reconstruction of the septum (see **Fig. 6.25**). Nasal dorsum, nasal base, and nasal tip can now be reconstructed around this newly created foundation. The nasal dorsal onlay graft, sculpted into a boat shape, is provided at its caudal end with a small notch that will later accommodate the columellar strut. A subperiosteal pocket, dissected exactly in the midline in the region of the nasal root, prevents any lateral displacement of the graft. The bone graft can be secured to the upper lateral cartilages over the cartilaginous nasal dorsum with a deep absorbable suture. This stitch not only prevents lateral displacement of the graft, but also prevents it from migrating caudally. In addition to the reconstruction of the correct level of the nasal dorsum with respect to the brow–tip aesthetic lines, the main aim of the dorsal onlay graft is the reconstruction or maintenance of adequate nasal length.

A columellar strut graft is now placed in front of the new caudal septal margin, between the medial crura of the lower lateral cartilages. It bears a notch to fit the dorsal onlay graft. The medial crura of the lower lateral cartilages are then secured to the strut with an absorbable suture and the domes of the lower lateral cartilages are clearly elevated (3–4 mm) above the level of the dorsal onlay graft. After circumscribed elevation of the vestibular skin from the undersurface of the lower lateral cartilages in the dome region, the lower lateral cartilages should cover the dorsal onlay graft. The domes are shaped with sutures and secured to each other (see **Fig. 6.60**).

A perioperative course of prophylactic antibiotics is advised, given the extensive amount of cartilage grafting.

Rules, Tips, and Tricks

If the soft-tissue envelope is poorly vascularized and contracted by scars, then overgenerous elevation may lead to skin necrosis. To expand the skin and to assess its resilience, it is recommended to insert a thick strip of sponge, or something similar, beneath the nasal dorsum immediately after degloving and to check perfusion at regular intervals during the further course of the operation. Sculpted costal cartilage grafts tend to buckle, especially if they

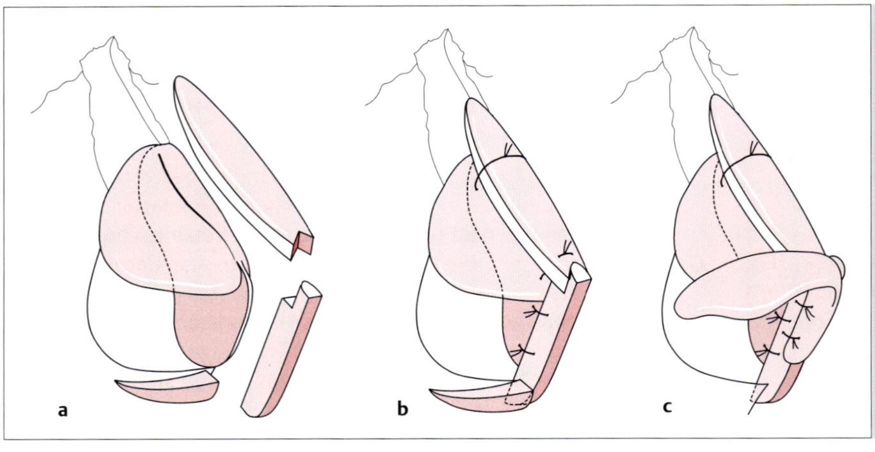

Fig. 6.51a–c Saddle-nose reconstruction after septal reconstruction: total reconstruction of the infrastructure.
a Grafts for the maxilla, nasal dorsum, and columella.
b Grafts in position and secured with sutures.
c Lower lateral cartilages secured to the columellar strut, dorsal onlay graft inserted "beneath" the lower lateral cartilages.

are taken from the cartilaginous parts of the costal surface. For this reason, entire costal cartilaginous segments should be harvested to obtain grafts from the medial cartilaginous parts with as stable a form as possible. Buckling is not entirely ruled out even then, but it usually occurs during the first 30 minutes after dissection and does not advance any further after that. The sculpting of the costal cartilage grafts should therefore be done immediately after harvesting, and they should then be put aside in saline solution. If buckling has occurred before insertion, then the graft should be re-sculpted. The following should be borne in mind:

Rules, Tips, and Tricks

Cartilage bends away from the cut surface. This rule should be kept in mind if additional cartilage is removed with the scalpel.

With marked hypoplasia of the cartilaginous nose and maxilla (nasomaxillary dysplasia, Binder syndrome), the lack of soft tissue may considerably hinder adequate elevation of the nasal tip and nasal dorsum. It is therefore preferable to aim for a suboptimal result for the sake of avoiding skin necrosis of the nasal dorsum and columella.

With a low radix, epicanthic folds result from the excess skin in the region of the medial canthus. They normally disappear after insertion of the dorsal onlay graft. Direct procedures to the skin in the form of Z-plasties or the like should be avoided.

A saddle-nose deformity will often make the bony pyramid appear wide. Narrowing by osteotomies should be avoided if possible, however, because the inserted grafts exert considerable pressure from above and could possibly push the mobilized bony walls apart again. If at all necessary, osteotomies should be done in a second operation after 6 months (e.g., percutaneously).

Optimal preparation of the nasal dorsum is decisive for an uneventful healing of a dorsal onlay graft. Removal of irregularities is necessary to ensure a smooth surface for the graft.

Any residual elevations of the nasal dorsum may result in the dorsal onlay graft being tilted down like a seesaw, particularly in the nasal tip area, and its cephalic end lifted up to appear as a palpable step-off at the nasal root. This can be avoided by ensuring an exact fit of the upper surface of the nasal dorsum and the undersurface of the dorsal onlay graft, together with a stable caudal support for the graft.

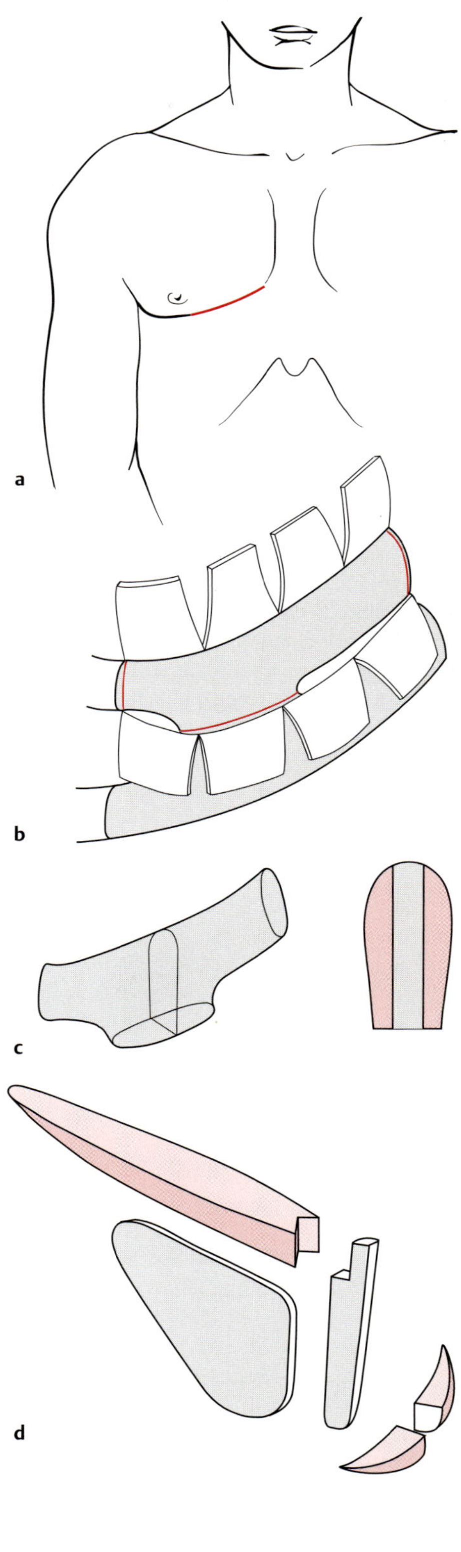

Fig. 6.52a–d Harvesting and sculpting the costal cartilage graft.
a Medial approach along the inferior margin of pectoralis major.
b H-shaped incisions of the perichondrium of the 6th rib and exposure of the cartilage. Medial and lateral chondrotomies and division of a synchondrosis with the 7th rib are marked.
c Removal of a complete segment (cross-section shown). Removal of the outer surfaces (red) leaves behind a central "well-balanced" graft (gray).
d The required cartilaginous graft is sculpted from the three segments. Septal and columellar grafts are taken from the central parts of the cartilage.

Narrowing of the nasal base by resection of skin from the floor of the vestibule is necessary only in extremely rare and exceptional cases. On the contrary, this skin and parts of the "long upper lip" are required to compensate for the absent length of the columella. Premature resection of skin from the alar–facial grooves may therefore put the entire operative result at risk.

! Risks and Complications

Postoperative buckling of the cartilage grafts can be prevented by taking into account the measures mentioned above. Any prominences of the graft at the root of the nose can be corrected by removal with a scalpel through an endonasal approach 6 months after surgery at the earliest. This also applies for minor irregularities of the dorsal onlay graft. Significant distortions necessitate its complete replacement, however, if necessary with renewed harvesting of further costal cartilage via the original chest incision. If skin necroses are impending over the nasal dorsum and columella, the inserted graft will have to be removed to take tension off the skin. The immediate replacement of the graft, reduced in size, is possible.

Transeptal absorbable mattress sutures are required to stabilize the septal graft and the columellar strut. These should not be placed too close together, to avoid skin and mucosal necrosis. Should circumscribed necroses still develop, however, then healing by secondary intention should be awaited while ensuring regular coverage of the wound with ointment. Given that the grafts are autologous cartilage grafts, they usually become covered with tissue in the course of secondary healing and thus survive. Any foreign material that becomes exposed in the course of wound-healing problems, however, inevitably leads to further tissue necrosis and will be rejected.

Postoperative Care

Since osteotomies are not usually performed, a plaster dressing applied in layers with additional pressure over the supratip area is sufficient. Provided the course is uneventful, no specific form of postoperative care is required.

Nasal Tip and Nasal Base

Preoperative Analysis (Fig. 6.53)

From an aesthetic point of view, the nasal tip forms the end of the brow–tip lines when viewed from the front. It appears aesthetically acceptable when the domes are well formed and close together (recognizable by the light reflections). In profile, tip projection should slightly exceed the level of the nasal dorsum ("supratip break"). The columella should lie caudal to the alar–facial junction.

With thin skin, the form of the nasal tip is determined by the angle between the lateral and medial crura of the lower lateral cartilages in the domal region, as well as by their distance apart. The domes of a bulbous nose with its round broad tip do not have an acute angle and are wide apart.

Important terms and definitions for analyzing the nasal base are nasal tip projection and nasal tip protection. Nasal tip projection is determined by the nasofacial angle (see **Fig. 6.39**). Roughly speaking, it corresponds to one-half of the nasal length (**Fig. 6.53c**). Actual nasal length represents the distance between nasal root and nasal tip. Rotation of the nasal tip upward shortens nasal length, at the same time enlarging the nasolabial angle (see **Fig. 6.57**). Nasal tip protection refers to the stability of the position of the nasal tip under external pressure and is

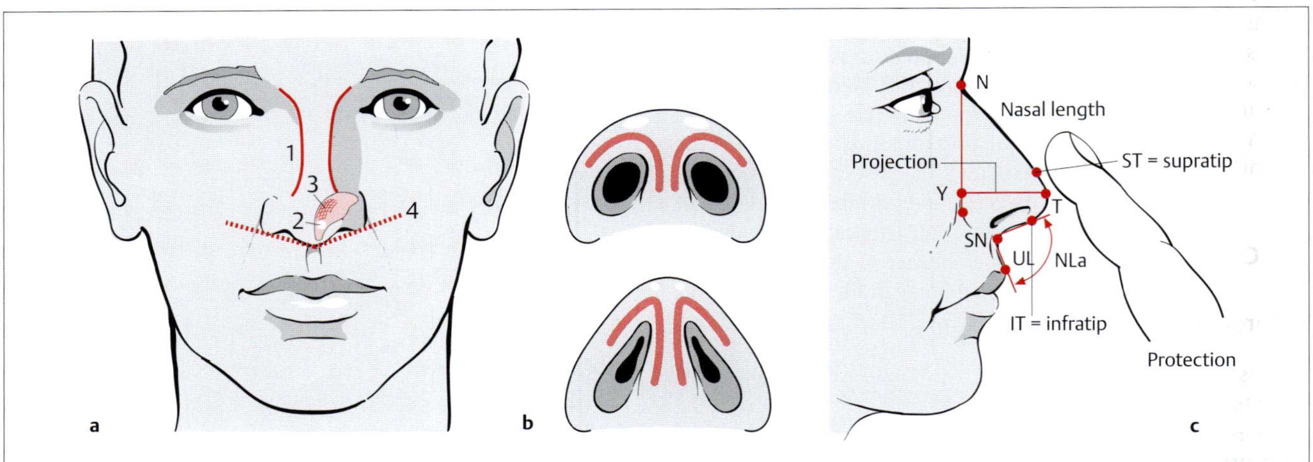

Fig. 6.53a–c Preoperative analysis for nasal tip and nasal base corrections.

a Frontal view.
1 brow–tip aesthetic line: interruption in the contour?
2 nasal tip: domes recognizable from the light reflections? Distance?
3 supratip region: fullness of the upper lateral cartilage?
4 nasal base: V-shaped contour?

b Basal view. Lower (normal situation): acute-angled dome with defined light reflections of the skin; short distance: Upper (broad tip): ptotic tip with increased dome angle and correspondingly widened light reflections at a wider distance; broad base, short columella, round nostrils.

c Profile view. Assessment of projection (distance Y–T) and protection of the nasal tip; projection Y–T/nose length N–T = ½. Nose length and nasolabial angle NLa. Double break (angulation) of the infratip region (IT) and supratip break (depression) of the supratip region (ST).

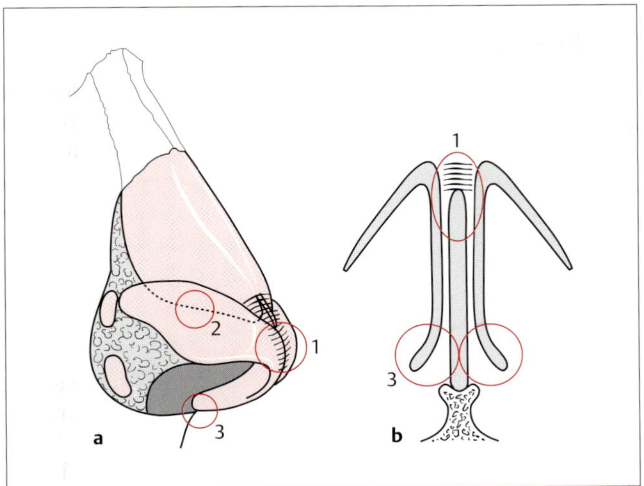

Fig. 6.54a, b Protection of the nasal tip.
a Oblique view.
b Basal view.
1 fibrous tissue between the domes around the anterior inferior septum corner
2 lateral connection between upper and lower lateral cartilages
3 junction between medial crura of the lower lateral cartilages and caudal septal margin

usually provided by the nasal septum (**Fig. 6.54**). The septum supports the fibrous tissue between the domes from below and this represents the major suspension mechanism of the lower lateral cartilages. Further fixation points for the lower lateral cartilages are the connection of the lateral crura with the upper lateral cartilages and the connection of the medial crura with the caudal septum. The latter two anchorages are detached by hemitransfixion or transfixion and by intercartilaginous incisions, with the possibility of the fibrous tissue between the domes slipping over the anterior inferior septal corner, and coming to lie anterior to the caudal septal margin. This mechanism plays a major role in the development of a polly beak deformity (see **Fig. 6.42**).

Correction of Nasal-Tip Projection

Surgical Principles

In case of moderate overprojection, detachment of the fixation points of the lower lateral cartilages. Cartilage resection at the domes and at the superior septal margin to correct significant overprojection of the dome. Insertion of a cartilage strut and dome sutures for underprojection.

Indications

Overprojection of a tension nose with vestibular stenosis. Underprojection of a saddle-nose deformity or nasomaxillary dysplasia with a short columella.

Contraindications

No division of the cartilage at the dome should be undertaken in the presence of extremely thin nasal tip skin or skin atrophy secondary to previous surgery, otherwise there is a risk of creating visible cartilage edges.

Enhancement of projection by insertion of a columellar strut via an external approach in the presence of a short columella: danger of skin necrosis if the columellar suture is under tension.

Specific Points Regarding Informed Consent

A relative excess of soft tissue after lowering the nasal tip can temporarily result in a mild swelling of the nasal tip, but this usually settles after 6 months. Cartilage sutures in the dome may result in asymmetries and visible step-offs. Similar deformities can also arise after elevation of the tip of the nose.

Operative planning

If there is only mild overprojection of the tip, then the approach to the nasal dorsum itself can lead to lowering of the tip by ca. 2 mm during the wound-healing phase as a result of the transfixion and intercartilaginous incisions. If there are very strong cartilages and obvious overprojection, however, then this effect is not usually enough and cartilage resections are necessary. The implanted cartilaginous frame needs to be stable to increase projection and should usually be harvested from the nasal septum. If a sufficient amount of cartilage is no longer available there, then an auricular sandwich graft is an option. An endonasal approach with delivery of the lower lateral cartilages is possible in principle (see **Fig. 6.61**), but symmetrical operating is more likely to be guaranteed by an open approach.

Surgical Technique

Dome resection for *over*projection (**Fig. 6.55**) can be accomplished by delivery of the lower lateral cartilages as well as by using an open approach. After removing a strip of cartilage from the nasal dorsum (septum and parts of the upper lateral cartilages), a roof-shaped segment is resected from the medial and lateral crura, with inclusion of the dome and preservation of the vestibular skin. The stumps of the medial crura of the lower lateral cartilages may be stabilized with a columellar strut. The level of the trimmed edge will determine the new nasal tip projection. The lateral crura of the lower lateral cartilages are now adapted to the medial crura with an absorbable suture (5/0) to prevent the development of any step-offs.

For *under*projection (**Fig. 6.56**), a cartilage graft, which may initially be overlong, is inserted into a pocket created between the medial crura of the lower lateral cartilages. The medial crura are then secured in a stepwise manner from below upward. The rounded domes are formed using a nonabsorbable, U-shaped, transdomal suture, ensuring that the knot comes to lie medially. The fibrous connection between the domes, which had been previously released, is repaired with an interdomal, nonabsorbable suture.

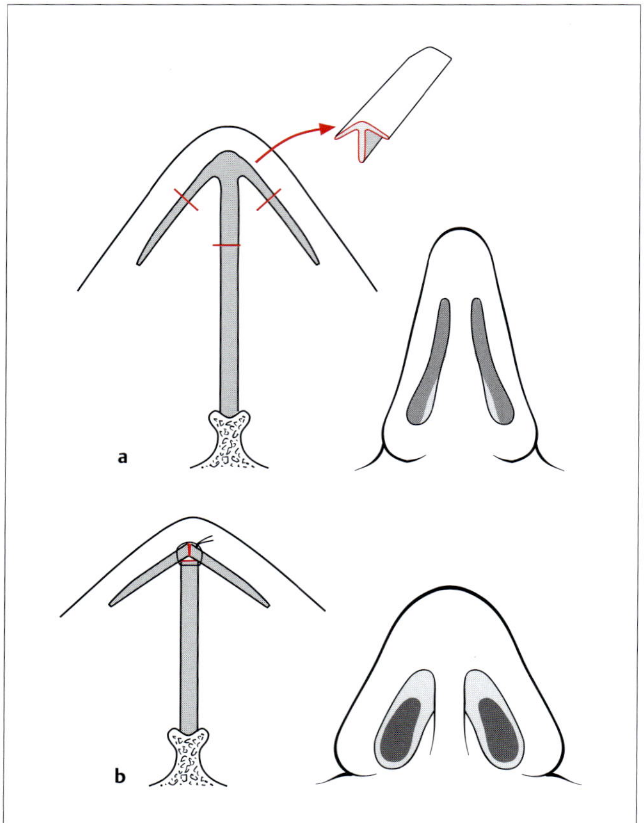

Fig. 6.55a, b Correction of an overprojection of the nasal tip.
a Resection of the dome and dorsum.
b Normalization of the nasal base after reconstruction of the domes by suturing; widening of the nasal valve angle.

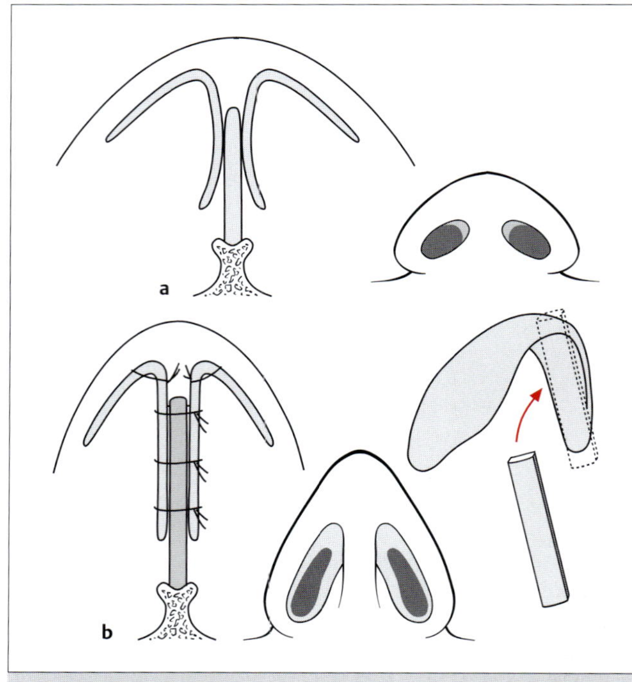

Fig. 6.56a, b Correction of an underprojection of the nasal tip.
a Preoperative situation: loss of the supportive function by an "overly short" caudal septal margin.
b New nasal tip support with the aid of a columellar strut, independent of the nasal septum. Refinement of the domes using "transdomal sutures."

Rules, Tips, and Tricks

When employing an endonasal approach with exposure of the lower lateral cartilages using the delivery technique, both domes are best delivered out of one nostril to form the domes exactly, both for overprojection and for underprojection. This procedure requires experience, otherwise asymmetries can easily arise from the lateral displacement of the lower lateral cartilages. Marginal incisions and intercartilaginous incisions required for delivery should therefore be made as long as possible to achieve enough freedom of movement.

! Risks and Complications

Suture fistulae resulting from nonabsorbable monofilament stitches for the lower lateral cartilages are extremely rare, especially if the knots are buried medially in the depths. If they do occur, however, then the sutures must be removed. Skin excision from the columella for excess tip projection after using an open approach is an absolute exception. Any redundant skin will shrink during the healing phase.

Correction of Nasal Length

Surgical Principle

Rotation of the nasal tip. A stepwise approach should be adopted to avoid over-rotation.

Indications

Ptotic nasal tip (e.g., due to aging) or a nose that has become relatively too long after hump reduction in the presence of a nasolabial angle of less than 100°.

Contraindications

An existing nasolabial angle of 110° or greater.

Specific Points Regarding Informed Consent

With inadequate stability of the tissue, the nasal tip may droop again. Ptosis may, however, be simulated if the base of the columella retracts after rhinoplasty.

Operative Planning

Rotation of the nasal tip always also results in a change in the position of the long axis of the nostril rim. A rotation should therefore only be done if the nasolabial angle is less than 110°.

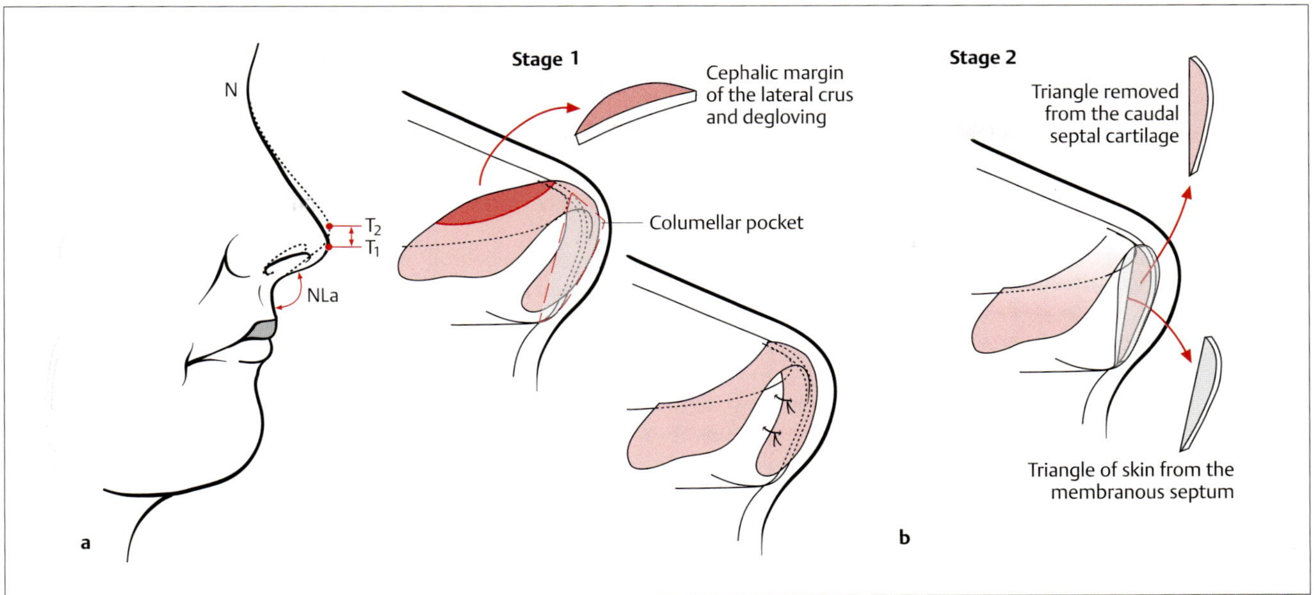

Fig. 6.57a, b Rotation of the nasal tip (multistage concept).
a Operative goal: to shorten nasal length and increase the nasolabial angle NLa by rotating the tip from T_1 to T_2.
Stage 1: columellar pocket is developed in the anterior region to accommodate the anterior inferior septal corner; degloving and resection of the cephalic margin of the lateral crus of the lower lateral cartilage; rotation achieved with septocolumellar sutures.
b *Stage 2:* triangular resection of cartilage from the caudal septum with/without resection of excess vestibular skin.

Otherwise over-rotation of the tip will result, with the subsequent formation of a short nose. When assessing the nasolabial angle, it should be kept in mind that this depends not only on the position of the nasal tip, but also on the position of the columellar base. A retracted columella is associated with a reduction of the nasolabial angle, even if the nose is not too long. Increasing the angle by rotating the tip would be contraindicated in this case; on the contrary, it is the columella retraction that needs to be addressed (see **Fig. 6.58**).

Surgical Technique (Fig. 6.57)

Since resections of cartilage and skin cannot be reversed, a stepwise approach to address the rotation is recommended.

- Transfixion, bilateral intercartilaginous incisions, and the creation of a columella pocket: Transfixion and intercartilaginous incisions separate the lower lateral cartilages from the rest of the pyramid and allow them to be moved in relation to it. A columellar pocket created between the medial crura of the lower lateral cartilages up to the level of the upper nostril rims allows rotation of the tip after the caudal septum has been inserted into the columellar pocket. This technique achieves shortening of the nasal length by 2–3 mm, which is quite adequate in many cases. After resection of the triangle of excess skin from the membranous septum produced by the rotation, the medial crura of the lower lateral cartilages and the caudal septal margin can be anchored together with deep mattress sutures. The connection between the lower lateral cartilages and the upper lateral cartilages may block the rotation movement, so a circumscribed resection of cartilage from the cephalic end of the lower lateral cartilage with degloving of the skin over the dorsum is very helpful.
- Only if the rotation using this technique is still not sufficient, then an additional resection of a triangular piece of cartilage from the caudal septal margin, with the base of the triangle in the direction of the nasal tip, should be considered. But resection here should be approached very conservatively to avoid producing too much rotation and a blunting of the infratip region (between the nasal tip and the upper nostril rims).
- Rotation is facilitated and maximally augmented if an additional triangular segment of cartilage is resected from the lateral crura and the cephalic gap thus created in the cartilage is re-approximated with a suture. With this relatively aggressive approach, a circumscribed resection of excess skin from the membranous septum is also necessary.

Rules, Tips, and Tricks

A stepwise approach is imperative for successful rotation of the tip and reduction of nasal length. Only real excesses of the membranous septum should be resected; if in doubt, then "less is more." Triangular resection from the lower lateral cartilages is reserved for exceptional cases and should only be considered as an additional measure after completing the other operative steps. Degloving is part of the rotation, even if no further surgery to the nasal dorsum is required. Without degloving, the skin of the supratip region would bunch up, which then tends to push the nasal tip back down again.

Risks and Complications

The main risk is excessive shortening by resections due to inadequate preoperative planning. Excessive shortening of the nose is one of the most common reasons for patients bringing law suits, and is difficult to correct surgically.

Retracted Columella

Surgical Principle

Caudal displacement of the columella by inserting a cartilaginous graft in front of the caudal septal margin (caudal septal extension graft).

Indications

The retracted columella decreases the nasolabial angle (<90°) and creates the impression of a ptotic nasal tip. The soft tissue at the ends of the medial crura of the lower lateral cartilages is no longer under tension; the footplates of the medial crurae diverge. The result is a wide columella base with reduced distance to the alae (**Fig. 6.58a**). The increased airflow during inspiration can result in increased negative pressure at this narrow point, sucking in the alae at the columella (alar collapse). In this case, the columella should not be narrowed by resection of fibrous tissue between the medial crura and re-approximated with a suture, as this would not eliminate the retraction. On the contrary, the columellar base is displaced caudally by a cartilaginous graft and the tissue is thus once more placed under tension.

Surgical Technique (Fig. 6.58b)

After hemitransfixion, a cartilage strut is harvested from the nasal septum and a not too deep columellar pocket is created. The cartilage strut is now inserted into this columellar pocket with two guide sutures. The lower of these two sutures is the important one, exiting through the columellar skin exactly at the deepest point of the columella retraction (see **Fig. 6.24b**). The two guide sutures are now held exactly, so that the columella is placed in the desired position. If the cartilaginous graft in the columella is large enough, it will now slightly overlap the caudal septal margin. This excess is removed precisely with the scalpel to bring the extension graft and the septum edge to edge. The ends of the cartilage are then secured to each other with a figure-of-eight absorbable suture. To avoid suturing under tension, incomplete septal tunnels should be created to allow the membranous septum to be more easily displaced caudally.

Rules, Tips, and Tricks

The extension graft is usually placed so that it lies caudal to the nasal spine to achieve a satisfactory effect. To avoid retraction back into the created septal tunnels, they should be well closed with bunching absorbable mattress sutures. It may be very helpful to suture in septal splints for 4–5 days to stabilize the cartilaginous construction.

Correction of the Form of the Nasal Tip

Successful correction of the nasal tip presupposes that an exact distinction is made as to which type of deformity is present (**Figs. 6.59** and **6.60**):

- Wide lateral crurae (widening of the supratip region, **Fig. 6.59a**) → cephalic lateral crura trimming.
- Bulbous nasal tip (blunt alar cartilage domes, **Fig. 6.60a**) → transdomal sutures.
- Broad nasal tip (increased interdomal distance, **Fig. 6.60b**) → interdomal sutures.

A combination of these three alterations to the lower lateral cartilages may be necessary, depending on the presenting deformity, and may be accomplished by an endonasal approach (delivery technique) or via an external approach.

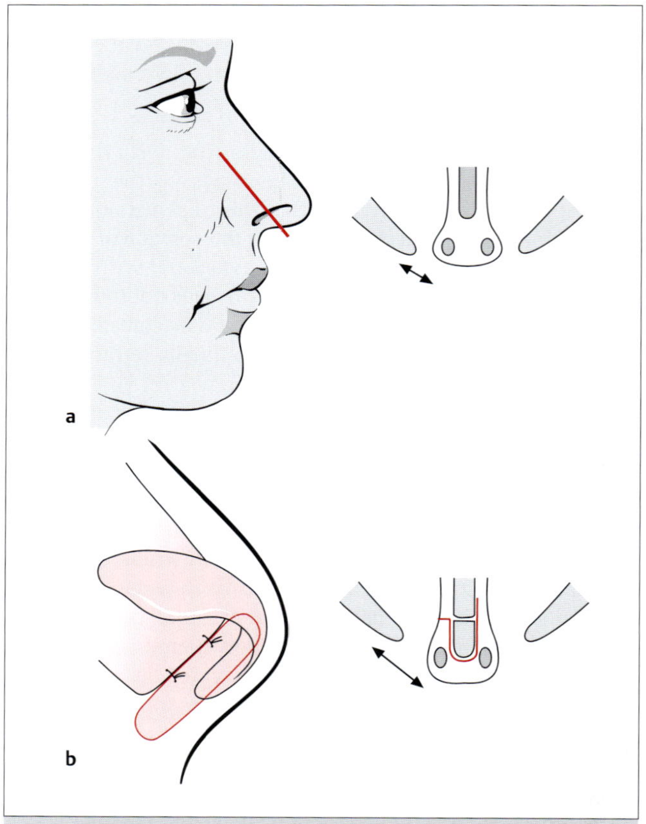

Fig. 6.58a, b Correction of a retracted columella.
a Retracted and wide columellar base with a narrow nasolabial angle and vestibular stenosis (double arrow: short distance between alar–facial groove and columella, risk of alar collapse; red line: cross-section).
b Caudal displacement of the columella with the aid of a graft: widening of the vestibulum (double arrow) and narrowing of the columellar base.

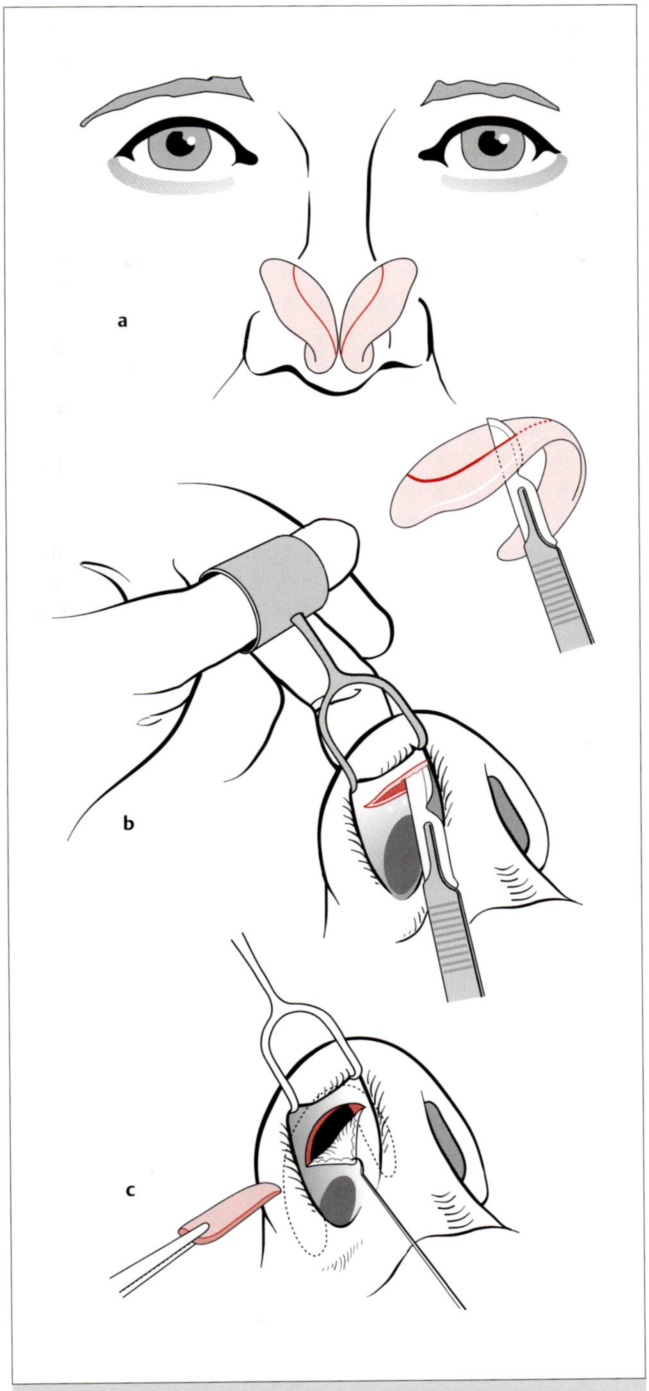

Fig. 6.59a–c Nasal tip correction: broad supratip region.
a The distance between the domes is normal, only the supratip region is prominent as a result of wide lateral crura of the footplates of the medial crurae. The cartilage incision has been marked and is made from an endonasal approach.
b Endonasal transcartilaginous approach: the vestibular skin is everted with the aid of a ring elevator, the external skin is protected by the middle finger; the incision divides skin first, then cartilage.
c The cephalic part of the cartilage is removed, together with the attached subcutaneous fibrous tissue of the external skin, leaving behind a stable caudal strip of cartilage. The vestibular skin is preserved; it is approximated with a suture.

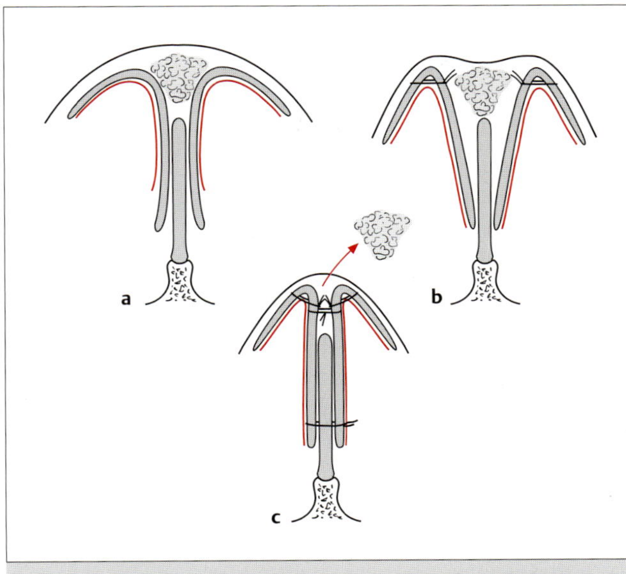

Fig. 6.60a–c Nasal tip correction: form of the domes and distance between them.
a Round, broad tip resulting from undefined domes with a wide distance; the gap is filled with fibrous and fatty tissue.
b Transdomal sutures to lend the domes form and definition (light reflections); the knots of the U-stitches come to lie medially.
c After resection of the fibrous tissue, an interdomal suture in placed to narrow the tips; the columellar base is narrowed by a suture.

Surgical Principle

Narrowing of the lower lateral cartilages by resection of a cephalic strip of cartilage, definition and approximation of the domes by suturing.

Specific Points Regarding Informed Consent

Asymmetries, irregularities. Only a limited narrowing effect is achieved with thick skin that is rich in sebaceous glands.

Operative Planning

Assessment of the widening at the supratip region, mainly by palpation. Assessment of the form of the domes and their distance apart with the aid of the light reflections.

Surgical Technique

If the domes are well defined and are situated close together, cephalic trimming of the lateral crura alone may suffice for broadness of the tip in the *supratip region*. This is done via an endonasal approach using a *transcartilaginous* incision (**Fig. 6.59b, c**): The vestibular skin is infiltrated with local anesthetic on the undersurface of the lower lateral cartilages to detach them more gently. The very thin skin is incised at the level of the desired cartilage resection site, beginning laterally and extending as far as the dome region; the underlying cartilage is not yet divided, however. The skin is then elevated off the cartilage with fine pointed scissors and the junction with the upper lateral cartilage identified. The stability of the remaining cartilage is important for the amount of cartilage resection. The intended cartilage incision and the amount of resection can either be estimated by palpation or marked with needles inserted from the outside. Next, the cartilage is incised and resected, together with the overlying subcutaneous fibrous tissue. The incision of the vestibular skin is re-approximated with an absorbable suture.

Surgery to the domes is performed via an external or an endonasal approach (**Figs. 6.60** and **6.61**). The external approach allows good exposure of the lower lateral cartilages. Cephalic excisions are done under direct vision. Here stability of the remaining cartilaginous struts is more readily assessed than with the transcartilaginous approach. It is usually necessary to excise the fibrous tissue between the domes to bring wide domes together. Dome angles are created using monofilament, nonabsorbable U-shaped sutures 5/0 (*trans*domal sutures). They are then secured together with *inter*domal sutures. These sutures must strictly lie beneath the vestibular skin, otherwise suture fistulas will develop.

Rules, Tips, and Tricks

The question repeatedly arises as to how much cartilage from the lateral crus may be removed without putting stability at risk. But how much has been removed is not important; rather, one should ask: *What is left of the lower lateral cartilages?* A remaining cartilaginous frame 2–3 mm wide with a very strong cartilage may suffice to guarantee enough stability for the vestibule. Very thin cartilage will require correspondingly more conservative resections.
The transdomal sutures should not pass too far laterally through the cartilage, otherwise they may cause buckling of the lower lateral cartilage and thus give the nasal tip a "pinched" look. The interdomal sutures should also not achieve a maximal approximation of the newly formed domes, but rather leave a gap of ca. 2 mm, which will result in natural, separated light reflections on the skin of the nasal tip.

! Risks and Complications

Corrective surgery of the lower lateral cartilages is only noticeable externally if the skin envelope is thin enough. Thick skin with abundant sebaceous glands is poorly adaptable to cartilage reduction. The skin can only be thinned out in the region of the subcutaneous fibrous tissue, which is found mainly in the supratip region. Any further thinning of the skin at the level of the dermis only leads to skin atrophy and livid discoloration, which should be avoided.

Alternatives

Narrowing and reshaping of the lower lateral cartilages may also be done via an endonasal approach. For this purpose, the lower lateral cartilages are delivered out of the nostrils (the so-called "delivery technique"; **Fig. 6.61**). Marginal incisions and intercartilaginous incisions, joined together by a transfixion, are required for this. After elevation of the skin envelope and detachment of the fibrous tissue between the medial crura and the domes, the lower lateral cartilages and the vestibular skin are delivered out of the respective nostril as medial and lateral bipedicled flaps and the domes supported with an instrument. This technique allows both resection at the cephalic segment and reshaping of the domes with transdomal sutures to be achieved under direct vision. Placing the interdomal su-

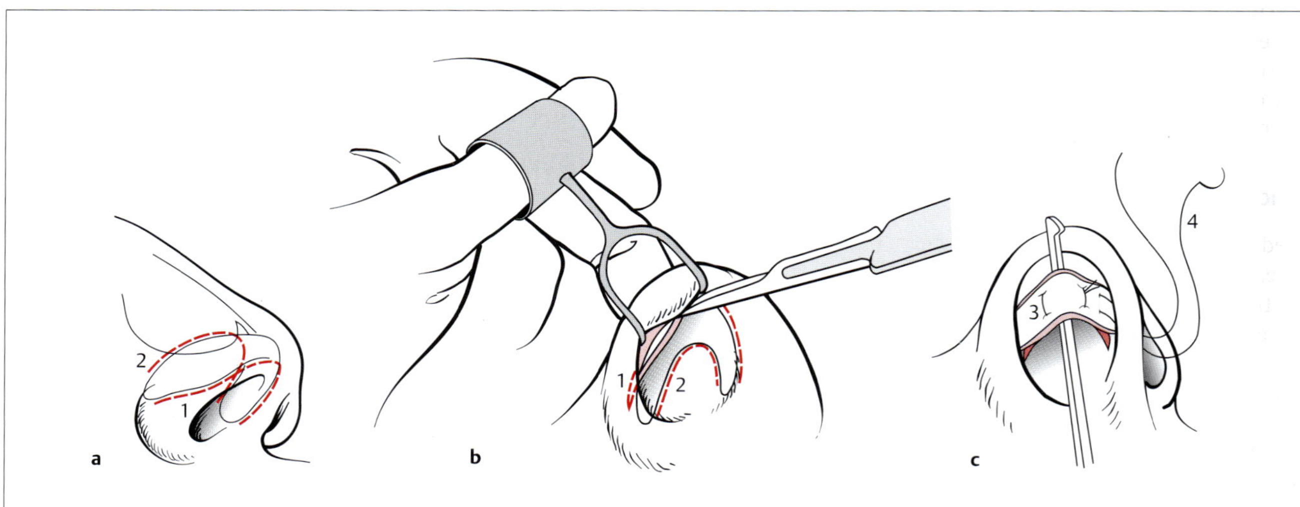

Fig. 6.61a–c Domal sutures after delivery of the lower lateral cartilages.
a Endonasal incisions.
1 caudal marginal incision
2 intercartilaginous incision
b Endonasal incision after eversion of the vestibular skin with the ring elevator; the "soft triangle" (corresponding to the position of the No. 15 scalpel blade) must be preserved.
c The chondrocutaneous bipedicled flap is delivered out of the nostril and supported with an elevator. The dome is formed with a transdomal suture (3) and an interdomal suture is placed (4).

ture is slightly more difficult and is done either after delivering both domes out of one nostril or with a suture, which is placed separately for each nostril through the medial crus of the lower lateral cartilage, medial to the dome, and then knotted "blind." Because all anchorage points of the lower lateral cartilages are detached with the delivery technique, the additional insertion of a columellar strut may be very useful in preventing later drooping of the nasal tip.

Symmetrical work on the lower lateral cartilages is difficult using the delivery technique and requires experience.

Correction of Alar Collapse

The nasal vestibule is the space between the nostril margin and the nasal valve area. It is tent-shaped and consists of a medial wall (columella and membranous as well as caudal septum), lateral wall (lateral crus of the lower lateral cartilage and connective tissue, filling the "empty triangle" at the piriform aperture), and floor (soft tissue between nostril margin and piriform crest). The lower lateral cartilages, with their tension in the dome area, are the main stabilizers of these walls, together with the attaching nasal muscles and their corresponding fibrous bands. Collapse of the nasal vestibule from negative pressure during inspiration occurs in particular when the distance between medial and lateral wall is too short (tension nose, retracted and broad columella, dislocation of the caudal septal margin), the ala is too soft or protruding medially, or the vestibular floor is elevated by scar webbing. Tension nose, septum deviation, and broad columella require correction using the techniques already described. Here, stabilization of the lateral wall of the vestibule is described.

Surgical Principle

The weak and medially convex or protruding lateral crura of the lower lateral cartilages are supported from below by a stable cartilaginous frame. This cartilaginous frame is supported on both ends like a bridge on firm riverbanks: laterally on the bony aperture and medially on the superior septal margin.

Indications

Medial convexity of the lateral crus of the lower lateral cartilage, especially at its distal part with approximation to the nasal septum. Significant collapse of the nostril during *normal* (not forced) inspiration.

Contraindications

Collapse only during strong inspiration (which happens to almost everyone and is physiological in the widest sense).

Specific Points Regarding Informed Consent

Usually there is already a noticeable depression of the lateral aspect of the ala, which is corrected by cartilage stabilization and thus "normalized." Occasionally, however, the placement of the cartilaginous graft on the piriform aperture may produce a slight swelling there.

Surgical Technique (Fig. 6.62)

Cartilage grafting may be done via an endonasal approach. The vestibular skin is infiltrated with a local anesthetic to facilitate dissection. A marginal incision is then made and extended beyond the dome to connect medially as an incomplete transfixion incision. Then the vestibular skin is elevated off the undersurface of the lower lateral cartilages. The anterior inferior septal corner, the caudal end of the upper lateral cartilage and, laterally, the piriform aperture are identified. The bend in the lateral crus of the lower lateral cartilage should now be quite recognizable and correctable by pressure with an instrument in a lateral direction. A cartilaginous frame from the nasal septum, with a width of ca. 4 mm, should be long enough to bridge the gap between piriform aperture and caudal superior septal margin. These two fixation points represent the stable supports for the "bridge construction."

At first, one end of the cartilaginous graft is inserted into a small periosteal pocket lateral to the piriform aperture, where it is secured with an absorbable suture from an endonasal access. The medial fixation of the graft is then placed under mild tension, bending it outward where the upper lateral cartilage is attached to the septum. The graft thus pushes the lateral crus laterally from below, causing the latter to bend slightly outward in a convex fashion. The vestibular incision is then suture-repaired and the vestibulum loosely packed for 1–2 days.

Rules, Tips, and Tricks

Instead of a septal cartilage graft, a convex concha cartilage from the auricle can in principle be used. However, it is less stable, which is why preference is given to septal cartilage.

! Risks and Complications

The cartilage should not be placed under so much tension that it breaks. Nor should it be too thick, since its volume might otherwise negate any widening of the vestibule gained.

Alternatives

If the deformed lateral crus of the lower lateral cartilage is sufficiently stable, then it may be divided 1–2 mm lateral to the dome, turned 180° around its longitudinal axis and sewn back to the dome with an overlap. This will maintain tension in the dome as well as transforming the medial convexity into a lateral convexity. For this to succeed, however, it is necessary to completely separate the vestibular skin from the lateral crus of the lower lateral cartilage as well as to secure it after this upside-down technique using deep mattress sutures. This approach will produce a slight widening in the region of the dome.

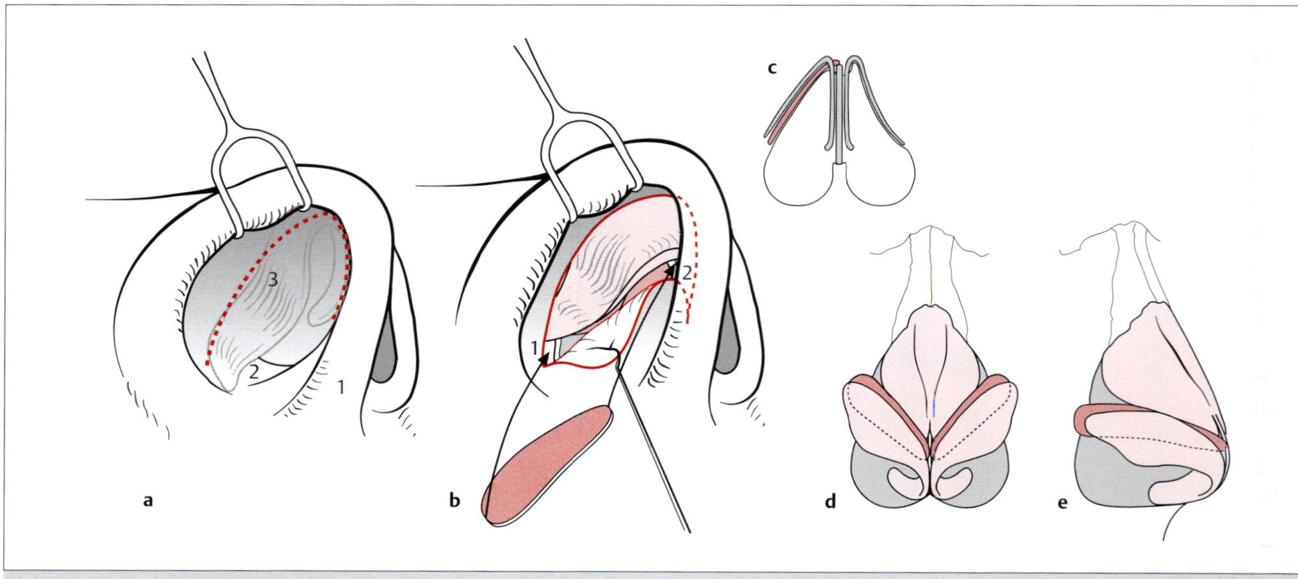

Fig. 6.62a–e Correction of collapsing nasal alae by insertion of a cartilaginous support.

a Analysis of the three walls of the vestibulum.
1 columella and caudal septum
2 vestibular floor
3 ala

This case presents a stenosis due to medial convexity of the lateral crus of the lower lateral cartilage.

b Incision of the vestibular skin caudal to the strongest convexity and elevation of the undersurface of the lower lateral cartilage. The supporting surfaces for the cartilaginous grafts are demonstrated:
1 lateral surface of the piriform aperture
2 anterior inferior corner of the septum

c The principle of converting convexity into concavity by insertion of the underlying cartilaginous graft.

d, e Position of the cartilaginous grafts with medial and lateral support.

Malformations

Nasal Fistulas and Cysts

With these congenital malformations, the fistula opening lies in the midline, usually in the region of the nasal dorsum, but also occasionally on the nasal tip or even at the columella. The fistula tract runs along the upper lateral cartilages, beneath the nasal bones, and leads into a cyst-like expansion, which can extend as far as the dura of the anterior skull base (foramen cecum). It is advisable to request a preoperative sagittal MRI scan to assess the situation.

Surgical Principle

Complete excision under good visualization. Reconstruction of deformities resulting from the fistulas and the avoidance of aesthetically unfavorable scars.

Indications

Established fistula, especially when several inflammatory episodes with swelling in the nasal dorsal region or even meningitis have already occurred.

Contraindications

Acute inflammation with the formation of granulation tissue, because this renders the identification of the epithelium difficult, which has to be completely removed.

Specific Points Regarding Informed Consent

The possibility of recurrence if the epithelium is not removed completely. Scarring of the skin, deformity, and disturbances of growth of the nose. Cerebrospinal fluid leak and meningitis in cases of extension as far as the dura.

Surgical Technique (Fig. 6.63)

Clear visualization is imperative for successful and reliable removal. The fistula, which runs along the nasal dorsum, must be well identified and it must be possible to follow it as far as the anterior skull base. An open approach via a columellar incision is best suited to achieve this. An additional incision is made in the RSTL around the external fistula opening. The beginning of the fistula in the small skin island is left behind on the cartilaginous nasal dorsum, after which the entire skin over the nasal dorsum is elevated (degloving). Clear exposure up to the nasal root is essential. The fistula lies in a groove over the superior septal margin and has often flattened out the cartilaginous nasal dorsum into the form of a trough. At the K-area it runs beneath the nasal bones. The bony nasal dorsum must therefore be cut with an osteotome or a fine drill and levered open or temporarily removed. The end of the fistula becomes visible, flaring as it does into a bulb-shaped form. It should be removed without injuring the wall of the cyst. Should this expose the dura of the anterior skull base, or if there is even evidence of a cerebrospinal leak, then the area will need to be covered, e.g., with autogenous fascia (fibrin glue), and endonasal packs inserted for 10 days.

After replacing the bone flap, which does not usually require any special fixation, the flattened-out cartilaginous nasal dorsum needs to be narrowed in most cases. If it is only slightly widened, then a stitch to re-approximate both upper lateral cartilages is all that is required. This will at the same time also raise the level of the cartilaginous nasal dorsum somewhat. If there is considerable widening, then it may be necessary to resect cartilage in the midline and then reunite the cut edges.

Rules, Tips, and Tricks

The marginal incisions must extend far enough laterally to provide sufficient visualization. The bone flap must also be made as wide as possible to reach lateral extensions of the nasal cyst also. It may be useful to fill the cyst with methylene blue, but this can become problematic. If a tear is inadvertently made during surgery, then the dye leaks into the surrounding tissue and renders identification of the epithelium almost impossible.

! Risks and Complications

See "Specific Points Regarding Informed Consent" for risks involving the frontal skull base. If dissection does not succeed in keeping to the right layer and the epithelium is only removed piecemeal, then a recurrent fistula is almost inevitable. It is then recommended to perform regular postoperative ultrasound scans and possibly MRI follow-up checks before undertaking revision surgery via the same approach should a recurrence become evident.

Occasionally a cyst may also develop deep in the nasal septum where it borders directly on the endonasal mucosa. Separation of the two epithelial layers can be difficult and requires gradual dissection with meticulous hemostasis using bipolar cauterization.

Growth of the nose may be retarded by both cyst and surgery (hypoplasia), in which case definitive reconstruction should be undertaken at about the age of 16 years.

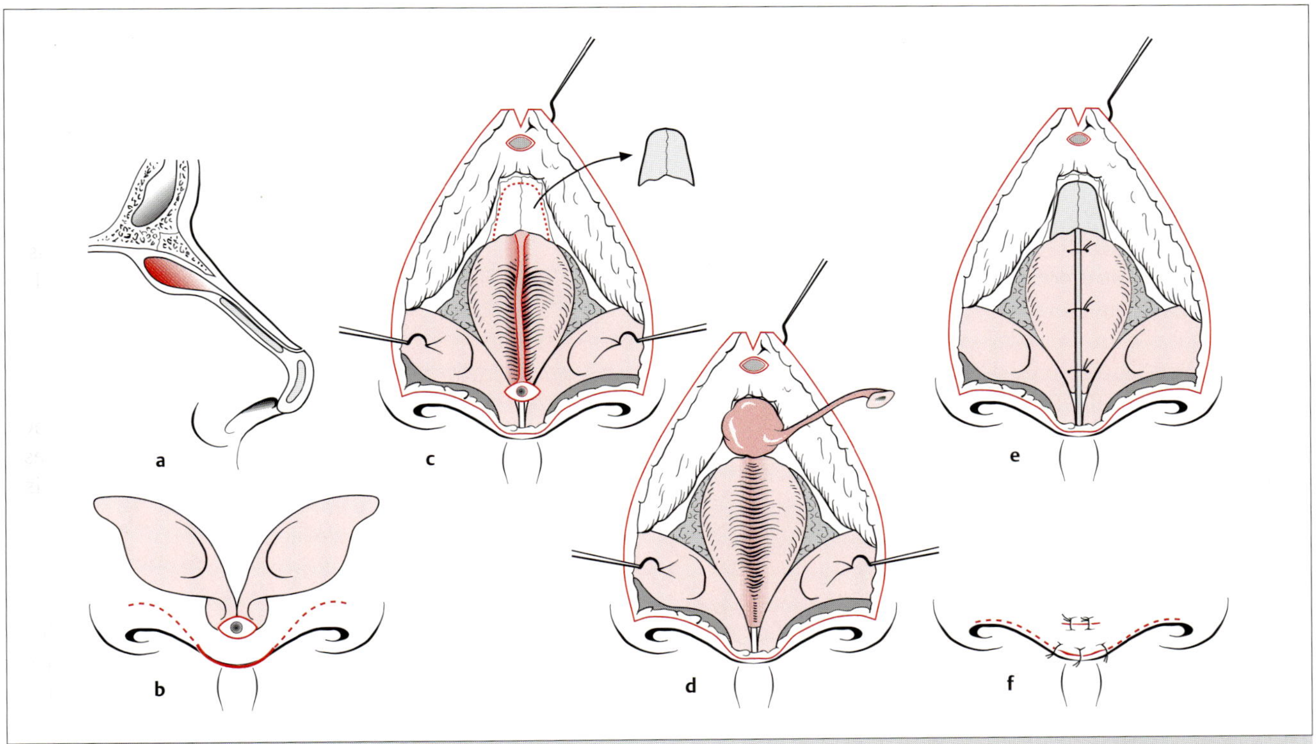

Fig. 6.63a–f Excision of a midline nasal fistula.
- **a** Course of the fistula from the nasal tip to beneath the nasal bones. In this case, there is no connection to the foramen cecum.
- **b** Elliptical incision around the fistula and external approach to the nasal dorsum using a columellar incision and marginal incisions.
- **c** The skin island is drawn through after elevating the nasal dorsal skin. The fistula tract is exposed as far as the piriform aperture and the osteotomies are marked. Usually the fistula has formed a wide trough between the upper lateral cartilages.
- **d** The bone flap is temporarily removed and the fistula sac exposed.
- **e** Reconstruction of the nasal dorsum after excision of the fistula: the bone flap is replaced and the upper lateral cartilages are sutured together to achieve narrowing.
- **f** Appearance after wound closure.

Choanal Atresia

Congenital choanal atresia is rare, predominantly unilateral (late onset of symptoms with unilateral rhinorrhoea), and in 80% of cases is caused by a persistent bony plate. It may also be associated with other malformations (e.g., CHARGE syndrome [**c**oloboma of the eye, **h**eart defects, **a**tresia of the choanae, **re**tardation of growth and/or development, **g**enital and/or urinary abnormalities, and **e**ar abnormalities and deafness]).

Bilateral choanal atresia is a life-threatening condition for the newborn; the infant has difficulty feeding and is asphyxiated. In this case, after establishing the diagnosis by gently blowing air into each nasal cavity with a Politzer bag, sounding with a soft suction catheter or by nasal endoscopy, early surgical opening has to be performed.

Surgical Principle

Surgical removal of the atresia plate while maximally protecting the mucosa to achieve rapid epithelialization. Partial resection of the vomer to widen the choanae. An endonasal approach is usually sufficient.

Indications

Bilateral bony or membranous choanal atresia (newborn). Unilateral atresia in older children.

Contraindications

Life-threatening situation due to other malformations that need to be treated primarily.

Operative Planning

Horizontal CT, if possible, to display the topography of the nasopharynx, pterygoid processes, and the position of the pterygopalatine fossa, which can be displaced medially (risk of vascular injury). Distinction between bony and membranous atresia.

Special Instruments and Implants

Use of a microscope (self-retaining speculum) or endoscope. Hand drill with protective sleeve to avoid injury to the skin of the nostril.

Surgical Technique (Fig. 6.64)

After achieving maximal decongestion of the mucosal membranes and lateral fracture of the inferior turbinate, the junction between nasal floor and nasal septum is identified, where the choana is opened. Its posterior wall is protected by inserting a pledget swab into the nasopharynx. The mucosa is incised and elevated in all directions and as far as possible *not* resected. If a bony atresia is present, it is now opened with a fine diamond drill. The opening thus created is either widened with the drill, or the bone is removed with a fine punch. Resection must include the posterior margin of the vomer to make the choana wide enough. It is important to ensure that the bony surface is covered by replacing the mucosal flap. Use of fibrin glue may be considered. Otherwise the circular wound area may result in the formation of a concentric scar and constriction.

A U-shaped breathing tube may counteract this development (**Fig. 6.65**). For this purpose, a silicone tube as thick as possible is selected, bent into a U shape, and slit at the kink. It is drawn through the mouth into the nasal lumina via the nasopharynx with the aid of two suction drains inserted transnasally and secured in front of the columella. It is removed after approximately 6 weeks, when any granulation tissue at the choanal margins is also resected. In case of a wide choana as a result of surgery however, the U-shaped tube should be abandoned.

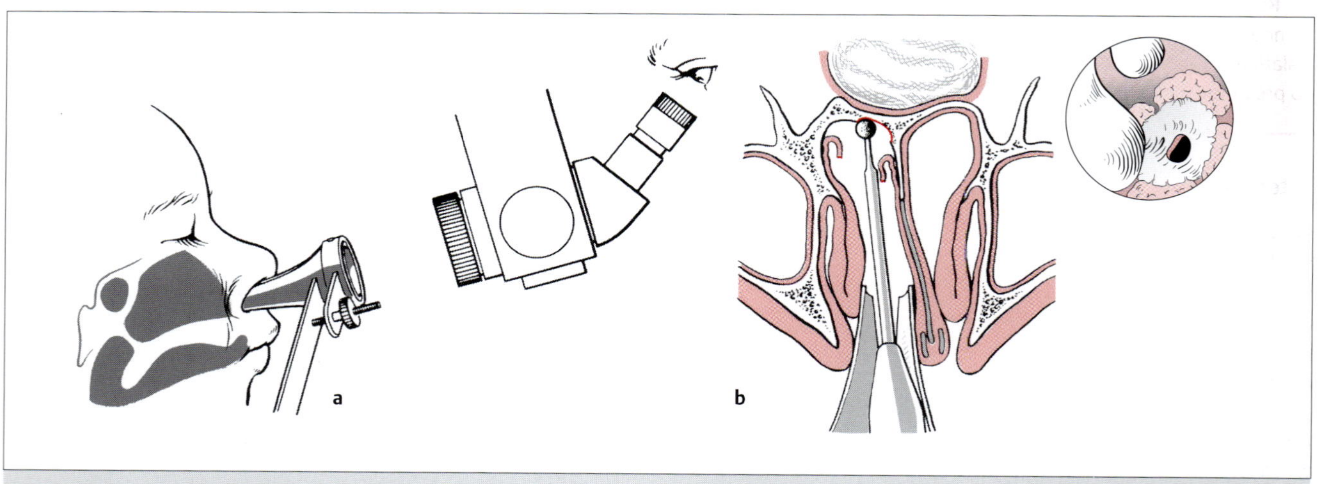

Fig. 6.64a, b Endonasal resection of a bony choanal atresia.
a Self-retaining nasal speculum and microscope.
b After elevating a mucosal flap, perforation is achieved with a diamond burr in the corner between septum and nasal floor. The nasopharynx is protected by inserting a swab.

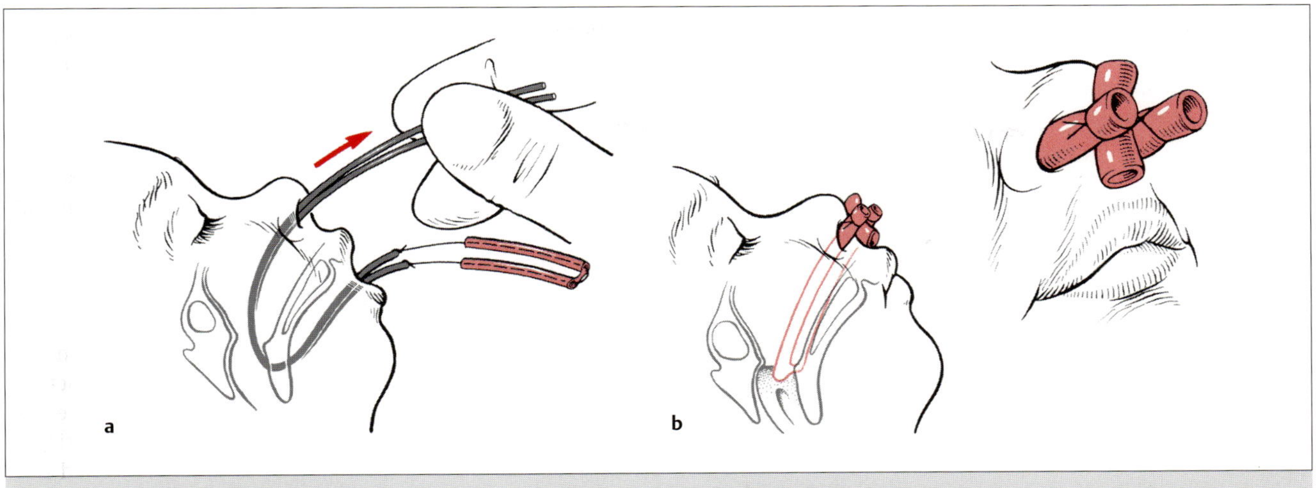

Fig. 6.65a, b Insertion of a spacer.
a U-shaped tube is drawn into the nasopharynx via a catheter inserted into the mouth and brought out through the nose.
b The spacer is secured in position over the columella. Look out for pressure sores of the columella.

Rules, Tips, and Tricks

Widening of the choana from a lateral and cranial approach is often limited by the medial displacement of the pterygoid processes and the low position of the sphenoid bone. Widening should therefore be achieved mainly from a medial aspect by resecting the vomer.

A purely membranous choanal atresia can also be easily perforated without the problem of bleeding with the aid of a CO_2 laser. However, this also tends to form a stenosis due to the circular wound surface and requires removal of the posterior margin of the vomer with other surgical instruments. Widening in the direction of the nasal floor with subsequent perforation of the palate must be avoided.

! Risks and Complications

Danger of vascular injury, particularly in the region of the pterygopalatine fossa, perforation of the palate, columellar necrosis due to pressure ulcers from the U-shaped tube.

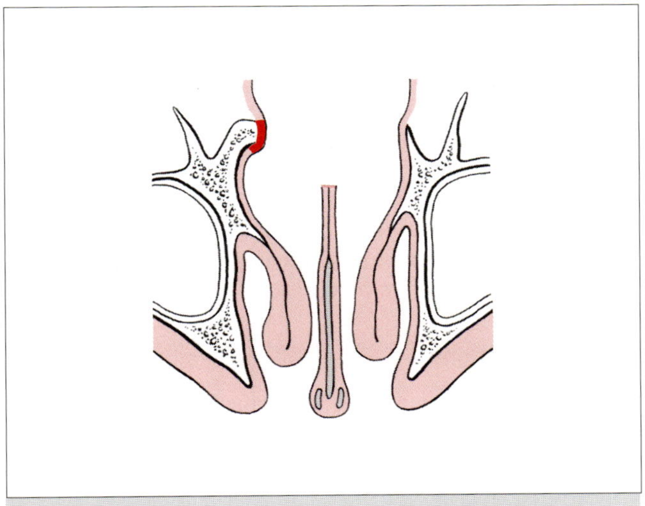

Fig. 6.66 Perforation of a unilateral choanal atresia.
The dorsal bony septal components are resected via an endonasal trans-septal approach, thus creating a large common choana. Mucosa will need to be mobilized to cover any raw bone (red area).

Alternatives

Instead of inserting a spacer, planned revision surgery to clear the choanae may be undertaken ca. 2–3 weeks after the initial operation. This involves the removal of granulation tissue to encourage epithelialization. This may need to be repeated at intervals, depending on the tendency to form stenoses, until the wound surface has completely epithelialized.

Instead of a transnasal approach, the operation may also be done via a transoral–transpalatine access. After separating the soft from the hard palate and removing a part of the hard palate and the vomer, the bony atresia plate may be resected under direct vision. This operation is associated with a high degree of morbidity. Disturbances of growth secondary to partial resections to the palate are discussed controversially.

A *unilateral* choanal atresia is usually operated on when a child is of school age. Here a trans-septal approach is appropriate, given that this facilitates removal of the posterior margin of the vomer (**Fig. 6.66**). The mucosa overlying the atresia plate is initially protected and only after sufficient removal of the bone is it resected so that the choana is widely opened and no significant wound surfaces remain.

Turbinates

Hypertrophy and deformities are indications for surgery of the turbinates. Septoplasty without accompanying surgery of the turbinates is often not possible because the space required to straighten the nasal septum is not available. Furthermore, turbinate reduction is often the only option for helping patients with chronic abuse of nose drops. The space adjacent to a concave side of a septal deviation is often filled with a pneumatized middle nasal turbinate (so-called concha bullosa). It must be understood that septoplasty only equalizes the passages of both nasal cavities. It does not necessarily create additional volume for breathing. Turbinate surgery, in contrast, reduces the volume of the turbinates, thus increasing the volume of the nasal passage.

Surgical Principle

Volume reduction of enlarged lower nasal turbinates, if necessary with lateral displacement by partial resection or fracture of the conchal bone. Lateralization of a concha bullosa after resection of the lateral part of the turbinate. Maximal protection of the mucosal membranes must be ensured and extensive scar formation avoided (drying and crusting, disturbance of mucociliary transport).

Indications

Obstructive hypertrophy of the inferior turbinate, possibly with additional evidence of a relevant "mucosal factor" on rhinomanometry. Prevention of the straightening of the nasal septum by an overly large inferior or middle turbinate.

Contraindications

Pre-existing wide nasal cavity with mucosal atrophy and scar formation secondary to previous surgery or long-term therapy with topical steroids.

Specific Points Regarding Informed Consent

Postoperative bleeding, dry nose, drying and crusting of the posterior wall of the pharynx, olfactory dysfunction.

Operative planning

If there is a large and thick conchal bone in addition to hypertrophy of the turbinate mucosa, then it will require partial resection or fracture. A concha bullosa may be assumed purely from the aspect of an enlargement of the middle turbinate, which is possibly recognizable on CT scans (CT examination is not obligatory for concha bullosa).

Special Instruments

Cutting (angled scissors) and punching instruments (Blakesley punch) are appropriate for turbinate reduction. Narrow bridges of tissue after partial resection of segments of the inferior and middle turbinates are best divided using a nasal snare.

Surgical Technique

Inferior Turbinate

Excess turbinate tissue can be recognized after maximal decongestion. Simple turbinectomy along the inferior margin, possibly with the additional removal of a strip of bone, leaves behind a large wound surface, which granulates over a long period of time and has a tendency to secondary hemorrhage. Exposed bone may become necrotic. This method is therefore only suitable to a limited degree (**Fig. 6.67**).

Inferior turbinoplasty is therefore better because it maximally protects the mucous membranes and leaves only a longitudinal narrow scar along the lateral surface of the turbinate (**Fig. 6.68**). After a vertical incision of the mucosa of the head of the inferior turbinate down to bone contact, the mucosa is undermined subperiosteally, medial to the conchal bone, as far as the posterior end of the turbinate using an elevator (e.g., the sharp end of a Cottle elevator). One blade of an angled scissors is inserted into this tunnel and the mucosa split along the free inferior margin of the turbinate. This allows the mucosa to be reflected upward on its cranial pedicle to expose the medial surface of the conchal bone. The lateral mucous membrane, and possibly part of the conchal bone, are now resected with scissors. The resulting wound surfaces can be cauterized by bipolar coagulation. The mucosa is then returned to its original position to cover the wound surface. Its re-approximation is accomplished with a loose pack for 1–2 days.

If the conchal bone is situated too far medially, then it may either be removed subtotally or osteotomized at its lateral attachment (**Fig. 6.69**). This allows the entire turbinate to be easily displaced laterally, providing sufficient distance to the nasal septum.

Sometimes the choanal area is partially blocked by an enlarged lobed posterior end of the inferior turbinate. Often this does not cause any significant impairment of nasal breathing,

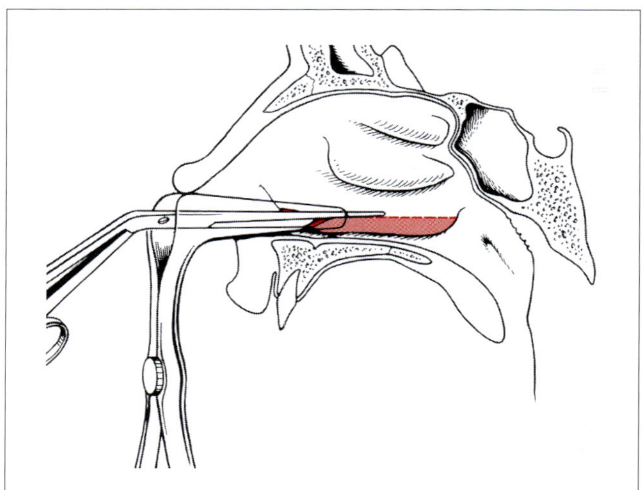

Fig. 6.67 Turbinate resection along the inferior margin of the lower turbinate. Simple removal of redundant mucosa.

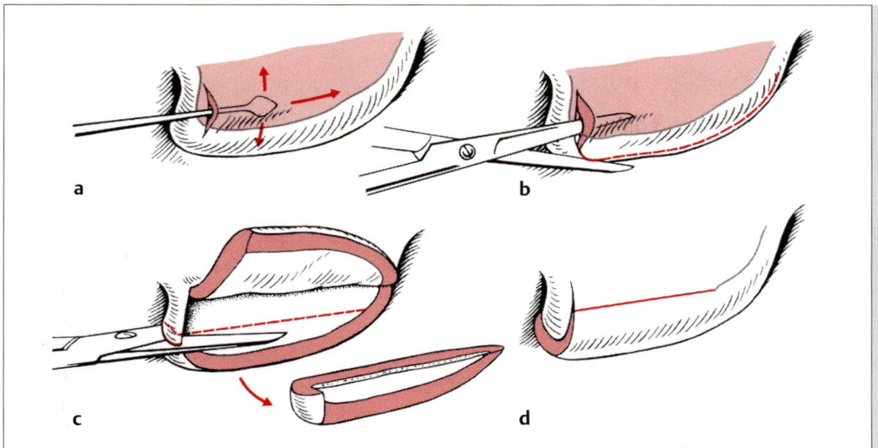

Fig. 6.68a–d Reduction of the inferior turbinate (turbinoplasty).
a Incision at the head of the turbinate; creation of a tunnel beneath the periosteum medial to the bone.
b A mucosal flap is elevated by incising the free margin using nasal scissors.
c The superiorly based mucosal flap is elevated and mucosa and bone of the lateral part of the turbinate are excised.
d The mucosal flap is returned.

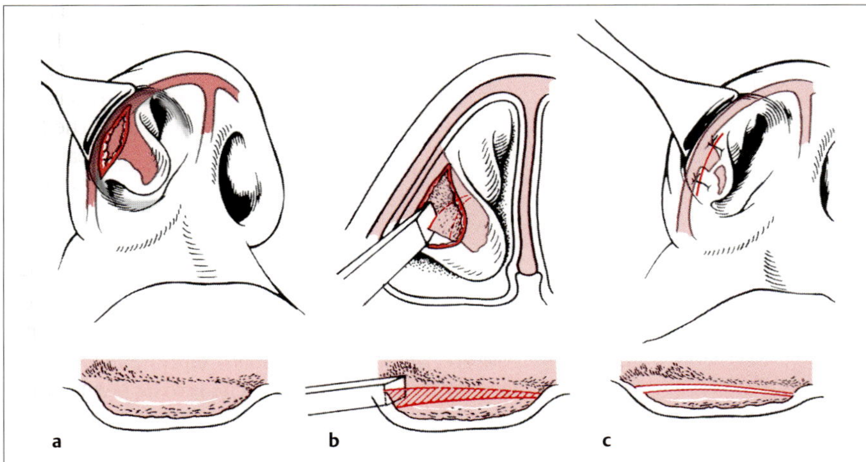

Fig. 6.69a–c Lateral displacement of the inferior turbinate with partial excision of the conchal bone.
a Vertical incision of the mucosa at the head of the inferior turbinate and subperiosteal exposure of the conchal bone.
b Osteotomy with wedge-shaped excision of the conchal bone.
c Lateral displacement of the turbinate, secured with an approximation suture.

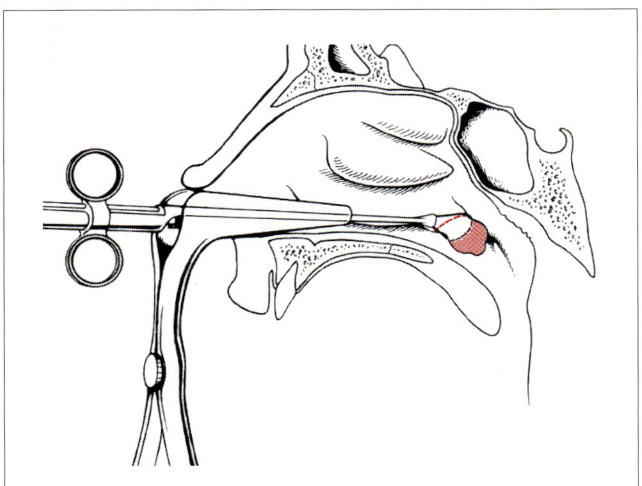

Fig. 6.70 Removal of a hyperplastic posterior end of the turbinate. A snare is placed around the posterior (bone-free) end of the turbinate, which is then resected. It is essential to identify and protect the pharyngeal ostium of the eustachian tube.

but hypertrophy of the posterior end of the turbinate is supposed to be partially responsible for bothersome postnasal drip. It may be removed with the aid of a nasal snare (**Fig. 6.70**).

Pneumatized Middle Turbinate (Fig. 6.71)

For inferior turbinoplasty, the head of the middle turbinate is incised vertically, dividing the very thin bone at the same time. This allows access to an air-filled cavity, which is normally lined with healthy mucous membrane. Here too, the free margin is incised with angled scissors as far as the attachment with the sphenoid sinus (basal lamella). The lateral wall is then detached via a cranial incision until it is only attached dorsally. The temptation to extract it with grasping forceps should be resisted, however, as the middle turbinate is very fragile and can easily be avulsed from the skull base. It is better to remove it with the aid of a nasal snare or a punch. The rest of the turbinate together with the thin medial bone can now be easily fractured laterally after the resection site has been cauterized, anterior to the sphenoid sinus.

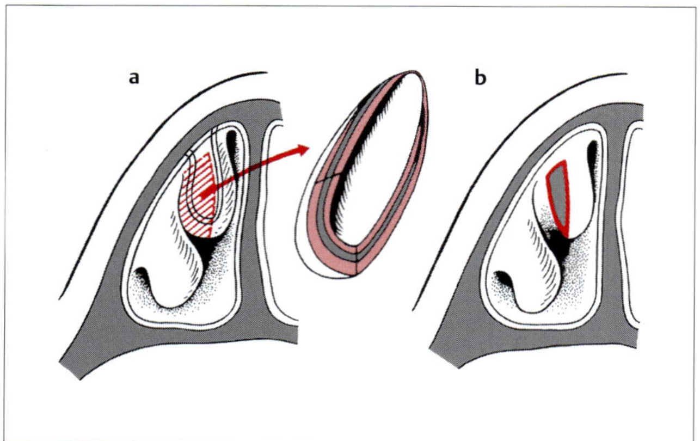

Fig. 6.71a, b Partial resection of a pneumatized middle turbinate (concha bullosa).
a Resection of the lateral part of the turbinate.
b Appearance after resection: the lateral mucosal surface (the original medial wall of the air cell) of the remaining turbinate is preserved to prevent adhesions to the lateral nasal wall.

Rules, Tips, and Tricks

Removal of the free edge of the inferior turbinate should be done parallel to the nasal floor, as otherwise there is a tendency to deviate upward, leaving only the head of the inferior turbinate remaining at the end of the maneuver.

Detachment of the mucosa off the bone can be difficult, especially in the middle parts of the inferior turbinate where it is very thin and can tear easily. The bone also protrudes medially at this point and the elevator may perforate the mucosa behind the prominence. It is therefore essential to ensure bone contact of the instrument here.

Risks and Complications

Removing the inferior turbinate too extensively can result in an "empty nose syndrome." Loss of a functioning mucous membrane means that the turbinate can no longer carry out its task of warming, humidifying, and filtering the inspired air. The result is recurrent infections, crusting and pharyngitis sicca. A ozaena-like disorder may develop. Ozeana is a separate entity, however, and has nothing to do with the sequelae of surgery to the turbinates. It not rare that after turbinate reduction and subsequent objectively wide nasal airways, patients still have the feeling of obstructed nasal breathing and want further surgery. They should be strongly advised against this. The feeling of obstructed nasal breathing can be the result of a disturbance of cold–warm sensation due to scar formation, especially if the mucosa is extensively scarred. Under normal circumstances, cooling of the mucous membrane during inspiration is associated with good nasal patency—an effect which can arise from peppermint and other essential oils, without any objective improvement of nasal respiration being actually present. This physiological temperature difference is no longer experienced in the presence of extensive scar formation.

Alternatives

The volume of the mucosa may be reduced thermally (**Fig. 6.72**). This can be done by monopolar cautery after inserting a needle (e.g., radiofrequency ablation). This technique is particularly useful when the erectile tissue of the nasal septum immediately in front of the head of the middle turbinate is to be reduced (so-called septal turbinate, intumescentia septi).

Various laser modalities have similar effects and offer the advantage of a simple operation under topical anesthesia. It should be borne in mind, however, that laser treatment leaves a scar at the site of penetration, which no longer consists of healthy mucosa. Problems may arise when larger areas are affected by scars secondary to laser treatment (see above).

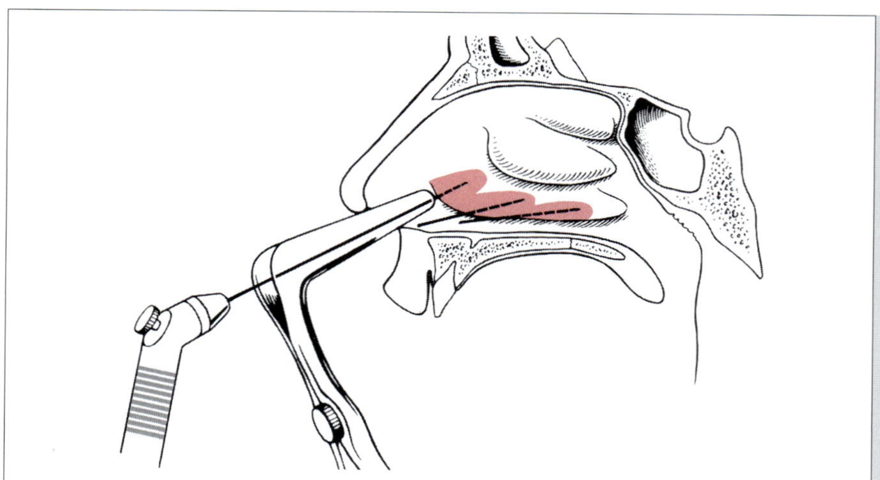

Fig. 6.72 Electrocautery of the lower turbinate.
The monopolar cautery tip is inserted in the hyperplastic turbinate mucosa and the submucous erectile tissue is cauterized.

Surgical Management of Epistaxis

Spontaneous epistaxis, or bleeding from the nose, often affects elderly patients with hypertension and receiving anticoagulant treatment. Minor bleeding usually originates from a vascular network located in the caudal septal mucosa (Little area, Kiesselbach plexus) and is usually amenable to bipolar cautery after a short period of packing. More significant hemorrhage from the posterior nasal cavity often originates from branches of the sphenopalatine artery, rarely from the anterior or posterior ethmoid artery. The primary objective is initially to control bleeding by packing. In cases of more significant bleeding, the flow of blood into the nasopharyngeal cavity must be initially prevented with a balloon catheter or a suitable pneumatic nasal tamponade. This is followed by anterior packing, e.g., using layers of gauze ribbon. The objective is either the direct compression of the bleeding site or the reduction and packing of the area immediately adjacent to the bleeding point. Once this area has filled with blood, the bleeding point is automatically compressed. The causes of the bleeding are subsequently addressed (hypertension, warfarin). If bleeding recurs after 2–3 days of packing and subsequent removal, then hemostasis by operative means is indicated.

Hereditary telangiectasia (Osler–Rendu–Weber disease) is characterized by severe nasal bleeding, which is difficult to control despite the fact that the bleeding point is usually located in the anterior nasal cavity. Endonasal packing is required as an initial measure. A rubber finger stall or a pneumatic tamponade is preferably used because otherwise removal of the pack always results in renewed hemorrhage if the blood clot that has formed is subsequently removed by the rough surface of a gauze pack.

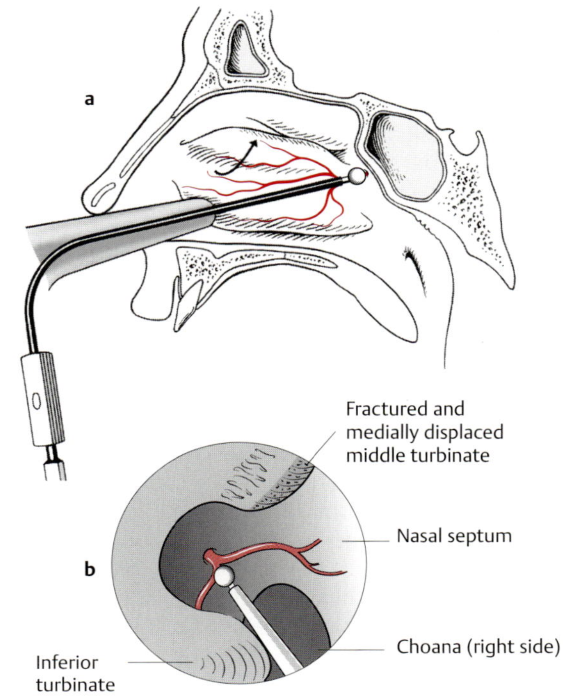

Fig. 6.73a, b Cauterization of the sphenopalatine artery
a Identification of the sphenopalatine foramen after lateral middle turbinate displacement. The monopolar suction cautery is used.
b Endoscopic view of the foramen, showing the medial and lateral branches of the artery.

Surgical Principle

Cauterization or occlusion of the bleeding vessel, as near to the bleeding point as possible.

Contraindications

Other life-threatening causes.

Operative Planning

Endonasal approach. Severe hemorrhage may require the transmaxillary approach to the maxillary artery in the retromaxillary space.

Surgical Technique (Fig. 6.73)

The bleeding point should be identified, which is sometimes only possible after raising the blood pressure and placing the patient in the head down position. Vessel stumps, in particular the anterior ethmoid artery, may be cauterized directly under endoscopic vision. It may be necessary to approach this artery after anterior ethmoidectomy with identification of the skull base.

Bleeding from the sphenopalatine artery requires exposure of the sphenopalatine foramen, lateral to the attachment of the middle turbinate, and identification of the artery as it exits the foramen with its septal and conchal branches. The artery is cauterized using bipolar diathermy between the bleeding site and foramen. Ongoing hemorrhage may obstruct the view; in such cases a monopolar suction cautery can be very helpful.

Rules, Tips, and Tricks

If the view is rendered difficult by an obstructing deviated septum, septoplasty may have to be done first, once the bleeding site has been temporarily packed. The sphenopalatine foramen is occasionally difficult to identify. After the maxillary cavity has been opened in the middle nasal meatus, the foramen lies medially, along the extension of the roof of the maxillary sinus.

If a definite bleeding point cannot be identified, it is advisable after previous severe bleeding to prophylactically cauterize the sphenopalatine artery of the affected side.

Alternatives

If the sphenopalatine artery is large in diameter, cauterization alone is often not enough and ligation or clipping is often impossible for technical reasons. In such cases, the maxillary artery located behind the maxillary sinus is addressed (**Fig. 6.74**). Through a transmaxillary approach, the mucosa is elevated superiorly and posteromedially and the posterior antral wall is partially removed. The fatty tissue behind it is then spread apart to expose the maxillary artery. The artery is clipped proximal to its division into the sphenopalatine and palatine arteries. Once the bleeding has ceased or clearly decreased, the endonasal bleeding point may be additionally cauterized.

In rare cases, hemorrhage from the anterior ethmoid artery is inaccessible from an endonasal approach because the vessel has retracted into the orbital cavity. Here there is the risk of a retrobulbar hematoma developing, resulting in blindness from the intraorbital rise in pressure. In this case, the vessel stump will need to be located in the orbital cavity via a medial eyebrow incision and cauterized with bipolar forceps.

In case of an emergency, endonasal coagulation of the sphenopalatine artery in the foramen is the standard in posterior nasal bleeding. The transmaxillary approach is rarely necessary, but it should not be forgotten, as it can be essential in life-threatening situations. The ligation of the anterior ethmoidal artery is generally a bipolar or monopolar coagulation and hardly ever necessary because of epistaxis. It is primarily indicated in paranasal sinus surgery, when the artery is disrupted and retracts into the orbit.

There is no bleeding into the nasal cavity but into the orbit. So the symptom is not epistaxis but exophthalmus.

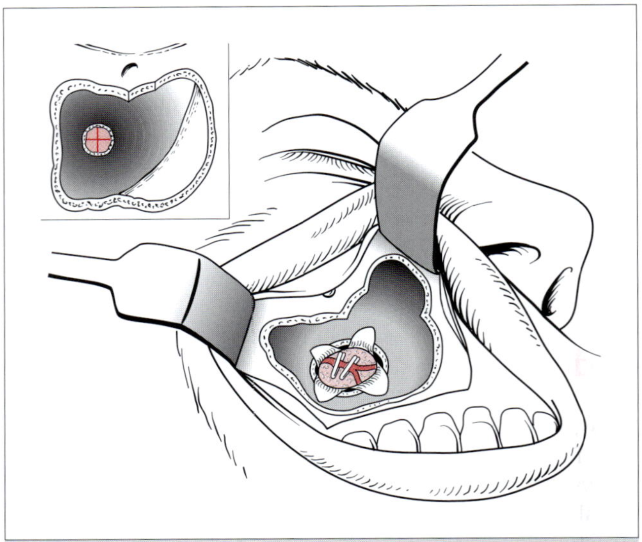

Fig. 6.74 Transmaxillary ligation of the maxillary artery. Transoral exposure of the maxilla after removal of the anterior wall while protecting the infraorbital foramen. Circumscribed removal of the mediocranial surface of the posterior maxillary wall. Cruciate incision of the periosteum and opening of the retromaxillary fossa. The maxillary artery is clipped proximal to its division into the palatine and sphenopalatine arteries.

7 Surgery of the Paranasal Sinuses and Their Adjacent Structures

C. Rudack

Endonasal Surgery of the Paranasal Sinuses

Today, endonasal surgery of the paranasal sinuses involves the use of optic systems—endoscopes and/or microscopes—and so allows the use of operative techniques that incorporate functional aspects of mucosal physiology and related anatomical structures. These procedures can therefore also be classified as functional operations. A distinction is made between *endoscopic surgery of the paranasal sinuses*, also referred to as functional endoscopic sinus surgery (FESS), and a *combined microscopic and endoscopic technique*. FESS comprises the circumscribed opening of the paranasal sinus system and the removal of its contents, as determined by the presenting pathology. Unlike earlier surgical procedures, this technique is minimally invasive: for example, the radical removal of mucous membranes from the paranasal sinus is avoided.

Indications

- Acute or chronic ethmoid, maxillary, frontal and/or sphenoid sinusitis, polyposis of the nose and sinuses.
- Orbital complications of ethmoiditis.
- Surgical approach to the orbit.
- Drainage of mucoceles, pyoceles, and pneumatoceles.
- Tumors of the lateral nasal wall and of the paranasal sinus system.
- Fractures involving the paranasal sinus system, midface, orbit, and optic nerve.
- Management of the dura secondary to injuries to the roof of the ethmoid.

Anatomical Aspects of the Paranasal Sinus System

The four paranasal sinuses—the *maxillary sinus*, *ethmoid sinus* (ethmoidal labyrinth), *frontal sinus*, and *sphenoid sinus*—represent paired lateral outgrowths from the main nasal cavities. The medial border of the main nasal cavity is the septum, while the lateral nasal wall bears the nasal turbinates (**Fig. 7.1a**). The three turbinates divide the lateral nasal wall into three distinct airspaces: the superior, middle, and inferior meatus. The paired *ethmoid sinuses* contain 10–15 air cells, which are lined with respiratory epithelium. Medially, the ethmoid is bordered by the middle turbinate. Superiorly it closes off the frontal bone, which is also referred to as the anterior roof of the ethmoid (**Fig. 7.1b**). The entire roof of the ethmoid extends from the planum sphenoidale to the frontal bone and can have various anatomic configurations, knowledge of which is of great importance for surgery of the sphenoid. Embedded in the cribriform plate of the ethmoid is the *crista galli*, a crest like elevation which extends into the anterior cranial fossa (**Fig. 7.1c**). The lateral border of the ethmoid sinus is formed by the *lamina papyracea* (**Fig. 7.1c**), a thin, bony structure separating the orbit from the paranasal sinuses. The lamina cribrosa fits into the ethmoid notch. The olfactory nerves pass through the lamina cribrosa from the olfactory region into the olfactory bulb. Basically, various types of ethmoid roof configurations are described, which develop according to the length of the lateral lamella of the lamina cribrosa. The longer the lateral lamella, the deeper is the olfactory groove (= "risky ethmoid"). This means that there is an increased risk of injury to the bone of the skull base as compared with a flat ethmoid roof (**Fig. 7.1d**).

The basal lamella of the middle turbinate divides the *ethmoid complex* anatomically into an anterior and a posterior ethmoid cell (**Fig. 7.2a**). The course of the basal lamella can be described in three parts as it extends between its endpoints (the ethmoid crest of the maxilla and the ethmoid crest of the perpendicular process of the palatine bone):

- An anterior vertical part at the lateral edge of the lamina cribrosa.
- A middle frontal part, lateral to the skull base and extending to the lamina papyracea.
- A posterior horizontal part, forming the roof of the posterior third of the middle meatus.

Anterior ethmoidal complex. The ostium of the *maxillary sinus* drains into a narrow funnel-shaped space, the *maxillary infundibulum* (**Fig. 7.1c**), which runs in a sagittal direction in the lateral nasal wall. Cranially the maxillary infundibulum drains into the *ethmoid infundibulum* (anterior ethmoid), which continues medially and dorsally into the *hiatus semilunaris*. The inferior hiatus semilunaris is a two-dimensional gap, which, when opened from a medial dorsal access, leads into the ethmoid infundibulum (**Fig. 7.2a, b**). Further anteriorly, the medial wall of the infundibulum is formed by the *uncinate process* (a sickle-shaped process, which corresponds to the rudiment of the first lamella in the middle meatus). Its anterior margin attaches to the lacrimal bone and the orbital surface (facies orbitalis) of the maxilla. Small processes extend out to the roof of the maxilla, with further connections fusing with processes of the palatine bone and the turbinate bone. This bony labyrinth

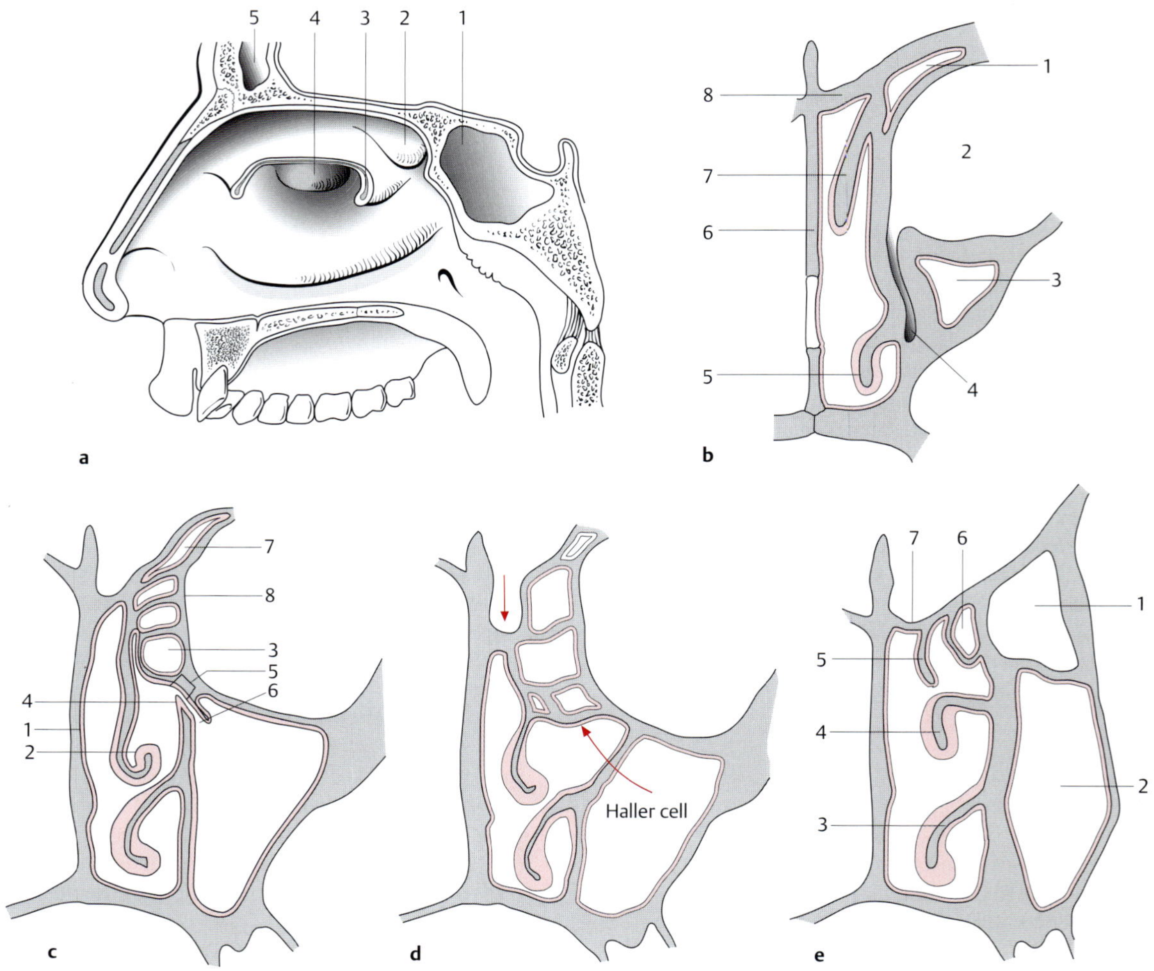

Fig. 7.1a–g Anatomical relationships of the paranasal sinuses.
a Lateral nasal wall.
1 right sphenoid sinus
2 superior turbinate
3 middle turbinate
4 inferior turbinate
5 right frontal sinus
b Coronary section through the nasolacrimal duct.
1 frontal sinus
2 orbit
3 maxillary sinus
4 nasolacrimal duct
5 inferior turbinate
6 septum
7 middle turbinate
8 ethmoid roof
c Coronary section through the maxillary sinus ostium.
1 middle turbinate
2 turbinate sinus
3 ethmoid bulla
4 uncinate process and medial infundibular wall
5 ethmoid infundibulum
6 maxillary sinus ostium
7 frontal recess
8 lamina papyracea (lamina orbitalis)
d Low-lying lamina cribrosa and Haller cell.
e Coronary section through the posterior ethmoid sinuses.
1 orbit
2 maxillary sinus
3 inferior turbinate
4 middle turbinate
5 superior turbinate
6 posterior ethmoid cell
7 lamina cribrosa
f–g see next page

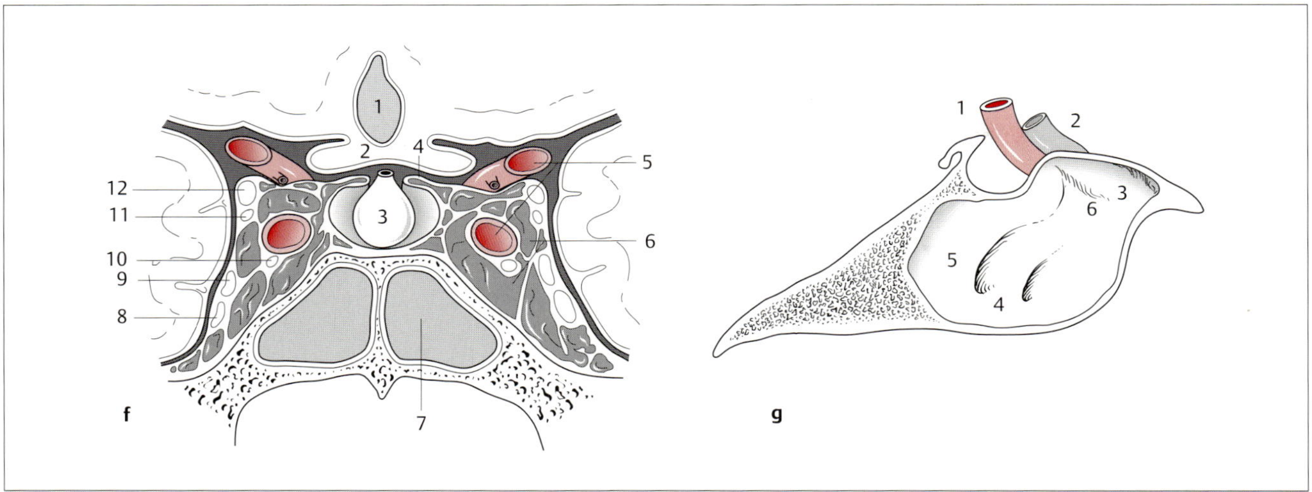

Fig. 7.1f–g
f Coronary section through the sphenoid sinus.
1 third ventricle
2 optic chiasma
3 pituitary
4 sellar diaphragm
5 internal carotid artery
6 cavernous sinus
7 sphenoid sinus
8 maxillary nerve
9 ophthalmic nerve (first branch of the trigeminal nerve, CN V)
10 abducens nerve (CN VI)
11 trochlear nerve (CN IV)
12 oculomotor nerve (CN III)
g Lateral view of the sphenoid sinus.
1 internal carotid artery
2 optic nerve
3 prominence of the optic nerve
4 prominence of the maxillary nerve
5 prominence of the internal carotid artery
6 infraoptic recess

is covered medially by nasal mucosa and laterally by mucosa of the maxillary sinus. The ethmoid infundibulum can merge without interruption with the frontal recess in a ventral and cranial direction, depending on how the uncinate process bends and attaches to the lamina papyracea. This makes it difficult to distinguish the ethmoid infundibulum from the frontal recess. The natural maxillary ostium is located at the junction between the middle and dorsal third of the ethmoid infundibulum, which is why it is often hidden in the middle meatus.

The second lamella in the anterior ethmoidal complex is formed by the *ethmoid bulla* (**Fig. 7.1a**), which extends as far as the lamina papyracea and finally continues onto the medial roof of the maxillary sinus as the frontal crest. An anterior ethmoid cell, known as the *agger nasi cell* or *cellula lacrimalis*, often takes its origin from the superior aspect of the ethmoid infundibulum or the frontal recess, descends into the agger nasi, and abuts on the lacrimal fossa.

Sometimes one or two cells drain into the lateral infundibular wall, just under the ethmoid bulla, and extend into the medial orbital floor; these are known as *Haller cells* (**Fig. 7.1d**). Clefts in the anterior ethmoid complex, which are situated above and behind the ethmoid bulla, are referred to as *suprabullar and retrobullar recesses* and are synonymous with a *lateral sinus* (**Fig. 7.2a, b**).

The *frontal infundibulum* is a funnel-shaped protrusion from the floor of the frontal sinus, caudally toward the natural frontal sinus ostium. From an anatomical view, the frontal infundibulum lies within the frontal sinus itself. The frontal recess is located caudal to the frontal infundibulum and to the natural frontal sinus ostium (**Fig. 7.2a, b**). It is shaped like a reversed funnel and forms the most anterior part of the anterior ethmoid sinus. It can be considerably narrowed by anatomic variations of the uncinate process, the ethmoid bulla, and the agger nasi cells. A knowledge of the anatomy and the course of these variations facilitates the search for the natural ostium of the frontal sinus during surgery.

The caudal part of the middle turbinate may be significantly curled downward laterally, especially in the middle part, or it may even appear as an almost horizontally and laterally bent crest. Its concave lateral surface forms the turbinate sinus. Cavities are frequently found in the middle turbinate; the best known of these is a cell in the anterior part known as the *concha bullosa*.

Posterior ethmoidal complex. The *posterior middle meatus* is formed medially by the first posterior ethmoid cell and by the superior meatus, which often indents into the middle turbinate. The posterior ethmoidal complex therefore projects medially slightly beyond the anterior ethmoid (**Fig. 7.1e**). Cranially the optic nerve lies against the lateral wall of the sphenoid sinus (**Fig. 7.1g, h**) and below it is found the anterior genu of the internal carotid artery. Onodi cells are posterior suprasphenoidal ethmoid cells, which can displace the location of the sphenoid cavity far laterally (**Fig. 7.3**). The optic nerve and the internal carotid artery then also run in the lateral wall of these cells. It should be borne in mind that in ca. 4% of cases the bony cover of the optic nerve, and in ca. 8% of cases of that of the internal carotid artery, is dehiscent.

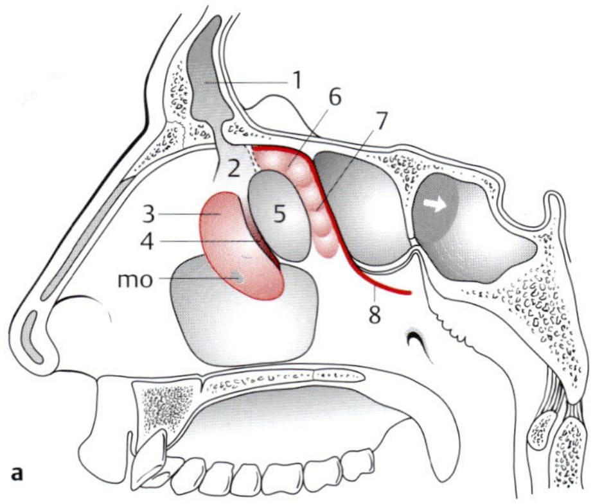

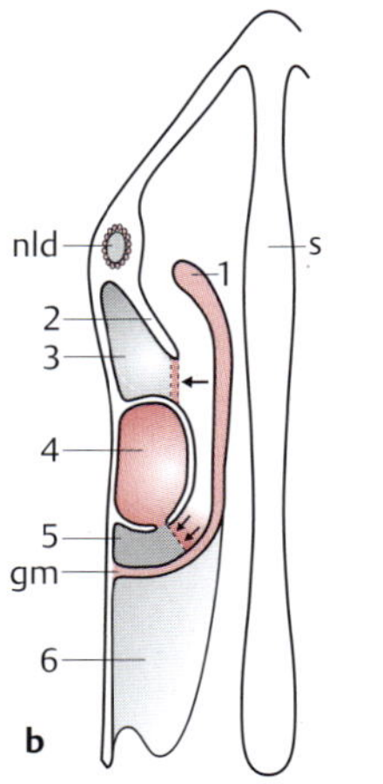

Fig. 7.2a, b Longitudinal and horizontal sections through the lateral nasal wall and the paranasal sinus system (modified after A. Hambrosch, Graz University, Austria).

a Highly schematized presentation of a paramedian longitudinal section through the lateral nasal wall and the paranasal sinus system. The red area shows the insertion line of the middle turbinate to the lateral nasal wall and skull base. For reasons of perspective, the anterior fifth of this insertion is not shown.

1 frontal sinus
2 frontal recess
3 uncinate process
4 hiatus semilunaris (inferior)
5 ethmoid bulla
6 suprabullar recess
7 retrobullar recess
8 insertion line of the middle turbinate (basal lamella), which separates the anterior ethmoid cells from the posterior ethmoid cells.
mo maxillary sinus ostium

b Schematic presentation of a horizontal section through the lateral nasal wall just above the horizontal course of the dorsal third of the middle turbinate.

s septum
nld nasolacrimal duct
gm frontal part of the basal lamella of the middle turbinate, which separates the anterior ethmoid cells from the posterior ethmoid cells.
1 cut edge: vertical part of the middle turbinate
2 uncinate process
3 ethmoid infundibulum
4 ethmoid bulla
5 retrobullar recess
6 posterior ethmoid cell
→ hiatus semilunaris (inferior)
⇉ hiatus semilunaris (superior)

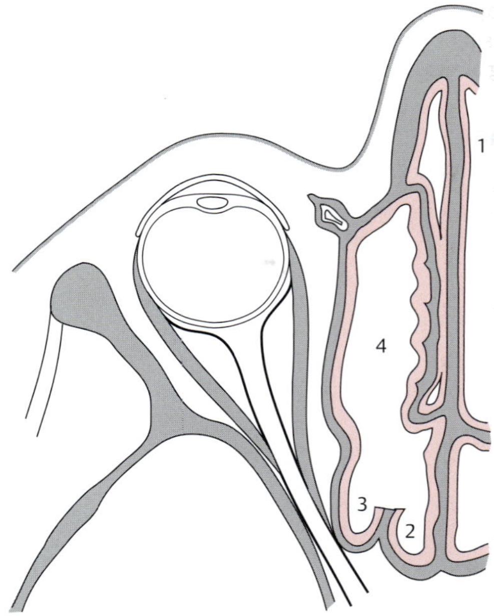

Fig. 7.3 Sphenoethmoid cell: Onodi cell.
1 septum
2 sphenoid sinus
3 Onodi cell
4 cleared ethmoid cells

Preparation for Endonasal Surgery of the Paranasal Sinuses

Preoperative Measures to Achieve Decongestion

Tapered sponge or ribbon gauze soaked in lidocaine and epinephrine (1:1 000) for approximately 10 minutes (ratio 5:1 lidocaine to epinephrine 1:1 000).

Local Anesthesia

Inject 1% lidocaine and epinephrine 1: 200 000 beneath the mucosa of the uncinate process and agger nasi. Additional infiltration of the insertion of the middle turbinate. Peripheral block of the ethmoid nerves if required: depot injection of 2 mL at a depth of 1–2 cm.

Surgery of the Maxillary Sinus

Endoscopy of the Maxillary Sinus (Sinuscopy, Antroscopy)

Surgical Principle

Transnasal puncture of the maxillary sinus with a trocar via the lower meatus, or *transoral* puncture through the canine fossa.

This allows exploration of the entire maxillary sinus using fine rigid scopes with various viewing angles. Tissue biopsies may be taken using instruments introduced either through the sleeve or using a combined transnasal and transoral approach.

Indications

- Culture swab for suspected mycosis or immune suppression.
- Biopsy for suspected malignancy.
- Cyst excision.

Contraindications

As a rule, the transnasal route should be adopted in children to avoid damage to the unerupted teeth.

Anesthesia

Local anesthesia. *Transnasal* decongestion of the nose. Lidocaine spray to the middle turbinate and in the lower meatus. A ribbon gauze soaked in local anesthetic is placed in the lower meatus. *Enough time (ca. 5 minutes) should be allowed for the onset of action.* An additional depot of 1 mL 1 % lidocaine may be administered to the nasal floor for a vasoconstrictive effect.

Depot injection of 1 % lidocaine with the addition of a vasoconstrictor *transorally* into the canine fossa.

Positioning is semi-supine or supine.

Instruments

Square-end trocar for children and adults. Sinoscopes with 0°, 25°, 30°, 70°, and 120° viewing angles, biopsy grasping forceps if required, flexible forceps, small scissors, and pediatric scopes.

Surgical Technique

Transnasal approach (**Fig. 7.4a–d**). The head of the inferior turbinate is visualized and displaced with the speculum. The trocar is inserted into the *inferior meatus to its highest point, roughly in the middle*. Careful pressure is exerted in the direction of the lateral canthus until the bony lamella is perforated. The heel of the operating hand is supported on the patient's cheek, while the other hand applies counter-support to the patient's head.

Transoral approach (**Fig. 7.4e**). The lip is raised laterally over the canine tooth. The upper border of the canine fossa is identified by palpation with the left index finger (ca. 1 cm below the infraorbital nerve). Here the trocar pierces the mucous membrane and is drilled into the facial maxillary wall using *rotary movements in a strictly sagittal direction*. The heel of the hand is simultaneously supported on the cheek. The trocar sleeve is then advanced a little further with twisting movements. Then as in the transnasal approach.

Postoperative Care

The patient should avoid nose-blowing with occlusion of both nostrils for 2–3 days and press the hand against the cheek during any inadvertent sneezing.

> **! Risks and Complications**
> - Injury to the wall of the maxillary sinus, orbit, retromaxillary space with bleeding, abscess formation, phlegmon, thrombophlebitis, and eye symptoms.
> - Air emboli have never been reported, although they cannot be completely ruled out.
> - Surgical emphysema, paraesthesias, hypaesthesias and neuralgia in the distribution of the second branch of the trigeminal nerve, buccal phlegmon, and abscess formation after using the transoral approach.

Endonasal Enlargement of the Maxillary Ostium

Surgical Principle

Endonasal enlargement of the maxillary ostium to the middle meatus for aeration and improvement of drainage.

Indications

- Incipient complication of an acute maxillary sinusitis.
- Acute recurrent maxillary sinusitis.
- Chronic maxillary sinusitis.
- Cysts and mucoceles.

Specific Points Regarding Informed Consent

- Postoperative bleeding.
- Injury to the nasolacrimal duct.
- Paraesthesias in the region of the canines and incisors from an opening created too far forward, damage to the unerupted teeth in children.

Operative Planning

Nasal endoscopy, conventional radiography of the paranasal sinuses, CT if appropriate.

Anesthesia

Local anesthesia or general endotracheal anesthesia.

Special Instruments and Implants

Endoscopes (0°, 30°, 45°, 70°) (**Fig. 7.5**), microscope (250- or 300-mm lens), ethmoid or Blakesley forceps, forward- and backward-oblique bone punches, Freer elevator, and microdisk knife.

Endoscopic Technique for Endonasal Enlargement of the Maxillary Ostium

Positioning. The head is not reclined and the upper body of the patient is slightly elevated. The surgeon sits or stands on the right of the patient.

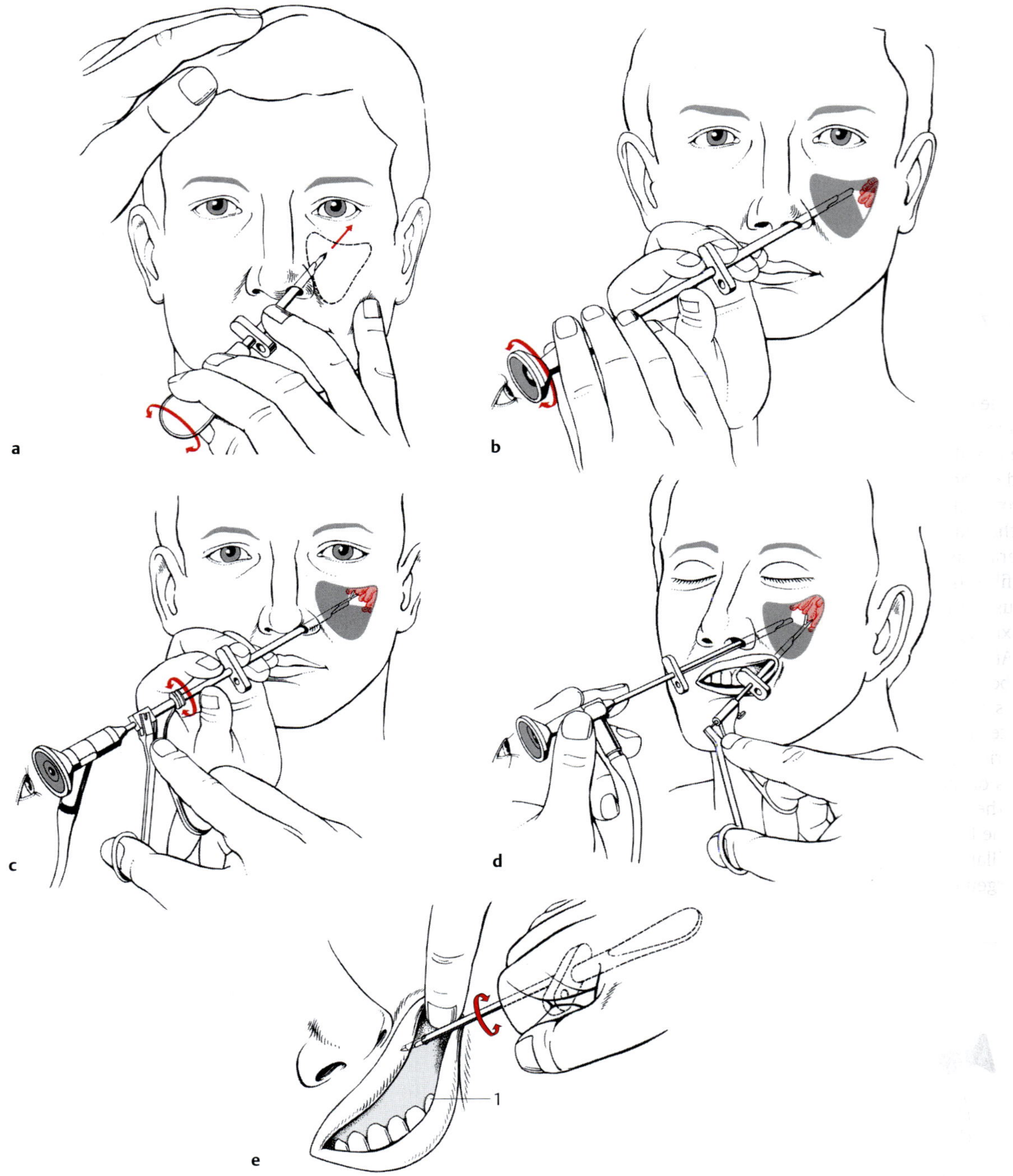

Fig. 7.4a–e Transnasal and transoral sinuscopy.
a Perforation of the lateral nasal wall using short counter-rotating movements. The hand is supported on the cheek.
b Inspection of the maxillary sinus after turning the optical trocar.
c Polypectomy in the maxillary sinus using rigid optical forceps.
d Biopsy of the maxillary sinus using a combined approach. Optical trocar nasal; forceps transoral.
e Transoral sinuscopy. Sagittal approach in the lateral canine fossa and above the canine tooth (1).

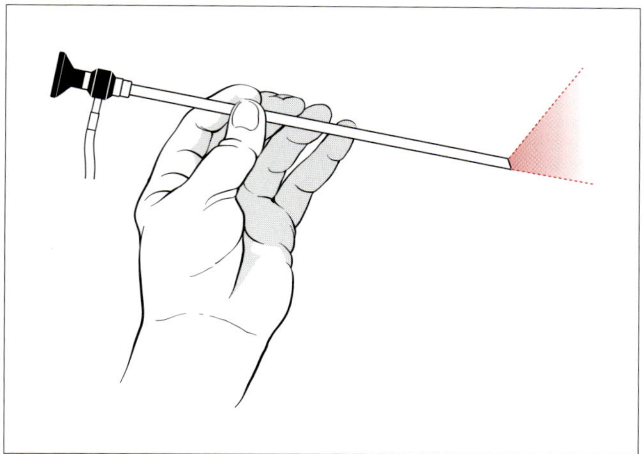

Fig. 7.5 Holding the endoscope.

The middle turbinate is displaced medially under endoscopic vision without fracturing it. The posterior fontanelle region of the maxillary sinus is identified dorsally, just above the dorsal end of the uncinate process (**Figs. 7.6** and **7.7b**). The fontanelle is covered medially by nasal mucosa and laterally by the mucosa of the maxillary sinus, and as such is a bone-free region of the lateral nasal wall. The two mucous membranes are connected by fibrous tissue. Accessory ostia also drain into the maxillary sinus via the fontanelle and may also be used to enlarge the maxillary ostium (**Fig. 7.7a, b**).

After gently penetrating the fontanelle with an angled suction probe or an angled Blakeley forceps, the lumen of the maxillary sinus becomes visible, allowing it to be enlarged with an appropriate punch (backward-oblique bone punch, **Fig. 7.8**) superiorly, anteriorly, and inferiorly. By using various scopes (30°, 70°), all areas of the lumen of the maxillary sinus can now be assessed and the pathological lesion removed with appropriate forceps.

The hiatus semilunaris is left untouched when enlarging the maxillary ostium. If an accessory maxillary ostium is present, the enlargement should be accomplished via the accessory ostium.

The creation of a second enlarged ostium should be avoided, otherwise recirculation of mucus via both ostia will occur.

A loose nasal pack is inserted at the end of the operation.

Microscopic Technique for Enlargement of the Maxillary Ostium

The patient is positioned supine on the operating table. After displacement of the middle turbinate (without fracturing it), the medial wall of the maxillary sinus is gently penetrated between the back end of the lower turbinate over the region of the fontanelle with a curved suction probe or an angled Blakesley forceps. The further procedure is identical to that of the endoscopic operation.

! Risks and Complications

- Postoperative bleeding from the sphenopalatine artery after enlarging the ostium too far dorsally.
- Injury to the nasolacrimal duct.
- Paraesthesias in the region of the canine and incisor teeth, from enlarging the ostium too far anteriorly.
- Damage to the unerupted teeth in children, which must be avoided.

Surgery of the Ethmoid

Surgical Principle

The contents of the ethmoid sinus are removed using an endonasal approach after dislocating the middle turbinate in a medial direction. An *infundibulotomy (partial ethmoidectomy)* involves only the anterior parts of the ethmoid.

A complete sphenoethmoidectomy (pansinus operation) involves removing all pathological mucosa from the entire ethmoid cell system, including the sphenoid sinus, the maxillary sinus, and the access to the frontal sinus (**Fig. 7.9**). The optimal

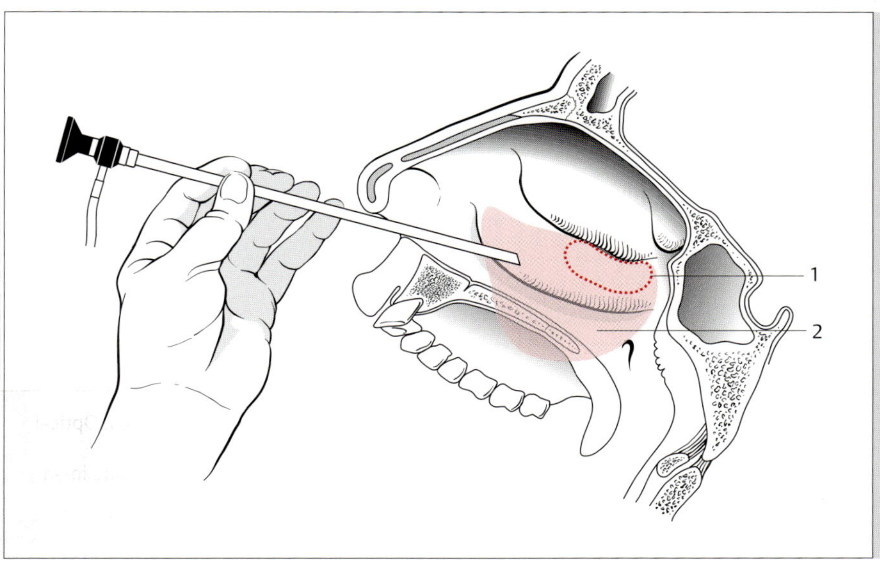

Fig. 7.6 Endoscopic enlargement of the maxillary sinus ostium.
1 location of the enlarged maxillary sinus ostium (shaded red)
2 extent of the maxillary sinus

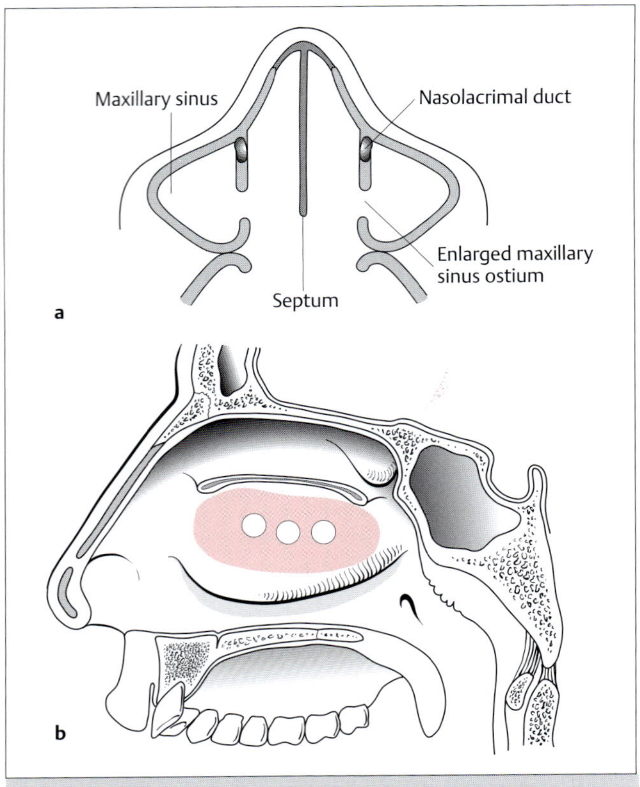

Fig. 7.7a, b Position of the enlarged maxillary sinus ostium.
a Position is axial to the nasolacrimal duct.
b Position of the fontanelle and the accessory ostia after resection of the vertical part of the middle turbinate.

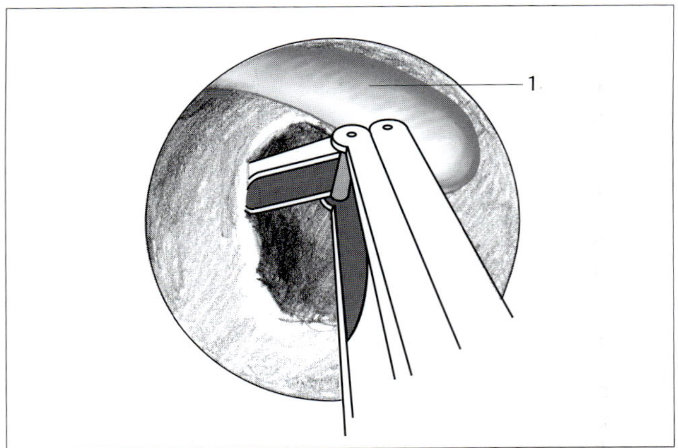

Fig. 7.8 Widening of a maxillary sinus ostium on the right with a back-biting punch. View through the endoscope.
1 posterior end of the middle turbinate

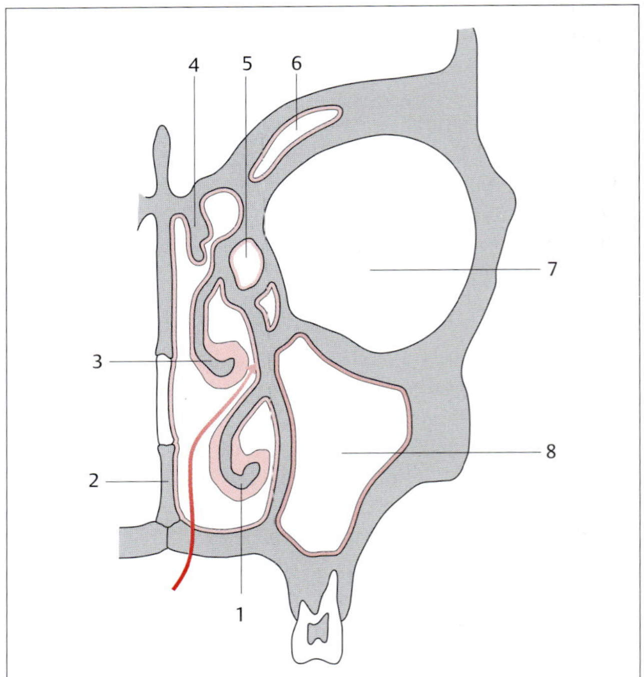

Fig. 7.9 Endonasal approach to the ethmoid cells.
1 inferior nasal turbinate
2 nasal septum
3 middle nasal turbinate
4 superior nasal turbinate
5 ethmoid cells
6 frontal sinus
7 orbit
8 maxillary sinus

preservation of healthy mucous membrane is essential, which is why the use of punching instruments is important.

Infundibulotomy

Surgical Principle

Endonasal enlargement of the ethmoid infundibulum by removing the uncinate process, and if necessary opening the ethmoid bulla to aerate and drain the downstream paranasal sinuses. Maximal protection of affected mucous membranes is essential, especially at anatomical bottlenecks.

Indications

- Acute, acute recurrent, and chronic nasal parasinusitis, especially in the region of the anterior ethmoid cells and the frontal and the maxillary sinuses without any significant changes to the mucous membranes.
- Mucoceles.

Contraindications

- Pronounced nasal polyposis involving the entire paranasal sinus region.
- Bleeding tendency and coagulopathies that are irreversible or therapy-resistant.

Specific Points Regarding Informed Consent

See Risks and Complications (p. 117).

Anesthesia

Local anesthesia with a topical anesthetic or general endotracheal anesthesia.

Instruments

Microscope, rigid scopes, ethmoid forceps, bone punches, curette, Freer elevator.

Endoscopic Surgical Technique

After decongestion of the nose, the free edge of the uncinate process is exposed and an incision is made around it. Starting cranially, just below the insertion of the middle turbinate, the incision is extended dorsally to the level of the maxillary sinus ostium (**Fig. 7.10a**). The medial wall of the infundibulum is then removed. From here, any obstructing processes, such as a medial-leaning uncinate process or infundibular wall, are corrected.

If the ethmoid bulla is protruding and thus causing an obstruction (**Fig. 7.10b**), it is gently penetrated with a blunt ethmoid forceps and its wall removed. Any more far-reaching polyposis is pursued into the ethmoid sinus. The prevailing mucosal appearance and the anatomical situation will determine whether a supraturbinal fenestration of the maxillary sinus is indicated.

A pack attached to a thread is then inserted into the middle meatus and left for a day.

Endoscopic–Microscopic Infundibulotomy

After decongestion of the nose, the middle turbinate is retracted medially with the speculum. A self-retaining speculum is then inserted (**Fig. 7.11**). The free edge of the uncinate process is easily identified under the microscope. As with the endoscopic operation, an incision is made around the uncinate process with

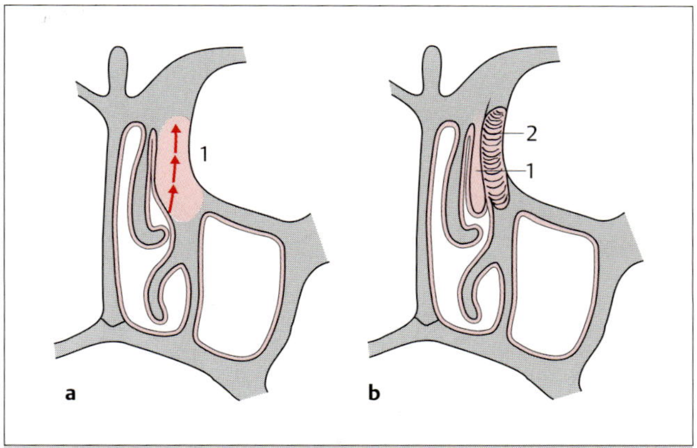

Fig. 7.10a, b Schematic presentation of an incision around the uncinate process (**a**). Direction of the incision (1). The ethmoid bulla becomes visible further dorsally (**b**).
1 uncinate process displaced to one side
2 ethmoid bulla

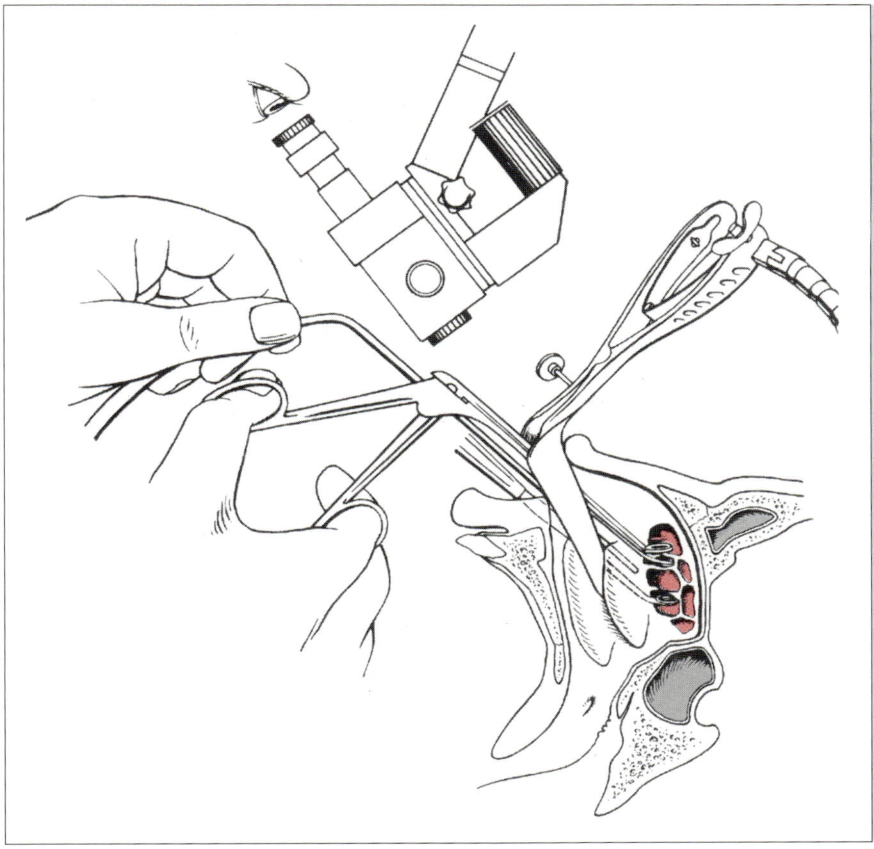

Fig. 7.11 Endoscopic surgery of the paranasal sinuses using the microscope. Endonasal surgery of the ethmoid. Removal of the contents of the cell system under the microscope using the double-spoon forceps and Volkmann curette.

a Freer elevator (**Fig. 7.12**) and it is removed with a Blakesley forceps. After removal of the uncinate process, residual parts of the ethmoid infundibulum now lie exposed cranially.

A pack attached to a thread is then inserted into the middle meatus and left for a day.

Endonasal Surgery of the Ethmoid

Surgical Principle

Removal of the contents of the ethmoid cells via an endonasal approach within their anatomical borders: ethmoid roof, medial turbinate, orbital roof, and lamina papyracea (**Figs. 7.13** and **7.14**).

The anterior ethmoid is exposed as far as the basal lamella of the middle turbinate, whereas the posterior ethmoid is accessible only after penetrating the basal lamella.

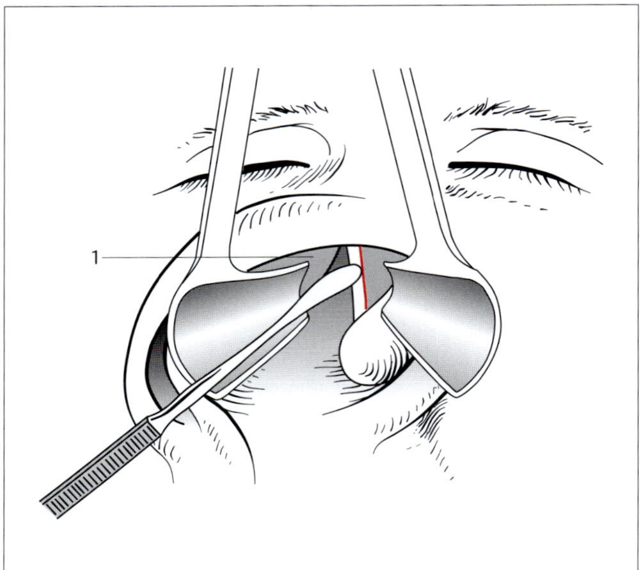

Fig. 7.12 Microscopical incision around the uncinate process using a Freer elevator.
1 middle turbinate retracted medially.

Indications

- Acute and chronic sinusitis.
- Orbital complications of sinusitis.
- Intracranial complications of sinusitis.
- Drainage of muco-, pyo-, and pneumatoceles.
- Trauma: extensive fracture of the ethmoid, fracture of the anterior cranial base, and/or decompression of the optic nerve.
- Tumors.
- Access to the orbit.

Endoscopic Surgical Technique

Positioning and preparation. As for an endoscopic operation. The patient is positioned supine with the upper part of the body slightly raised (20°). The surgeon sits or stands on the right of the patient, while the scrub nurse is positioned on the left side of the patient.

The middle turbinate is identified with a 0° or 25° scope, a crescent-shaped convex incision is made around the uncinate process, which is then removed using rotary movements to avoid tearing the mucosa in a caudal or cranial direction. The ethmoid bulla, which bulges out antero-inferiorly, is opened using a Blakesley forceps and the lumen is displayed (see Infundibulotomy, p. 118). The retrobullar recess and the suprabullar recess may be found dorsal to and above the bulla, respectively.

To open the posterior ethmoid sinus, the basal lamella of the middle turbinate is perforated anteriorly, ca. 3–4 mm above the dorsal third of the basal lamella. The individual ethmoid cells, which are bordered by a few bony septa, are then removed with a curved Blakesley forceps or with ethmoid punches. The roof

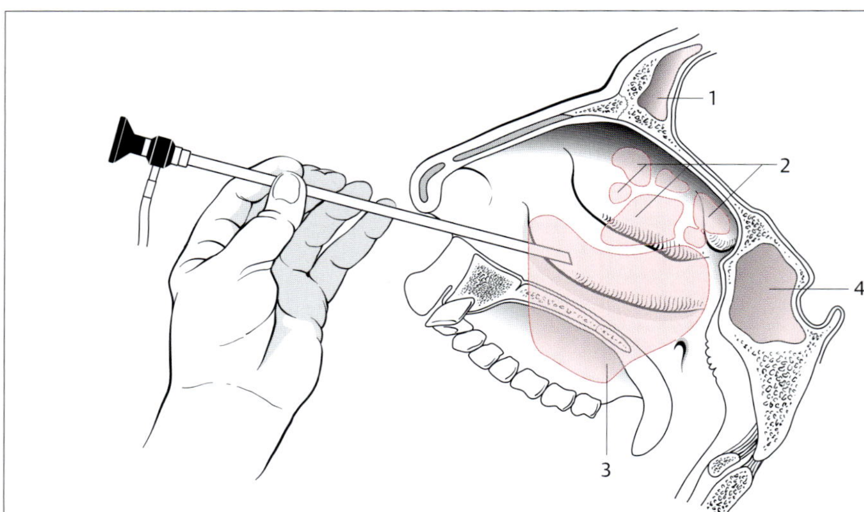

Fig. 7.13 Projection of the paranasal sinuses onto the lateral nasal wall.
1 frontal sinus
2 ethmoid sinus
3 maxillary sinus
4 sphenoid sinus

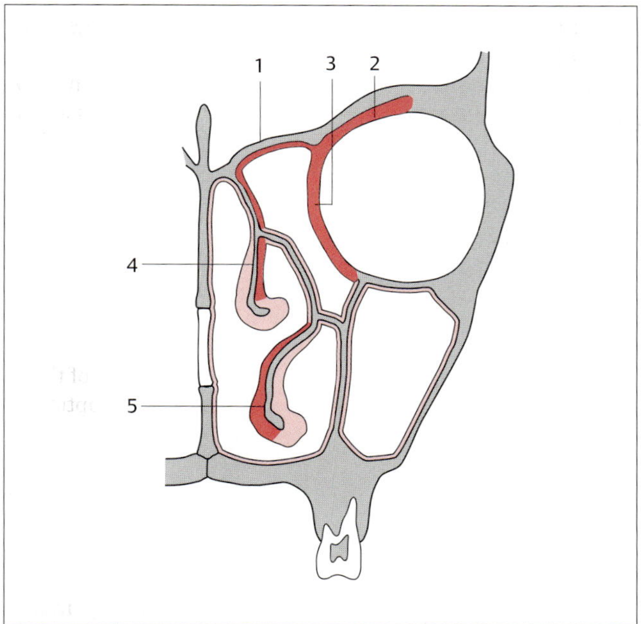

Fig. 7.14 Boundaries of surgery of the ethmoid.
1 ethmoid roof
2 orbital roof
3 lamina papyracea
4 middle nasal turbinate
5 low nasal turbinate

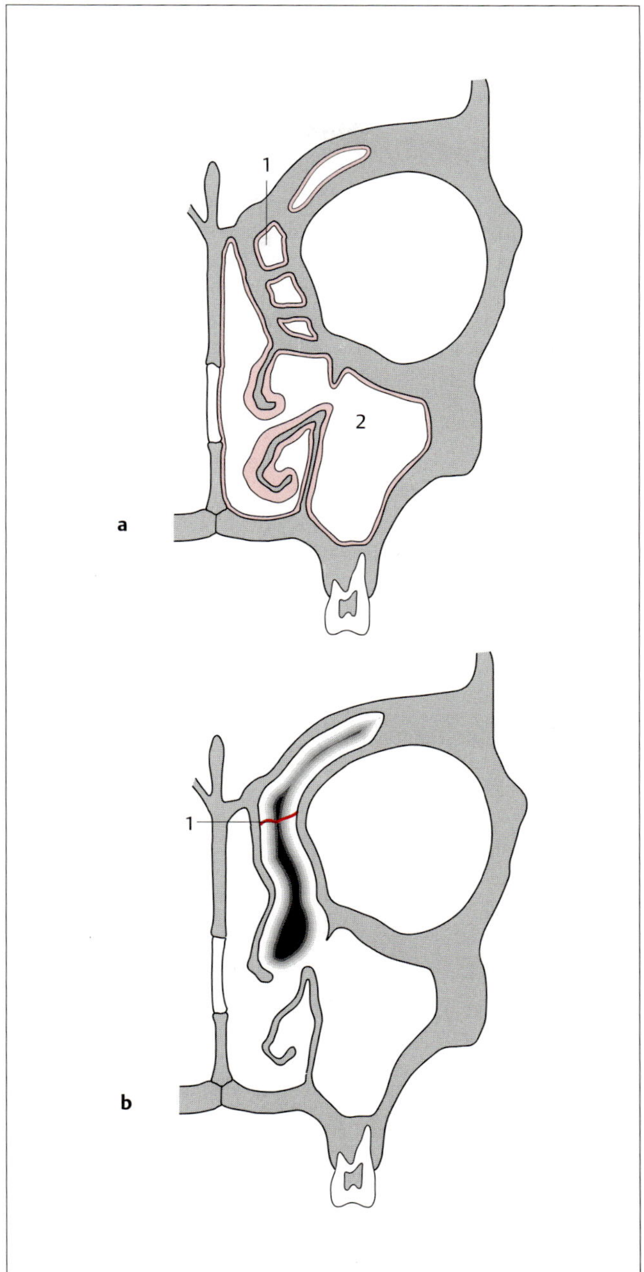

Fig. 7.15a, b Principle of endonasal ethmoidectomy.
a Wide enlargement of the maxillary sinus ostium and opened ethmoid bulla.
1 ethmoid cells
2 enlargement of the maxillary sinus ostium
b Ethmoid cells after removal of their contents.
1 anterior ethmoid artery in projection

of the ethmoid is then identified, paying due regard to the bony landmarks—the middle turbinate medially and the lamina papyracea laterally (**Fig. 7.15a, b**).

Attention should be directed to a possible attenuated lamina papyracea or to ethmoid cells, which extend far dorsally, so-called suprasphenoid Onodi cells. In the presence of Onodi cells, the ethmoid sinus will need to be identified further medially to protect the optic canal.

When removing the contents of the ethmoid cells anteriorly, care should be taken to identify the ethmoid arteries, which run transversely across the roof of the ethmoid.

After the contents of the ethmoid sinus are removed, the frontal sinus ostium can be identified ventral to the anterior ethmoidal artery, which runs horizontally (see Surgery of the Frontal Sinus, p. 123). A pack is inserted for 1 day.

Microscopic Surgical Technique

Positioning and preparation. The patient is positioned supine, with the head slightly lowered. The surgeon sits below the head on the contralateral side; depending on the direction of access, the patient's head will need to be turned toward or away from the surgeon (see Infundibulotomy, p. 118). For work on the anterior ethmoid region it is important that the head is reclined as far as possible.

As a rule, it is recommended that surgical landmarks and anatomical borders are identified when performing microscopic surgery of the ethmoid, as well as for endoscopic ethmoid surgery.

Surgery of the Sphenoid

Endonasal Opening of the Sphenoid Sinus

Surgical Principle

Removal of the anterior wall of the sphenoid sinus converts it into a wide open secondary nasal sinus. Removal of the mucous membranes is undertaken only to the extent that is absolutely necessary, and should also be performed extremely conservatively in the region of the optic nerve. Access to the sphenoid sinus can be endonasal, trans-septal, or transethmoidal.

Indications

- Acute and chronic isolated sphenoid sinusitis.
- Acute and chronic parasinusitis.
- Irradication of the underlying focus of ocular complications (retrobulbar neuritis, optic neuritis, cavernous sinus thrombosis).
- Exploration and biopsies for suspected tumors.
- Mucocele formation in the region of the sphenoid sinus.
- Cerebrospinal fluid (CSF) fistula in the sphenoid region.

Operative Planning

Thin-slice CT or MRI.

Special Instruments

Mushroom punch (see below) and other punches.

Anesthesia

General endotracheal anesthesia.

Surgical Technique

Transethmoidal approach. At first the contents of the entire ethmoid sinus are removed. Next, the anterior wall of the sphenoid sinus is identified, further medial and caudal to the ethmoid cells which have already been opened and emptied of their contents. The ethmoid cells are gently perforated with an elevator or grasping forceps. Use of an angled punch or a mushroom punch is recommended for the removal of further parts of the anterior wall (**Fig. 7.16**).

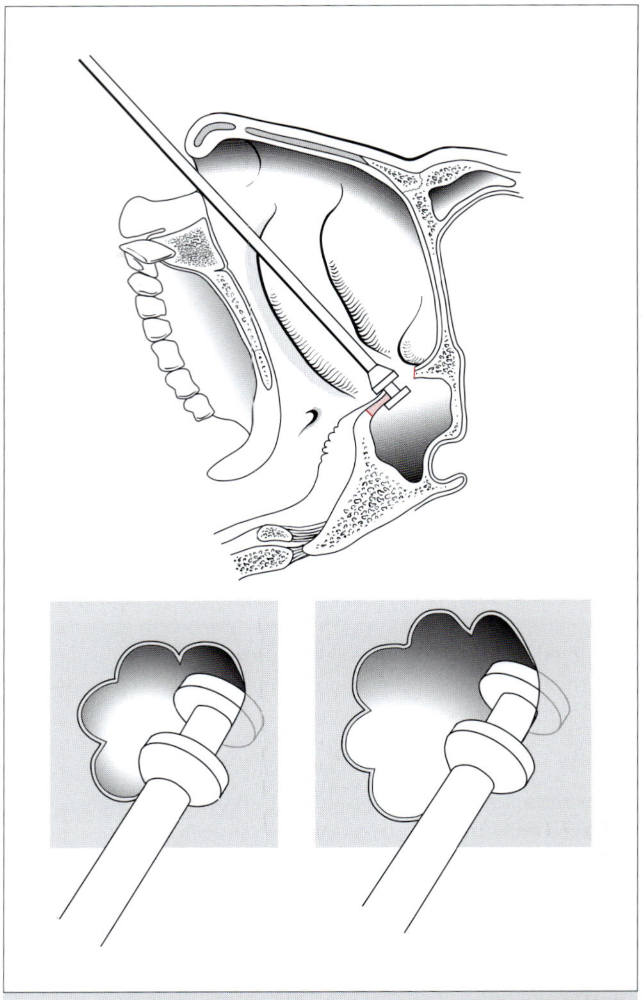

Fig. 7.16 Schematic illustration of transethmoidal enlargement of the sphenoid sinus ostium (modified after Stammberger). Removal of the anterior wall of the sphenoid sinus with a mushroom punch.

Transnasal approach. Decongestion of the nose. The posterior part of the middle turbinate is retracted laterally under direct endoscopic view (**Fig. 7.17**). The mucosa is swept off the anterior wall of the sphenoid sinus. The sphenoid sinus ostium is identified. The anterior wall of the sphenoid sinus is gently penetrated with light pressure ca. 1 cm above the turbinate, lateral to the septum. The anterior wall of the sphenoid sinus is then removed piecemeal with a punch.

Trans-septal approach. The trans-septal approach to the sphenoid sinus initially requires the temporary removal of the bony nasal septum and resection of the superior part of the vomer. After careful elevation of the mucous membranes off the vomer, the vomerine plate is mobilized by careful movements to and fro with forceps or Blakesley forceps, and removed. The anterior wall of the sphenoid sinus is mobilized with a careful horizontal tap of the chisel ca. 5 mm below the nasal roof, and a further blow ca. 1 cm lower and parallel. The two fracture lines are joined with two cuts placed at right angles to them to remove the bony plate, which is now mobile (**Fig. 7.18**). The pathological lesion is now removed via this opening in the anterior wall.

When removing the anterior wall of the sphenoid sinus, care should be taken not to remove it too far laterally and posteriorly, as it is possible to injure the internal carotid artery or the optic nerve, which both run here. Nor should the anterior wall be removed too far caudally and laterally, because of the course of the sphenopalatine artery.

A pack is then inserted.

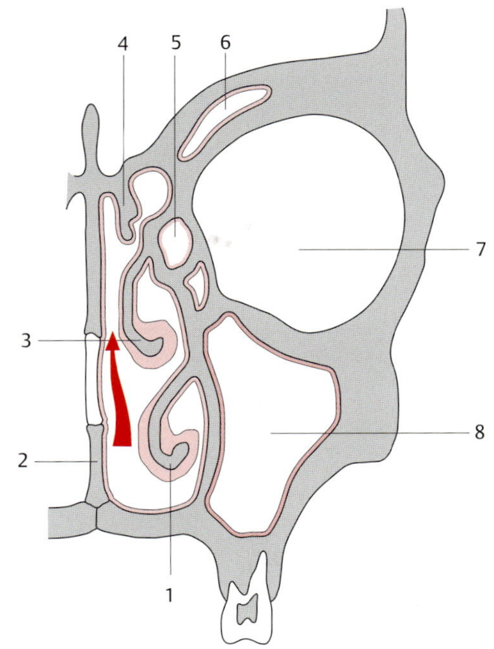

Fig. 7.17 Enlargement of the sphenoid sinus ostium; transnasal approach.
1 inferior nasal turbinate
2 nasal septum
3 middle turbinate
4 superior turbinate
5 ethmoid cells
6 left frontal sinus
7 orbit
8 maxillary sinus

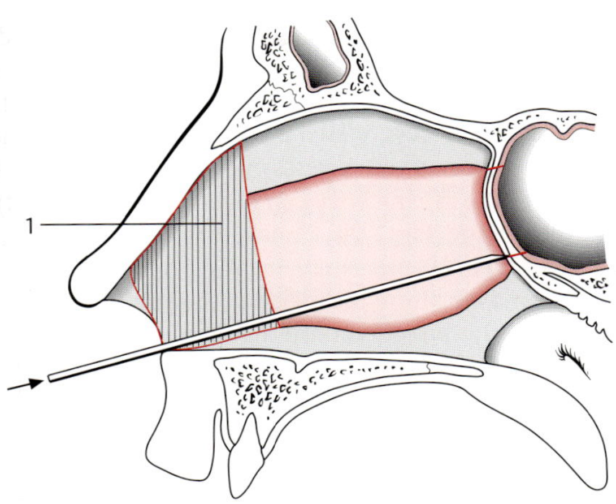

Fig. 7.18 Trans-septal enlargement of the sphenoid sinus ostium. The cartilaginous septum (1) remains intact.

Surgery of the Frontal Sinus

Endonasal Surgery of the Frontal Sinus

Surgical Principle

Transethmoid. Surgery in the region of the frontal recess to identify the frontal sinus ostium is usually performed during a *pansinus operation under endoscopic view* using curved punches, small forceps, and angled scopes, with as little traumatization as possible.

Apart from endoscopic operations, endonasal drainages of the frontal sinus (three types) using *Draf's micro-endoscopic surgical technique* are also described. The principle of *simple drainage of the frontal sinus (Draf Type 1)* involves the identification of the frontal recess, removal of its contents, and identification of the frontal sinus ostium.

The *Draf Type 2 extended drainage procedure* involves the removal of those parts of the frontal sinus that are obstructing the ostium (type 2A), and the removal of the floor of the frontal sinus, from the medial border of the orbit to the nasal septum, anterior to the level of the posterior wall of the frontal sinus (type 2B).

Draf Type 3 endonasal median drainage consists of the additional removal of the parts of the septum adjacent to the frontal sinus floor as well as the floor of the contralateral frontal sinus.

Indications

- Draf Type 1: Simple drainage of the frontal sinus for uncomplicated disturbances of aeration of those frontal sinuses with a wide natural ostium.

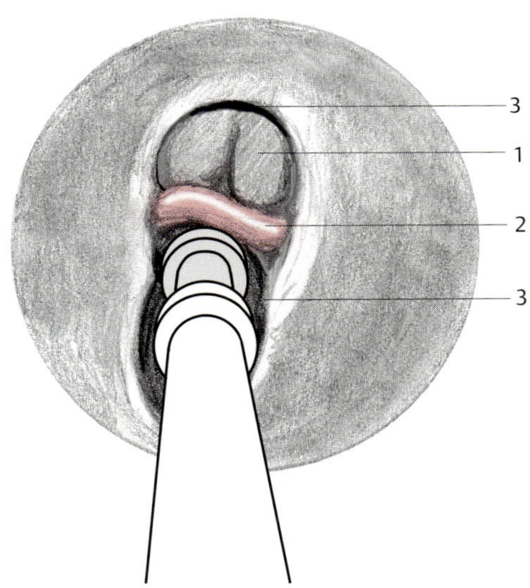

Fig. 7.19 Endonasal enlargement of the frontal sinus ostium. View through the endoscope.
1 frontal sinus ostium
2 anterior ethmoid artery
3 bone to be removed, cranial and posterior

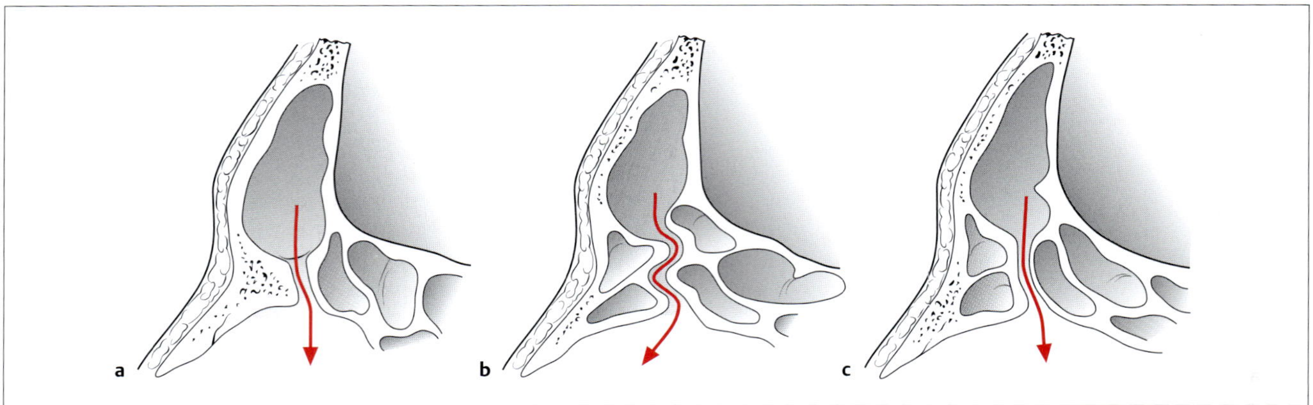

Fig. 7.20a–c Variations of development and position of the frontal recess (nasofrontal duct).

- Draf Type 2A: Removal of ethmoid cells obstructing the frontal recess to produce a natural wide funnel.
- Draf Type 2B: For recurrences and narrow ethmoid, small natural frontal sinus ostium.
- Draf Type 3: Reserved for revision surgery after acute and chronic sinusitis, mucoceles located far medially, and endocranial complications of sinusitis (cautious indication).

Anesthesia

General endotracheal anesthesia.

Instruments

Diamond burr, endoscope, operating microscope.

Surgical Technique

Endonasal. After removal of the uncinate process and, if appropriate, the ethmoid bulla, the frontal recess, which represents the uppermost front part of the anterior ethmoid sinus, is visualized. After identification of the frontal sinus ostium, which merges cranially into the infundibulum of the frontal sinus, the anterior ethmoid artery can be visualized, marking the limits of dissection. The anterior ethmoid artery usually runs in a bony canal across the roof of the ethmoid and through the ethmoid fovea toward the lamina cribrosa, dorsal to the frontal sinus ostium. The ostium should not be looked for too far medially, to avoid injury to the lamina cribrosa (skull base defect) (**Fig. 7.19**).

Any soft tissue obstructing the frontal sinus ostium should be removed with an angled forceps. Angled circular punches are also suitable for opening and enlarging a frontal sinus ostium obstructed by scarring. Removal of the mucous membrane lining the frontal sinus should be avoided as far as possible, to prevent the formation of circular scars.

Draf Type 2 drainage. According to Stammberger, there are three potential causes leading to obstruction of the frontal recess: the ethmoid bulla, agger nasi cells, and uncinate process. An uncinate process extending far cranially (terminal recess) may obstruct the frontal recess, as can an agger nasi cell aerated via the frontal recess. They can thus form a tubular duct located within the frontal recess, which is referred to as a nasofrontal duct. In these cases curved curettes or even circular punches are suitable for removing the bony cap together with the diseased mucous membrane (**Fig. 7.20**) ("uncapping the egg"; type 2A).

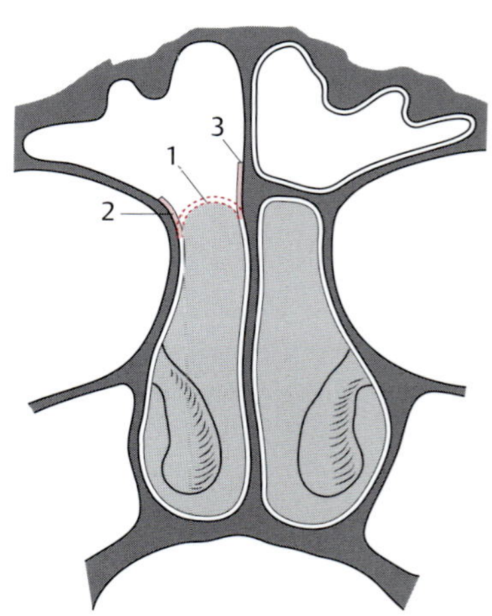

Fig. 7.21 Boundaries of frontal sinus drainage type 2B.
1 nasal roof
2 lateral cut edge of the mucosa
3 medial cut edge of the mucosa

The Draf Type 2B procedure involves removing the bone with a diamond burr from the region of the ethmoid infundibulum in an anterior direction until the floor of the frontal sinus has been opened. The anterior ethmoid artery runs transversely and should not be injured. If necessary, it should be microcauterized (**Fig. 7.21**).

Draf Type 3 drainage. With bilateral frontal sinus operations, access via the nose may be extended by removing the interfrontal septum, the medial parts of the floor of the frontal sinus, and the superior part of the nasal septum (**Fig. 7.22**). After completely removing the anterior wall of the frontal sinus situated in front of the duct, the interfrontal septum is trimmed

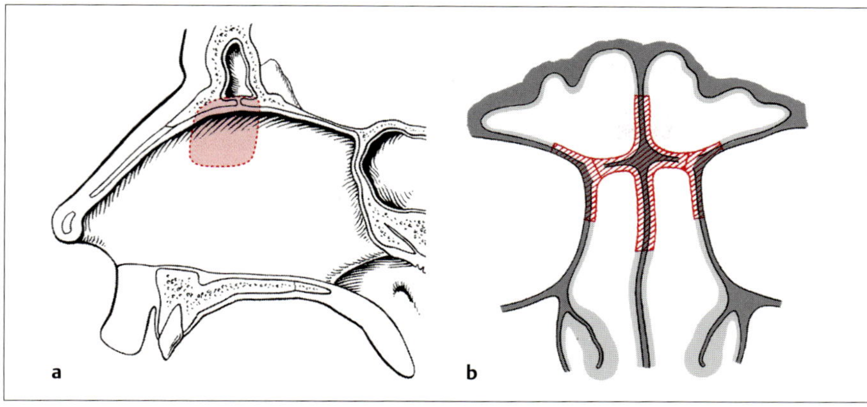

Fig. 7.22a, b Boundaries of endonasal midline drainage type 3.
a Lateral resection area.
b Frontal resection area.

off and the anterior wall of the frontal sinus is smoothed down with a burr. Then the uppermost part of the nasal septum is elevated along a submucous plane, excised, and the elevated septal mucosa is incised and inset as a rotation flap over the posterior and anterior bony parts of the thus created funnel.

! Risks and Complications

"Risky sphenoid" with displacement of the intersinus septum.

Rules, Tips, and Trickss

Dealing with Surgical Problems of Endonasal Surgery of the Paranasal Sinuses

- A CT scan of the paranasal sinus system must be obtained before surgery of the ethmoid and/or sphenoid sinus to assess the anatomic structures and determine the extent of the inflammatory process. Particular attention should be paid to:
  - location of the lamina cribrosa in relation to the ethmoid.
  - pneumatization of the ethmoid bulla to avoid perforating the lamina papyracea in the absence of pneumatization.
  - location of the bony optic canal (dehiscence in the bony encasement).
  - location of the internal carotid artery (dehiscence in the bony encasement).
  - variations of pneumatization.
- The eye is not covered during any surgery of the paranasal sinuses and the pupil is repeatedly checked during the operation. A palpatory and visual assessment is also recommended, to verify whether the globe demonstrates appropriate movement with traction or pressure with forceps.
- Any severe bleeding will require interruption of the operation and the insertion of a hemostatic tamponade.
- Globe protrusion secondary to a retrobulbar hematoma (avulsion of the anterior or posterior ethmoid artery). The anterior ethmoid artery runs across the roof of the ethmoid, in a small bony canal dorsal to the frontal recess. Avulsion of the anterior ethmoid artery may result in the orbital end of the artery retracting back into the orbital fat pad and so cause bleeding into the orbit. The posterior ethmoid artery runs across the roof of the ethmoid, in front of the wall of the sphenoid sinus. Injury to this artery can also cause retraction of the vessel stump, thus leading to the development of an intraorbital hematoma. The development of globe protrusion should prompt the immediate decompression of the orbit with release of the periorbita, given that intraorbital hemorrhage can lead to limited ocular motility and reduction or loss of visual acuity. An ophthalmological consultation is mandatory in this case.
- Injury to the lamina papyracea. Nose-blowing with occlusion of both nostrils should be strictly avoided.
- Dural defects. Dural defects identified by a postoperative CSF leak, should be managed immediately by dural repair (see Injuries to the Anterior Cranial Base, p. 145). However, not all defects are recognized immediately by a CSF leak. If the patient reports severe headache after surgery, a CT scan is indicated to exclude a pneumocephalus.
- Deterioration of visual acuity. Injury to the optic canal in the presence of so-called Onodi cells is a possibility. An Onodi cell is a posterior ethmoid cell extending far dorsally and cranially, in the lateral part of which the optic nerve runs. The sphenoid sinus is displaced further medially by the Onodi cell. A progressive deterioration of visual acuity postoperatively or pupillary dilation intraoperatively should prompt immediate evaluation of the optic canal and optic nerve decompression.
- Polyps in the olfactory groove medial to the middle turbinate. Polyps are not removed in their entirety from the olfactory groove, but are preferably sharply excised, carefully and gradually, until the superior meatus is visible (do not pull).
- Injury to the internal carotid artery within the roof of the sphenoid sinus. Immediate extensive packing of the operative site, compression on the ipsilateral carotid artery at the neck, and angiographic imaging of the course of the vessel. Depending on the angiographic results, ligation of the internal carotid artery may be necessary.
- Injury to the sphenopalatine artery. The sphenopalatine artery is at risk if removal of the anterior wall of the sphenoid cavity is extended too far laterally, caudal to the sphenoid. An attempt at coagulation may be made in an effort to stop the bleeding.
- Excision of the middle turbinate. Only indicated for:
  - concha bullosa: lateral hollow enlargement of the middle turbinate
  - a curl in the free edge of the middle turbinate in a lateral direction
  - polypoid changes to the head of the turbinate; the vertical part of the turbinate is preserved.

! Risks and Complications

Specific Points Regarding Informed Consent for Endonasal Surgery of the Paranasal Sinuses

- Bleeding into orbit and brain; bleeding from the internal carotid artery, or the anterior or posterior ethmoid artery.
- Orbital hemorrhage, postoperative bleeding.
- Deterioration of visual acuity to the extent of blindness, diplopia.
- Dural tear with CSF rhinorrhoea, meningitis, cerebral abscess, olfactory dysfunction or loss, dry nose.
- Injury to the nasolacrimal duct.
- Recurrence; formation of muco-, pyo-, or pneumatoceles; revision surgery.

Postoperative Care for Endonasal Surgery of the Paranasal Sinuses

- Perioperative IV antibiotics; continuing oral or IV antibiotics postoperatively depends on the initial findings.
- Regular suction of the wound cavity.
- Inhalation and application of a nasal ointment for approximately 8 days postoperatively to soften crust formations.
- Saline nasal irrigations.
- Prevention of the formation of synechiae.
- Topical steroids should be applied for up to 8 weeks postoperatively to treat underlying chronic inflammatory disorders.

Surgery of the Paranasal Sinuses, Combined with Extranasal Approaches

Transfacial Approach to the Maxillary Sinus

Surgical Principle

The Caldwell–Luc procedure has now been rendered obsolete by the further development of functional endoscopic sinus surgery. Nowadays only a modified form of transfacial osteoplastic maxillary sinus surgery is used. Diseased tissue is removed from the maxillary sinus after trephination of its facial wall, with partial preservation of the mucous membrane in the maxillary sinus.

Indications

- Recurrence after a Caldwell–Luc procedure.
- Multiple recurrences after endonasal surgery.
- Depressed fracture of the maxillary sinus.
- Ligation of the maxillary artery.
- Encapsulation of the maxillary sinus by mucocele formation.
- Cysts of the maxillary sinus: radicular and follicular dental cysts.
- Transmaxillary surgery of the pituitary gland.
- Access to the pterygopalatine fossa during transmaxillary surgery of the ethmoid/sphenoid sinus.
- Tumors of the maxillary sinus.

Contraindications

Children up to the end of the second dentition because of the danger of damage to the unerupted teeth.

Operative Planning

- CT.
- Sinuscopy.
- Nasal endoscopy.

Anesthesia

- General endotracheal anesthesia.
- Infiltration anesthesia using 1% lidocaine with the addition of a vasoconstrictor applied in the gingivolabial sulcus and from there in a fan-shaped pattern via the canine fossa as far as the infraorbital foramen. Additional injection in the region of the agger nasi around the maxillary ostium, after opening the maxillary sinus medially.

Instruments

A Langenbeck–Brüning or Hayek maxillary sinus retractor, Sternberg commissure retractor, rasp, drill with handpiece, hammer and chisel, Feldmann reciprocating saw or Lindemann burr.

Surgical Technique

Positioning. Upper part of the body flat or slightly elevated. The surgeon stands on the side that is to be operated on.

The assistant retracts the upper lip. A sublabial incision is made in the gingivolabial sulcus—over the alveolar ridge of the edentulous maxilla—extending from the second molar to the incisor. The scalpel is directed obliquely in order later to overlap the wound margins when closing. The periosteum is divided and raised with a broad elevator as far as the area medial and lateral to the infraorbital foramen, or if necessary slightly higher (as far as the base of the frontal process of the maxilla).

Rules, Tips, and Tricks

Dealing with Intra-operative Problems

The elevated soft tissues of the cheek should be held up with narrow retractors without crushing or stretching the infraorbital nerve.

A bony window is excised with a saw (alternatively, a round bony plate of approximately 1 cm diameter is chiselled out in the region of the canine fossa, ca. 1.5 cm below the intraorbital foramen). A bone flap is sawn out of the facial wall of the maxillary sinus using a reciprocating saw. First, two drill holes are created at diagonally opposite corners of the intended bone flap. Two cuts are made from each drill hole and the bone flap is removed in its entirety, to be replaced later and secured with sutures inserted through auxiliary drill holes. The objective is to prevent scar retractions of the cheek tissue *(Feldmann's osteoplastic operation of the maxillary sinus)* (**Fig. 7.23a–c**).

Via the transantral facial access, only areas of mucosa that appear irreversibly damaged are selectively grasped with forceps and removed. Any larger areas of mucosa that require removal are excised first. The remaining mucous lining prevents any subsequent tendency for scar contractures and new bone formation to develop. Damage to the alveolar nerve plexus with sensory dysfunction of the teeth is also avoided. Furthermore, the facial window is kept small and not created too far medially and superiorly to avoid endangering the anterior alveolar branch, which is situated in the bone of the anterior wall. If necessary, a window is created to gain access to the inferior and middle nasal meatus.

Rules, Tips, and Trickss

Dealing with Intra-operative Problems

- The primary incision in the oral vestibule must not be made too far caudally, otherwise there will not be enough mucous membrane available for closure.
- The infraorbital nerve is protected by gentle traction on the retractor and the avoidance of hematomas.
- The window to the inferior nasal meatus, if required, should made large enough, given that there is a tendency for considerable postoperative contracture.
- Closure is accomplished by passing the suture through both mucosa and periosteum.

! Risks and Complications

- Paraesthesias of the maxillary teeth, which are frequent (but sensory loss is not to be equated with loss of viability).
- Buccal hematoma, massive hemorrhage from the operative site (transmaxillary ligation of the maxillary artery and the sphenopalatine artery necessary).
- Buccal soft-tissue abscess or thrombophlebitis of the angular vein, inflammatory processes in the pterygopalatine fossa (the posterior wall of the maxillary sinus will need to be opened).
- Lacrimal drainage obstruction at the ostium of the nasolacrimal duct.
- Osteomyelitis of the maxilla.
- Transient, as well as persistent, trigeminal neuralgia.
- Anesthesia and paraesthesia in the distribution of the maxillary branch of the trigeminal nerve.
- Fistula formation in the region of the oral vestibule.
- Mucoceles of the maxillary sinus.
- Enophthalmus secondary to scar contracture (rare).
- Injury to the orbit due to penetration of the orbital wall.
- Scar contracture in the oral vestibule with dental problems secondary to contracture of the gingivolabial sulcus.

Postoperative Care

- See Postoperative Care for Endonasal Surgery of the Paranasal Sinuses.
- Do not allow maxillary dentures to be replaced until after the suture line has healed.

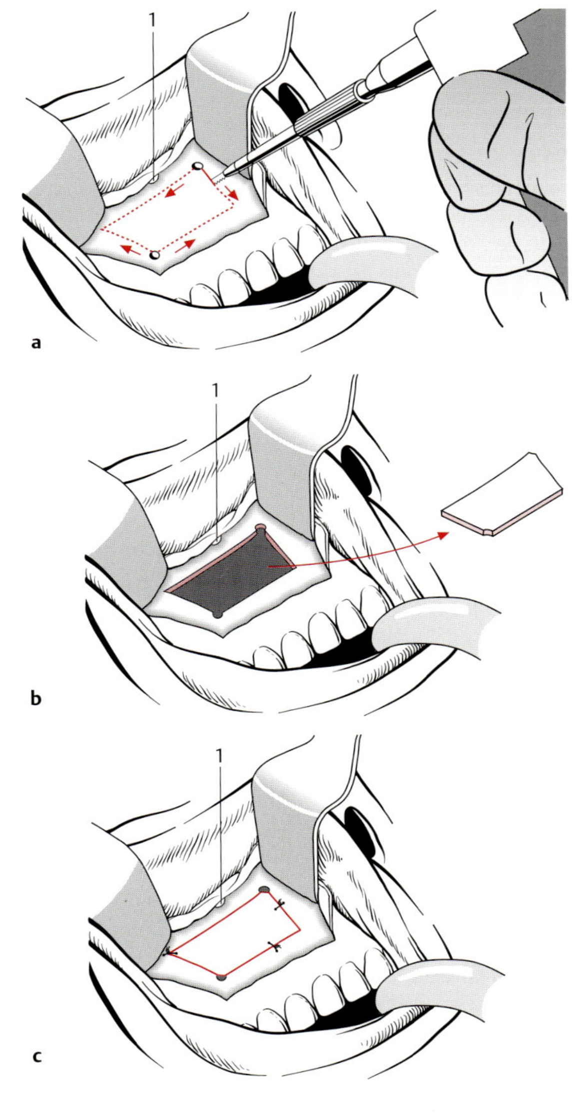

Fig. 7.23a–c Feldmann's transfacial osteoplastic operation of the maxillary sinus.
1 infraorbital foramen with infraorbital nerve

7

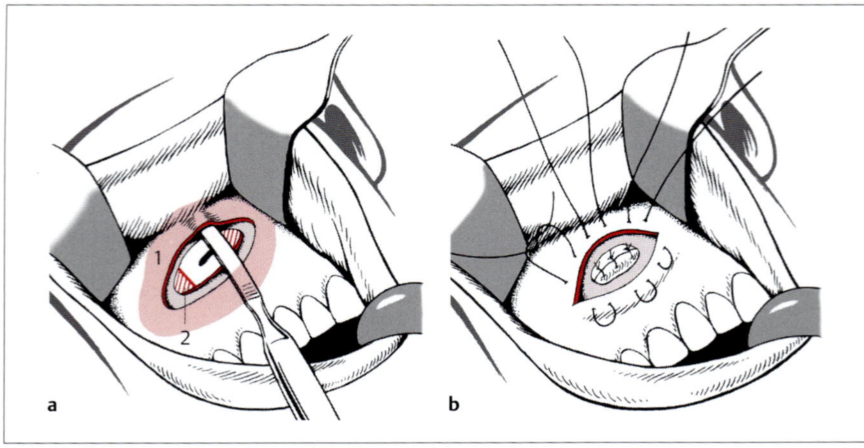

Fig. 7.24a, b Closure of an oral–maxillary sinus fistula.
a Elliptical excision.
1 extent of undermining
2 excisions
b Coverage of the buried fistula after undermining the surrounding mucosa.

7

- The patient should have soft foods for 8 days and should refrain from nose-blowing for 8 days.

Surgery of Oro-Antral Fistulas

According to their anatomical location, distinctions are made between the following forms of maxillary sinus fistula:

- *Oral–maxillary sinus fistula* between the maxillary sinus and the vestibulum (usually after surgery of the maxillary sinus.
- *Palatinal–maxillary sinus fistula*, usually after tooth extraction.

Fistula closure requires a careful plastic surgical approach with proper drainage, if required. The cause of the initial fistula within the maxillary sinus should always be removed.

Closure of an Oral–Maxillary Sinus Fistula

A asymmetrical spindle-shaped incision is made around the fistula, extending in a more superior direction. The incised mucous membrane is undermined as far as the edge of the fistula (**Fig. 7.24**). The lateral ends of the spindle are excised and the two sides of the flap are folded over and sutured together over the fistula with absorbable material. The outer margins of the excision are generously mobilized. The mucosa is advanced to cover the first line of sutures and closed with mattress sutures.

Closure of a Palatinal–Maxillary Sinus Fistula Using a Cheek Rotation Flap

Surgical Principle

Fistula coverage using a cheek rotation flap. The inner layer is formed from the incised oral mucosa next to the fistula. A rotation flap is elevated from the adjacent buccal mucosa to finally close the fistula. It is important to create a supraturbinal nasoantral window to aerate the maxillary sinus.

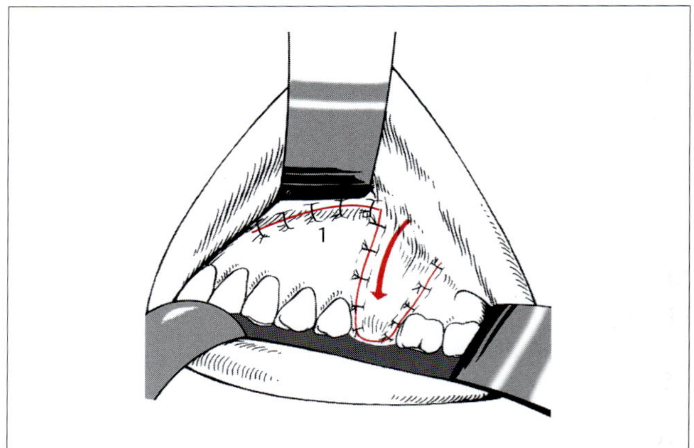

Fig. 7.25 Closure of a palatinal–maxillary sinus fistula with a cheek rotation flap (90°).
1 suture closure of the donor site

Indications

Persistent palatinal–maxillary sinus fistula.

Anesthesia

Local anesthesia; general endotracheal anesthesia for extensive removal of the initial cause of the fistula within the maxillary sinus.

Surgical Technique

Incision around the fistula. The edges of the fistula are undermined, the flaps are folded inward, and secured with inverted sutures.

A mucosal rotation flap is incised from the buccal mucous membrane, running toward the alveolar ridge, and elevated together with the periosteum (**Fig. 7.25**). A Burrow triangle is excised at the lateral end to allow the flap to be inset over the fistula without tension.

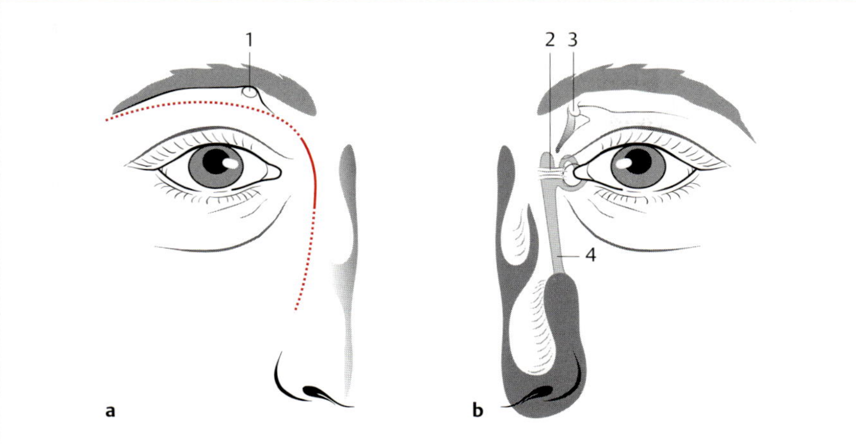

Fig. 7.26a, b External approach to the ethmoid.
a Incision and options for extending the incision.
b Important anatomical structures to be protected.
1 supraorbital nerve
2 medial palpebral ligament (medial canthal tendon)
3 trochlea and tendon of the superior oblique muscle
4 lacrimal drainage pathways with lacrimal duct and sac

Postoperative Care

- Enteral nutrition for a few days of to protect the suture, followed by liquid–semisolid food.
- Antibiotics.

Surgery of the Ethmoid Sinus Using an External Approach (Transfacial)

Surgical Principle

Access to the ethmoid sinus via the lateral nasal pyramid.

Indications

Access via the lateral nasal pyramid:
- Orbital and intracranial complications secondary to an ethmoiditis.
- Revision surgery after previous endonasal operations.
- Simultaneous surgery of the maxillary sinus from an external approach.
- Osteomas.
- Surgery with difficult anatomical conditions involving the ethmoid sinus.
- Extensive trauma to the ethmoid sinus (medial blow-out fracture, fracture of the anterior cranial base).

Operative Planning

High-resolution CT using axial and coronary slice orientation.

Anesthesia

General endotracheal anesthesia.

Surgical Principle

Removal of the contents of the ethmoid sinus and creation of a single sinus, with access via the bony nasal pyramid. This provides the best possible visualization of the ethmoid and allows extensive removal of its contents. There is less risk of collateral damage. The visible scar is a disadvantage.

Operative Planning

CT, image guidance if appropriate.

Special Instruments and Implants

Reciprocating micro-saw, hammer, chisel, operating microscope. A diamond drill is recommended in addition to the usual ethmoid forceps, punches, and chisels. Otic microscope and ear instruments.

Anesthesia

Usually general endotracheal anesthesia, plus the additional infiltration of a vasoconstrictor into the surgical area. The internal nose should be decongested with ribbon gauze soaked in xylometazoline. Positioning is supine and flat. The surgeon stands next to the patient on the side to be operated on, or alternatively at the head end with the head hyperextended.

Surgical Technique

The skin incision is a lateral rhinotomy incision, extended immediately below the medial lower angle of the eyebrow and slightly curved to the level of the lower orbital margin, with a possible further extension laterally (**Fig. 7.26**). Vessels are cauterized, especially the angular artery. The soft tissue, together with the periosteum, is raised with an elevator as far as the dorsum of the nose and the nasolacrimal duct, which can be mobilized out of the lacrimal fossa by releasing the medial palpebral ligament. A globe protector is then inserted. The anterior part of the periorbita is displaced off the lamina papyracea. Dissection is extended superiorly only as far as the trochlea, which is not detached. An oval window, corresponding to the size of the soft-tissue incision, is created in the bone using a burr or punch (the bone in the lacrimal fossa is gently penetrated) (**Fig. 7.27**). An alternative option is to saw out a bone flap. A rounded, straight, or curved forceps is inserted into the opened ethmoid and gradually advanced down to the base. The further removal of the ethmoid contents is always done parallel to the skull base. Here too, the use of a microscope deep within the operating field offers a significantly better degree of visualization and greater safety during this types of operation. Removing the bony septa will create a cavity that is bordered medially by the medial turbinate and laterally by the globe and the orbital plate of the ethmoid bone.

Special care is required for the subsequent removal of the contents of the periorbital ethmoid cells between the orbital roof and the lesser wing of the ethmoid, because of the close proximity of the optic nerve. When a microscope is used, significantly better visualization may be achieved by moving it to the contralateral side. Before removal of the bony septa between the ethmoidal air cells, it is recommended to first explore the walls and recess by palpation with a probe. Thorough removal of the contents of the anterior ethmoid cells will allow exposure of the access to the frontal sinus. The bony flap is replaced in the manner described above for the osteoplastic maxillary sinus procedure. If no bone flap is elevated, a periosteal suture should be placed for better stability. Deep subcutaneous sutures are then inserted using absorbable material. The skin is closed using either an intracutaneous suture or 5/0 monofilament suture material. Loose packing is applied via the nose.

Extranasal Surgery of the Frontal Sinus

Of all the frontal sinus operations using an external approach, and the various conventional methods used for surgery of the frontal sinus, the Jansen–Ritter technique and the osteoplastic frontal sinus procedure are now regarded as standard. The creation of median drainage requires a special indication. Riedel's radical frontal sinus operation is practically never used nowadays.

Surgery of the Frontal Sinus Modified after Jansen–Ritter

Surgical Principle

A sub-brow incision is made. The bony floor of the frontal sinus is removed and the anterior wall in the region of the supraorbital margin is bevelled. The contents of the ethmoid cell system are removed. If the mucous membranes do not appear irreversibly damaged (i. e., only certain areas are affected), then only a partial removal is indicated and the remaining mucosa is left untouched. Irreversible damage to the mucous membranes will require their complete removal. A wide drain is placed and brought out through the nose.

Indications

- Refractory chronic frontal sinusitis.
- Mucoceles, pyoceles, orbital complications secondary to a frontal sinusitis.
- Depressed fractures and fractures of the anterior cranial base, small osteomas of the floor of the frontal sinus and in the region of its excretory duct.

Operative Planning

Thin-slice CT.

Anesthesia

General endotracheal anesthesia.

Special Instruments and Implants

Chisels, punches, forceps, probes, elevator, curette, diamond burr, loupes, microscope.

Surgical Technique

Positioning. Supine and flat. Do not shave the eyebrows, and leave the eye uncovered.

A curvilinear incision is made below the eyebrow, beginning medial to the supraorbital foramen, continuing over the middle of the lateral nasal wall and ending at the level of the infraorbital margin (**Fig. 7.26**). The incision also divides the periosteum. The incision line should be marked beforehand; vessels are coagulated or ligated. Using a rasp, the periosteum is swept off the frontal process of the maxilla and the nasal bone, as well as the lower part of the anterior wall over the floor of the nasal sinus, as far as the midline. The medial palpebral ligament is released with the rasp. The lacrimal sac is dissected out as far as its entry into the nasolacrimal duct. A globe protector is placed on the lateral wound margin. The anterior lamina papyracea is exposed using a rasp. A trephination is made in the floor of the

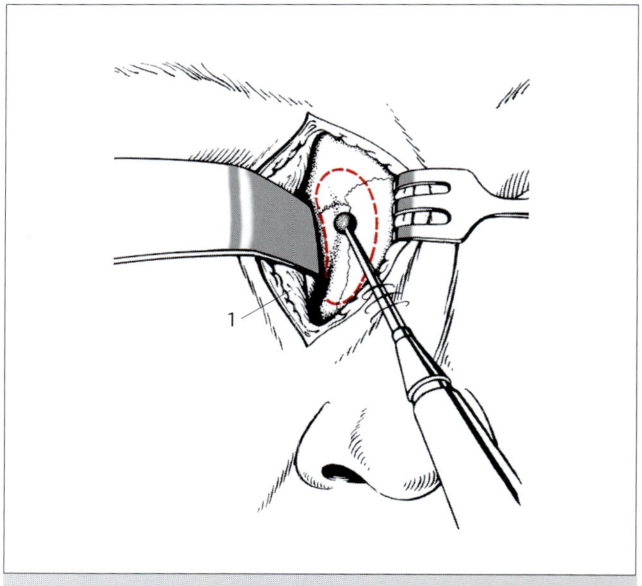

Fig. 7.27 Surgery of the ethmoid from an external approach. Mobilization of the nasolacrimal duct (1) and the periorbita. Trephination over the ethmoid bone.

frontal sinus in the inner angle of the orbit with a chisel or a burr and the floor is extensively removed with a Brüning punch (**Fig. 7.28**). The frontal process of the maxilla and the nasal bone are removed almost to the midline. Only a narrow margin of bone remains preserved inferiorly along the piriform aperture. The lacrimal bone and, if appropriate, the anterior part of the orbital lamina are removed using a punch, while the anterior border of the bony margin of the frontal bone is bevelled. The mucosa beneath the nasal bone and the frontal process of the maxilla is preserved. Using an elevator, the mucous membrane of the frontal sinus is carefully detached, as far as possible in one piece, beginning at the edge of the bone. Attention should be paid to any recesses that may be present and an endoscopic assessment should be considered. Any bony septa between the air cells, which are otherwise inaccessible, should be removed with a burr. If the mucosa only appears reversibly altered, then the operation may be restricted to removing any polyps or more severely degenerated areas and the remaining mucosa left intact.

If the ethmoid sinus demonstrates similar alterations, then removal of its contents follows that of the sphenoid. The cells in the region of the junction between frontal sinus and ethmoid should also be removed along the base. A large diamond burr is used to smooth out any bony protrusions in the proximity of the dura.

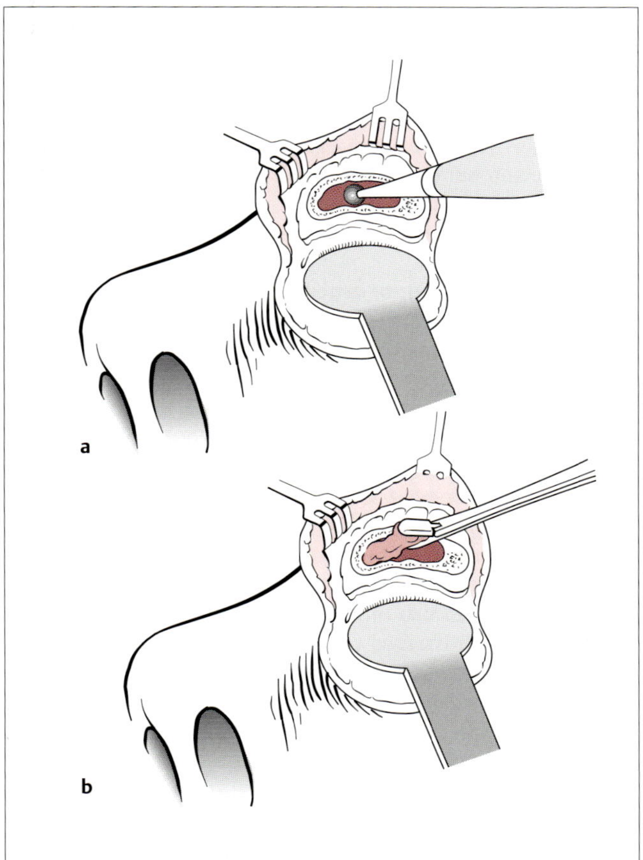

Fig. 7.28a,b Jansen–Ritter operation of the frontal sinus.

! Risks and Complications

- Injury to the dura of the posterior wall, especially there is a "risky frontal bone." The interfrontal septum is displaced laterally, next to which the protrusion of the olfactory crest is visualized. Any dural tear is repaired immediately. Diplopia arises as a result of detachment of the trochlea and may require later reconstruction.
- Orbital lesions, as with surgery of the ethmoid.
- Injury to the lacrimal duct.
- Anesthesia in the supraorbital region, secondary to division of the nerve.
- Neuralgias in the distribution of the supraorbital nerve.
- Keloid formation in the region of the scar; undesired scar development.
- Recurrent suppuration, ductal stenosis with the development of mucoceles and pyoceles.
- Scar contracture of the anterior wall of the frontal sinus secondary to too extensive resection of the anterior wall.
- Rejection of inserted spacers, largely because of the associated increased scar formation.

Postoperative Care

As for endonasal surgery of the paranasal sinuses.

Riedel's Radical Frontal Sinus Operation

Surgical Principle

Complete obliteration of the frontal sinus by removing the entire anterior wall and simultaneously removing the contents of the ethmoid.

Rare Indication

Osteomyelitis of the frontal bone.

! Risks and Complications

Considerable cosmetic impairment due to the forehead defect.

Rules, Tips, and Trickss

Dealing with Intra-Operative Problems

- Exact preoperative radiological assessment, given that the surgical interventions are decided by the size of the frontal sinuses.
- Special care should be taken with the surgical approaches to protect the lacrimal ducts and the supraorbital nerve.
- The frontal sinus should be explored with a probe after opening.
- Burrs should be used for the meticulous removal of the contents of the deeper and lateral recesses of the frontal sinuses.

- When temporarily detaching the trochlea and the obliquus superior tendon, it is recommended to detach the trochlea together with a fragment of bone and to reflect it medially. The advantage here is that at the end of the operation the displaced piece of bone can be refixated together with the trochlea. This measure avoids the postoperative development of diplopia.

Osteoplastic Surgery of the Frontal Sinus

Surgical Principle

Wide opening of the frontal sinus (good cosmetic result from the temporary removal of the entire anterior wall of the frontal sinus, which can either be removed completely or left pedicled on the periosteum). The mucosa of the draining ostium should remain untouched. There are several principal options for the initial incision.

Indications

- Surgically indicated management of intractable chronic rhinosinusitis of large frontal sinuses.
- Mucopyoceles *in large frontal sinuses.*
- Osteomas in the frontal sinus region.
- Extensive fractures of a large frontal sinus with dislocation of the bony fragments.
- Rhinogenic and endocranial complications.

Contraindications

Small frontal sinuses, comminuted fracture of the anterior wall of the frontal sinus.

Operative Planning

- High-resolution CT.
- Radiological assessment of the borders of the frontal sinus, using a plain radiograph to prepare a template of the shape of the sinus.

Anesthesia

General endotracheal anesthesia.

Special Instruments and Implants

Fine and standard burrs (with protective sleeve if appropriate), reciprocating saw, Raney clamps.

Surgical Technique

Positioning. With the patient flat and supine, the head is supported in a headrest. The surgeon stands or sits at the head end. With a bicoronal incision, consider shaving a hairless zone of 0.5–1 cm width along the incision.

Incision. *Sub-brow incision:* A curvilinear incision is made below the eyebrow, beginning medial to the supraorbital foramen (or possibly further laterally), continuing over the middle of the lateral nasal wall and ending at the level of the infraorbital margin. The incision also divides the periosteum. The incision line should be marked beforehand; vessels are coagulated and ligated (**Fig. 7.26**).

Bicoronal incision: Behind the hairline, extending from the pre-auricular region of one ear to the other at the level of the vertex. Hemostasis is achieved with Raney clamps, which also grasp a 2-cm margin of the drape. Spurting blood vessels are immediately ligated. *Do not divide the periosteum.* The galea is elevated beyond the supraorbital margins, partially by blunt dissection and protecting the insertion of the temporalis muscle. The supraorbital and frontal nerves are protected, while their bony foramina may be opened, leaving a cuff of bone around the nerves. This then allows the scalp to be mobilized still further in a caudal direction (**Fig. 7.29a**).

Dissection of the bone flap. The borders of the frontal sinus are marked out using either a wire pattern or a previously cut template following the occipitofrontal radiograph. The periosteum is incised with a 1–1.5 cm margin around the sinus borders thus determined, and elevated just beyond the markings. It is left untouched along the inferior margin of the frontal sinus (**Fig. 7.29**).

Drill holes are placed in the same manner as for raising the bone flap for the osteoplastic maxillary sinus operation and are then connected using the reciprocating saw. Alternatively, the frontal sinus may be opened inferomedially with a diamond burr and the bone flap elevated via this opening in a superior direction and back down again to the inferolateral end. Depending on the instruments available, a burr or a reciprocating saw is used to make an oblique cut (**Fig. 7.29d**), which will later provide the bone flap with an underlying shelf as support. A probe is used to sound out which direction the wall of the sinus takes. At the supraorbital margin, the burr cut is directed on either side another 0.5 cm into the base of the bone flap, which can then be elevated and prised out with a sturdy elevator. The bone flap remains hinged to the periosteum along the orbital margin.

The further procedure depends on the findings. Osteomas and mucoceles are removed, while protecting the mucosa. The nasofrontal duct remains untouched. During the osteoplastic frontal sinus procedure using a superior approach, removal of the contents of the ethmoid sinus can usually only be achieved in the region of the supraorbital cells. If required, any further removal must be done from an endonasal access.

The *osteoplastic obliteration of the frontal sinus*, with the complete removal of the mucosa, is only very rarely indicated. After radical removal of the mucosa, the frontal sinus is ground out with a diamond burr and thus de-epithelialized. The mucous membrane is also removed from the bone flap. The nasofrontal duct is dissected out, displaced toward the nose, inverted, and secured in position with fibrin glue. The cavity can now be obliterated with fat harvested from the abdominal wall via a periumbilical incision.

The bone flap is then returned to its original position. There then follows either a periosteal suture or the flap is secured with several Vicryl stitches after placing several appropriate drill holes.

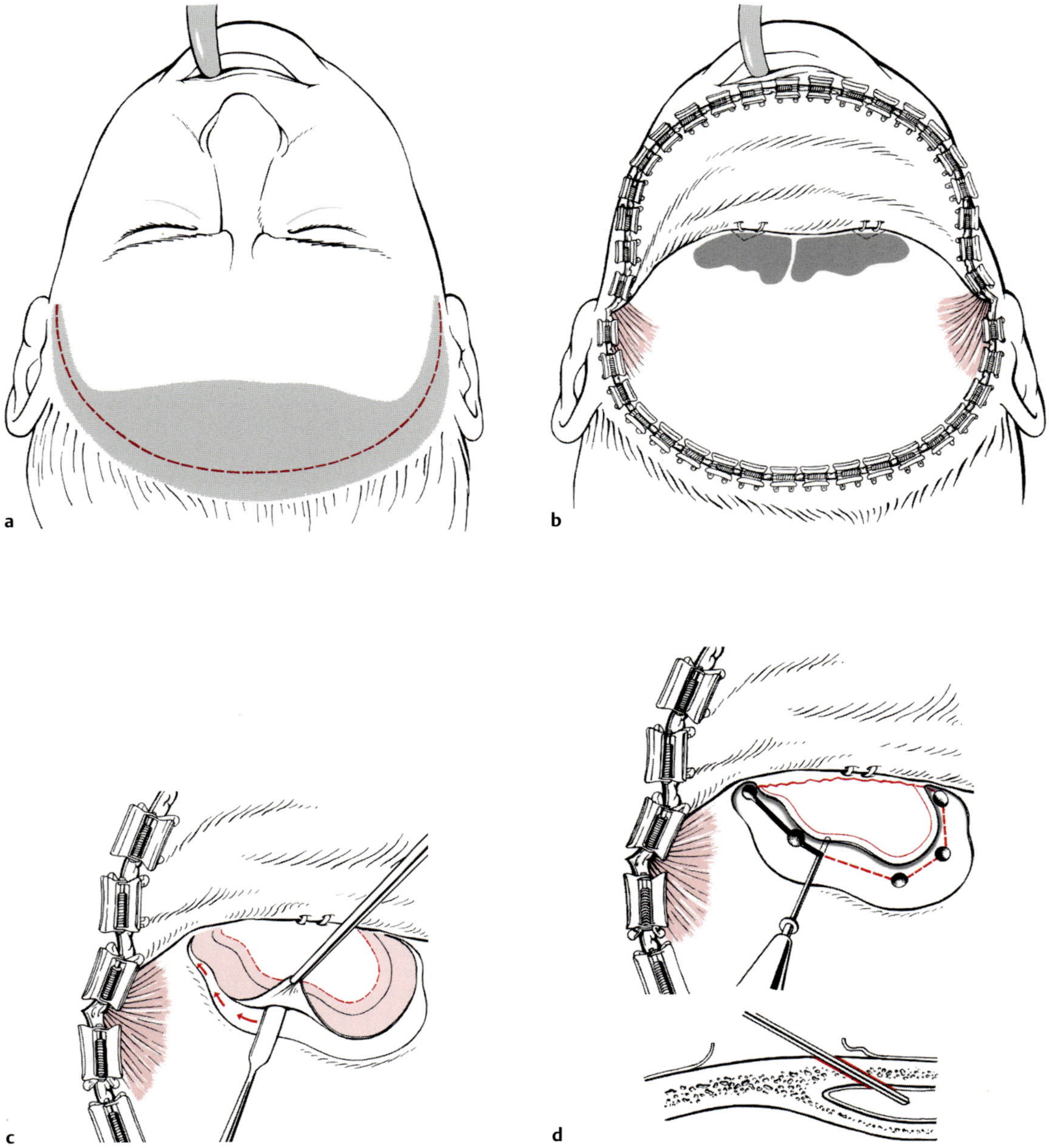

Fig. 7.29a–d Osteoplastic operation of the frontal sinus via a bicoronal incision.

a Positioning with reclined, slightly lowered head. Surgeon at the head end. Incision starts from a preauricular point behind the frontal hair line.

b Mobilization of the supraorbital and frontal nerves by burring the bony canals free.

c The periosteum is incised lateral to the borders of the frontal sinus and elevated to just medial to the margins of the frontal sinus (shaded area).

d After placing drill holes in the frontal sinus, the bone flap is elevated by directing the saw in a tangential direction.

Median Drainage

Surgical Technique

As with the endonasal approach, but with access using the osteoplastic frontal sinus procedure.

Postoperative Care

As for endonasal surgery of the frontal sinuses, gauze head dressing.

Rules, Tips, and Tricks

Dealing with Intra-operative Problems

- The frontal sinus borders must be identified preoperatively.
- Bicoronal incision is not advisable for patients with a tendency to baldness; the supraorbital nerve must be protected when elevating the flap.
- The burr or reciprocating micro-saw should be directed at an angle of ca. 30° when elevating the bone flap, to avoid injury to the posterior wall of the frontal sinus. Also, a burr with a blunt round head should preferably be used.

7

Surgery of Malignant Tumors of the Paranasal Sinus Region

The surgical procedure for, and the prognosis of, tumors of the paranasal sinuses is determined by the site of origin and location of the tumor, its extension, and invasion into contiguous structures. Sebileau differentiates between three levels of tumor location:

- Upper level: roof of the maxillary sinus, ethmoid (maxilloethmoid angle), frontal sinus.
- Middle level: maxillary sinus and lateral nasal wall.
- Lower level: alveolar process, palate, and floor of the maxillary sinus.

The prognosis is most favorable for the lowest level and worst for the highest level. It is also true that tumors lying anterior to the Öhngreen line (the line connecting the inner canthus and the angle of the jaw), have a more favorable prognosis than tumors situated behind this plane.

Furthermore, it is important when planning surgery to assess to what extent contiguous structures—the main nasal cavity, the nasopharynx, the oral cavity, the orbit, the soft tissues of the face, the pterygopalatine fossa, or the endocranium—are involved.

Operative Planning

- Biopsy.
- Endoscopy.
- Radiography, CT with bone and soft-tissue window setting.
- MRI (invasion of the brain, eye, muscles).
- Ophthalmological examination, neurological assessment and, if appropriate, dental pre-assessment with preparation of a cast for an obturator.

Special Instruments

Burrs and oscillating bone saws are needed in addition to the usual standard instruments required for paranasal sinus surgery.

Indications

The indication is determined from knowledge of the histological result and by the extent of the tumor as shown on CT and MRI.

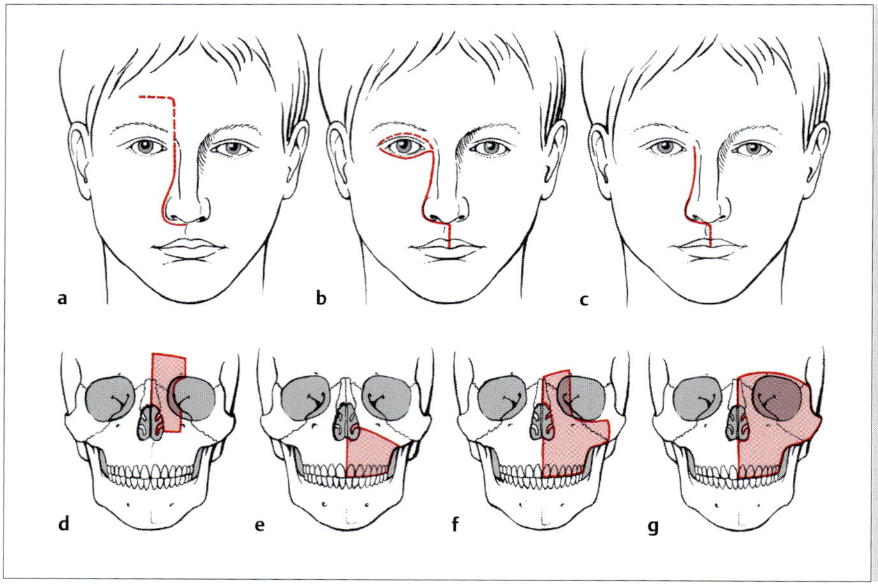

Fig. 7.30a–g Incisions for elevating the cheek flap for maxillary tumors.
a Lateral rhinotomy incision with the option of extension to the forehead.
b Lateral rhinotomy incision with extension to the cheek using a Zange subciliary incision and extension to the upper lip.
c Lateral rhinotomy incision with division of the upper lip.
d Area of bony resection for paranasal sinus tumors of the upper level.
e Tumours of the lower level.
f Maxillectomy.
g Maxillectomy with orbital exenteration.

Contraindications

Evidence of distant metastases, poor general condition.

Smaller anterior tumors located at the lower and middle levels can be removed with clear margins using appropriate methods of resection and good pre-operative diagnostics. With tumors extending more posteriorly at the upper level, removal with clear wide margins is not possible for anatomical reasons. Sometimes the main tumor must be removed first and then its extensions need to be further isolated.

Surgical Techniques

Tumors confined to the upper level are approached via a Moore incision, which can be extended to the forehead in the midline (**Fig. 7.30a**). Tumors confined to the ethmoid and the maxillo-ethmoid angle can be exposed via the Moore incision (lateral rhinotomy). Tumors located at the middle level are removed by resection of the maxilla and by reflecting back the upper cheek. Invasion into the orbit will require the subsequent extension of the excision and exenteration of the orbit. Tumors of the lower level can be demarcated after elevating the cheek flap (**Fig. 7.30**).

Lateral Rhinotomy Approach

Moore's lateral rhinotomy incision (**Fig. 7.30a**): The soft tissues are dissected and elevated on either side of the incision in front of the piriform aperture; the soft tissues are detached from the mucosa. The bone is carefully penetrated in the region of the ethmoid sinus. The trephination is extended to the maxillary sinus and/or frontal sinus. Depending on the finding, the tumor is encircled under direct vision (**Fig. 7.31**). Alternatively, a bone flap may also be sawn out temporarily, to be refixated later (depending on the findings).

Technique for Tumors of the Lower Level with Elevation of a Cheek Flap

A lateral rhinotomy incision is made, which runs around the ala and under the base of the columella, to be extended in the midline through the philtrum and the upper lip (midline upper-lip split incision) (**Fig. 7.30b, c**). The mucous membrane of the oral vestibule is divided. The cheek flap is elevated off the bone. Bone cuts are made around the tumor with the oscillating saw in the region of the facial maxillary sinus wall, the alveolar ridge, and the hard palate. The tumor is then extirpated (**Figs. 7.32** and **7.33**).

Technique of Total Maxillectomy

The incision is as already described, but is extended as a *Zange subciliary incision*: 1–2 mm below the lower lid margin (**Fig. 7.30b**), medial to the canthal tendon, skin and muscle fibers are divided down to the orbital septum, and the orbicularis oculi muscle is detached bluntly together with the skin flap. The periosteum over the lower edge of the orbit must be incised

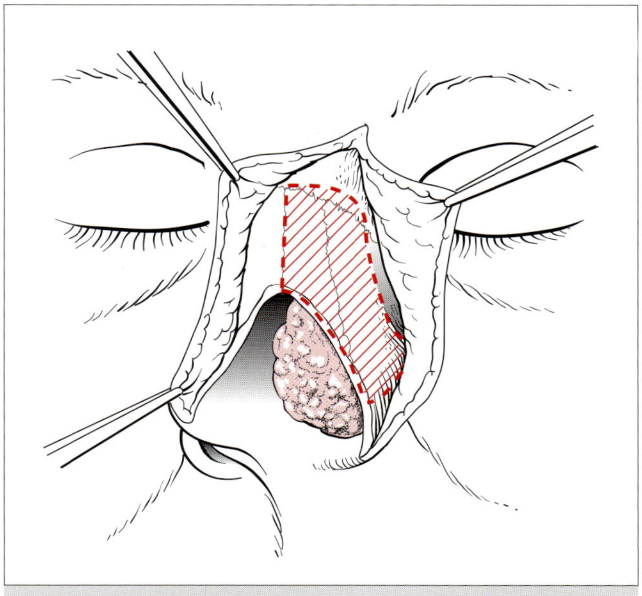

Fig. 7.31 Lateral rhinotomy.
Resection of the bone at the lateral nasal wall. Included is the entire nasal bone, as well as the frontal process of the maxilla, the frontal process of the frontal bone and the lacrimal bone.

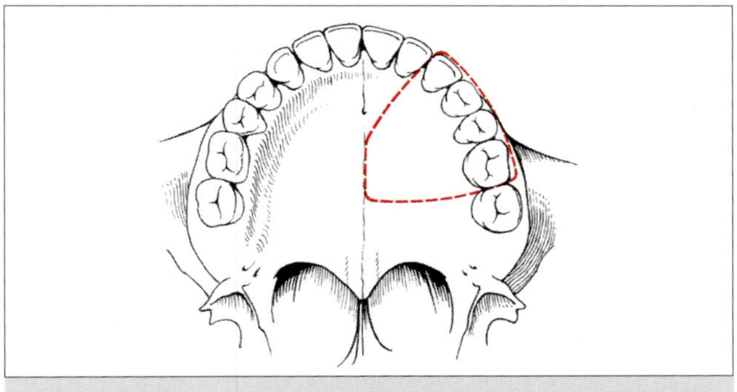

Fig. 7.32 Partial resection of the hard palate for tumors of the lower level.

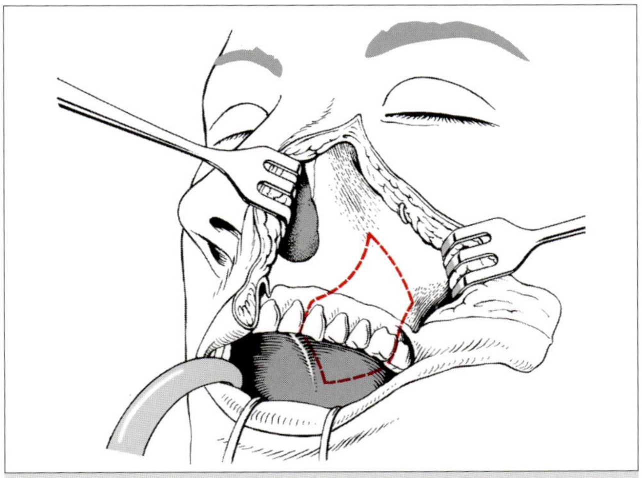

Fig. 7.33 Partial resection of the maxilla for tumors of the lower level.

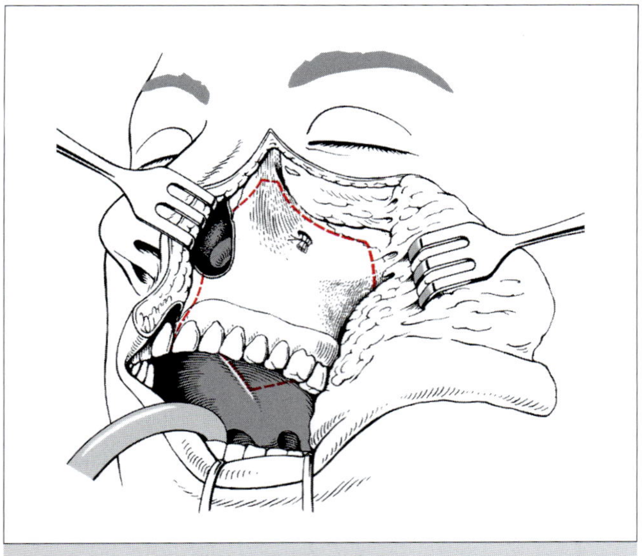

Fig. 7.34 Area of resection for maxillectomy (after Naumann).

sharply. After division of the infraorbital nerve, the superior part of the cheek is reflected back. The maxilla is then cut with an oscillating saw, first along the nose, then parallel to the inferior orbital margin and across the zygomatic body (**Fig. 7.34**). This is followed by a paramedian cut with the saw through the hard palate. The maxilla is then divulsed with a chisel, which is placed on the pterygoid process laterally behind the maxilla after carefully dissecting off the soft tissues. Drawing the block of bone forward allows the remaining medial and retromaxillary soft-tissue attachments to be sharply divided to complete the detachment. The maxillary artery is then ligated. Closure of the wound in layers completes the operation. Before that, either an interim prosthesis is inserted or the wound cavity is packed with a tamponade, which is brought out through the nose.

If tumor invasion of the orbit is discovered, then the operation may be extended as an *orbital exenteration (with preservation of the eyelid skin)* (**Figs. 7.35** and **7.36**). An incision is made along the upper eyelid, corresponding to the subciliary incision along the lower eyelid. The palpebral fissure may be closed with two sutures to place the eyelid skin under tension and facilitate the incision. The eyelid skin is undermined and elevated as far as the superior orbital margin. This preserved skin of the upper and lower eyelids may be used later to cover the bone in the orbital cavity. After incising the periosteum along the supraorbital rim, the orbital roof and the orbital floor are exposed in a subperiosteal plane using a broad elevator. The medial and lateral palpebral ligaments and the suspension apparatus of the lacrimal gland are sharply divided. Using the optic nerve as a pedicle, it is grasped with a clamp, flush with the optic canal, divided with scissors, and ligated.

! Risks and Complications

- Sequelae and risks depend on the extent of the operation. It must be confirmed prior to surgery that the remaining eye has adequate vision, especially when an exenteration is planned.
- Depending on the location of the tumor, all the other risks associated with surgery of the paranasal sinuses are also valid for the meninges. Furthermore, cosmetic repercussions from the incisions, cavities, and scar formation should also be kept in mind. An ectropion or problems with tear drainage may also result.
- Furthermore, partial loss of the maxilla produces dramatic changes to the masticatory system, which will later require prosthetic management. Difficulties with chewing, swallowing, and speech are possible. A significant amount of local nasal crusting may also develop.
- Dysfunction of the infraorbital nerve and olfactory loss may arise, depending on the extent of resection. Clearances undertaken in a posterior direction may also result in disturbances of aeration of the eustachian tube. A significant amount of blood loss during the operation and postoperative bleeding are also possible.

Technique of Midfacial Degloving

Surgical Principle

Midfacial degloving involves lifting the entire soft-tissue coverage of the midface and exposing the midface as far as the infraorbital rim and/or nasal root.

Indications

Tumor resection in the region of the midface, the nasal septum, the maxillary sinus, the main nasal cavity, and the paranasal sinus system; tumors of the sphenoid sinus and clivus; extensive fractures and comminution of the midface.

Tumors with expansion into the retromaxillary fossa (e.g., angiofibroma).

Contraindications

The anterior cranial base is not accessible via this approach.

Surgical Technique

This approach is selected when there is a need to create a very wide and clear access to the midface, the nasal pyramid, and the maxillary sinus as well as the adjacent orbits. A bilateral incision is made in the oral vestibule, below the mucogingival junction, and both incisions meet at the frenulum of the upper lip (**Fig. 7.37a, b**). Then a transfixion incision is made and extended on either side in a curvilinear fashion along the floor of the nasal vestibulum laterally to end in an intercartilaginous incision on the inside of the ala. The nostril is thus incised circumferentially. Then the soft-tissue coverage of the cheek and the entire nose, together with the lower lateral cartilages, may be reflected in a caudal-to-cephalic direction. In the region of the anterior wall of the maxillary sinus, dissection proceeds over the bone (**Fig. 7.37c, d**). The entire soft-tissue coverage of the midface can be elevated as far as the infraorbital margin and/or the nasal root. Which bony and cartilaginous parts are removed or temporarily displaced depends on the individual

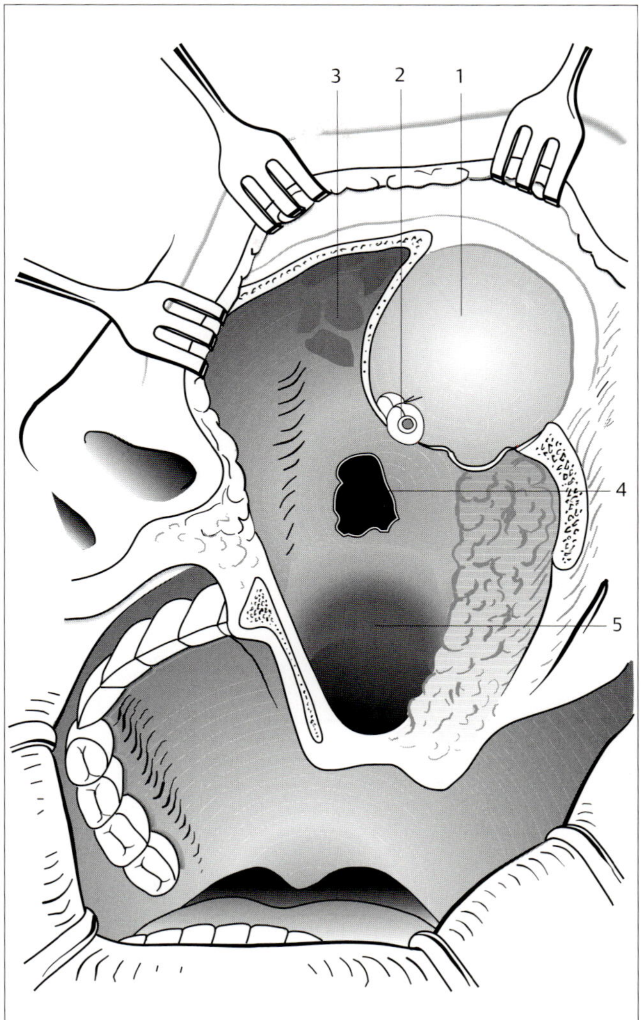

Fig. 7.36 Operative site after orbital exenteration and maxillectomy.
1 orbital roof
2 optic nerve and ophthalmic artery
3 ethmoid cells
4 sphenoid sinus
5 choana

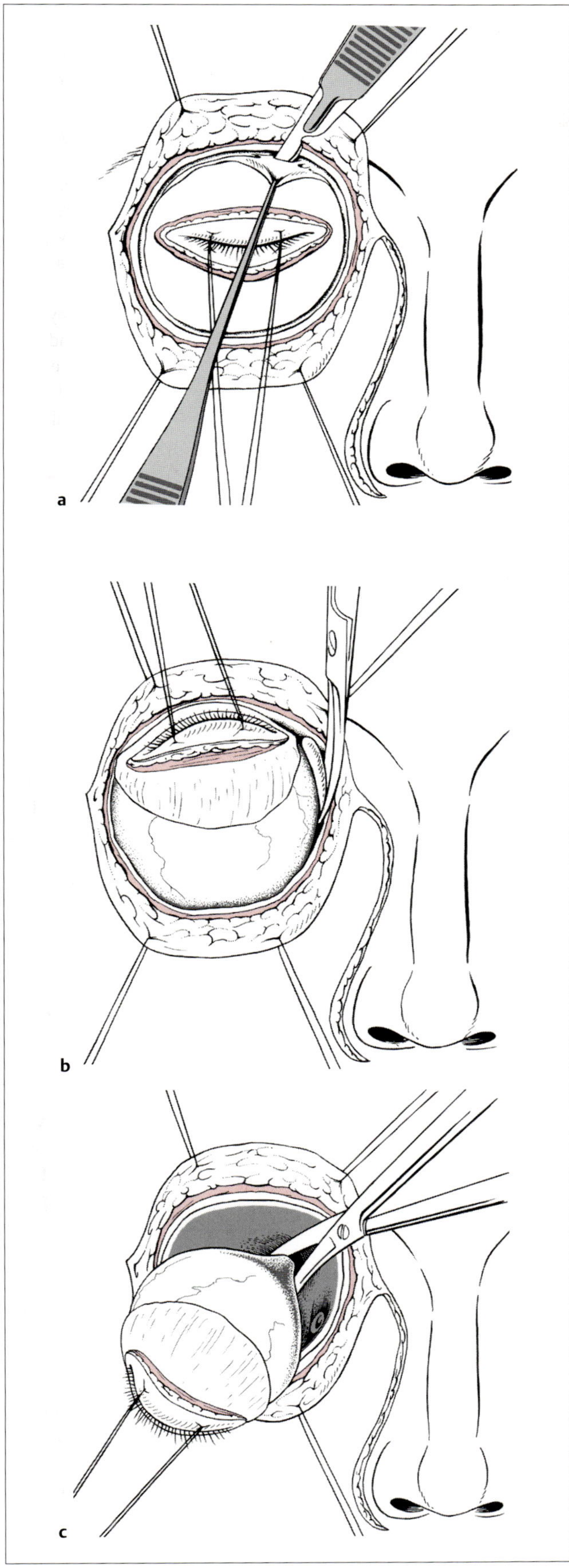

Fig. 7.35a–c Orbital exenteration.
a Periosteal incision over the bony orbital rim.
b Division of the lateral and medial palpebral ligaments.
c Trans-section of the optic nerve flush with the optic foramen.

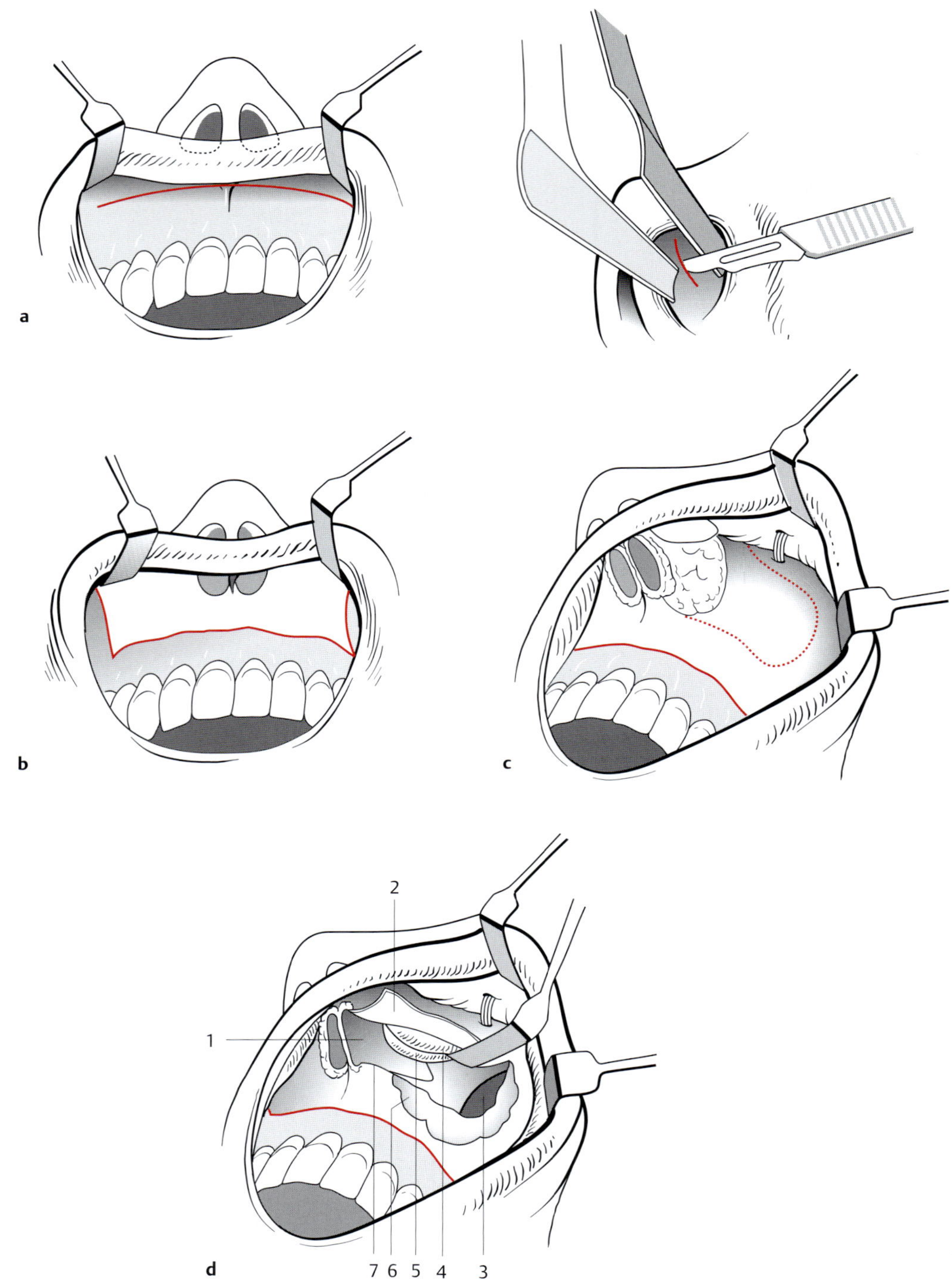

Fig. 7.37a–d Technique of midfacial degloving.
1 nasal septum
2 mucous membrane of the lateral nasal wall, elevated
3 choana
4 inferior turbinate
5 middle turbinate
6 maxillary sinus
7 lateral wall of the nasal cavity, incision line

case and on the extent of the pathological process (**Fig. 7.37**). First, a large window may be created in the maxillary sinus and then, depending on the presenting disease, the bony margin of the piriform aperture and the nasal wall of the maxillary sinus are resected, with division of the lacrimal duct. This access allows exploration of the orbital floor and the medial wall of the maxilla, while protecting the infraorbital nerves. After dissecting the lacrimal sac, the medial canthus may be exposed. The nasal septum is then disarticulated off the maxilla, elevated and, if affected by the tumor, partially excised. Removal of the bony nasal septum, and in particular parts of the vomer, allows access to the nasopharynx.

Rules, Tips, and Tricks
Dealing with Intra-operative Problems

- Exact preoperative assessment to determine the type of operation.
- Stenting of the lacrimal duct, if necessary.
- When coagulating tumor tissue, it should be kept in mind that tissue within a 1-cm radius of the coagulation becomes necrotic. The course of the internal carotid artery, the course of the optic nerve, and the location of the dura should be considered with this in mind.
- After exenteration of the orbit, the cavity is lined with a split-thickness skin graft. A bone-anchored epithesis is planned and, with partial resection of the maxilla, an obturator is fitted preoperatively. An impression is taken pre-operatively for a surgical obturator which is inserted at the end of the procedure.
- When removing the tooth-bearing part of the maxilla, the teeth adjacent to the bone cut should also be removed.
- Trismus secondary to damage to the muscles of mastication will require postoperative stretching with the aid of a spatula. If no improvement is achieved, then removal of the ascending branch of the mandible should be considered.

Postoperative Care

- Leave packs in place for approximately 1 week under antibiotic protection.
- Defects of the hard palate will require the fitting of an obturator.
- If screws are inserted intraoperatively to anchor an epithesis, the latter should be applied in a second step after the wound surfaces have healed.
- With involvement of the skull base, look out for the development of a nasal cerebrospinal fluid leak.
- Regular hygiene of the oral cavity is important.
- Rehabilitation and, if appropriate, postoperative plastic reconstructive measures must be considered.

Surgery of the Lacrimal Ducts

Endonasal Microscopic and Endoscopic Procedure for Dacryocystorhinostomy

Surgical Principle

Endonasal exposure of the lacrimal sac. Creation of an anastomosis with the nasal cavity above the stenosis.

Indications

Intrasaccal and postsaccal obstruction of the nasolacrimal duct.

Anesthesia

General endotracheal anesthesia or local anesthesia. Topical anesthesia of the nose. Infiltration with lidocaine and a vasoconstrictor in the region of the agger nasi and the outer parts of the nasal wall in the region of the piriform aperture.

Surgical Technique

A planned septoplasty should be performed first to correct any septal deviation or narrow anatomical conditions. Retract the middle turbinate. Using an angled disk knife, two mucosal flaps are outlined over the agger nasi, in front of the insertion of the middle turbinate. They are raised by the use of a elevator and reflected inferiorly and superiorly. The soft tissue is detached via the piriform aperture from the bone to the region of the lacrimal sac. The bone covering the lacrimal sac is removed with a burr or a punch (**Fig. 7.38**).

Alternatively, the suture line between the lacrimal bone and the frontal process is opened with an angled scalpel and the bone thus removed over the lacrimal sac (**Fig. 7.39**). This will also open some ethmoid cells at the same time. A probe is inserted into the lacrimal duct via the lacrimal punctum, over which the lacrimal sac is incised and, using a sickle knife, opened widely. A caudally pedicled flap may be elevated, which can be drawn downward, or alternatively the tissue may be discarded. The insertion of an Oggel probe, armed with a silicone thread, is also useful, but not essential. The nose is packed for 1 day.

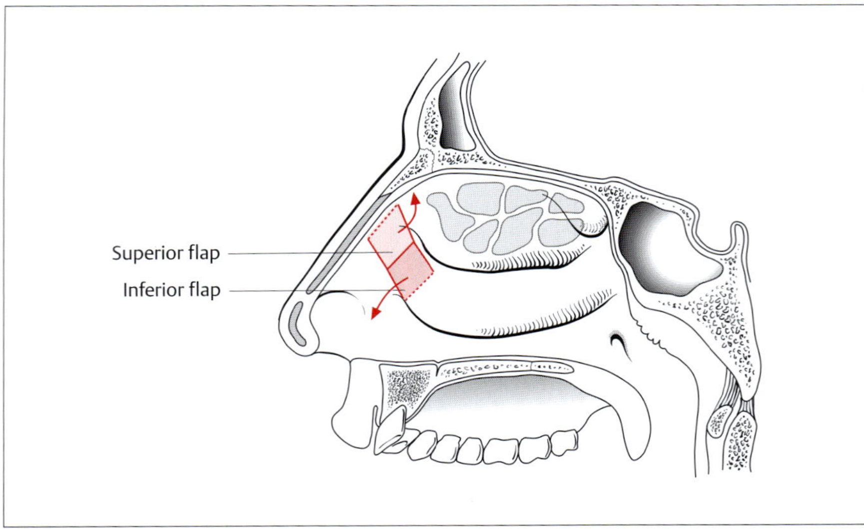

Fig. 7.38 Endonasal approach to the lacrimal sac.

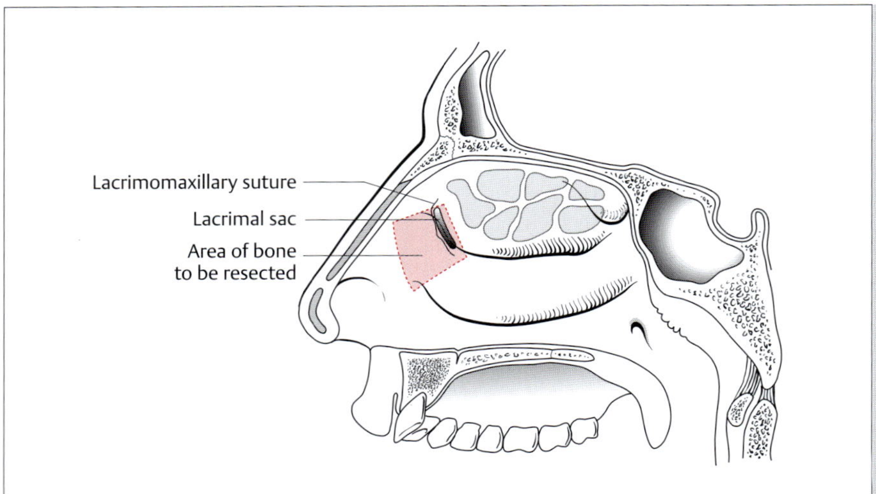

Fig. 7.39 Lateral view of the area of bone to be resected.

Surgery for Trauma to the Paranasal Sinuses, Orbit, and Anterior Cranial Base; and Surgery of Endocranial Complications

Approach to Fractures of the Zygoma

Surgical Principle

Reduction of the depressed zygoma and internal fixation using a miniplate secured over the frontozygomatic suture line.

Operative Planning

Radiographs of the paranasal sinuses and zygoma (jug-handle view of the zygomatic arch), high-resolution CT (axial and coronary views), ophthalmologic evaluation, evaluation of the sensory function of the infraorbital nerve.

Indications

Dislocated fractures of the zygoma with associated orbital symptoms and facial deformity.

Because complex maxillary zygomatic fractures also involve the orbital floor, this must be assessed separately via a second approach.

Anesthesia

General endotracheal anesthesia, infiltration of a vasoconstrictor.

Surgical Technique

Incision over the lateral end of the eyebrow. Spreading of the soft tissues will reveal the fracture gap in the frontozygomatic suture line. Reduction of the zygoma is accomplished by traction on a malar hook inserted percutaneously. Accuracy of reduction is confirmed by palpation of the lower and lateral upper orbital rim before internal fixation is achieved using a miniplate secured over the suture line. The plate is bent slightly for good adaptation (**Figs. 7.40** and **7.41**).

Postoperative Care

Radiography to verify improved alignment of the fracture.

> **! Risks and Complications**
> - Eye symptoms, diplopia.
> - Hypaesthesia or neuralgia in the distribution of the infraorbital nerve.
> - Unsatisfactory result due to cosmetic deformity following inadequate reduction or over-correction.
> - Trismus, problems with mastication.

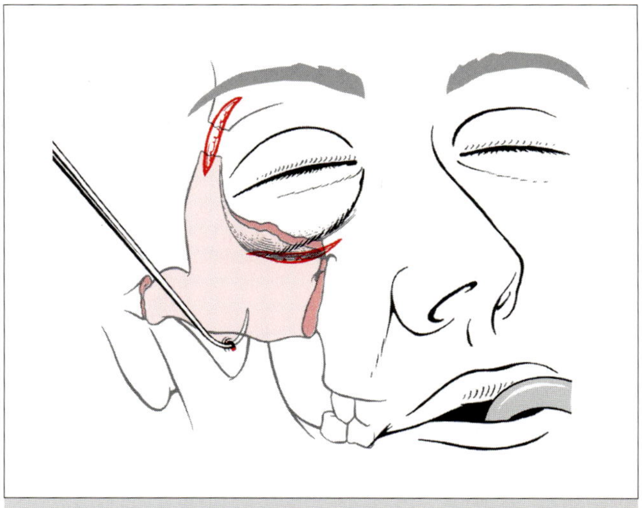

Fig. 7.40 Reduction of the zygomatic bone by percutaneous insertion of a malar hook, which is passed beneath the zygomatic arch: skin incision for internal fixation using a mini plate.

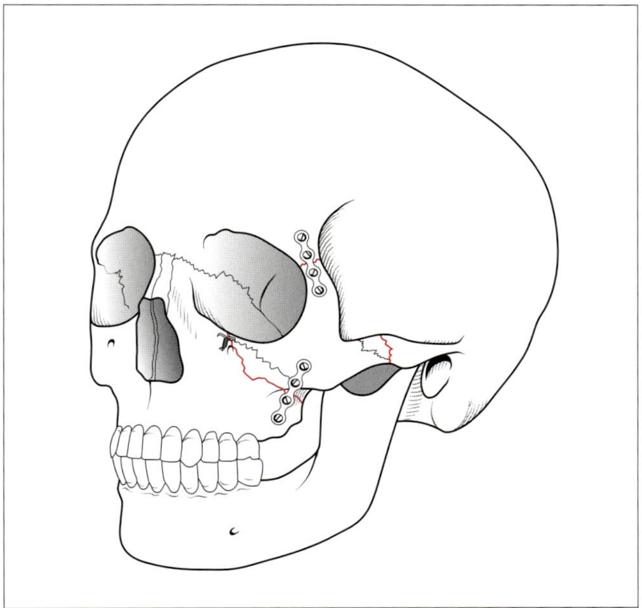

Fig. 7.41 Fracture of the zygomatic bone.
Internal fixation of the zygomatic bone using a miniplate over the frontozygomatic suture and, if appropriate, over the zygomatico-alveolar crest. An additional wire cerclage may be required in the region of the infraorbital canal.

Fractures of the Zygomatic Arch

Reduction is achieved by strong traction on a malar hook inserted percutaneously beneath the fragments. Usually the zygomatic arch snaps back well into place without re-displacing. If stabilization is not achieved because of comminution or an unfavorable fracture position, then the zygomatic arch and its fragments are undermined and exposed via a skin incision placed in a relatively far preauricular position, reduced and secured by suture and internal fixation with a miniplate. Reduction can also be accomplished via the oral vestibule, given that the fracture position is easily palpable externally (**Figs. 7.40** and **7.41**). Alternatively, reduction can also be achieved from a cranial direction via a bicoronal incision (which is safer for the facial nerve).

> **! Risks and Complications**
> - Problems with mastication and trismus may remain, in addition to inadequate reduction and the associated poor cosmetic result.
> - Any additional external incisions through the skin require protection of the frontal branch of the facial nerve. Sensory disturbances may persist in the distribution of the infraorbital nerve.

Fractures of the Orbital Floor

Surgical Principle

Reduction of the orbital contents, release of muscle entrapment, removal of penetrating bone splinters, and stabilization of the orbital floor. The approach is either a purely transmaxillary one or via external incisions (subtarsal, transconjunctival, subciliary), connected, if appropriate, between both cheeks.

Operative Planning

Conventional plain radiographs of the paranasal sinuses, high-resolution CT of the paranasal sinuses (coronary or axial views), ophthalmological assessment: enophthalmus, ocular mobility, diplopia, visual acuity, sensory disturbances in the distribution of the infraorbital nerve.

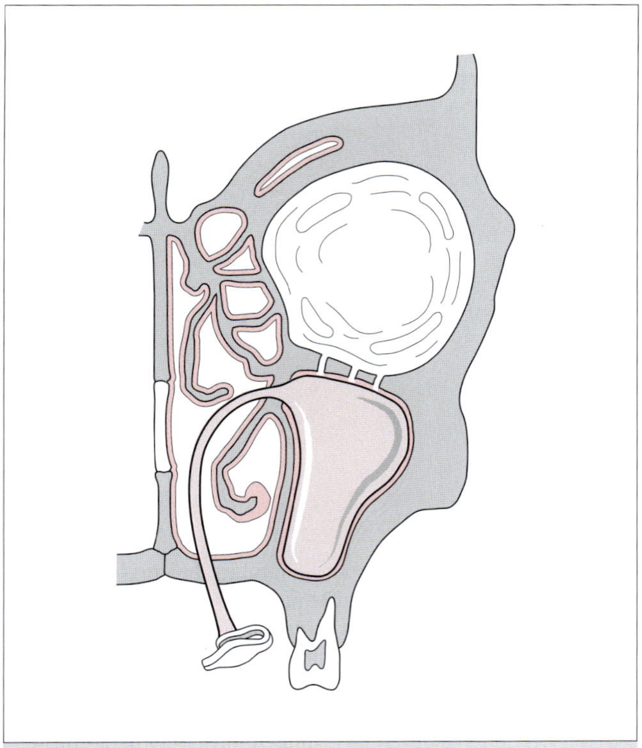

Fig. 7.42 Fracture of the orbital floor.
Transmaxillary approach. The reduced orbital floor is supported by an antral balloon catheter; the port is bought out through the maxillary window.

Indications

Fractures of the orbital floor with entrapment (diplopia, muscle dysfunction, enophthalmus secondary to herniation of orbital fat) within the first 2 days after injury.

Special Instruments and Implants

Fascia, poly-*p*-dioxanon (PDS) foil (0.25 mm), dura substitute, antral balloon catheter.

Surgical Technique

Transmaxillary Approach (Fig. 7.42)

Osteoplastic approach through the maxillary sinus. An incision is made in the mucosa with a disk scalpel across the roof of the maxilla, over the still, stable bone and around the prolapse. The incised mucous membrane is removed from the orbital fat prolapse. Bone splinters are removed using fine ear instruments. The cavity is supported with a Milewski antral balloon catheter, which is filled with saline and whose port is brought out through the nose. The intraoral vestibular incision is repaired with sutures and the catheter secured to the cheek or dorsum of the nose.

Transfacial Approach (Fig. 7.43)

Subtarsal incision. An incision is made in the middle of the lower eyelid along the relaxed skin lines from medial to lateral, dropping laterally below the line connecting the inner and outer canthus, ca. 5–6 mm below the eyelid margin (**Fig. 7.44**). The fibers of the orbicularis oculi muscle are separated and entered by blunt dissection in an inferior direction along the orbital septum. The periosteum is incised over the orbital margin and the periorbita elevated. The full extent of the fracture margins is identified and any bone splinters are removed. The orbital contents are carefully lifted with a blunt hook. Any smaller defect is bridged with fascia (fascia lata or temporal fascia) and an extensive orbital fracture is additionally supported from the maxillary sinus with an antral balloon catheter. Finally, the subtarsal incision is repaired.

Subciliary incision. The subciliary incision runs immediately below and parallel to the eyelid margin. It begins 2–3 mm below the inferior lacrimal punctum. After division of the often very delicate fibers of the orbicularis oculi muscle, dissection is continued along the tarsus in the direction of the inferior orbital margin and, after dividing the periosteum, down to the bony structures. The typical lower-eyelid incision uses the natural crease lines of the skin (**Fig. 7.45**).

Transconjunctival incision. First, a lateral canthotomy (blepharotomy) is made with straight scissors or a scalpel, beginning exactly at the lateral canthus and dividing the skin and underlying soft tissues. The lower eyelid is pulled downward with a lid retractor and the palpebral conjunctiva incised below the tarsal edge. The infraorbital margin is dissected in the plane between the orbital septum and the orbicularis muscle, creating a tunnel into which scissors can be inserted. The conjunctiva is then divided in a medial direction with scissors, ca. 0.3–0.5 cm

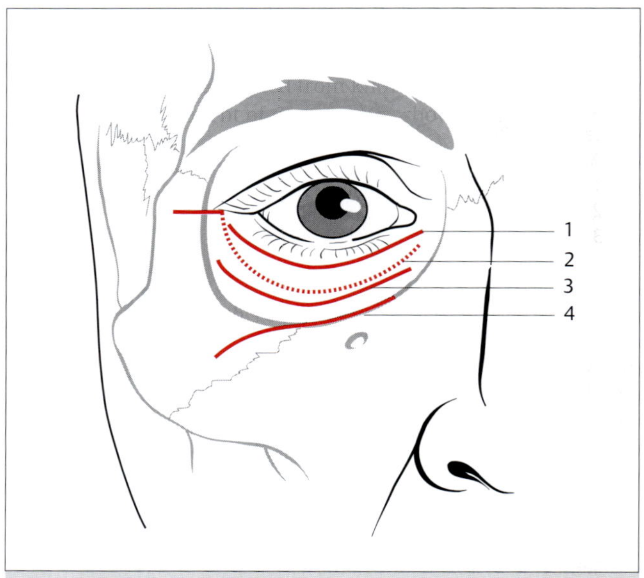

Fig. 7.43 Approaches to the orbital floor.
1 subciliary
2 transconjunctival incision
3 subtarsal incision
4 orbital rim incision

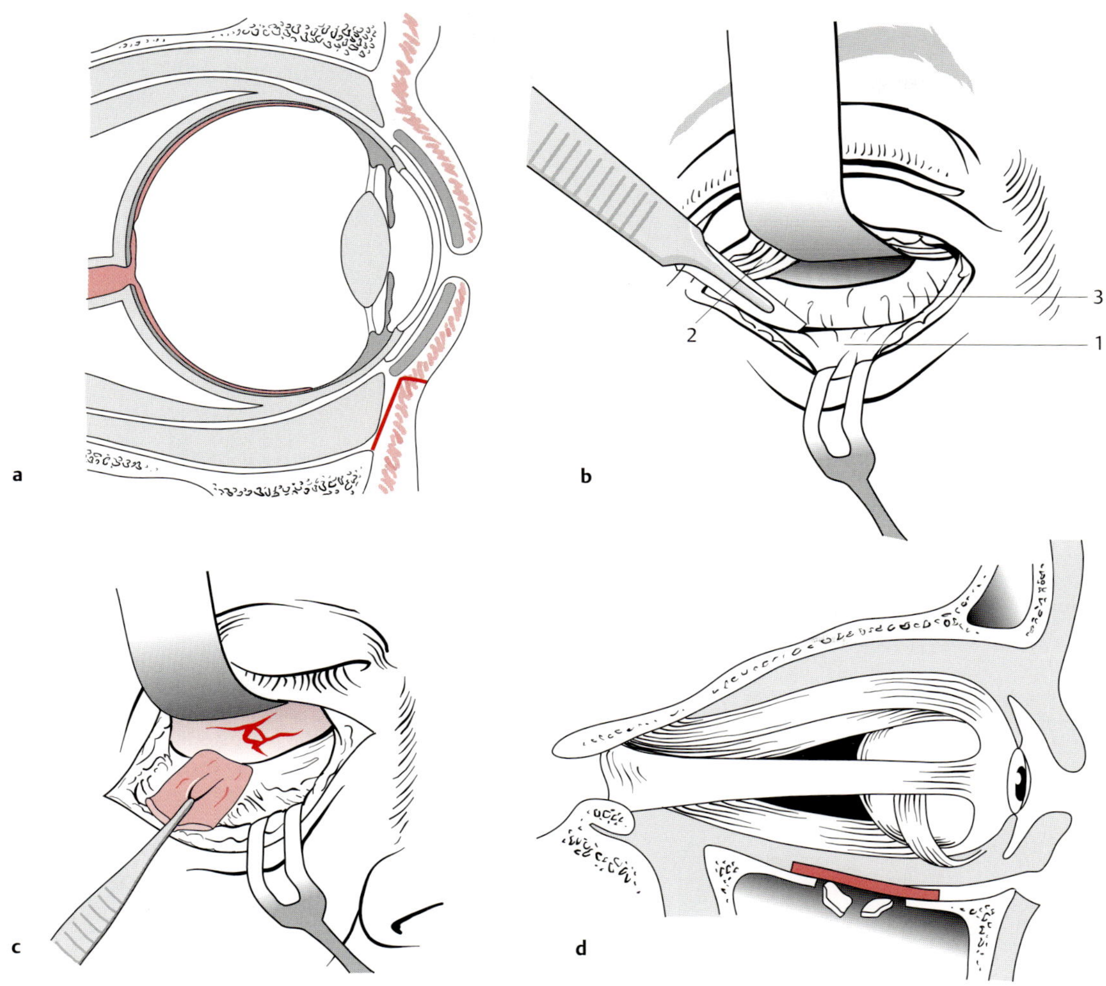

Fig. 7.44a–d Approach to the orbital floor. Subtarsal incision.
a Lateral view of the subtarsal incision.
b Approach to the orbital floor after the skin incision.
1 infraorbital margin, periosteum
2 orbicularis oculi muscle
3 periorbita
c Exposure of the orbital floor from the subtarsal incision; insertion of fascia.
d Position of the fascia over the defect in the orbital floor after a subtarsal approach.

above the conjunctival reflection and 0.5 cm away from the lacrimal punctum. The orbital margin is identified and the periosteum divided sharply (**Fig. 7.45**).

After repair of the orbital floor, the orbital septum is reconstructed. Suture of the conjunctiva is performed using a continuous 6/0 absorbable suture. Closure of the lateral canthotomy is done with two or three interrupted sutures.

Orbital rim incision. The orbital rim incision is made parallel to the orbital rim, extending caudally into the skin lines and carried down to the bone. A reported disadvantage of this incision is the prolonged edema of the lower eyelid (**Fig. 7.46**).

Postoperative Care

- The antral balloon is emptied and the catheter removed after 1–2 weeks.
- The lid sutures are removed after 4 days.
- Ophthalmological follow-up is required.

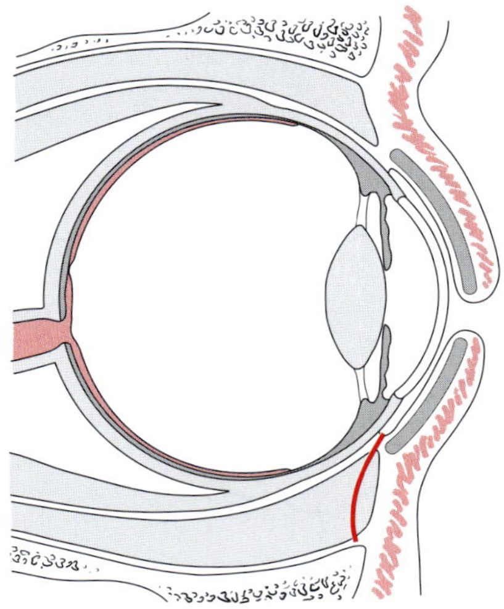

Fig. 7.45 Transconjunctival approach.

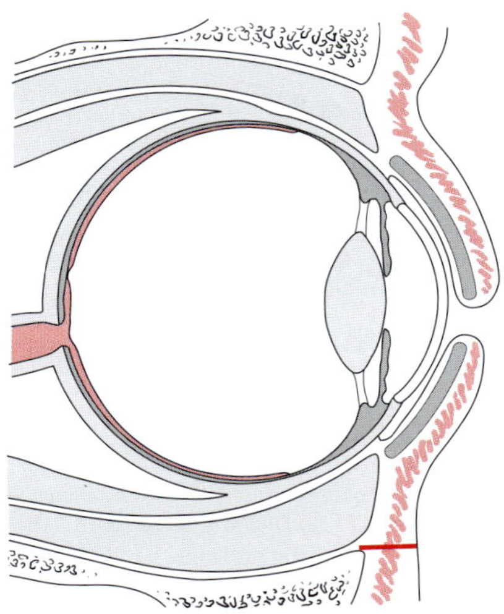

Fig. 7.46 Orbital rim incision.

Risks and Complications

- With a transmaxillary approach, risks and complications as for the Caldwell–Luc procedure.
- Eyelid edema and the risk of an ectropion after a subtarsal incision, transconjunctival incision, and ciliary incision.
- Diplopia may persist if mobilization is not complete, the development of fat necrosis may produce an enophthalmus, and disturbances of sensory function may arise in the distribution of the infraorbital nerve.

Rules, Tips, and Tricks

Dealing with Intra-operative Problems

- An intraoperative traction test provides the first indications of globe mobility. For this purpose, the inferior, superior, or lateral rectus muscle is grasped with fine forceps through the conjunctiva.
- Avoid too strong traction on the globe retractor to protect the globe from rupturing.
- Meticulous hemostasis to prevent an orbital hematoma.
- Mandatory repair of the divided periosteum to avoid ectropion.
- Vasoconstrictors should not be injected too deeply into the skin of the lower eyelid. The vasoconstrictive effect could extend intra-orbitally and result clinically in dilation of the pupil.

Approach to Fractures of the Orbital Rim

Surgical Principle

Debridement and reconstruction of the supraorbital margin.

Surgical Technique

Exposure of the fracture using a suitable incision. The eyebrow incision is suitable for fractures of the superior orbital rim. After exposure of the bone, the periosteum is elevated with a Freer elevator and the bony fragments reduced. The avulsed fragment can be fixated with a miniplate system.

Approach to Injuries of the Upper Paranasal Sinus/Orbital Region

Fractures of the Frontal Sinus Region without Injury to the Skull Base

Injuries confined to the pneumatic structures of the upper paranasal sinus region and not associated with the skull base and skull contents are approached according to the classic rules of paranasal sinus surgery, which allow more comprehensive procedures at any time. The choice of incision is determined by the extent of bony injury. Very extensive injuries require a bicoronal incision and an osteoplastic approach. It should be borne in mind, however, that simple elevation of a depressed anterior-wall fracture of the frontal sinus is often approachable via the laceration wound that may be present. Otherwise an incision below the eyebrow is used to lever out the fragment, together with the periosteum, with the aid of an elevator. More extensive fractures are managed by plate fixation.

As a rule, an exact preoperative radiographic assessment should be considered as an initial step to rule out further injuries. After exposing the paranasal sinuses, the posterior wall, the frontal sinus, and the roof of the ethmoid are inspected to avoid overlooking any fractures of the posterior wall. A dural tear may well be concealed behind barely dislocated fracture lines.

Injuries to the Anterior Cranial Base

Surgical Principle

The objective is the debridement of the fractures with generous exposure and demonstration of the contiguous paranasal sinus region together with the inspection of the skull base. If appropriate, cleansing of a skull-base defect and the watertight closure of the dura then follow. Access is gained via the usual incisions for surgery of the fontal sinus, via available open wounds, a bicoronal incision or by using an endonasal microscopic approach.

Indications

A distinction is made between vital, absolute, and relative indications:

Vital indications—immediate emergency treatment without any further diagnostic assessment:

- Life-threatening rise in intracranial pressure secondary to an intracranial hemorrhage.
- Life-threatening hemorrhage from the paranasal sinus region.

Absolute indications:

- Open brain injury.
- Closed brain injury with CSF leak, pneumatocele.
- Traumatic infectious meningitis.
- Cerebral abscess, epidural abscess.
- Late complications following injury to the dura.
- Iatrogenic injury to the dura.
- Orbital complications with deterioration of visual acuity, amaurosis, disturbances of ocular motility.

Relative indications:

- Fractures of the region of the upper paranasal sinuses and the basal skull region without suspected dural tear.

Contraindications

Shock, provided there is no vital indication.

Special Instruments and Implants

Galea–periosteal flap, fascia lata or even dura substitutes, miniplates (absorbable, nonabsorbable), fibrin glue, gelatin sponge (e.g., Gelitta).

Operative Planning

- High-resolution cranial CT.
- Neurological, neurosurgical, and ophthalmological assessments.

Anesthesia

General endotracheal anesthesia.

Surgical Technique

Isolated and endoscopically accessible defects. The *endoscopic management* of dural defects is preferable. Iatrogenic injuries during paranasal sinus surgery of the roof of the ethmoid are particularly suitable for management from an endonasal approach under microscopic and endoscopic vision.

Open cranio-cerebral injuries. An external approach should be chosen, depending on the location and extent of the defect. A *sub-brow incision*, which may be extended by a *bilateral external ethmoidectomy incision with a connection across the glabella*, or a *bicoronal incision*, is suited for this. Bone splinters should be debrided, with larger fragments preserved for later reconstructive measures. If appropriate, the *anterior wall of the frontal sinus should be removed using plastic surgical techniques*. Removal of the floor of the frontal sinus and the further procedure are initially undertaken as for the Jansen–Ritter operation.

With both approaches (endonasal and external), the frontal sinus, the ethmoid, and the roof of the ethmoid as well as the sphenoid sinus should first be examined for fractures *microscopically or endoscopically*. *Splinters are removed from any fracture gaps, which are then carefully opened up* if they are gaping and tend to give. The dura is assessed for tears. *Larger mobile parts, especially the crista galli, are left, provided there are no dural tears.* All reasonable effort should be made to preserve the lamina cribrosa region.

A galea–periosteal flap, fascia lata, or even dura substitutes (e.g., Tutopatch, Tachocomb) are suitable for the *closure of dural fistulas*. Even a (free) mucoperiosteal flap, with or without bone, taken from the middle turbinate, is available as a resurfacing material. When an open approach is used for the region of the posterior wall of the frontal sinus, fixation of the graft can be achieved with a suture. For surgical technical reasons, however, a suture is not possible in the region of the ethmoid and sphenoid. Here it is recommended to use fibrin glue for fixation.

To close the fistula, the dura must be *released sufficiently widely* all around the bone defect with a disk knife, so that the graft can be *inserted in between bone and dura* and fixated (underlay technique). For the overlay technique, suitable coverage is with a mucoperiosteal flap, which can be harvested from the septal mucosa or the turbinate mucosa (**Fig. 7.47**).

After removing the mucous membranes, dural fissures in the sphenoid region are closed by lining the sphenoid sinus with a fascia graft coated externally with fibrin glue. This graft is first folded like a tobacco pouch and filled with gelatin sponge (**Fig. 7.48**). A cerebral prolapse through the fistula into the paranasal sinus region is carefully removed with a sucker under low suction pressure. The operation is completed after applying gelatin sponge onto the graft. Nasal packs are left as usual for 5 days. Fragments temporarily removed from the anterior wall of the frontal sinus are replaced and secured with bone fixation plates or with suture wires. After undergoing a Riedel operation, a comminuted fracture of the anterior wall will later require plastic reconstruction of the defect.

Postoperative Care

Careful monitoring, antibiotic coverage, removal of packs after 5 days.

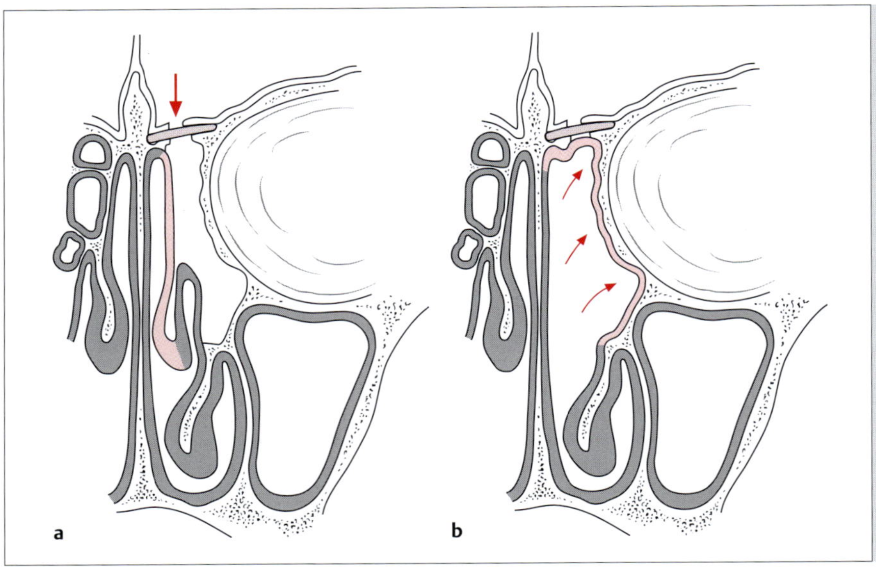

Fig. 7.47a, b Closure of dural defects.
a Underlay technique.
b Combined underlay and overlay technique after resection of the middle turbinate.

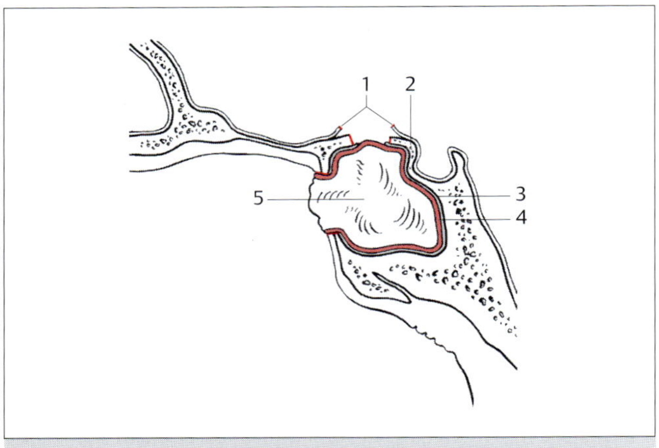

Fig. 7.48 Closure of a sphenoid sinus fistula. Lining of the cavity with fascia, which covers the fracture gap. The cavity is filled with fibrin foam.
1 dura
2 bone of the anterior cranial base
3 fibrin glue
4 fascia
5 gelatin sponge

Watch out for signs of increased intracranial pressure, signs of meningitis, and CSF leak.

! Typical Surgical Risks and Sequelae of Surgery of the Frontal Sinus

- In particular, there is a risk of endocranial complications.
- Cosmetic impairment in the region of the frontal sinus is possible, depending on the location of the bony defect and scar formations.
- The sense of smell usually remains intact, unless damaged by the primary injury.

- A recurrent CSF fistula may develop in the postoperative phase and will require revision surgery. However, the sequelae of endocranial injuries are often of greater concern.

Optic Nerve Decompression

Surgical Principle

Decompression of the optic nerve from the orbital apex to the sphenoid cavity (as far as the internal carotid artery).

Indications

- Traumatic compression of the optic nerve with deterioration of visual acuity or blindness.
- Inflammatory compression of the optic nerve with deterioration of visual acuity or blindness.

Operative Planning

- Thin-slice CT using axial slice orientation.
- Ophthalmological assessment.

Instruments

Burr, operating microscope, endoscope, sickle knife, disk scalpel.

Surgical Technique

Transethmoid–trans-sphenoidal approach. Access to the ethmoid and to the sphenoid sinus may be gained either from an endonasal or an extranasal approach (endoscopic or microendoscopic). After complete removal of the contents of the ethmoid, the anterior wall of the sphenoid sinus is removed and the course of the optic nerve and the prominence of the carotid

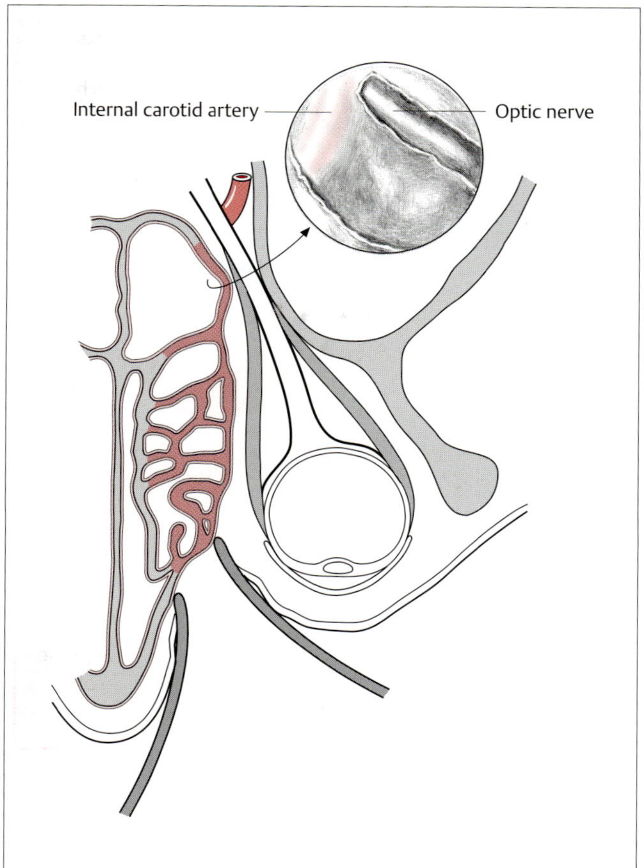

Fig. 7.49 Optic nerve decompression.

artery are identified (**Fig. 7.49**). About 1 cm in front of the optic nerve tubercle, the lamina papyracea is removed and the optic canal thinned out over the optic nerve tubercle with a diamond burr. Any fracture lamellas present are removed with a disk knife. The optic nerve should be exposed over the entire medial region. Releasing the optic nerve sheath is controversial. If done, the fibrous reinforcement of the nerve sheath at the optic foramen should also be divided. Postoperative packing should be avoided, if at all possible.

Rules, Tips, and Tricks

Dealing with Intra-operative Problems

- In 4 % of cases the bony cover of the optic nerve in the sphenoid sinus is dehiscent, and in ca. 8 % of cases that of the internal carotid artery.
- Minor hemorrhage may be dealt with by the insertion of tapered sponges soaked in naphazolin nitrate. Coagulation of the roof of the sphenoid sinus should, however, certainly be avoided.
- If CT has already demonstrated a fracture crossing the course of internal carotid artery, extreme caution is advised when removing any bony lamella for fear of injury to the artery.

Approach for Orbital Complications of Acute Sinusitis (Orbital Subperiosteal Abscess)

Surgical Principle

Endonasal incision and drainage of a subperiosteal abscess secondary to ethmoidectomy.

Indications

Subperiosteal abscess and phlegmon of the orbit associated with an acute sinusitis.

Anesthesia

General endotracheal anesthesia.

Operative Planning

- Thin-slice CT using axial slice orientation.
- Ophthalmological assessment.

Instruments

Burr, operating microscope, endoscope, sickle knife, disk scalpel.

Surgical Technique

The contents of the ethmoid sinus and the other affected paranasal sinuses are removed with preservation of the middle turbinate, as already described in the sections on endonasal surgery of the paranasal sinuses. After identification of the landmarks, the lamina papyracea is identified and then removed. This will already result in the discharge of abscess fluid in the presence of a subperiosteal abscess (**Fig. 7.50**). Gentle pressure on the globe with a finger from the outside will allow more purulent fluid to empty from the abscess cavity.

If removal of the lamina papyracea has not yet opened the abscess cavity, then the periorbita may be further exposed and then incised with a sickle knife.

! Complications

- Intraorbital hemorrhage.
- Injury to the ocular muscles with persistent diplopia.

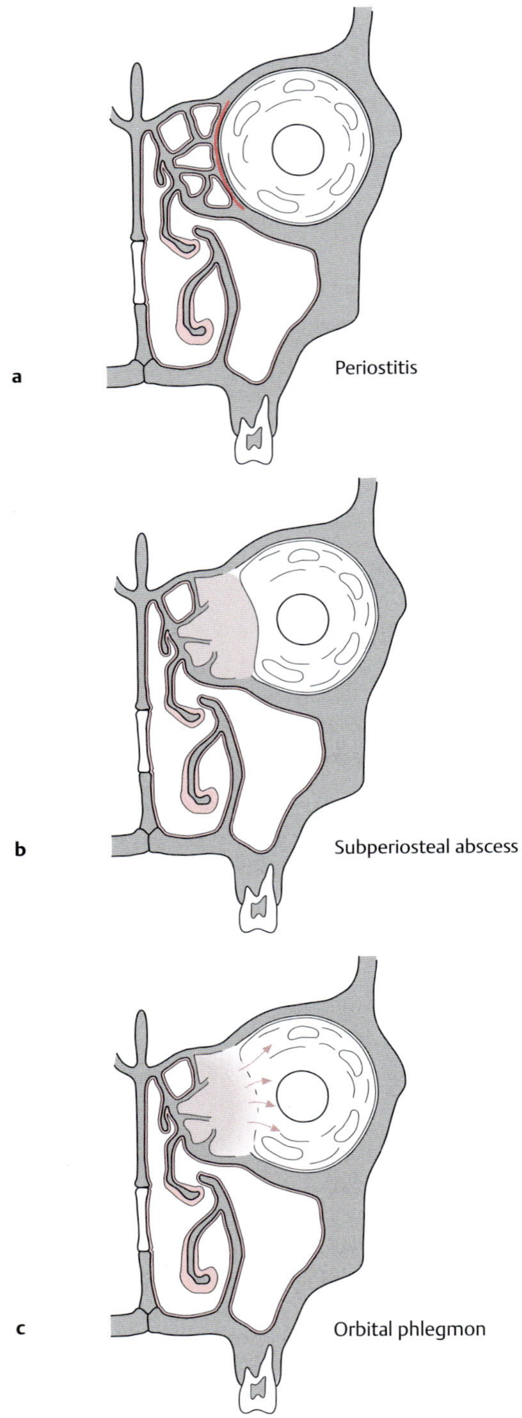

Fig. 7.50a–c Staging system for orbital complications
a Periostitis.
b Subperiosteal abscess.
c Orbital phlegmon.

8 Surgery of the Epipharynx

Adenoidectomy

Surgical Principle

Curettage of the lymphadenoid tissue of the nasopharynx.

Indications

Significant hyperplasia of the pharyngeal tonsil associated with:

- Nasal airway obstruction, mouth breathing, snoring, obstructive sleep apnea syndrome.
- Recurrent sinusitis, chronic purulent rhinitis, nasopharyngitis.
- Recurrent middle ear effusion (otitis media, glue ear), serous or mucoid otitis media.
- Recurrent laryngitis or tracheobronchitis.

Contraindications

- Overt, operated or submucous cleft palate.
- Hypernasal speech (rhinolalia aperta) (phoniatric assessment).
- Bleeding disorder or coagulopathy.
- An urgent indication in children only before their second year of life.
- Suspected juvenile nasopharyngeal fibroma.

Specific Points Regarding Informed Consent

- Risk of postoperative bleeding, risk of aspiration with subsequent extremely rare risk of hypoxia.
- Damage to teeth.
- Transient, in exceptional cases permanent, hypernasal voice.
- Nasopharyngeal stenosis secondary to scar formation.
- Scar formation at the orifice of the eustachian tube with subsequent recurrent otitis, conductive hearing loss.
- Cervical lymphadenopathy or prevertebral fasciitis with subsequent torticollis.
- Risk of recurrence.
- Revision surgery.
- Outpatient surgery: specific instructions regarding postoperative behavior and observation.

Operative Planning

- Nasopharyngoscopy/endoscopy. Identification of indirect signs such as serous otitis media, marked nuchal lymphadenitis.
- Blood count and clotting profile.

Anesthesia

General anesthesia with orotracheal intubation or larynx mask.

Special Instruments

Beckmann ring knife or appropriate instrument of various sizes, Jurasch forceps, curved suction tube with spherical tip, conchotome (triangular jaw), mouth gag (e.g., McIvor gag), nasolaryngoscope or angled scope, bipolar diathermy, suction cautery.

Surgical Technique

- Positioning: head-down position achieved by lowering the head rest or placing padding beneath the shoulders; reclination (**Fig. 8.1**).
- Introduction of the McIvor blade: A closed blade corresponding in size to the anatomy of the mouth is introduced, placed over the oral intubation tube (which is placed in the midline), and then opened after being supported on the canines.
- The pharynx is inspected using the nasolaryngoscope or angled scope.
- A ring knife, appropriate in size to the patient's age, is passed beneath the soft palate and up to the roof of the pharynx, behind the margin of the vomer.
- The knife is then drawn downward with mild pressure, keeping the blade *straight and strictly in the midline*. An approach that is controlled and not too abrupt will avoid injury to the arch of the atlas, the prevertebral fascia, or the mucous membrane of the oropharynx (**Fig. 8.2**).
- The pharyngeal recesses are curetted after removal of the adenoids. The ring knife is again held in the midline, advanced parallel with the blade straight into the pharyngeal recess and, while maintaining light contact with the tissue, is then drawn back again in a strictly craniocaudal direction (**Fig. 8.3**).

- Remaining remnants of mucosa and residual adenoid tissue over the lower curetted margin are removed with the conchotome (**Fig. 8.4**).
- The nasopharynx is checked with the laryngoscope/endoscope or by palpation with a finger or ring knife. Residual adenoid tissue is re-curetted or removed under direct vision with the Jurasch forceps.
- Hemostasis is achieved by inserting a swab, *attached to a thread* and possibly soaked with nose drops, into the nasopharynx for 3 minutes; *it is imperative to confirm its removal (risk of bolus obstruction)*. Any bleeding that still continues is then directly coagulated with a bipolar diathermy or by suction cautery under endoscopic vision after drawing the soft palate forward.
- The pharynx is suctioned before extubation.

Rules, Tips, and Tricks

- All adenoidal tissue must be removed, otherwise there is the danger of postoperative bleeding and the risk of recurrence.
- Check the nasopharynx for any retained swabs. If more than one swab is used, always insert the swab attached to a thread first, to be subsequently removed last. Do a swab count.
- Residual tissue may also be removed transnasally with forceps under endoscopic guidance, or by endoscopy via the nose, removing the tissue transorally.

! Risks and Complications

- Persistent bleeding during the operation:
  - Usually due to retained pharyngeal tonsil tissue.
  - In rare cases due to an unrecognized coagulopathy.
  - In extremely rare cases due to injury to ectopic branches from the external carotid artery region. Kinking of the internal carotid artery is regarded as a most extreme rarity. Severe arterial hemorrhage initially requires firm packing, followed by revision of the carotid sheath from an external approach.
- Postoperative bleeding:
  - Residual adenoid tissue, unrecognized coagulopathy: re-curette, clotting profile, consider blood component replacement therapy, exclude aspiration.
- Intra- or postoperative aspiration of coagulated blood: if suspected, then undertake immediate bronchoscopy.
- Wound infection, acute otitis media: antibiotics, nose drops.
- Postoperative nasal/pharyngeal suppuration with obstructed nasal breathing: this is suggestive of a retained swab.
- Injury to the orifices of the eustachian tubes: decongest and insufflate the tubes, administer corticosteroids.
- Stenosis or atresia of the nasopharynx secondary to extensive mucosal injury or massive wound infection: antibiotics, corticosteroids, consider plastic surgical measures.
- Injury to the prevertebral fascia with torticollis (atlantoaxial subluxation, Grisel syndrome) or injury to the arch of the atlas with osteitis/osteomyelitis: antibiotics.
- Hypernasal speech (rhinolalia aperta)/secondary to velopharyngeal insufficiency. A hypernasal voice after removal of a very large pharyngeal tonsil is not too rare, but disappears again spontaneously and quickly.
- Mistaking a nasopharyngeal fibroma for adenoids: apply diagnostic imaging techniques when suspected, e. g., CT and MRI.

Postoperative Care

- Monitor breathing and circulation carefully (recovery unit).
- Check the wound bed for *postoperative bleeding (indirect signs: epistaxis, hemoptysis, increased swallowing reflex, urge to cough, hematemesis, signs of shock)*.
- Keep the patient nil by mouth for about 4 hours, then allow tea, later rusks, etc.; in the evening a light meal, ice cream. Normal diet on the first postoperative day.
- Check the wound on the first postoperative day, with subsequent follow-ups depending on findings.
- Outpatient surgery will require arranging for supervision at home.

Alternatives

Shave resection of the adenoids using an angled endoscopic shaver under direct vision after drawing the soft palate forward with a retractor or rubber slings.

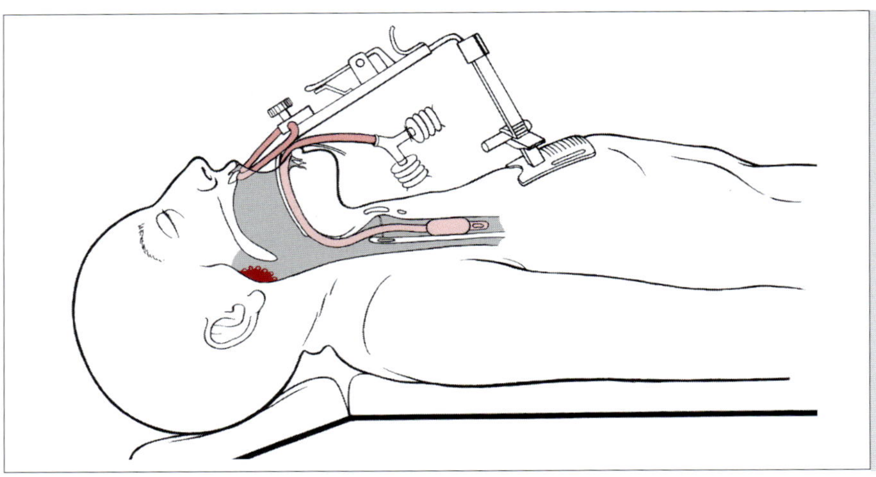

Fig. 8.1 Adenoidectomy. Positioning: head slightly lowered and reclined.

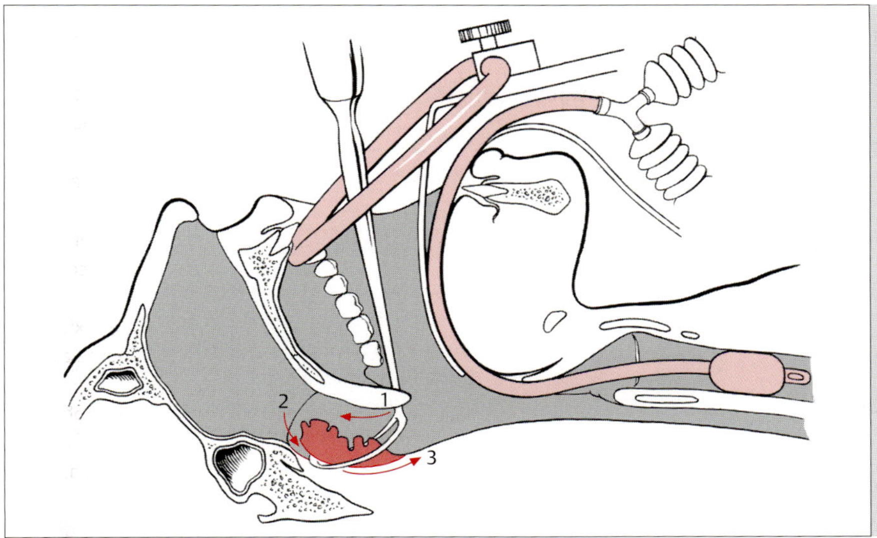

Fig. 8.2 Adenoidectomy.
The ring knife is introduced behind the soft palate and moved upward (1), placed in position behind the margin of the vomer (2), and then drawn downward (3).

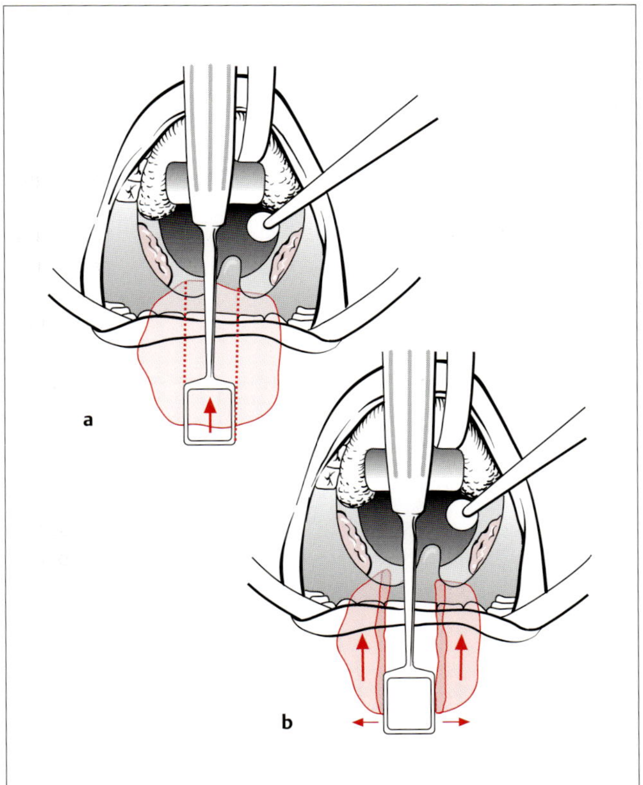

Fig. 8.3a, b Adenoidectomy.
a Curettage of the nasopharynx.
b The pharyngeal recesses are curetted by drawing the knife in parallel lines along the roof of the pharynx.

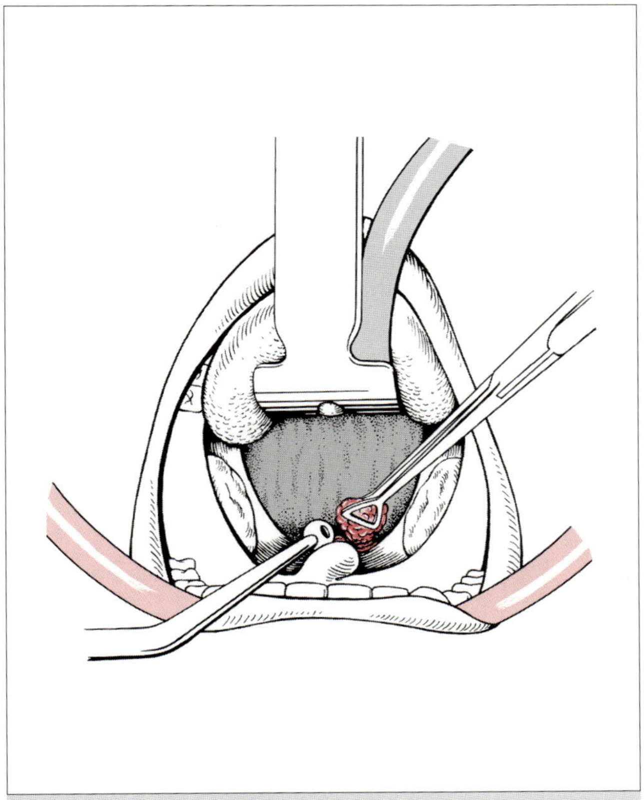

Fig. 8.4 Adenoidectomy.
The residual tissue over the lower wound margin is removed with the triangular jaw conchotome.

Biopsy of the Nasopharynx

Surgical Principle

Transnasal, transoral, or combined scope-guided tissue sampling.

Indications

Equivocal tissue hyperplasia in the nasopharynx.

Contraindications

- Suspected nasopharyngeal fibroma without the possibility of continuing the operation.
- Bleeding disorder or coagulopathy.

Specific Points Regarding Informed Consent

- Hemorrhage or postoperative bleeding.
- Revision surgery.
- Instructions regarding behavior following outpatient surgery.

8

Anesthesia

- Topical anesthesia applied in spray form to the nose and pharynx. Before this, the nose should be decongested. Atropine should be administered for hypersalivation.
- General anesthesia with intubation or larynx mask.

Special Instruments

Slender scopes of 0–90°; straight or curved forceps; suction cautery; straight or curved optic forceps.

Surgical Technique

- Positioning: the patient should be seated when a transnasal or transoral approach is used under topical anesthesia; flat and supine when surgery is performed under general anesthesia; head-down for transoral access.
- The optic forceps is introduced through the wider nostril or through the side nearer the lesion (**Fig. 8.5** [1]).
- Excision under direct vision; if scope and forceps are being used, they should be introduced separately, one in each nostril.
- Transoral access: after inserting the blade, e.g., of a McIvor gag, the soft palate is drawn forward with a rubber sling or a velum retractor, and tissue is sampled under guidance of the scope (**Fig. 8.5** [2]).
- Hemostasis is achieved under guidance of the scope using suction cautery; if appropriate, a swab soaked in nose drops and attached to a suture should be inserted into the nasopharynx. It is essential to confirm its later removal.

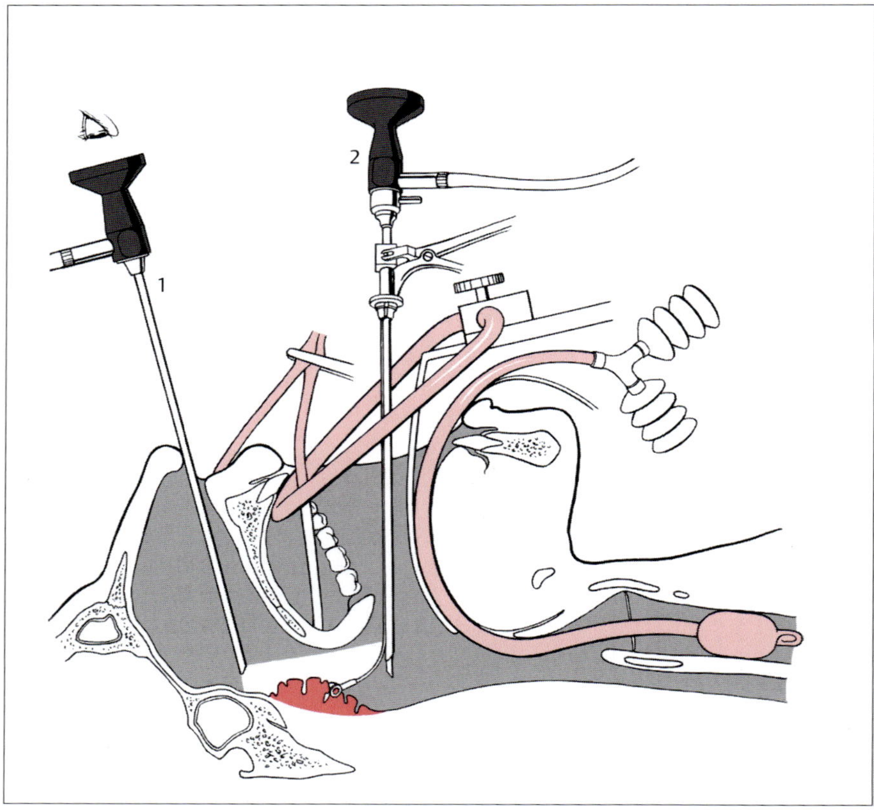

Fig. 8.5 Biopsy taken from the nasopharynx.
1 transnasal introduction of the scope
2 peroral access using the optic forceps

Rules, Tips, and Tricks

- The nose and nasopharynx should be adequately decongested, for better visualization and less tendency to bleed.
- Topical anesthesia should not be applied until adequate decongestion has been achieved.
- When using the transoral approach under topical anesthesia, atropine should be used to reduce the production of saliva.

! Risks and Complications

- Persistent intraoperative hemorrhage.
- Unrecognized nasopharyngeal fibroma (imaging, consider angiography with embolization).
- Postoperative bleeding.

Postoperative Care

- Post-surgical monitoring for bleeding.
- Postoperative clinical examination.

Surgical Technique for Nasopharyngeal Angiofibroma

Surgical Principle

Identification and radical removal of the tumor via lateral rhinotomy or midface degloving with simultaneous ligation of the afferent vessels near the lesion.

Indications

Nasopharyngeal angiofibroma in the nose, nasopharynx, paranasal sinuses, pterygopalatine fossa, and in the margins of the orbita.

Contraindications

- Invasion of the temporal fossa, the endocranium, the retromaxillary space / cavernous sinus (radical removal impossible).
- Coagulopathy.
- Severe underlying general disorder with serious limitation of operability.

Specific Points Regarding Informed Consent

- Severe intraoperative hemorrhage with all its secondary risks, blood transfusion, postoperative bleeding.
- Visible external scar (depending on the approach), scar contracture of the eyelid (edema), lip, nasal vestibule (stenosis).
- Depression of the contours of the nasal wall or the cheek.
- Sensory disturbances or pain (trigeminal or glossopharyngeal neuralgia) of forehead, cheek, lip, maxilla, teeth.
- Obstruction of lacrimal drainage with tearing.
- Disturbances of ventilation of the eustachian tube.
- Dry nose with crust formation.
- Olfactory dysfunction.
- Obstruction of a paranasal sinus secondary to scar formation (cele formation).
- Disturbances of vision with loss of visual acuity, disturbances of ocular mobility/diplopia.
- Cerebrospinal fluid fistula, meningitis, cavernous sinus thrombosis.
- Tendency for recurrence.

Operative Planning

- CT, MRI, digital substraction angiography possibly with embolization.
- Endoscopy.
- Clotting profile.
- Autologous blood donation.

Anesthesia

General endotracheal anesthesia.

Special Instruments

Paranasal sinus instruments with endoscopes, microscope, burrs, silver clips with clip applicator.

Surgical Technique

Lateral Rhinotomy

Skin incision. Moore's lateral rhinotomy incision, beginning immediately next to the inner canthus and proceeding along the base of the nasal pyramid, around the alar attachment and down to the philtrum. The periosteum is swept off the facial wall of the maxillary sinus and the lateral nasal wall, as far as the piriform aperture. The inner mucoperiosteum is detached from the lateral nasal wall beyond the piriform crest.

Extension. Large tumors will require the additional elevation of an upper cheek flap via a marginal incision around the eye (resection of the infraorbital nerve) and a medial division of the upper lip.

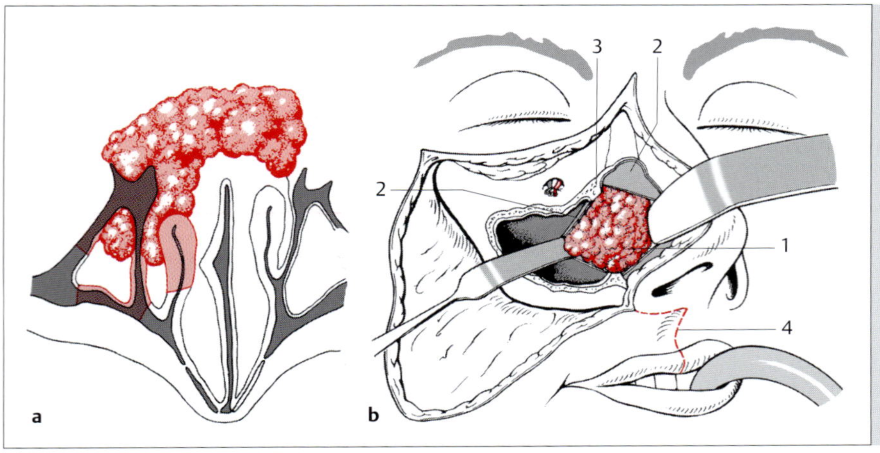

Fig. 8.6a, b Nasopharyngeal angiofibroma.
a Area of resection of the bony wall of the maxillary sinus.
b Removal of the tumor.
1 tumor
2 mucosa of the lateral nasal wall
3 bony edge of the posterior lateral nasal wall
4 optional extension of the skin incision

Removal of the lower piriform aperture and the facial wall of the maxillary sinus, preservation of the mucous membrane, trephine of the posterior wall of the maxillary sinus medially using a diamond burr, division of the periosteum, identification of the maxillary artery, and placement of clips on the lateral afferent branch and the medial efferent branches (**Fig. 8.6a**).

Removal of bone from the medial wall of the maxillary sinus. A full-thickness vertical incision is made through the soft-tissue layer of the lateral nasal wall, immediately behind the nasolacrimal canal, which has been cleared of bone. The anterior part is retracted firmly anteriorly, while the posterior lateral nasal wall is divided at the floor and displaced laterally (**Fig. 8.6b**).

Depending on the findings, the posterior wall of the maxillary sinus, the medial lamella of the pterygoid process, as well as the posterior septum, the ethmoid cells, and the sphenoid sinus may also require removal.

The tumor is then identified, encircled, detached using a dissecting swab, elevator, and digital pressure and removed in its entirety.

Antral balloon catheter. Closure in layers.

Rules, Tips, and Tricks

- The risk of recurrence and postoperative bleeding make the radical removal of all tissue essential.
- The excised tumor should be examined for completeness.
- Preoperative embolization is necessary.
- Afferent vessels must be clipped close to the tumor.
- When suturing, ensure exact approximation of the muscle stumps at the medial canthus and upper lip.

Risks and Complications

- Profuse intraoperative bleeding.
- Risks relating to the eye (amaurosis, diplopia, obstruction of the lacrimal duct).
- Meningitis, cerebrospinal fluid fistula, anosmia.
- Injury to the internal carotid artery, hemiplegia, cavernous sinus thrombosis.
- Injury to the eustachian tube.
- Wound breakdown and problems with scar formation.
- Paralysis of the trigeminal and glossopharyngeal nerves.
- Recurrence.

Alternatives

- Endoscopic microinvasive approach.
- Midfacial degloving.
- Transmandibular approach.
- Radiotherapy for recurrence / residual tumor.

9 Surgery of the Oral Cavity and Oropharynx

Surgery of the Tonsils

Tonsillectomy

Surgical Principle

Complete removal of the tonsillar tissue with its crypts along the capsular plane.

Indications

- Recurrent tonsillitis: the indication for surgery should be considered most carefully for children under 4 years of age.
- Chronic tonsillitis with local symptoms, halitosis, or cervical lymphadenopathy.
- Peritonsillar abscess.
- Tonsillar sepsis or deep neck infection.
- Infection with suspected tonsillar focus (rheumatic fever, endocarditis, certain forms of glomerulonephritis, palmar plantar pustulosis).
- Excessive tonsillar hyperplasia with obstructive sleep apnea syndrome, difficulty in swallowing.
- Monocytic angina with considerable obstruction causing breathing and swallowing difficulties.
- Suspected tumor of the tonsils (biopsy for histological examination).
- Suspected tonsillar primary lesion of tuberculous cervical lymphadenopathy.

Contraindications

- Cardiovascular compromise, severe hypertension.
- Severe general disease.
- Leukemia, agranulocytosis.
- Hepatic failure.
- Coagulopathy: in exceptional urgent indications, special techniques (fibrin glue, replacement of blood components, laser surgery) may allow surgery after hematological preassessment.
- Overt, repaired, or submucous cleft palate: deterioration in speech is possible despite meticulous protection of the muscles; a speech and language therapist should be consulted if the indication is still clinically urgent.
- Singers: a change in voice is possible due to postoperative alterations to the resonating cavity secondary to scar formation.
- Severe atrophic pharyngitis.
- Polio vaccination: interval of 6 weeks.

Specific Points Regarding Informed Consent

- Severe intra- and postoperative hemorrhage with the risk of aspiration and hypoxia, hypovolemic shock.
- Inflammatory complications—infection of the wound bed, cervical lymphadenopathy, retro- and parapharyngeal abscess, deep neck infection, thrombosis of the jugular vein, and mediastinitis.
- Disorders of taste, difficulty in swallowing, reduction of tongue mobility.
- Damage to teeth, damage to the temporomandibular joint, velopalatine insufficiency, disturbances in swallowing and speech (change in voice).

Operative Planning

- Any (family) history of bleeding or coagulation problems.
- PT, PTT, INR, platelet count, blood count, bleeding time test.
- Perioperative antibiotics if appropriate, e.g., prophylaxis against endocarditis.

Special Instruments

- Mouth gag, e.g., McIvor gag, in various sizes.
- Blunt curved tonsil scissors.
- Pointed long scalpel or long angled scissors.
- Henke tonsil elevator.
- Tonsil snare, Röder loop.
- Long clamp, long needle holder, and long forceps.
- Tonsil grasping forceps.
- Tonsil sucker.
- Conchotome (round jaw).
- Bipolar coagulation forceps.
- Fenestrated tongue depressor.

Anesthesia

- General anesthesia with intubation or laryngeal mask, or alternatively local anesthesia.
- General anesthesia is appropriate for:
  - children up to the age of 14
  - adults with intellectual or autonomic lability or epilepsy
  - abscess tonsillectomy
  - hypertensive patients or patients with coagulopathy (more meticulous hemostasis).

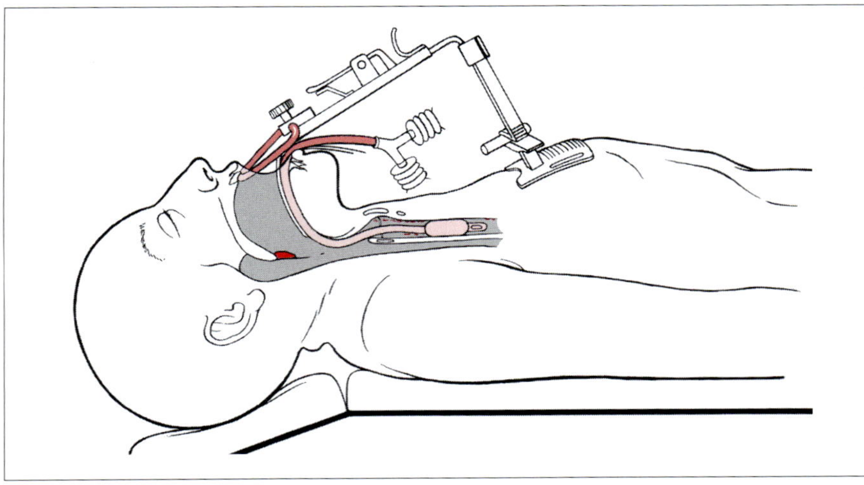

Fig. 9.1 Tonsillectomy under general anesthesia.
The surgeon sits at the head of the patient, which is slightly lowered and reclined.

Surgical Technique

Positioning. The surgeon sits at the head of the patient, slight head-down position, reclination (**Fig. 9.1**) ("hanging head" or Rose position).

Exposure. The oral intubation tube, fixed exactly in the middle of the lower lip, is fixed in the groove of the McIvor blade. While remaining closed, the McIvor gag is advanced carefully deeper, levering slightly (correct blade size: largely covering the tongue, but not touching the mandibular arch, teeth or posterior pharyngeal wall). The frame of the mouth gag is supported between the canines and the incisors (**Fig. 9.2**). The *gag* is carefully opened *(risk of overstretching the temporomandibular joint, pressure palsy of the hypoglossal or lingual nerves, kinking of the tube)*. The tonsil must nevertheless still be visible as far as the glossotonsillar sulcus. The chest support or holder is attached.

Incision. The tonsillar tissue is grasped by its superior pole and drawn medially and downward. The mucous membrane is incised with nasal scissors or scalpel along the edge of the anterior soft palate (recognizable by moving the tonsil to and fro) (**Fig. 9.3**). Careful tangential spreading and retraction of the muscles with the scissors in a lateral direction will allow identification of the capsule, shining through as a grayish-white layer (**Fig. 9.4**). The tissue is spread apart along the subcapsular plane to allow incision of the anterior pillar down to its attachment to the tongue (**Fig. 9.5**).

Superior pole. While continuous traction is maintained on the tonsil in a medial and downward direction, the superior pole is exposed, using the curved tonsil scissors and keeping strictly to the subcapsular plane (**Fig. 9.6**). The posterior pillar is undermined with spreading movements in a downward direction. The posterior pillar is then incised (**Fig. 9.7**).

Dissection. The grasping forceps are placed on the tonsil tissue and drawn firmly down in a medial direction. The peritonsillar tissue is swept off using the Henke rasp, small gauze dissector, or tonsil scissors (**Fig. 9.8**); dissection is always directed away from the tonsil. Readjusting the grasping forceps will keep the tonsillar tissue under tension.

Resection. The tonsil is pedicled beyond the triangular fold down to the base of the tongue, to be then resected beneath the inferior pole using the tonsil sling (**Fig. 9.9**).

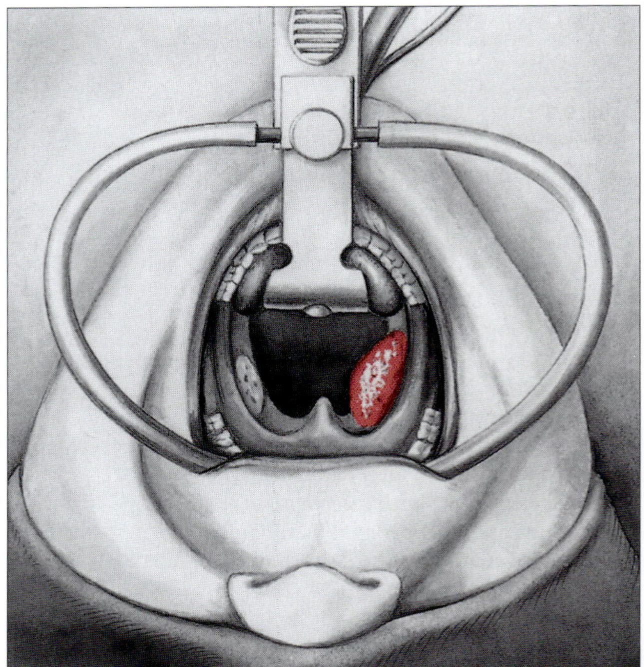

Fig. 9.2 Tonsillectomy under general anesthesia.
Exposure of the tonsils (after Theissing in Naumann HH. Kopf- und Hals-Chirurgie [Head and Neck Surgery]).

Hemostasis. Important: when operating on individuals with Down Syndrome, special attention must be paid to a very careful procedure, because they are particularly prone to subluxation of the cervical spine if they are hyperextended.

Larger spurting vessels are grasped with forceps, the tissue cone is drawn laterally, a clamp is passed beneath it (**Fig. 9.10**) and the tissue is ligated (either a Röder loop is used or the knot is drawn down with a clamp or slider) (**Fig. 9.11**) or secured with a suture ligation. When passing the needle for the suture ligation, adequate traction must be placed on the clamp before the needle is inserted tangentially at the base of the tissue to avoid collateral damage in the depths (**Fig. 9.12**). Minor bleeds can be coagulated with the bipolar diathermy forceps (**Fig. 9.13**).

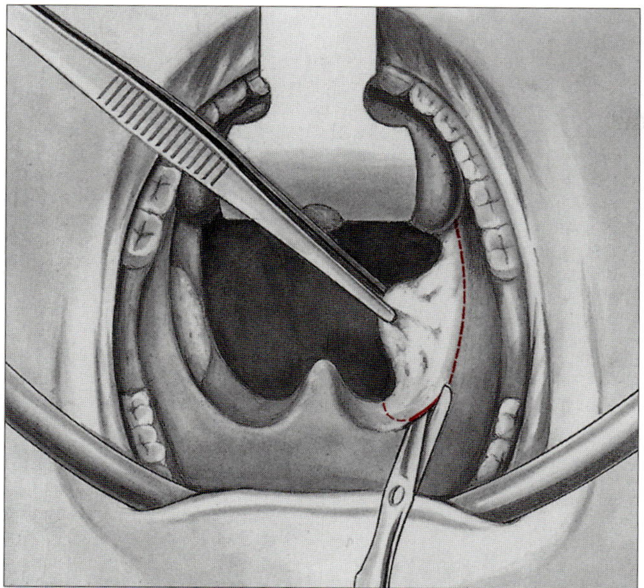

Fig. 9.3 Tonsillectomy under general anesthesia.
Incision of the mucosal margin of the anterior pillar, the position of which is confirmed by repeated medial traction (after Theissing in Naumann HH. Kopf- und Hals-Chirurgie [Head and Neck Surgery]).

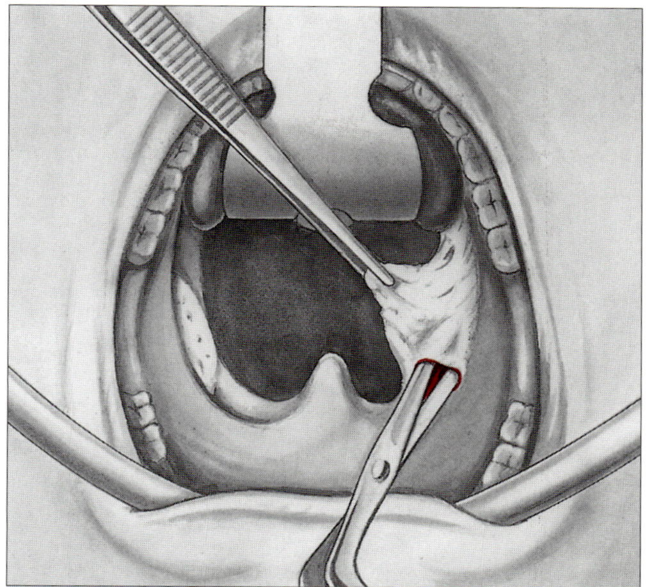

Fig. 9.4 Tonsillectomy under general anesthesia.
Identification of the capsule by spreading and retracting the muscles (after Theissing in Naumann HH. Kopf- und Hals-Chirurgie [Head and Neck Surgery]).

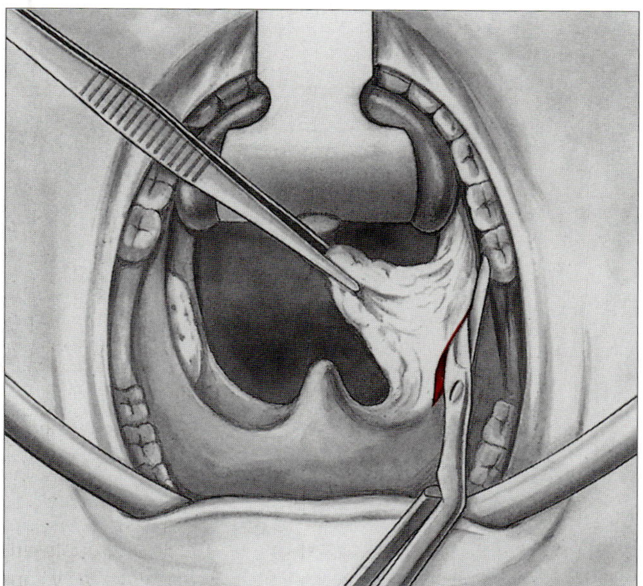

Fig. 9.5 Tonsillectomy under general anesthesia.
Incision of the anterior pillar as far as the attachment of the tongue (after Theissing in Naumann HH. Kopf- und Hals-Chirurgie [Head and Neck Surgery]).

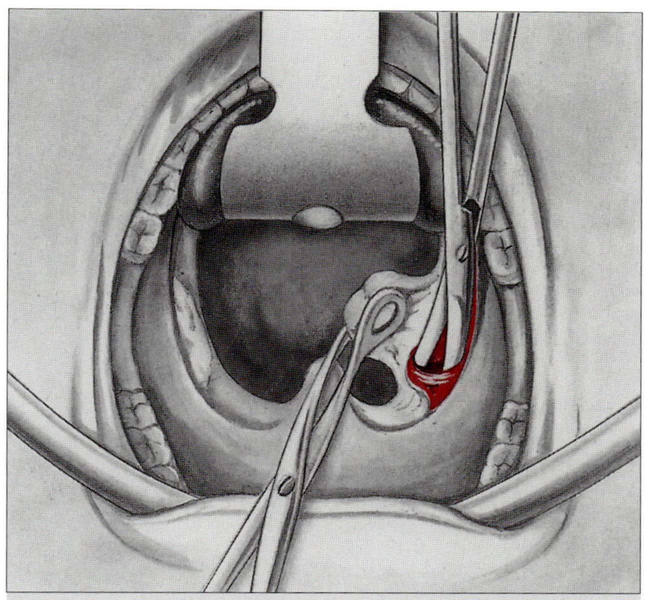

Fig. 9.6 Tonsillectomy under general anesthesia.
Exposure of the superior pole by undermining along the plane of the capsule (after Theissing in Naumann HH. Kopf- und Hals-Chirurgie [Head and Neck Surgery]).

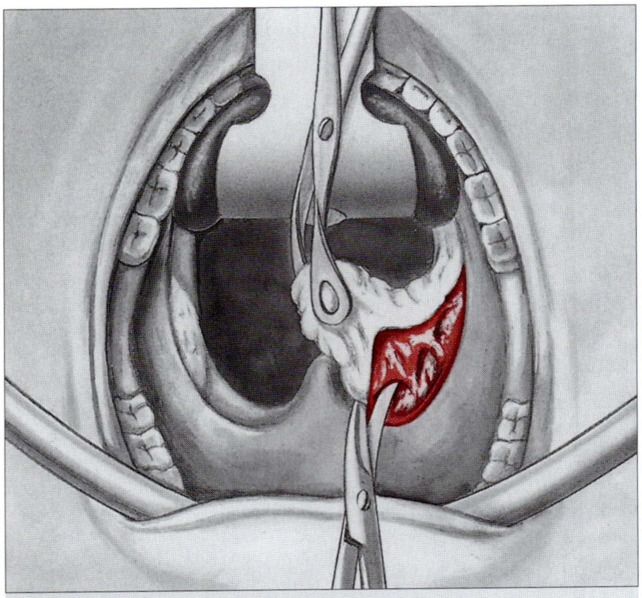

Fig. 9.7 Tonsillectomy under general anesthesia. Incision of the posterior pillar (after Theissing in Naumann HH. Kopf- und Hals-Chirurgie [Head and Neck Surgery]).

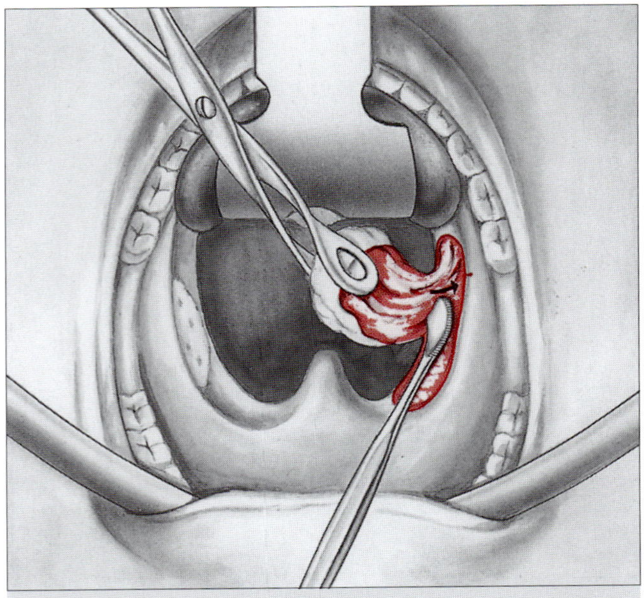

Fig. 9.8 Tonsillectomy under general anesthesia. Dissection of the tonsils by sweeping off the peritonsillar tissue with the Henke rasp (after Theissing in Naumann HH. Kopf- und Hals-Chirurgie [Head and Neck Surgery]).

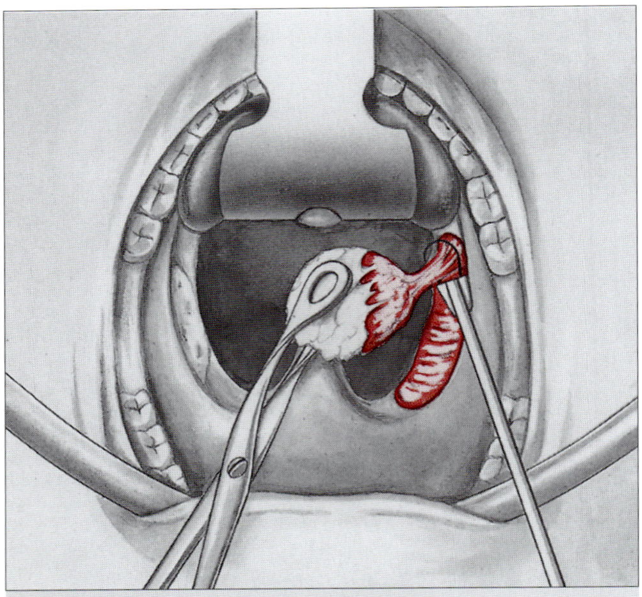

Fig. 9.9 Tonsillectomy under general anesthesia. Removal of the tonsils at the base of the tongue using a tonsil snare (after Theissing in Naumann HH. Kopf- und Hals-Chirurgie [Head and Neck Surgery]).

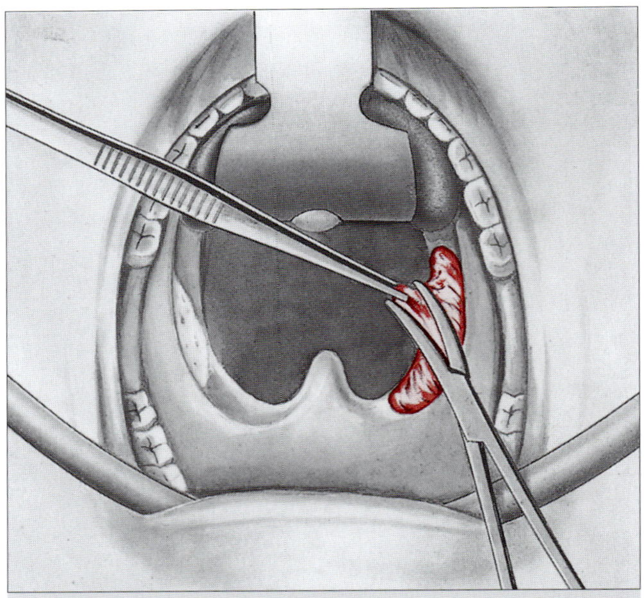

Fig. 9.10 Tonsillectomy under general anesthesia. An artery clip is placed after applying traction to the tissue (after Theissing in Naumann HH. Kopf- und Hals-Chirurgie [Head and Neck Surgery]).

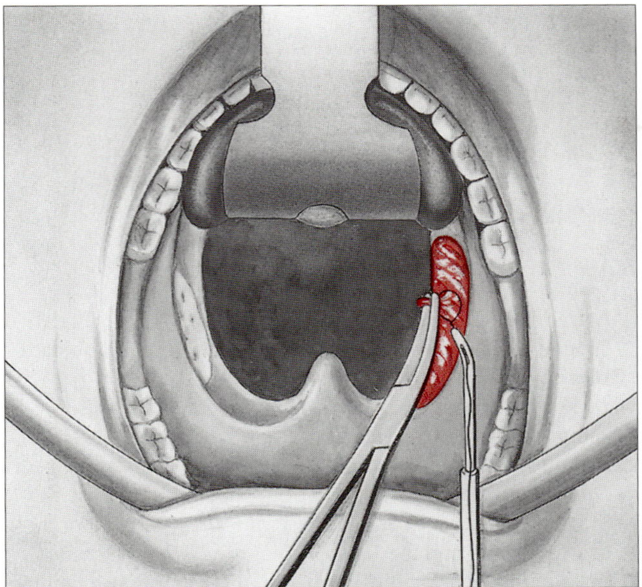

Fig. 9.11 Tonsillectomy under general anesthesia.
Vessel ligation using a Röder loop (after Theissing in Naumann HH. Kopf- und Hals-Chirurgie [Head and Neck Surgery]).

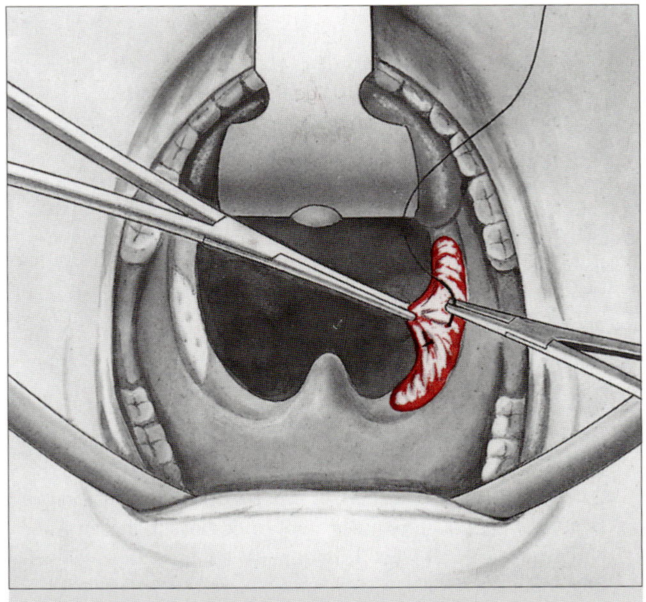

Fig. 9.12 Tonsillectomy under general anesthesia.
Suture ligation. The needle is inserted superficially through the tissue (after Theissing in Naumann HH. Kopf- und Hals-Chirurgie [Head and Neck Surgery]).

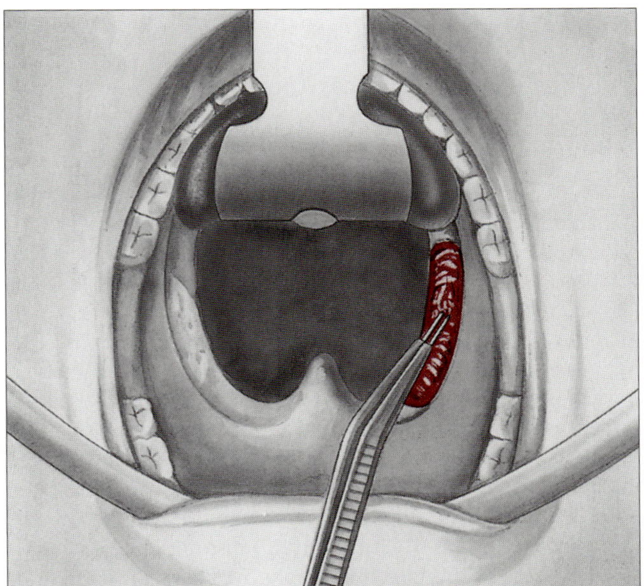

Fig. 9.13 Tonsillectomy under general anesthesia.
Cauterization using a bipolar forceps (after Theissing in Naumann HH. Kopf- und Hals-Chirurgie [Head and Neck Surgery]).

Rules, Tips, and Tricks

- Always dissect within the correct plane along the tonsillar capsule. If the capsule is inadvertently breached, then it is identified again, more laterally and caudally, using the same principle.
- In the region of the inferior tonsillar pole/triangular fold, the layer sometimes retracts medially and can be lost. The grasping forceps should therefore be placed close to the plane of dissection and the tissue held well under tension in a medial and downward direction. Bipolar hemostasis should be secured during dissection to achieve better visualization. Remains of the triangular fold are removed with the conchotome.
- To avoid leaving behind remains of the inferior pole and the triangular fold—which may become the initial site of recurrent local inflammations—incision of the anterior and posterior pillars is continued as far as the glossotonsillar sulcus.
- The wound bed should be well exposed when securing hemostasis to enable adequate visualization of the source of bleeding. Avoid pulling on the grasping clamp and placing suture ligations with large bites, otherwise there is the risk of injuring adjacent structures or breaking off the needle.
- The pharynx should be carefully suctioned before extubation.

! Risks and Complications

- Severe intraoperative hemorrhage from abnormal vessels extending to the tonsillar bed (branches of the external carotid artery, ascending and descending pharyngeal artery, descending palatine artery, lingual artery and, in exceptional cases, the internal carotid artery due to kinking). Strong pulsations of the pharyngeal walls or the tonsils after exposing the pharynx are indications of abnormal courses of the vessels. If a severe hemorrhage cannot be controlled by a suture ligature from an internal access, then the carotid sheath must be exposed from an external approach. If there is any suspicion of injury to the internal carotid artery then a vascular surgeon should be involved.
- Injury to the glossopharyngeal nerve, which runs near the tonsils in the inferoposterior pillar: this results in disturbances of taste and swallowing and can be caused by transsection, overgenerous suture ligation, or hypertrophic scar formation. Dissection should therefore be performed close to the capsule and suture ligatures with big bites in the region of the inferoposterior pillar should be avoided.
- Postoperative bleeding: most commonly on the day of the operation, on the first postoperative day, as well as between the fifth and seventh postoperative days in the form of a delayed bleed. Postoperative bleeding may occur as late as 14 days after surgery, and in exceptional cases even later.
  Basic measures:
  - exclude aspiration, if necessary intubate and perform bronchoscopic suction
  - check hemoglobin, blood pressure, and pulse
  - venous access, infusion, if necessary transfusion
  - clotting profile.

  Local measures:
  - suck away coagulated blood, infiltrate the source of bleeding with a vasoconstrictor and local anesthetic
  - bipolar diathermy or suture ligation of the source of bleeding, under general anesthesia if necessary
  - cover the wound bed with a collagen fleece soaked in fibrin glue in the presence of coagulopathy.

  Locally persistent arterial bleeding:
  - After packing the wound bed and pharynx, ligation from an external approach. Skin incision over the sternocleidomastoid, identification of the carotid sheath, ligation of the facial and retromandibular veins, follow the course of the branches of the external carotid artery, lingual artery, facial artery, ascending pharyngeal artery and ligate as peripherally as possible.
  - Alternatively, consider the occasional option of performing an angiography and embolizing the damaged vessel.
- Para- and retropharyngeal abscess, wound-bed infection, thrombosis of the jugular vein, deep neck infection, suppurative cervical lymphadenopathy.
- Disturbances of taste, which are rarely permanent (the administration of glucocorticoids may be tried) and are more common in the first postoperative day when they are short-term and disappear spontaneously.
- Scar contracture of the soft palate with velopalatine insufficiency and disturbances of swallowing or hypernasal speech (rhinolalia aperta).
- Injury to the hypoglossal nerve secondary to pressure from the McIvor blade.
- Damage to teeth or disturbances of the temporomandibular joint from the mouth gag.

Postoperative Care

- Close postoperative monitoring with inspection of the wound bed and attention to signs of internal hemorrhage (hemoptysis, increased swallowing reflex, urge to cough, stridor, aspiration, signs of hemorrhagic shock and hematemesis).
- Analgesia (*no salicylic acid derivatives*) especially 20–30 minutes before meals, ice pack applied to the neck.
- Antibiotics for focal or acute inflammatory reactions.
- Nutrition: only tea on the day of the operation, then a soft diet. Fruit and juices may burn significantly because of their acidity. More solid food may be resumed from the second postoperative week. If children are not drinking sufficiently, consider an IV infusion.
- Initially, patients should avoid washing the hair and taking hot baths.
- Patients should avoid physical exertion completely for 2 weeks and not resume sports until after 3 weeks.

Alternatives

Tonsillectomy under Local Anesthesia

Local Anesthesia

Timely premedication with sufficient atropine administration (salivation interferes with the topical anesthesia and is a hindrance during the operation).

Topical anesthesia is sprayed onto the tongue, tonsillar pillars, and posterior wall of the pharynx.

Infiltration anesthesia with 20 mL 1% lidocaine plus epinephrine (1:200 000). The mouth-gag blade is placed directly next to the tonsil to allow the triangular fold to be also placed under tension. Subcutaneous infiltration of the mucosa of the pillars as far as the tongue (**Fig. 9.14**). The tonsil is displaced medially with forceps and the peritonsillar tissue is infiltrated with three depots of 2 mL each into the groove that then comes into view (**Fig. 9.15**). The tonsil itself must not be injected. Always aspirate before injecting. Apply 2 mL each to the inferior pole and in the region of the triangular fold. Wait 5–10 minutes to allow for better vasoconstriction.

Surgical Technique

- Positioning: semi-seated. The surgeon stands at the side, next to the patient's upper body.
- Spatula insertion: begin with the tonsil that was anesthetized first. The tongue is displaced downward and toward the contralateral side with the self-retaining spatula. The glossotonsillar sulcus must be visualized.

9

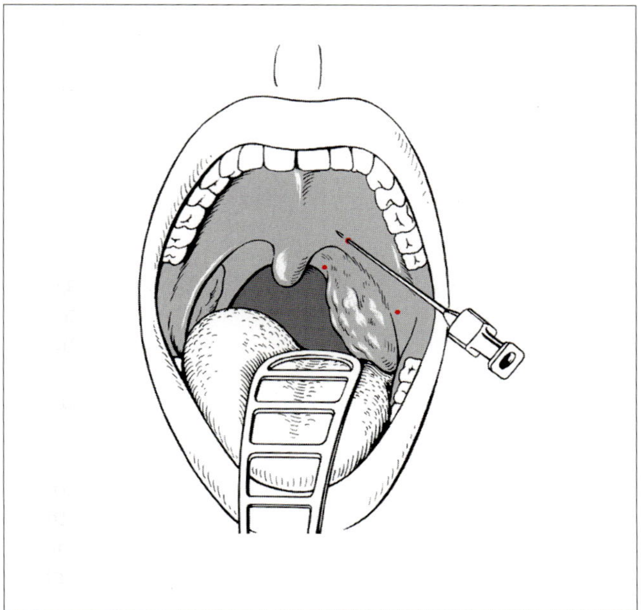

Fig. 9.14 Tonsillectomy under local anesthesia. Subcutaneous infiltration of the mucosa.

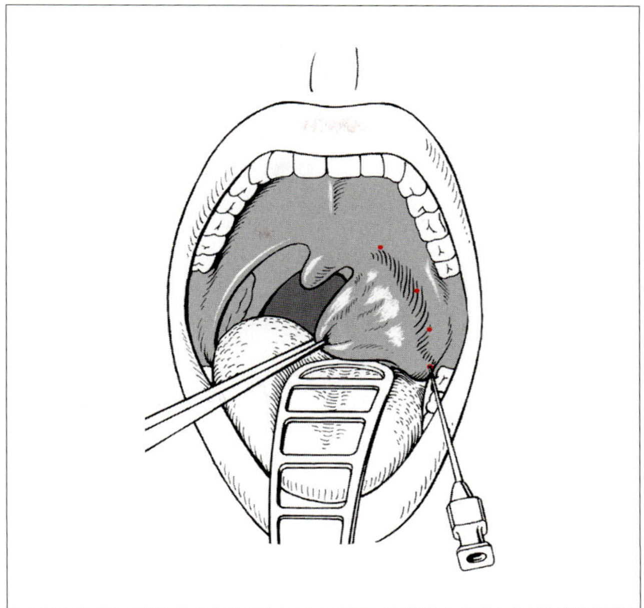

Fig. 9.15 Tonsillectomy under local anesthesia. Peritonsillar infiltration.

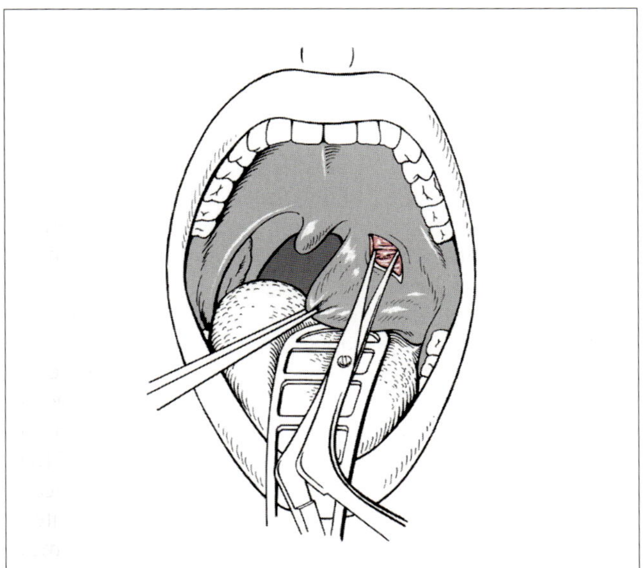

Fig. 9.16 Tonsillectomy under local anesthesia. Incision of the mucosa and identification of the tonsillar capsule.

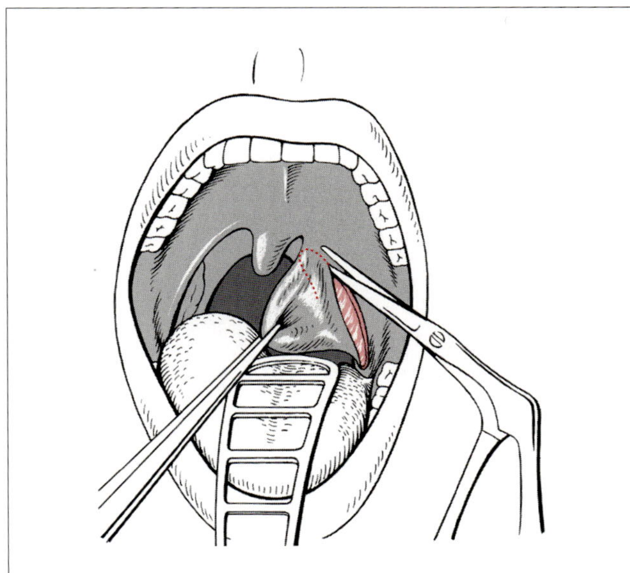

Fig. 9.17 Tonsillectomy under local anesthesia. Incision along the anterior tonsillar pillar.

- The steps for dissection are the same as for surgery under general anesthesia, except that they are performed in the opposite direction: incision of the margin of the anterior pillar after drawing the tonsil forward. The capsule is identified with spreading movements (**Fig. 9.16**).
- The anterior pillar is undermined and the superior pole of the tonsil is detached using the spreading curved tonsil scissors. The posterior pillar is also undermined and incised (**Fig. 9.17**).
- The peritonsillar tissue is detached by dissecting the muscularis layer from the capsule, pedicled to the base of the tongue (**Fig. 9.18**) and removed using the tonsil snare (**Fig. 9.19**).
- The assistant can suction during dissection to avoid aspiration and gagging.

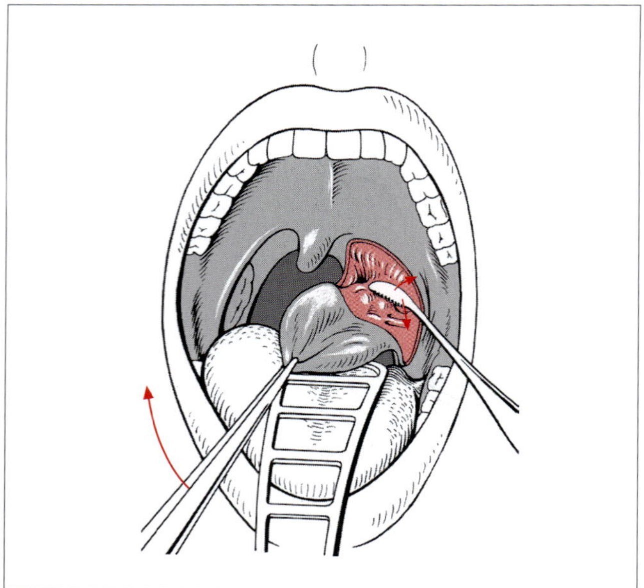

Fig. 9.18 Tonsillectomy under local anesthesia.
Detachment of the peritonsillar tissue from the capsule using the rasp.

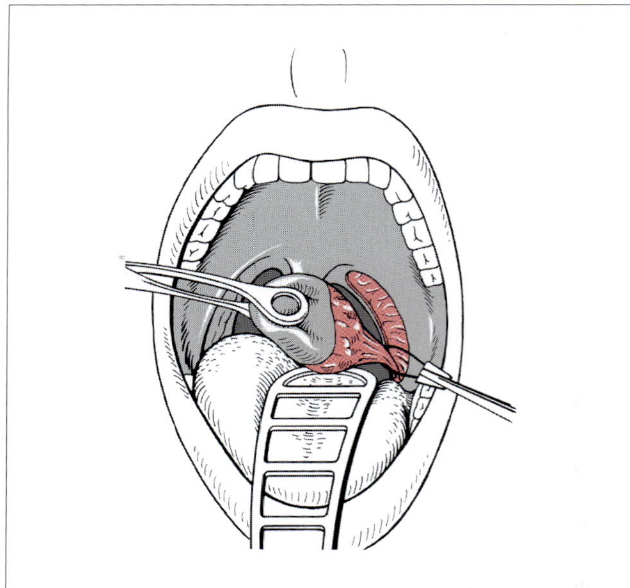

Fig. 9.19 Tonsillectomy under local anesthesia.
Ligation below the inferior pole of the tonsil using the tonsil snare.

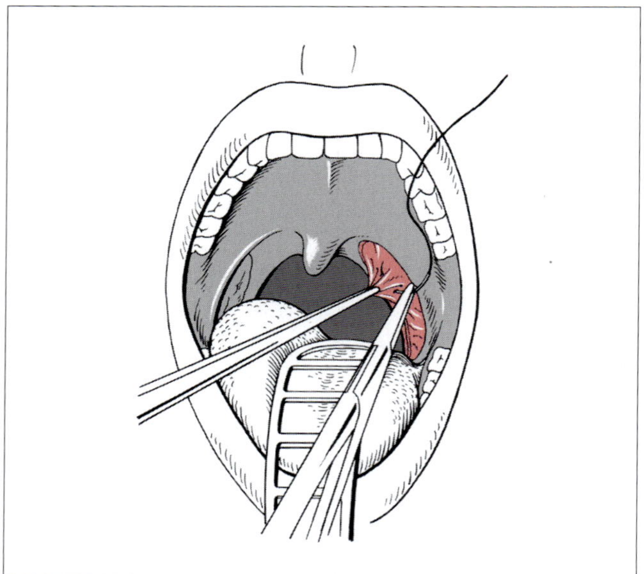

Fig. 9.20 Tonsillectomy under local anesthesia.
Suture ligation of a vessel.

- More profuse bleeding should be controlled immediately by bipolar diathermy or suture ligation (**Fig. 9.20**).

Adenotonsillectomy

The procedure is the same as for tonsillectomy under general anesthesia and adenoidectomy. If adenoidectomy is done first, the nasopharyngeal pack for hemostasis may be left during tonsillectomy. This saves an additional waiting period while performing hemostasis in the nasopharynx. Removal of the swabs at the end of the operation must be ensured.

Laser Tonsillectomy

Instead of the conventional blunt-sharp dissection using instruments, the tonsils may also be dissected using a laser. Nd:YAG and potassium titanyl phosphate (KTP) lasers are preferred, in addition to the CO_2 laser.

Basically, laser tonsillectomy is associated with less bleeding, although the larger vessels that are disrupted nevertheless require bipolar coagulation. The frequency of postoperative bleeding is the same as in the conventional technique, while wound healing appears to be slightly delayed; usually a somewhat stronger edema of the uvula develops. Postoperative pain lasts slightly longer.

Guidelines for laser protection must be followed: protect the tube from igniting, protect the posterior wall of the pharynx from inadvertent radiation by covering it with a damp swab layer, use safety glasses, etc.

The technique follows the same steps as for the conventional approach. More traction is needed on the superior tonsil pole to bring the tissue more into the surgical site for dissection because the laser only cuts in a straight line.

For tonsillar hypertrophy in infants, where the part of the tonsil that extends beyond the anterior and posterior pillars is resected tangentially, *laser tonsillotomy* has recently been once again propagated as an alternative to tonsillectomy. Genuine long-term follow-ups, which have led to abandonment of the once-customary tonsillotomy using cutting instruments because of the significant late complications, are so far not available.

Tonsillectomy Using the Argon-Plasma Coagulation Dissector

Argon-plasma coagulation (APC) is a special technique for applying high-frequency radiation for thermal dissection and coagulation. When using Bergler APC dissector, the technical procedure is the same as when using conventional instruments. Operating time is supposed to be shorter because there is less intraoperative bleeding.

Surgery for Inflammatory Complications Originating from the Tonsils

Incision and Drainage of a Peritonsillar Abscess

Surgical Principle

Incision and drainage of peritonsillar accumulations of pus.

Indications

Para- (supra-, retro-, intra-) tonsillar abscesses.

Contraindications

- Deep neck infection.
- Hidden (infra- or retrotonsillar) site of the abscess (indication for abscess tonsillectomy).
- Bleeding disorder (relative contraindication, consider just needle aspiration).

Specific Points Regarding Informed Consent

- Aspiration.
- Hemorrhage.
- Vascular injury.
- Abscess tonsillectomy, if indicated.
- Postoperative care, including repeat spreading of the wound.

Operative Planning

- Laryngoscopy to exclude a life-threatening glottis edema.
- Possible administration of cortisone, e.g., 250 mg prednisolone (decongestion of the glottis edema, pain reduction, better localization of the abscess).
- Antibiotics.
- Exclusion of a deep neck infection or thrombosis of the jugular vein.
- Bleeding and coagulation history.
- PT, PTT, INR, blood count.

Special Instruments

- Syringe with an attached large-bore needle.
- Scalpel or sharp spreading forceps.
- Dressing forceps or slightly curved long tonsil clamp.
- Round-headed sucker.

Anesthesia

- For children, general anesthesia.
- For adults, apply local anesthesia using a topical anesthetic and inject lidocaine plus epinephrine intracutaneously into the mucous membrane.

Surgical Technique

Needle drainage. Use a syringe with an attached large-bore needle. The needle is inserted directly above the superior pole of the tonsil, in the middle of an imaginary line between the base of the uvula and the superior wisdom tooth, or at the most prominent site. Under continuous aspiration, the needle is advanced deeper in an exactly sagittal direction until pus is encountered.

Incision and drainage. From the aforementioned puncture site, an incision is made obliquely downward from medial–superior to lateral–inferior for a distance of 1.5 cm; the incision is also deepened in a sagittal direction to a depth of 1.5 cm with a scalpel or dressing forceps or a tonsil spreader and widened until the abscess cavity is completely drained. The pus is removed by suction (**Fig. 9.21a, b**).

Rules, Tips, and Tricks

- The prior administration of cortisone facilitates identification of the abscess.
- Premedication with atropine administration improves anesthesia in the highly inflamed tissue.
- Working down in a strictly sagittal plane avoids deviating toward the lateral-running vessels.
- Retro- and infratonsillar abscesses are difficult to identify and are better managed by abscess tonsillectomy.

! Risks and Complications

- Vascular injury with considerable hemorrhage.
- Aspiration of pus into the lungs resulting in secondary pneumonia.
- Glottis edema.
- Deep neck infection or jugular vein thrombosis.

Postoperative Care

- Daily opening of the wound until only small amounts of serous fluid are drained.
- Antibiotics.
- Consider proceeding to tonsillectomy after 3–5 days ("tonsillectomy à tiède").
- Abscess tonsillectomy in the presence of severe bleeding or an abscess which is difficult to identify.

Abscess Tonsillectomy

Surgical Principle

Removal of the tonsils along the subcapsular plane with the simultaneous drainage of the abscess.

Indications

- Late presentation or delayed healing of incised abscesses.
- Deep or parapharyngeal abscesses, when drainage by incision is not possible.
- Septic conditions arising from the tonsils associated with peritonsillar inflammation.
- Persistent bleeding after abscess incision.
- Peritonsillar abscess in infants.
- Peritonsillar abscesses, as an alternative to abscess incision, especially if there have been previous abscesses or a relevant history provides the indication for tonsillectomy anyway.

Contraindications

As a rule, the same as for tonsillectomy (see p. 155); imminent complications such as sepsis, thrombosis of the jugular vein, necrotizing fasciitis, or septic necrosis of the carotid artery, however, outweigh the relative contraindications.

9

Specific Points Regarding Informed Consent

As for tonsillectomy (see p. 155).

Operative Planning

- Any (family) history of bleeding or coagulation problems.
- PT, PTT, INR, platelet count, blood count, if appropriate bleeding time test.
- Inspection of the larynx and pharynx, if appropriate using fiber-optic methods.
- Ultrasonography of the neck, including the carotid sheath and tonsil region.

Special Instruments

As for tonsillectomy under general anesthesia.

Anesthesia

As a rule, general endotracheal anesthesia. Be aware of intubation problems; consider fiber-optic intubation.

Surgical Technique

The approach is basically the same as for tonsillectomy under general anesthesia.

The mucosal incision is oriented along the base of the uvula and the triangular fold. Suture repair of any incision from a previous abscess incision will avoid tearing it further.

Because of the brittleness of the tissue, the capsule and superior pole must be identified without any significant traction on the tonsillar tissue and without pressure on the peritonsillar tissue. This is done by blunt dissection and without abrupt spreading with the tonsil scissors. The curve of the scissor blades lies against the tonsil when releasing the superior pole and the lateral and anterior surfaces of the tonsil. This type of dissection leads inevitably to the abscess cavity. A culture swab for bacteriological examination is taken from the cavity.

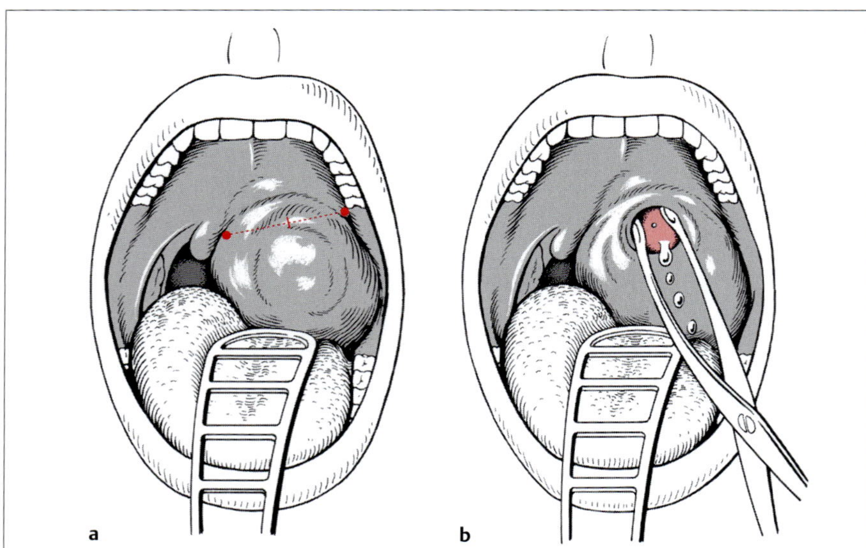

Fig. 9.21a, b Peritonsillar abscess.
a Site for needle drainage/incision.
b Spreading open the incision wound.

The lateral abscess capsule should not be injured, as this otherwise results in significant bleeding.

Any significant bleeds are secured by suture ligation, and any minor bleeding is easily controlled by bipolar coagulation. A swab placed temporarily into the tonsillar recess will also stop any oozing.

The contralateral tonsil is generally removed as well.

Rules, Tips, and Tricks

- Careful identification of the capsular plane by dissecting with the inverted Henke rasp (V-shaped gouge).
- Careful bipolar coagulation provides better visualization in the surgical field.

! Risks and Complications

- As for tonsillectomy (see p. 160).

Postoperative Care

As for tonsillectomy (see p. 160).

Alternatives

- Peritonsillar abscess incision and drainage.
- Laser tonsillectomy.
- Parapharyngeal abscesses extending to the carotid sheath require the additional revision of the neck from an external approach.

Incision and Drainage of a Retropharyngeal Abscess

Surgical Principle

Wide drainage of the abscess.

Indications

Any retropharyngeal abscess.

Specific Points Regarding Informed Consent

- Hemorrhage, aspiration with hypoxia.
- Aspiration of pus into the lungs with secondary pneumonia or pulmonary emphysema.
- Risks involved with the spontaneous course of a retropharyngeal abscess: mediastinitis, thrombosis of the jugular vein, obstruction of the larynx, vascular rupture.

Operative Planning

- Any (family) history of bleeding or coagulation problems.
- PT, PTT, INR, platelet count, blood count, bleeding time test.
- Positioning for general anesthesia is supine and flat, head reclined and hanging down (Rose or “hanging head” position).
- Perioperative antibiotics.
- Lateral soft-tissue neck radiography.

Anesthesia

Usually general anesthesia, but local anesthesia is also an option for adults.

Surgical Technique

- Exposure: McIvor mouth gag as for tonsillectomy with hanging-head position.
- Aspiration using a large-bore needle.
- Strictly sagittal incision running along an inferior to superior line until the abscess cavity is reached, simultaneous suctioning of the pus with the round-head aspirator, culture swab.
- To improve drainage, the incision wound should be opened up, or converting it into a cruciate incision may be considered; nasogastric tube.

Rules, Tips, and Tricks

- In cases of difficult intubation: consider endoscope-assisted intubation or use a Negus rigid emergency endoscope.
- Care is also needed during extubation: secure patent airways, suction pharynx well.

! Risks and Complications

- Injury to the ascending palatine artery and ascending pharyngeal artery: if necessary the vascular stump should be ligated with a suture. If this is impossible, the carotid sheath can be exposed from an external approach.
- Aspiration pneumonia.
- Mediastinitis or jugular vein thrombosis.

Postoperative Care

Generally as for tonsillectomy; consider enteral nutrition initially. Adjust antibiotics according to the swab results. Open up the incision wound again if there is retention of pus.

Surgery for Deep Neck Infection Originating from the Tonsils and for Tonsillar Sepsis

Surgical Principle

Elimination of the source of infection (tonsillectomy), the focus of hematogenous spread, and abscess material with exposure of the carotid sheath.

Indications

- Chills, rigor, septic temperatures during the course (not at the beginning) of a tonsillitis or peritonsillar abscess, or after apparent healing:
  - with intense tenderness and swelling along the jugular vein
  - sonographic evidence of jugular vein thrombosis
  - sharp increase of the inflammatory parameters.
- Prior treatment with antibiotics may result in a less fulminant clinical course, thus obscuring the clinical picture.

Contraindications

None, being a vital indication.

Specific Points Regarding Informed Consent

- For simultaneous tonsillectomy, see p. 155.
- Hemorrhage, postoperative bleeding; also consider blood transfusion and mention relevant risks.
- Progression of the thrombosis, embolic event, mediastinitis, septic emboli with possible vital threat or severe secondary functional impairment (e.g., cerebral).
- Functional sequelae of injury to the vagal, hypoglossal, and accessory nerves, and to the mandibular branch of the facial nerve and the phrenic nerve.
- Chyle fistula.
- Wound breakdown, scar formation, sensory dysfunction of the skin of the neck.

Operative Planning

- Local findings relating to the tonsils, mirror inspection of the larynx, e.g., for possible problems with intubation.
- Local findings from B-ultrasonography and Doppler of the neck.
- Measure temperature, blood cultures, white blood count, ESR, coagulation status.
- Broad-spectrum antibiotics.

Special Instruments

Standard neck instrument tray.

Anesthesia

General endotracheal anesthesia.

Surgical Technique

Exposure. Incision over the anterior margin of the sternocleidomastoid muscle, extending from the mastoid process to the sternal notch. Division of the subcutaneous fat, platysma, and superficial cervical fascia, ligating any traversing veins in the process. The anterior margin of the sternocleidomastoid is identified and retracted, while dissection continues bluntly down to the carotid sheath using dissecting forceps, scissors or dissector sponge, and nontoothed forceps.

Identification. If the tissue shows significant adhesions, the easily identifiable omohyoid muscle is chosen as an anatomic landmark and the jugular vein is traced from its crossing of the carotid sheath. The vessel is very vulnerable in the presence of a deep infection and must be dissected with the utmost care. The accessory, vagus, and hypoglossal nerves are also identified to avoid any inadvertent injury. Dissection proceeds parallel to the direction of the structures.

Ligation. In the presence of a jugular vein thrombosis (discoloration of the vein wall, absent venous pulse, hard to palpate), the vein itself is traced further in a cranial and caudal direction and ligated where it still appears normal, the vein wall is incised, and the thrombus extracted (**Fig. 9.22**). Even if the internal jugular vein is still conveying blood and is thus preservable, the retromandibular and facial veins must still be exposed as far as the tonsillar region and ligated. While tracing the inflammatory process, the deep neck spaces medial to the carotid sheath are opened over the prevertebral fascia up to the pharyngeal wall. Exposure and drainage of the upper mediastinum may also be necessary.

Progression of the thrombosis to the superior vena cava is managed by thrombolysis after ligating the jugular vein above the angulus venosus, the junction with the subclavian vein. Extension of the thrombosis into the sigmoid sinus is similarly treated, in addition to ligating the sinus and jugular bulb.

Wound closure. Primary wound closure with insertion of a suction drain is required only after purely phlebitic processes.

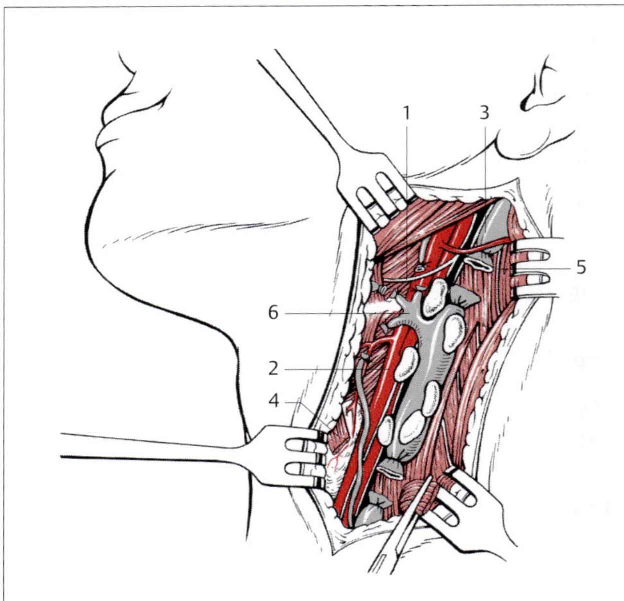

Fig. 9.22 Tonsillar sepsis.
Ligation of the jugular vein.
1 hypoglossal nerve
2 carotid bifurcation
3 superior stump of the jugular vein
4 stump of the omohyoid muscle
5 accessory nerve
6 facial and retromandibular veins

After a deep infection, open postoperative wound management with gauze packing or Penrose drain. Only the superior and inferior wound poles are reduced by sutures.

Tonsillectomy, if the tonsils are still present.

Rules, Tips, and Tricks

- Always ensure general endotracheal anesthesia to eliminate an air embolus.
- Veins are extremely vulnerable when inflamed; use only blunt dissection. If the vein does tear, apply pressure above and below with sponge-holding forceps. The vein wall should then be exposed distal to the lesion and ligated.
- If inflammatory scarring makes the identification of anatomic structures difficult, attempt dissection more peripherally and trace back.
- Watch out for the thoracic duct on the left side of the neck. If a chyle fistula develops, manage immediately by suture ligation.

! Risks and Complications

- Intra- and postoperative bleeding with all its secondary complications.
- Chyle fistula.
- Septic emboli.
- Injury to the vagus, hypoglossal, or accessory nerves or the mandibular branch of the facial nerve with the corresponding functional deficits.
- Conspicuous scar formation following healing by secondary intention; sensory dysfunction.

Surgery for Abscesses of the Oral Cavity

Lingual abscesses originate from infected injuries, inflammation of the lingual tonsil, and less frequently from inflammatory processes of adjacent structures (jaw, teeth, tonsils). They may be located superficially or deeply in the tip of the tongue, the body of the tongue, and the base of the tongue (**Fig. 9.23**).

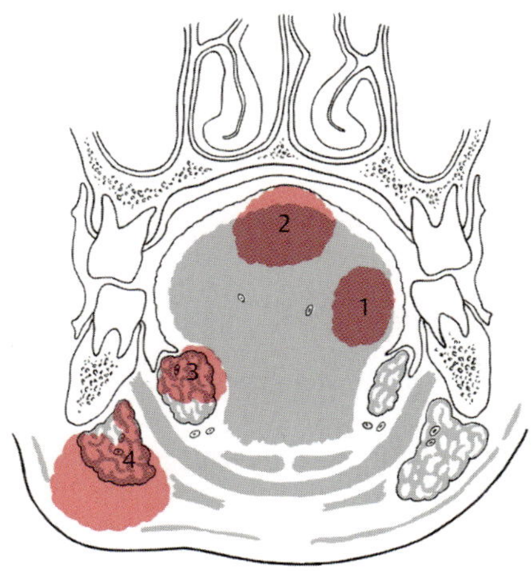

Fig. 9.23 Abscess formation in the region of the tongue and floor of the mouth (after Denecke 1980).
1 abscess of the lingual margin
2 superficial lingual abscess
3 abscess of the floor of the mouth
4 submental–submandibular abscess

Surgical Principle

Early incision and drainage of the abscess.

Indications

Any abscess.

Superficial Lingual Abscess

Anesthesia

Mainly topical and infiltration anesthesia for adults, general anesthesia for children.

Surgical Technique

Stab incision, after prior needle aspiration if appropriate, spread the wound open with a small dressing forceps, evacuate the contents by suction. Have the head leaning forward to prevent aspiration.

Abscesses situated laterally on the margin of the tongue are incised immediately below and parallel to the papillary margin (**Fig. 9.24**), while superficial abscesses of the base of the tongue are incised with a curved, protected blade under magnified laryngoscopic guidance.

Large abscesses are temporarily drained using a soft drain sutured to the incision margin.

Rules, Tips, and Tricks

- Prior corticosteroid administration allows better identification of the abscess by reducing the edema.
- With the tongue drawn forward by the patient or assistant, gently hold the abscess with the left hand, palpate, and stabilize while incising.
- Pus must not be aspirated into the lungs.

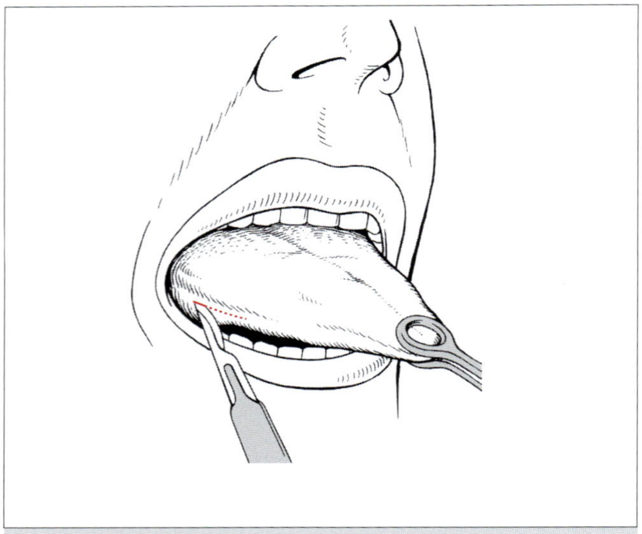

Fig. 9.24 Superficial abscess of the lingual margin. Incision placed laterally below the papillary border.

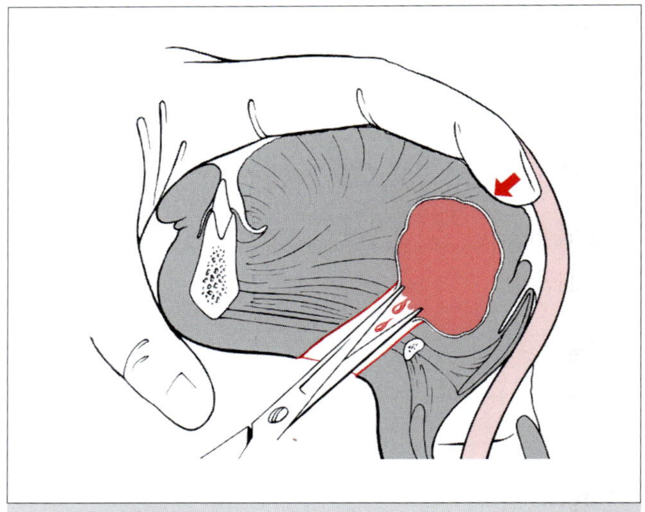

Fig. 9.25 Deep abscess of the base of the tongue. External incision while applying counter-pressure with the finger from within the mouth.

Risks and Complications

- Aspiration of pus into the lungs with secondary pneumonia.
- Collateral laryngeal edema, long-term intubation may be necessary, emergent tracheotomy.
- Severe hemorrhage (consider ligation from an external approach).

Postoperative Care

- Repeat opening of the wound.
- Antibiotics.
- Respiratory monitoring; monitoring for postoperative bleeding.

Deep Tongue Abscess

Surgical Principle

Incision and drainage always from an external approach.

Anesthesia

Usually general endotracheal anesthesia.

Surgical Technique

Incision. In the midline, two finger-breadths behind the chin, extending to a point over the hyoid bone, dividing the subcutaneous layer and midline between the genioglossus muscle.

Incision and drainage. The abscess is approached above the hyoid bone by blunt dissection using spreading movements with the dressing forceps or dissecting forceps. The abscess is stabilized with the index finger of the contralateral hand, which is introduced into the mouth to provide counter-pressure (**Fig. 9.25**). Alternatively, the abscess is aspirated with a needle, which is used as a guide, along which the incision and drainage are performed.

Placement of a Penrose drain or suction drain. Suture of the corner of the wound.

Rules, Tips, and Tricks

- Prior corticosteroid administration allows better identification of the abscess by reducing the edema.
- Identification of the body of the hyoid bone; the abscess is situated anterior to it, in the direction of the chin.
- Needle aspiration facilitates identification of the abscess, after which the soft tissue is spread open along the needle.

Risks and Complications

- Aspiration of pus into the lungs with secondary pneumonia.
- Collateral laryngeal edema, longer-term intubation may be necessary, emergent tracheotomy.
- Severe hemorrhage (if necessary, ligate the lingual artery, accessed from the carotid sheath).
- Scar formation.

Postoperative Care

- Repeat opening of the wound.
- Antibiotics.
- Respiratory monitoring, consider corticosteroid administration, monitoring for postoperative bleeding.

Abscesses of the Floor of the Mouth

Surgical Principle

Incision and drainage of infections originating from the tongue, floor of the mouth, salivary glands, gingiva, and apical dental infection of the mandible with perimandibular abscesses.

Indications

Any abscess.

Anesthesia

Superficial abscesses are managed under local anesthesia; those lying deeper require general anesthesia.

Surgical Technique

- Abscesses of the floor of the mouth, in the sublingual space, or on the inner side of the perimandibular region are incised from an oral approach, spread open, and drained (**Fig. 9.26**).
- Abscesses of the submental space: midline incision extending from the chin toward the hyoid bone, division of the raphe and spreading open of the tissues in the depths and then toward the lateral spaces beneath the muscles; consider initial needle aspiration for orientation.
- Abscess of the submandibular space: skin incision beneath the submandibular gland, two finger-breadths below the mandibular arch, deepened down through the platysma. Spread open the tissue in the direction of the abscess with digital counter-pressure applied from within the mouth, followed by drainage (**Fig. 9.27**).

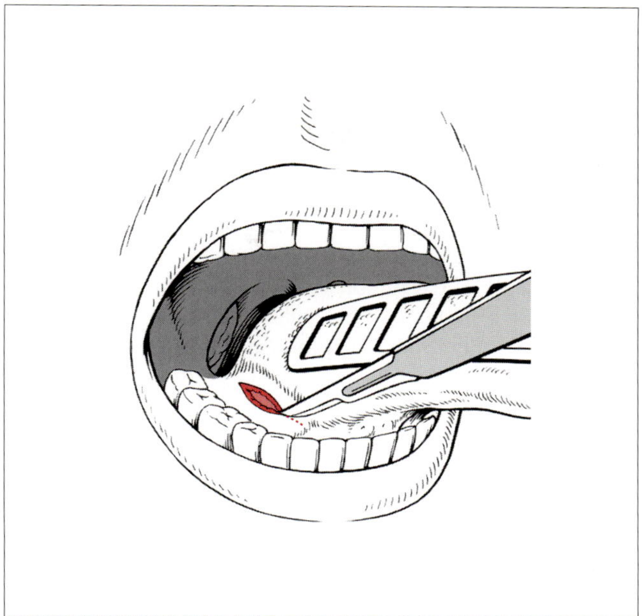

Fig. 9.26 Abscess on the floor of the mouth. Intra-oral incision.

! Risks and Complications

- Aspiration of pus into the lungs with secondary pneumonia.
- Collateral laryngeal edema, longer-term intubation may be necessary, emergent tracheotomy.
- Parapharyngeal abscess, deep neck infection, jugular vein thrombosis, mediastinitis.
- Severe hemorrhage (consider vessel ligation from an external approach).
- Scar formation.
- Division of the Wharton duct, injury to the lingual nerve.
- Injury to the marginal mandibular branch of the facial nerve.

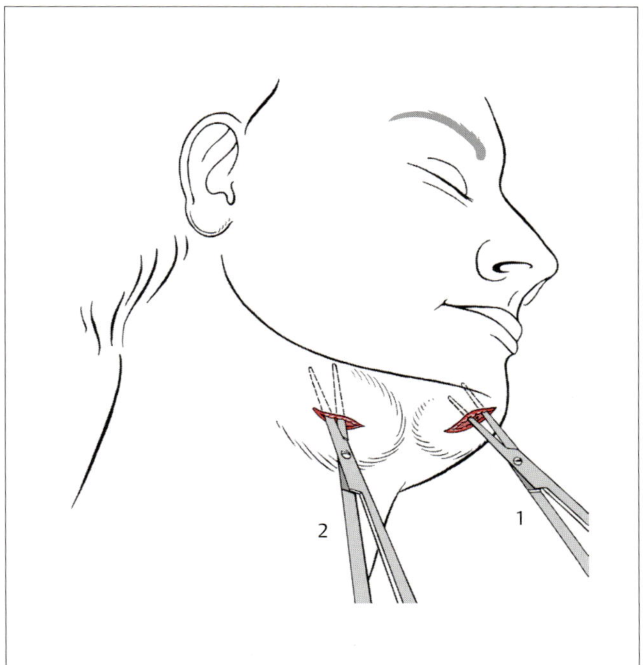

Fig. 9.27 Abscess of the submandibular space (2) and submental region (1). External incision.

Postoperative Care

- Repeat opening of the incision wound.
- Antibiotics.
- Respiratory monitoring, consider steroid administration, monitoring for postoperative bleeding.

Surgery for Benign Tumors and Cysts of the Oral Cavity and Oropharynx

Benign Lingual Tumors

Small fibromas and papillomas of the tongue (uvula, tonsillar pillars, tonsil). Incision around the base of the lesion under local anesthesia and primary wound closure.

Small lymphangiomas or hemangiomas of the tongue. Use of local anesthesia is rarely possible because of the considerable depth of the tumor; general anesthesia is better. The area of excision is exposed by placing stay sutures around the intended line of excision. The tumor region itself is placed under traction by further stay sutures. A suture ligature should be placed around the base of hypervascular tumors before removal. Wedge excision may be done either electrosurgically or by laser ablation (CO_2, Nd:YAG, KTP). Closure of the defect is accomplished by gathering the muscle together with deep stitches followed by deep sutures to approximate the mucosa (**Fig. 9.28a, b**).

Leukoplakia of the tongue, floor of the mouth, or inside of the cheek. These tumors are removed under topical and infiltration anesthesia plus epinephrine. The lesion must be excised completely within healthy tissue, so the incision margins should be marked with Bonney's blue before the local anesthetic is administered, as they become blurred after the injection. The lesion should be carefully exposed by placing the tissue under tension with tongue depressors or stay sutures. The entire thickness of the mucosal layer, down to the muscularis, is excised. As a precaution, the Stensen (parotid) or Wharton ducts may be marked with a stent. Laser is well suited for excision. Vaporization is also an alternative technique. The wound need not be resurfaced.

Cysts of the Floor of the Mouth

A ranula is a retention cyst of the sublingual gland and lies on the floor of the mouth or, rarely, projects through the mylohyoid muscle onto the chin side (plunging ranula). Occasionally dermoid cysts present at the same site.

Management of a Ranula

Surgical Principle

Enucleation of the cyst, if necessary together with all or part of the sublingual gland, using an oral approach.

Indications

Any ranula.

Specific Points Regarding Informed Consent

- Risk of recurrence.
- Sensory dysfunction of the tip of the tongue or floor of the mouth secondary to injury to the lingual nerve.

Special Instruments

Silver probe to identify the salivary duct.

Anesthesia

Topical anesthesia of the mucosa and infiltration anesthesia (with epinephrine).

Surgical Technique

- Mark the Wharton duct with a silver probe.
- Make the incision in the mucosa elliptically over the cyst. The mucosa of the floor of the mouth is carefully grasped and gently swept off the cystic sac.
- Detached the ranula from the sublingual gland—if this is impossible, then include the gland in the dissection; the identified duct and the sublingual nerve are separated by blunt dissection (**Fig. 9.29a, b**).
- Suture only if enough mucosa is available.

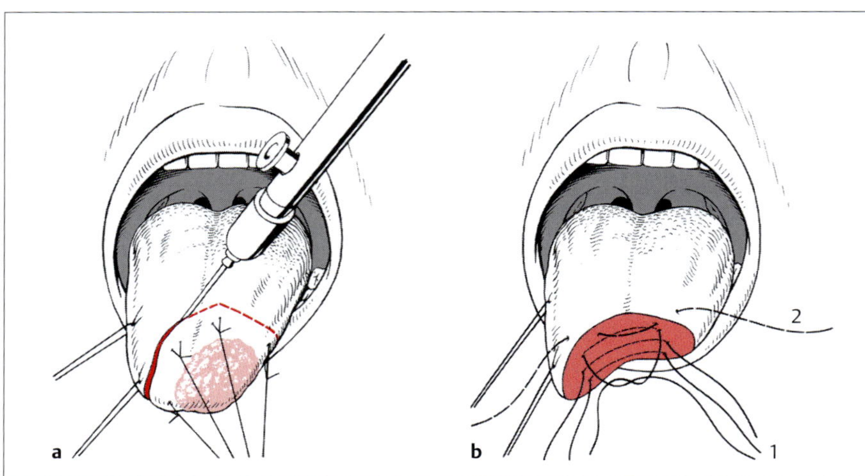

Fig. 9.28a, b Wedge excision of a tumor of the tip of the tongue.
a Area of resection is marked by stay sutures.
b Wound closure and reduction of the defect using deep sutures (1), followed by superficial sutures (2).

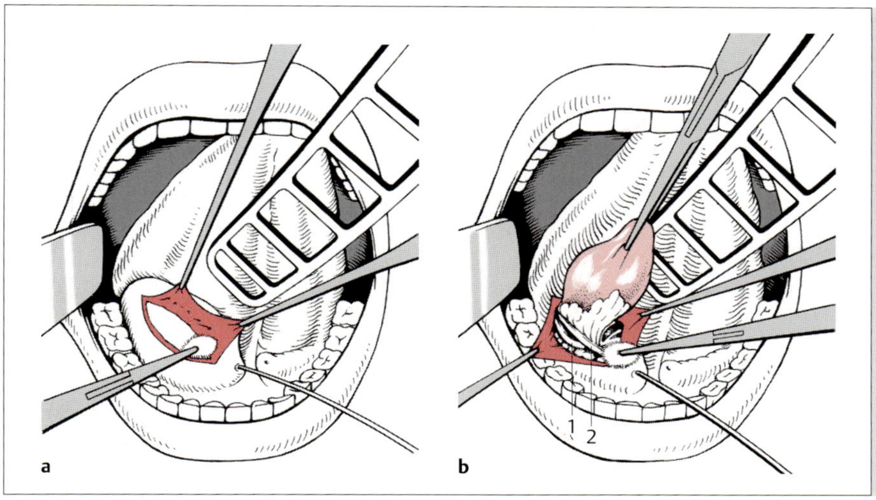

Fig. 9.29a, b Excision of a ranula.
a Elliptical incision of the mucosa after identifying the excretory duct with a probe.
b Blunt separation from the lingual nerve (1) and Wharton duct (2) traversing beneath (after Miehlke).

Rules, Tips, and Tricks

- A ranula can only be dissected out when it is full. If a tear occurs, then the operation should be converted to a marsupialization (see below); packing out the cavity, as otherwise done when dissecting a cyst, is impossible because the mucosa is extremely delicate.

! Risks and Complications

- Risk of recurrence, especially after incomplete enucleation.
- Injury to the lingual nerve.
- Retention of saliva secondary to suture ligation or scar formation of the Wharton duct.
- Keloid formation or injury to the mandibular branch of the facial nerve following an external approach.

Postoperative Care

Soft food, mouth washes, administer antibiotics for signs of infection.

Alternatives

Marsupialization

Surgical technique. Circular incision of the dome of the cyst, close to the transition of the bulge of the cyst and the mucosa of the floor of the mouth. The mucosa of the floor of the mouth and the incisional margin of the cyst are approximated with a few stitches. The floor of the cyst thus becomes a small secondary cavity of the oral cavity.

Management of a Plunging Ranula

Surgical principle. A plunging ranula, or a dermoid cyst of similar location, is enucleated from a submental approach and passed through to the oral cavity, where it is excised.

Anesthesia. General anesthesia.

Surgical technique. The incision is slightly curved and runs at least 1 cm medial and parallel to the mandibular arch. Skin, subcutaneous tissue and superficial facia are divided. The wall of the cyst is freed by blunt dissection using dissecting forceps or a small gauze dissector. It may be necessary to aspirate 3–5 mL of the cystic contents when approaching the level of the floor of the mouth to gain more room (**Fig. 9.30**). After passing the inferior portion of the cyst through the gap, detachment is continued from above as for dissection of a simple ranula. The operation is completed by the external closure of the wound in layers over a drain.

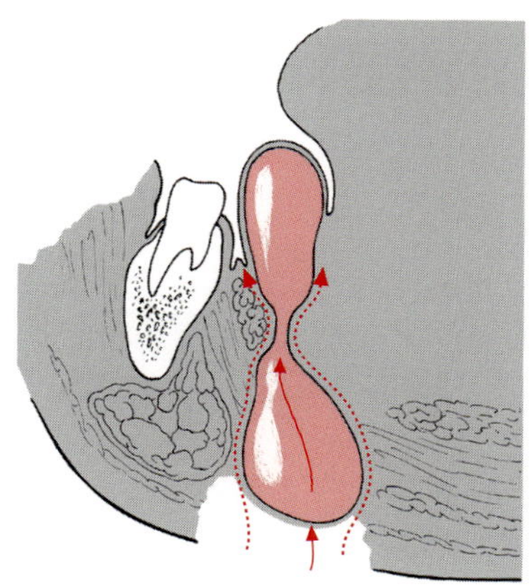

Fig. 9.30 Plunging ranula.
The cystic sac is carefully dissected from a submental approach and then passed up through the gap.

Surgery for Malignant Tumors of the Tongue, Floor of the Mouth, Tonsils, and Posterior Pharyngeal Wall

Tumors of the Tip of the Tongue, Margin of the Tongue, and Floor of the Mouth

Oral Approach

Surgical Principle

Excision of circumscribed tumors of the tip of the tongue, floor of the mouth, or margin of the tongue with adequate resection margins.

Indications

- T1 tumors, selected T2 tumors—the latter usually in combination with a neck dissection.

Contraindications

- Involvement of the Wharton duct.
- Fixation to the mandible, or too close to it.
- Locoregional metastatic spread.

Specific Points Regarding Informed Consent

- Risk of recurrence.
- Adjuvant neck dissection or radiotherapy.
- Sensory or motor dysfunction of the tongue, possibly with disturbances of speech, mastication, or swallowing.
- Postoperative bleeding, hematoma, or edema formation in the tongue as far back as the base of the tongue, in extreme cases resulting in the need for tracheotomy.
- Congestion and inflammation of the submandibular gland.
- Wound infection, healing by secondary intention, strictures secondary to scar formation.

Operative Planning

- Histological confirmation.
- Exclusion of synchronous tumors by endoscopy.
- Ultrasonography of the region around the primary tumor and its lymph draining area.
- Assessment of the tumor and lymphatic drainage by palpation, also bimanually.

Special Instruments

- Conventional technique using the scalpel, electrosurgery.
- Alternatively, CO_2 or Nd:YAG laser.
- Mouth gag.

Anesthesia

The operation may be performed under local or general anesthesia; the latter being obligatory for the simultaneous clearance of the lymphatic draining area and best done with nasotracheal intubation. When giving premedication for local anesthesia, ensure adequate administration of atropine to restrict salivation.

Surgical Technique

Exposure. This is achieved by drawing the tongue forward using stay sutures and using a tongue depressor to retract the lip and, if necessary, the tongue.

Marking the area of resection. This is done by placing several stay sutures at least 1 cm distant from the edge of the tumor, with which the operation site can be put on stretch and unfolded (**Fig. 9.31a**).

Resection. Excision is done under vision and with palpation using a scalpel or laser. Adequate resection margins should also be ensured at the deep margin. Smaller vessels are secured using bipolar diathermy, larger ones are suture ligated.

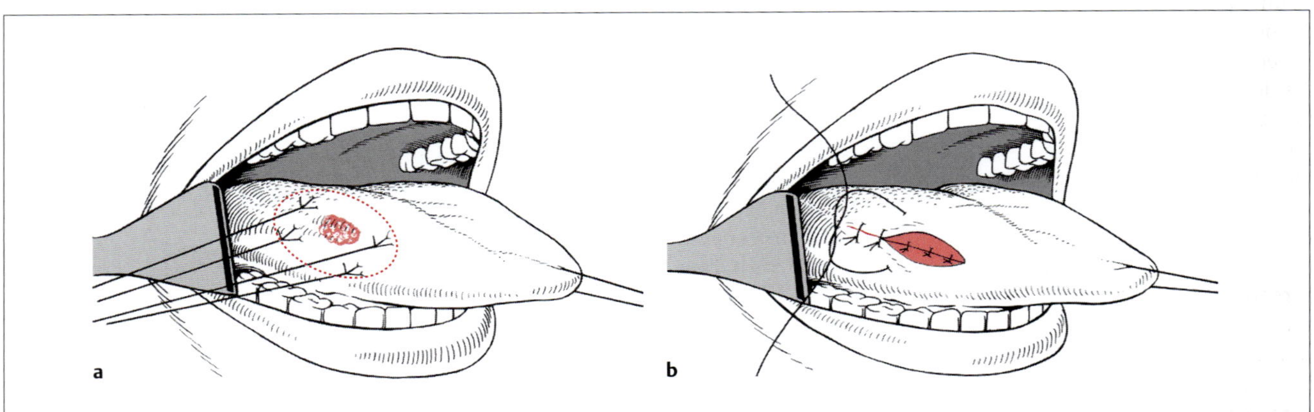

Fig. 9.31a, b Excision of a tumor of the margin of the tongue.
a Area of resection is marked with stay sutures.
b Wound closure.

Defect. The defect is usually left to secondary epithelialization when using laser resection, otherwise primary wound closure with sutures placed through the entire wall (**Fig. 9.31b**).

Rules, Tips, and Tricks

- The tumor tissue must be fully extended to ensure its safe removal. The stay sutures must be held well apart.
- The margins of the specimen must be clearly marked for unequivocal histological examination.

! Risks and Complications

- Risk of recurrence
- Injury to the lingual nerve.
- Postoperative bleeding, hematoma or edema formation in the tongue, base of the tongue, and larynx.
- Congestion and inflammation of the submandibular gland.
- Wound infection, healing by secondary intention.
- Scar contractures with reduction of tongue mobility.

Postoperative Care

- Enteral nutrition may be necessary for more extensive resections, otherwise soft foods or nutrition using a straw.
- Postoperative monitoring because of the risk of postoperative bleeding, aspiration, and breathing difficulties.
- Antibiotics.

Laser Surgical Resection of Carcinomas of the Oral Cavity

J. A. Werner

Laser surgical resection of carcinomas of the oral cavity and the oropharynx does not currently figure as prominently as laser surgery of the larynx and hypopharynx. Small carcinomas of the floor of the mouth (without creating a larger corresponding wound on the undersurface of the tongue), the lingual margin, the buccal mucosa, the soft palate and the tonsil can all be resected by laser surgical means, without the need to resurface the defect. However, laser surgery without subsequent defect coverage reaches its limits, e.g., when corresponding wound surfaces in the region of the undersurface of the mobile tongue and the floor of the mouth result in scars that limit movement of the tongue. More extensive resections of the soft palate without adequate defect coverage not only produce hypernasal speech, but also cause swallowing through the nose, which not infrequently necessitates defect coverage with the use of a free microvascular flap.

The operative steps for the management of well-defined carcinomas at an early stage are similar to those for tumors of other regions of the upper aerodigestive tract. The areas affected by the tumor are exposed with the aid of retractors and mouth gags. Special instruments are inserted to optimize access to the operative site.

Surgical Principle

Small carcinomas of the tongue (T1) are resected en bloc, but with a relatively wide excision margin of usually 10 mm. Care must be taken when excising the tumor to also ensure an adequate distance from the lesion in the deeper muscle layers. If the superficial extent of the tumor appears too great, or if there is any indication of deep infiltration, the tumor may also be excised in several portions using laser surgical technique, depending on its location and extent. When resecting carcinomas of the floor of the mouth by laser surgery, care must be taken to prevent adhesions to the mobile parts of the tongue. Remarks on tumor fragmentation using laser microsurgical technique are to be found elsewhere in this book (Chapter 10). Frozen section analysis of the specimen is mandatory in patients undergoing partial glossectomy.

Indications

T1, and occasionally T2, carcinomas of the tongue and anterior floor of the mouth without infiltration of the alveolar ridge. Should a superficial infiltration of the bone be discovered intraoperatively, then an additional partial (inner table) mandibulectomy would need to be performed.

Contraindications

Infiltration of the mandible as detected on imaging or even clinically.

Specific Points Regarding Informed Consent

- Hemorrhage, postoperative bleeding.
- Damage to teeth or even loss of teeth.
- Swallowing difficulties (dysphagia), nasogastric tube.
- Disturbances of speech and articulation.
- Possible need for tracheotomy with insertion of a cannula.
- Sensory disturbances and motor dysfunction of the tongue secondary to injury of the lingual and hypoglossal nerves or as a result of scar formation.
- Disturbances of taste due to injury to the glossopharyngeal nerve.

Operative Planning

Panendoscopy and histological confirmation, CT and, if appropriate, MRI to assess bony infiltration; multislice imaging (usually MRI) should be considered for carcinomas of the tongue to assess the extent of depth. Scintigraphy is now used less frequently than it used to be, being increasingly displaced by CT and MRI.

Special Instruments

Microscope with CO_2 laser attachment; dissection is also possible using the handpiece. Nd:YAG and KTP lasers are also suitable for this indication; not only is intraoperative bleeding less, but slice precision and assessment of the tissue appearance are also less than with a CO_2 laser.

Anesthesia

General endotracheal anesthesia, usually with nasotracheal intubation, laser tube if appropriate, otherwise cover the tube with a damp cotton swab (see also Chapter 10 for questions on laser safety).

Surgical Technique

Carcinomas of the Mobile Tongue and the Floor of the Mouth

- Exposure of the tumor area: the tumor is identified within the surrounding healthy tissue and exposed (**Fig. 9.32**).
- Positioning of the microscope, attached to the laser (**Fig. 9.33**).
- In the case of carcinoma of the floor of the mouth, two different situations must be considered. The first involves resection of the excretory ducts of the sublingual and submandibular glands together with the tumor; and the second is the modification of the procedure if the mandible is involved. The excretory ducts of the salivary gland may be either left intact or excised. With processes in the midline the question arises of whether the Wharton duct should be preserved at least unilaterally, i. e., whether it can occasionally be dissected out, mobilized, and then transposed. The tumor must, however, be removed with adequate resection margins—that is the absolutely essential point. The periosteum may be dissected using the laser or a rasp. The deep surface is marked with blue ink and sent for histological examination. If infiltration of the mandible is suspected, the involved bony area is excised using conventional surgical technique.

Carcinoma of the Buccal Mucosa, Soft and Hard Palate, and Uvula

Superficial carcinomas of the oral mucosa can be completely excised using laser microsurgical technique. Defect coverage is not necessary as these wounds heal without any significant functional impairment, although the healing process is delayed, as with all laser wounds. Resection of carcinomas of the oropharynx is undertaken in a similar manner. Deep infiltrating extensive carcinomas of the soft palate are usually amenable to conventional surgical excision, followed by appropriate defect coverage. The same applies for larger carcinomas of the hard palate.

Rules, Tips, and Tricks

Creating corresponding wound surfaces in the region of the undersurface of the tongue and the floor of the mouth should be avoided. Instead, primary reconstruction should be undertaken, e. g., with a free skin graft harvested from the groin.

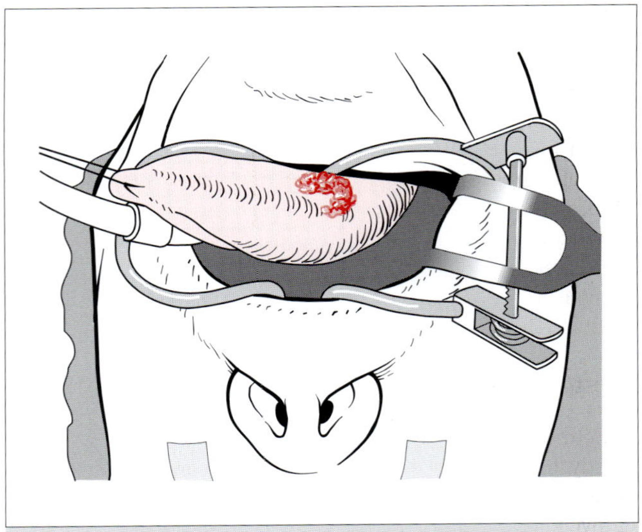

Fig. 9.32 Exposure of a tumor of the margin of the tongue for laser resection.

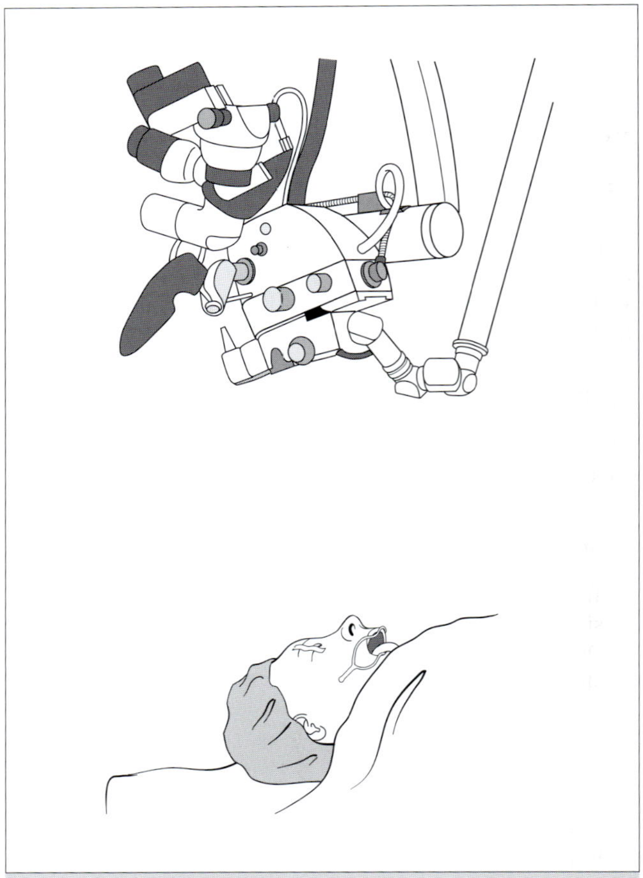

Fig. 9.33 Laser positioning for tumor of the tongue.

! Risks and Complications

Especially with the presence of corresponding wound surfaces, there is the risk of adhesions secondary to scar formation, resulting in impairment of speech and swallowing. Disturbances of sensation of the tongue and in the region of resection may arise. Wound breakdown, wound infection, mandibular osteomyelitis, and postoperative bleeding are also possible. Exceptional cases may develop relevant swelling of the tongue and the base of the tongue with obstruction of the airways.

Postoperative Care

Monitoring of the postoperative phase for bleeding, aspiration, and dyspnea. Nutrition tube for 1–2 days, administration of antibiotics adjusted to the bacterial flora of the mouth (e.g., clindamycin, cefuroxim). Any fibrin adhesions between the tongue and the floor of the mouth should be released with a cotton bud to prevent later tethering. Studies have not made sufficiently clear to what extent the local application of cortisone or mitomycin can prevent any tendency for adhesions here.

Alternatives

Transoral Approach with Marginal Mandibulectomy

Surgical Principle

T1 tumors in the region of the floor of the mouth near the mandible are excised with adequate resection margins after transoral, partial, marginal mandibulectomy (continuous resection), yet preserving the contours of the mandible.

Indications

T1 tumors near the mandible without fixation to the surrounding tissues and without obvious regional metastatic spread.

Contraindications

- Tumor fixation to the surrounding tissues, especially invasion of the mandible.
- Obvious regional metastatic spread (pull-through technique should be used for this).

Specific Points Regarding Informed Consent

- Severe intra- and postoperative bleeding with the risk of aspiration and hypoxia, hypovolemic shock.
- Inflammatory complications: wound bed infection, cervical lymphadenopathy, retro- and parapharyngeal abscess, deep neck infection, thrombosis of the jugular vein, and mediastinitis.
- Disorders of taste, swallowing difficulties, reduction of tongue mobility.
- Teeth damage, loss of teeth, prosthetic management, damage to the temporomandibular joint, trismus; velopalatine insufficiency, disturbances of speech and swallowing (alterations of speech quality).
- Wound breakdown, formation of salivary gland fistulas, possible sequelae of neck dissection.
- Risk of recurrence, possibility of adjuvant radiochemotherapy or revision surgery.
- Laser risks.
- Sensory or motor dysfunction of the tongue, teeth and the distribution of the mental nerve, possibly with disturbances of speech, mastication, or swallowing.
- Postoperative bleeding, hematoma, or edema formation in the tongue as far back as the base of the tongue, in extreme cases associated with the need for tracheotomy.
- Congestion and inflammation of the submandibular gland.
- Wound infection, secondary healing, strictures secondary to scar formation.
- Mandibular osteomyelitis with its corresponding sequelae.

Operative Planning

- Histological confirmation.
- Exclusion of synchronous tumors by endoscopy.
- Ultrasonography of the region around the primary tumor and its lymphatic drainage area.
- Assessment of the tumor and lymphatic drainage by palpation, also bimanually.
- Radiographic examinations, oblique view of the mandible, orthopantomograph of the mandible, high-resolution CT.

Special Instruments

- Conventional technique using the scalpel, electrosurgery.
- Alternatively, CO_2 or Nd:YAG laser.
- Mouth gag.
- Oscillating saw.

Anesthesia

General anesthesia, preferably with nasotracheal intubation. Infiltration of the surgical field with an epinephrine-containing solution.

Surgical Technique

Exposure. This is achieved by drawing the tongue forward using stay sutures and using a tongue depressor to retract the lip and, if necessary, the tongue.

Marking the area of resection. This is done by placing several stay sutures at at least 1 cm distance from the edge of the tumor, allowing the operation site to be put on stretch and unfolded.

Buccal dissection. The gingiva is incised at the level of the neck of the teeth and the buccal mucoperiosteum is elevated inferiorly as a flap.

Osteotomy cuts. These are made at right angles at either end of the tumorous region, then ca. 1.5 cm parallel to the inferior mandibular margin. This mobilizes the tumorous region in a lateral direction. Unless already divided during osteotomy, the

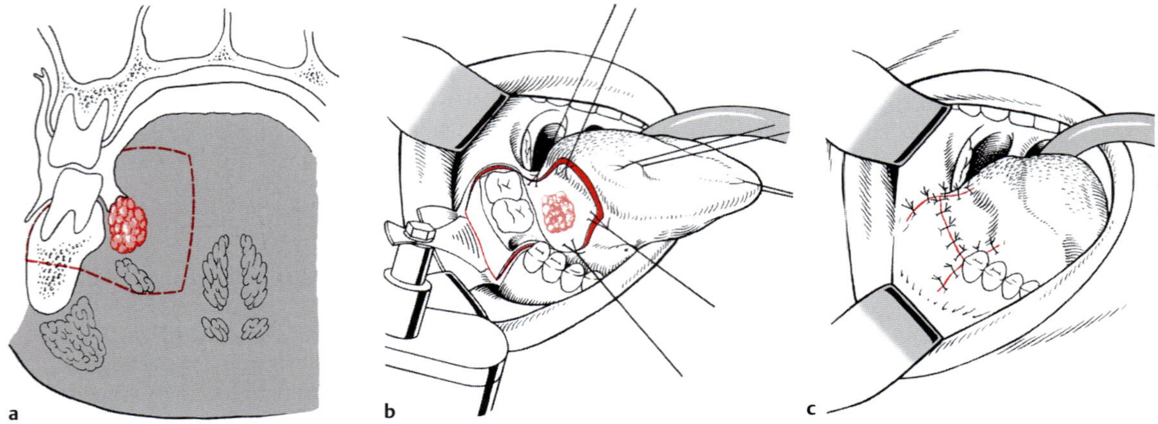

Fig. 9.34a–c Tumor of the floor of the mouth.
Transoral approach with marginal mandibulectomy (after Denecke).
a Area of resection.
b Mucosal and osteotomy incisions.
c Resurfacing of the defect.

lingual periosteum is divided from a medial direction during the subsequent resection of the tumor (**Fig. 9.34a, b**).

Resection. Excision is done under vision and palpation, using a scalpel or laser. Adequate resection margins should also be ensured at the deep margin. Smaller vessels are secured using bipolar diathermy, larger ones are suture ligated. The excised tissue is removed together with the attached bone.

Resurfacing. This is achieved by creating a tongue flap, which is approximated to the buccal gingiva (**Fig. 9.34c**). Because this often results in excessive fixation of the tongue, resurfacing with a platysma flap is an alternative to be considered.

Rules, Tips, and Tricks

- Do not extend the osteotomy cuts too deeply, to protect the alveolar nerve. Removing a tooth from the resection segment helps in gauging the depth of the cut. The horizontal cut need not be completed, as the final bridge of bone may be split with a chisel.
- The bony resection surface must be reliably covered to avoid the development of osteomyelitis. As in the approach for a Rehrmann technique, the buccal periosteum may be additionally incised at its inferior margin to allow further mobilization of the cheek flap.
- If the submandibular gland is not also removed during the operation, the Wharton duct must be marked with a silver probe.

! Risks and Complications

- Tethering of the tongue secondary to scar formation with subsequent impairment of speech, swallowing, and mastication.
- Sensory dysfunction in the distribution of the lingual and mental nerves.
- Wound breakdown with subsequent healing by secondary intention.
- Mandibular osteomyelitis.
- Postoperative bleeding, hematoma, and edema formation at the base of the tongue and the larynx.

Postoperative Care

- Antibiotics
- Enteral nutrition.
- Monitoring for postoperative bleeding, aspiration, and breathing difficulties.

Approach Using the Pull-Through Technique

Surgical Principle

Double-approach resection in monobloc technique: neck dissection, submandibular–submental clearance; peroral tumor excision, if necessary together with a marginal mandibulectomy plus removal of intermediate tissue and neck dissection. Defect coverage accomplished with a platysma myocutaneous flap or free microvascular radial forearm flap. A tracheotomy is occasionally required.

Indications

Deep infiltrating T1 tumors or, at the most, T2 tumors attached to the periosteum with regional metastatic spread.

Contraindications

T2 and T3 tumors with considerable fixation to the mandible, T4 tumors.

Specific Points Regarding Informed Consent

As for the transoral approach with a marginal mandibulectomy, considerably increased risk of fistula formation.

Surgical Technique

Curved incision from the tip of the chin to the mastoid, Y-shaped auxiliary incision along the anterior margin of the sternocleidomastoid muscle downward. Neck dissection with lymph-node clearance of the submental and submandibular regions, ligation of the lingual artery, elevation of the lingual aspect of the mandibular periosteum, detachment of the mylohyoid muscle. Dissection around the tumor from an oral access, working down to the submandibular area. Defect coverage.

! Risks and Complications

- Tethering of the tongue secondary to scar formation with subsequent impairment of speech, swallowing, and mastication.
- Sensory dysfunction in the distribution of the lingual and mental nerves.
- Wound breakdown with subsequent healing by secondary intention.
- Mandibular osteomyelitis.
- Postoperative bleeding, hematoma, and edema formation at the base of the tongue and the larynx.
- Tracheotomy and its sequelae.

Approach Using the Transmandibular Technique

Surgical Principle

After elevation of an inferior cheek flap, segmental resection of the mandible; if appropriate, hemimandibulectomy and monobloc resection of the tumor, neck tissue, and part of the mandible. Peroral defect coverage using a free microvascular radial forearm flap or free jejunal graft, or pectoralis major flap.

Indications

- T2 and T3 tumors of the floor of the mouth and body of the tongue with adherence to the mandibular periosteum.
- T4 tumors with invasion of the mandible if resectable.

Contraindications

- Extensive tumors, especially those crossing the midline, the resection of which would involve major functional defects with a poor prognosis.
- Untreatable regional metastatic spread, distant metastases.

Specific Points Regarding Informed Consent

- As for the transoral approach with marginal mandibulectomy.
- Considerably increased risk of fistula formation.
- Partial loss of the mandible, loss of teeth, swallowing difficulties, reconstruction with harvesting of a bone graft.
- Risk of graft failure, sequelae at the donor site.
- Adjuvant radiochemotherapy.
- Tracheotomy.
- Changes to the contour of the mandible.
- Injury to the mandibular branch of the facial nerve.

Surgical Technique

Incision made through the middle of the lower lip, across the tip of the chin and curving beneath the mandible to the mastoid; Y-shaped incision along the sternocleidomastoid muscle to the clavicle. Elevation of a lower cheek flap. After neck dissection, segmental resection of those parts of the mandible adjacent to the tumor or hemimandibulectomy. Peroral dissection of the tumor via the gap in the mandible under direct vision and with good exposure, and release of the tumor tissue in a caudal direction. Peroral defect coverage. Plate reconstruction of the mandible, if necessary using a bone graft. Tracheotomy.

Rules, Tips, and Tricks

- As for the pull-through technique.
- Changes to the contour of the mandible, dysfunction of the mandibular joint.
- Injury to the mandibular branch of the facial nerve, or the lingual, hypoglossal, or glossopharyngeal nerve.

9

Surgery for Tumors of the Tonsils, Base of the Tongue, and Pharyngeal Wall

Tumor Tonsillectomy

Surgical Principle

Transoral resection, lesions limited to the tonsil or T1 and T2 tumors, which are well defined with respect to the surrounding tissue, nowadays usually with the use of CO_2 or Nd:YAG laser. To achieve adequate resection margins, dissection is not along the capsule, unlike tonsillectomy, and, depending on the type of tumor, parts of the tonsillar pillars, the pharynx or the base of the tongue are also excised, with frozen-section examination used to assess the intraoperative resection margins. Lymph-node clearance is achieved by neck dissection, as either a one- or a two-stage procedure and without opening the oral wound bed in the process.

Indications

- Well-defined T1 tumors, limited to the tonsils.

- Well-defined, non-adherent T2 tumors, without extensive invasion of the base of the tongue or adherence to the mandible.

Contraindications

- T3 and T4 tumors, especially those with involvement of the mandible, invasion of the pterygopalatine fossa or those with direct transition to the cervical lymph nodes.
- Extensive and untreatable local, regional, or distant metastases.

Specific Points Regarding Informed Consent

- Severe intra- and postoperative bleeding with the risk of aspiration and hypoxia, hypovolemic shock.
- Inflammatory complications: wound bed infection, cervical lymphadenopathy, retro- and parapharyngeal abscess, deep neck infection, thrombosis of the jugular vein, and mediastinitis.
- Disorders of taste, swallowing difficulties, reduction of tongue mobility.
- Tooth damage, damage to the temporomandibular joint, trismus; velopalatine insufficiency, disturbances of speech and swallowing (alterations of speech quality).
- Wound breakdown, formation of salivary gland fistulas, possible sequelae of neck dissection.
- Risk of recurrence, possibility of adjuvant radiochemotherapy or revision surgery.
- Laser risks.

Operative Planning

- Histological confirmation.
- Assessment of the extent of the tumor by palpation, inspection, and endoscopy (also to exclude a synchronous tumor).
- CT, MRI, B-ultrasonography, and Doppler ultrasonography are each indicated depending on relevant findings.
- Chest radiograph, abdominal ultrasonography.

Special Instruments

As for tonsillectomy, laser if appropriate.

Anesthesia

General anesthesia, local anesthesia is possible in principle.

Surgical Technique

Neck dissection. Provided a two-stage approach is not planned, prior management of the lymphatic draining area has the advantage that the vascular bundle is already isolated, thus reducing the risks involved with extensive tumor resections. Furthermore, the lingual, ascending pharyngeal, or facial arteries may, if required, be ligated already and so render the operation less bloody and provide more visualization.

Exposure. As for tonsillectomy, with the blade of the mouth gag placed slightly to the side of the midline to better expose the base of the tongue.

Incision. The tonsil is stretched and rotated medially, creating a groove for the incision, which is placed behind the anterior pillar at an adequate distance from the tumor. It is extended as far as the ascending branch of the mandible in a superior direction, widely circumventing the upper pole of the tonsil, continuing back behind the posterior pillar, again ensuring adequate distance from the tumor (**Fig. 9.35a**).

Dissection. Unless the operation is done using laser—which optically allows good delineation between the tumor and the muscularis layer, despite the vaporization (which in fact disappears quite rapidly)—removal of the tonsillar tumor is accomplished using an elevator, tonsil scissors, and index finger, which conveys a good feeling for the distance to the tumor (**Fig. 9.35b**).

Removal. Under direct vision and employing manual and instrumental palpation, the tumor is divided at the base of the tongue, exposing and stretching the tissue of the triangular fold and the base of the tongue. Additional traction on the tumor and the adjacent tissue can be accomplished by placing stay sutures. Meticulous hemostasis. No defect coverage.

A specimen for frozen-section histology is taken from the critical marginal regions, followed, if necessary, by wider excision.

Rules, Tips, and Tricks

- Careful preoperative diagnostic workup: tonsillar tumors not infrequently go considerably deeper than at first expected on inspection. If doubts regarding extent cannot be excluded at the start, request the patient's consent for a possible extension of the operation via an external approach, with possible resections to the mandible, to allow for a possible change of plan during surgery.
- A one-stage approach is more advantageous for locating any residual tumor. As a rule, the transoral approach is advantageous because of its clearly lower morbidity rate (fewer functional deficits).
- Maintain an adequate distance from the tumor from the start. Subsequent resections may pose histological problems for grading and staging.
- Ensure unambiguous marking of the frozen-section specimen.
- Exact exposure at the base of the tongue is particularly difficult. Re-adjustment of the blade of the mouth gag is sometimes necessary. The insertion of additional blades serves to provide more traction on the tissue.

! Risks and Complications

- Severe intraoperative hemorrhage or postoperative bleeding (branches from the external carotid artery, ascending and descending pharyngeal arteries, descending palatine artery, lingual artery and, in exceptional cases, the internal carotid artery due to kinking, bleeding from the carotid artery secondary to erosion due to fistula formation).

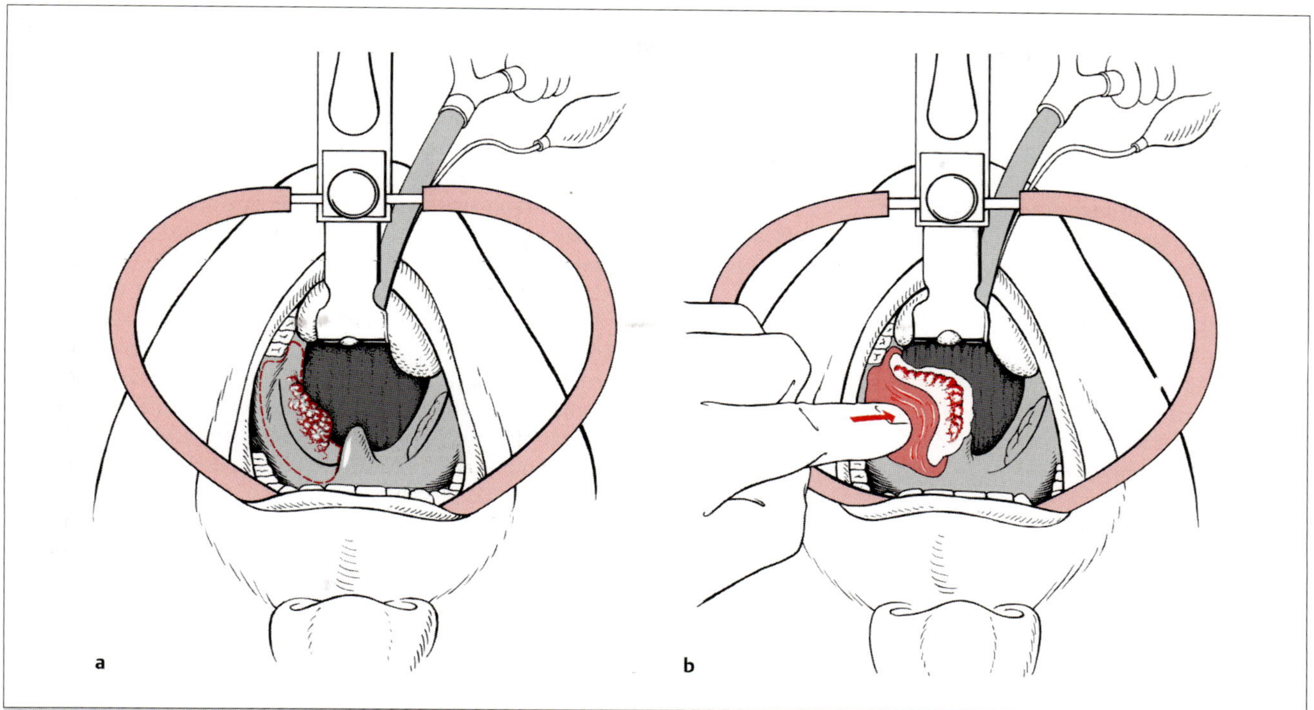

Fig. 9.35a, b Tumor tonsillectomy.
a Area of resection with inclusion of the pillar.
b Blunt dissection of the tonsil and the tumor using a finger.

- Injury to the glossopharyngeal or hypoglossal nerves, with subsequent disturbances of taste and swallowing, reduction of tongue mobility.
- Para- and retropharyngeal abscess, wound bed infection, thrombosis of the jugular vein, deep neck infection, cervical lymphadenopathy with abscess formation.
- Deformity of the tonsillar pillar from scar contracture with subsequent velopalatine insufficiency and disturbances of swallowing, regurgitation, or hypernasal speech.
- Damage to teeth or temporomandibular joint with subsequent trismus.
- Salivary gland fistula.
- Laryngeal edema with severe dyspnea.

Postoperative Care

- As for tonsillectomy.
- Monitoring for the development of laryngeal edema.
- Management of the lymphatic drainage system as a second stage operation, if appropriate.
- Adjuvant radiochemotherapy, depending on staging.

Laser Surgical Resection of Oropharyngeal Carcinomas

J. A. Werner

Tonsils, Glossotonsillar Sulcus, Tonsillar Pillars

See also preliminary remarks on laser surgical resection of carcinomas of the oral cavity, page 172.

Surgical Principle

The surgical approach for carcinomas of the tonsils differs from that for other regions. The different tissue structure and growth patterns of tumors in this region necessitate a particularly careful histological examination of the clearly marked specimen. Circumscribed lesions with a more superficial growth pattern can be excised en bloc using laser surgical technique. Larger tumors in the region of the tonsils may possibly be resected piecemeal.

Indications

Circumscribed carcinomas (T1 and, in selected cases, T2).

Contraindications

As a rule, preoperatively diagnosed evidence of infiltration of the alveolar ridge or hard palate; tumor invasion of the parotid bed or the soft tissues of the neck.

Specific Points Regarding Informed Consent

- Hemorrhage, postoperative bleeding.
- Damage to teeth, or even loss of teeth.
- Swallowing difficulties (dysphagia), nasogastric tube.
- Hypernasal speech.
- Disturbances of speech and articulation.
- Dyspnea, tracheotomy with insertion of a cannula.
- Reduction of tongue mobility secondary to injury to the hypoglossal nerve.
- Disturbances of taste secondary to injury to the glossopharyngeal nerve.
- Disturbances of sensation in the region of the tongue and the posterior pharyngeal wall.
- Temporomandibular joint problems.
- Injury to the lingual nerve.
- Delayed wound healing, wound infection.
- Fistula formation.

Operative Planning

Panendoscopy, histological confirmation, multisection imaging (usually CT) to assess infiltration into adjacent structures.

Surgical Technique

The question of the best exposure of the tumor is of particular importance for this indication. The cranial part of the carcinoma will not infrequently require exposure with the aid of the tonsillectomy retractor, while that part of the tumor caudally adjacent to the base of the tongue will need a short bivalved laryngoscope.

Hemostasis

Bleeding often obstructs visualization during the operation. Branches of the ascending palatine artery (from the facial artery) and the descending palatine artery (from the maxillary artery), as well as branches of the ascending pharyngeal artery, will need conventional ligation or vascular clips. The glossotonsillar sulcus is a region regarded as a high risk for serious hemorrhage. The lingual artery and the external carotid artery are particularly at risk. Other important structures in close proximity are the hypoglossal and glossopharyngeal nerves.

Carcinomas of the Posterior Wall of the Oropharynx

Technically, tumors of the posterior pharyngeal wall can often be completely resected without difficulty using a laser surgical technique. If tumor invasion into the hypopharynx or the nasopharynx has occurred, resection is extended accordingly. Expansion in a cranial direction can usually be exposed with the aid of palatal retractors. The bivalved laryngoscope is used for cases with caudal extension. Infiltration of the anterior longitudinal ligament of the cervical spine is problematic for laser surgical resection as it is usually no longer curable surgically. These cases need a preoperative workup using imaging studies (MRI).

Base of the Tongue and Vallecula

Several factors complicate laser resection of carcinomas of the base of the tongue. This particularly applies to those cases where exposure is not optimal, despite use of the bivalved oropharyngoscope. Furthermore, differentiation between carcinoma and normal tissue under the operating microscope can be particularly difficult in the region of the base of the tongue, because various types of tissue (mucosa, tonsil, muscle) occur in close proximity here. Nevertheless, assessment with the aid of the operating microscope is usually successful. Surgery can become particularly problematic if the bivalved oropharyngoscope slips and exact orientation is subsequently lost. It should once more be stressed that the tumor excision margins must be identified and precisely marked for the subsequent histological examination. This particularly applies to cases where the carcinoma is resected piecemeal.

Rules, Tips, and Tricks

Laser surgical resection of carcinomas of the floor of the tongue must be carefully planned, down to the individual operative stages. The oral part of the tumor must be exposed first and an incision made around it with an adequate safety margin using laser surgical technique. The bivalved oropharyngoscope is then advanced step by step to maintain orientation. Adequate paralysis of the patient is essential because any degree of dislocation of the blade of the mouth gag could mean that the plane of dissection is lost. Laser surgery of the floor of the mouth presupposes a particularly high level of experience on behalf of the surgeon.

Alternatives

Operations Using a Submandibular Approach

Surgical Principle

Exposure of the tumor via a lateral pharyngotomy approach. Monobloc resection with inclusion of the lymphatic draining area, if necessary with the additional resection from a transoral approach using the pull-through technique. As a rule, bilateral neck dissection, tracheotomy. If necessary, defect coverage is accomplished with a pedicled or free flap.

Indications

Stage T2 or T3 tumors of the tonsil, oropharynx, and base of the tongue that cannot be adequately exposed or encompassed from a transoral approach.

Contraindications

- T4 tumors with invasion of the mandibular bone (transmandibular approach).
- Invasion of the internal or common carotid artery, untreatable distant metastases.

Specific Points Regarding Informed Consent

- Risks of flap failure, sequelae at graft donor site.
- Tracheotomy.
- Injury to the mandibular branch of the facial nerve.
- Severe intra- or postoperative hemorrhage with the danger of aspiration and hypoxia, hypovolemic shock.
- Complications of infection: wound bed infection, cervical lymphadenopathy, retro- and parapharyngeal abscess, deep neck infection, thrombosis of the jugular vein, and mediastinitis.
- Disturbances of taste and swallowing, reduction of tongue mobility.
- Damage to teeth or temporomandibular joint, trismus; velopalatine insufficiency, disturbances of swallowing and speech (alterations of speech quality).
- Wound breakdown, formation of a salivary gland fistula with the risk of bleeding from the great vessels of the neck secondary to erosion.
- Sequelae of neck dissection.
- Risk of recurrence, possibility of adjuvant radiochemotherapy or revision surgery.

Surgical Technique

Skin incision. Curved incision from the tip of the chin to the mastoid, Y-shaped auxiliary incision along the anterior margin of the sternocleidomastoid muscle downward.

Neck dissection and submandibular clearance. The specimen is pedicled to the lateral pharyngeal wall. Ligation of the lingual, ascending pharyngeal, and facial arteries.

Opening the pharynx. This is done below the palpable margins of the tumor, usually in the region of the piriform sinus. Any extension in a cranial direction will require mobilization and displacement of the hypoglossal nerve. Excision is accomplished under vision and by palpation. An additional excision may be necessary from a transoral access. The resected tissue is then extracted in a caudal direction.

Wound closure. Either primary closure or by flap coverage, depending on the defect.

! Risks and Complications

- Injury to the mandibular branch of the facial nerve and the lingual, hypoglossal, and accessorial nerves.
- Disturbances of taste and swallowing, reduction of tongue mobility.
- Damage to the temporomandibular joint, trismus, velopalatine insufficiency.
- Formation of a salivary gland fistula with the risk of bleeding from the great vessels of the neck secondary to erosion.
- Severe intra- or postoperative bleeding with the risk of aspiration and hypoxia, hypovolemic shock.

Operations Using a Transmandibular Approach

Surgical Principle

Paramedian or midline mandibulotomy or partial mandibulectomy in the region of the ascending branch or at the insertion of the mandibular arch. After exposure and resection of the tumor, plate reconstruction of the mandible. Primary defect closure or resurfacing using a pectoralis major flap or a free microvascular flap. Bilateral neck dissection and usually also tracheotomy.

Indications

Unfavorably located T2, T3, and T4 tumors of the tonsil and oropharynx.

Contraindications

- Invasion of the tumor into the internal or common carotid arteries.
- Untreatable distant metastases.

Specific Points Regarding Informed Consent

- See submandibular approach.
- Partial loss of the mandible, osteomyelitis, changes of contour, loss of teeth, disturbances of mastication, reconstruction using a free bone graft.
- Risks of flap or graft failure, sequelae at graft/flap donor site.

Surgical Technique

The incision passes through the middle of the lower lip and over the tip of the chin, to curve beneath the mandible toward the mastoid, followed by a Y-shaped incision along the anterior margin of the sternocleidomastoid muscle toward the clavicle. Elevation of a lower cheek flap. After neck dissection and, if appropriate, tracheotomy, either a paramedian Z-shaped osteotomy of the mandible or, if the bone is involved, partial mandibulectomy of the infiltrated area. Excision of the tumor under direct vision and with palpation, closure of the pharynx either primarily or with the use of a free flap. Plate reconstruction of the mandible.

Surgery for Snoring and Obstructive Sleep Apnea Syndrome

Uvulopalatopharyngoplasty (UPPP)

Surgical Principle

Tightening of the tissue and widening of the lumen by resecting redundant mucosa in the region of the velopharynx, if appropriate together with a tonsillectomy.

Indications

- Site of collapse or cause of the snoring located in the velopharyngeal segment.
- Long uvula >10 mm, webbing of the posterior pillar >5 mm, soft palate longer than the hard palate.

Contraindications

- Poor general condition; cardiac, pulmonary, neurological or psychiatric comorbidity.
- Midface malformations.
- Posterior airway space (PAS) at the level of the mandible <10 mm.
- Obesity with a body mass index (BMI) >28.
- Considerable obstructive sleep apnea with an apnea–hypopnea index (AHI) >30.
- Presence of a further site of collapse.

Specific Points Regarding Informed Consent

- The outcome of the operation is not reliably predictable.
- Velopharyngeal insufficiency, nasal reflux, dys- and odynophagia, globus sensation, both temporary and permanent.
- Rhinolalia aperta (hypernasal speech), in rare cases also rhinolalia clausa (hyponasal speech), alterations of speech quality, pharyngitis sicca, xerostomia, hypersalivation, formation of viscous mucus, increased nasal secretion.
- Disturbances of taste, paraesthesias of the palate, disturbance of mobility and sensation of the tongue, increased gag reflex.
- Nasopharyngeal obstruction, disturbances of ventilation of the eustachian tube.
- Postoperative bleeding, wound infection.
- Reduced CPAP tolerance.

Operative Planning

- Polysomnography.
- Nasopharyngeal flexible endoscopy for topodiagnostic studies.
- Pressure measurements of the upper airways, if appropriate.
- CT and MRI, if appropriate.

Special Instruments

As for tonsillectomy.

Anesthesia

Usually general endotracheal anesthesia.

Surgical Technique

Exposure. As for a tonsillectomy with a hanging-head (Rose) position and use of a McIvor mouth gag. Traction on the uvula allows assessment of the degree of redundant mucosa.

Incision. Along the edge of the anterior tonsillar pillar, starting at the insertion of the triangular fold, across the base of the uvula to the contralateral insertion (**Fig. 9.36**). The muscle layer is preserved.

Tonsillectomy. In typical fashion, using bipolar diathermy if available.

Dissection of the mucous membrane. The mucosa of the posterior pillar is carefully elevated from the underlying muscle, either using the tonsillectomy incision margin or the incision margin of the anterior pillar. A parauvular incision is then made and deepened down to the muscle. The elevated layer of mucosa is drawn in an oral and lateral direction and the redundant mucosa is excised along the incision line of the anterior pillar (**Fig. 9.37**). Then the two layers of mucosa are approximated to each other using deep sutures (2/0).

Uvular resection. The uvula is excised obliquely at its base, preserving more of the posterior surface, which is then turned over and sutured anteriorly to the incision margin of the anterior pillar (**Fig. 9.38**).

Rules, Tips, and Tricks

- Preserve the muscles.
- Avoid radical resections.
- Protect the anterior tonsillar pillar.
- The indication must be clearly defined; in particular, exclude any contraindications.

! Risks and Complications

- Basically the same as for tonsillectomy.
- In addition:
  - velopharyngeal insufficiency, nasal reflux, dys- or odynophagia, globus sensation, both temporary and permanent
  - nasopharyngeal obstruction, disturbances of ventilation of the eustachian tube
  - pharyngitis sicca, xerostomia, hypersalivation, formation of viscous mucus, increased nasal secretion
  - reduced CPAP tolerance.

Postoperative Care

- Prolonged recovery phase or intensive care unit due to the risk of apnea.
- No sedatives.

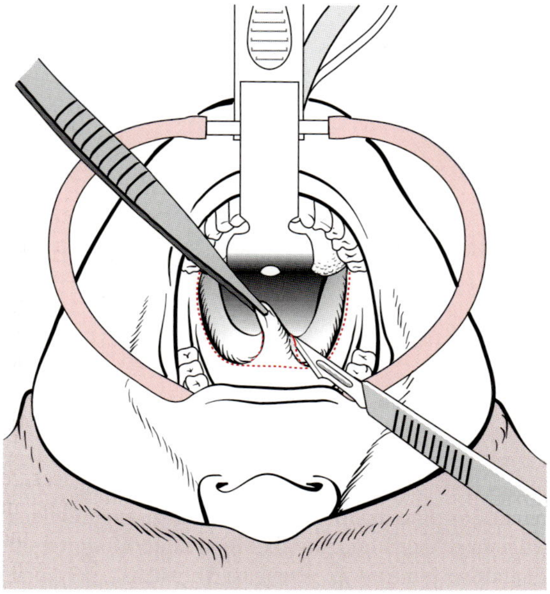

Fig. 9.36 Uvulopalatopharyngoplasty.
Incision of the mucosa in the region of the anterior pillar and para-uvular incision in the region of the posterior pillar.

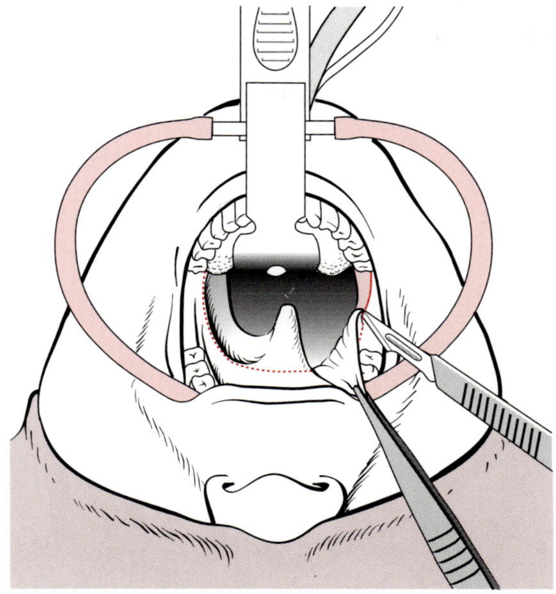

Fig. 9.37 Uvulopalatopharyngoplasty.
Removal of the detached posterior mucous membrane as far as the incision margin of the anterior pillar.

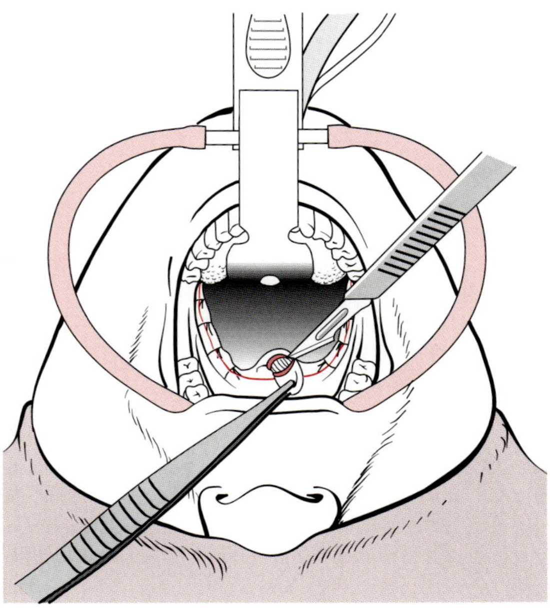

Fig. 9.38 Uvulopalatopharyngoplasty.
Resection of posterior surface of the uvula mucosa, while preserving the mucularis. This cut surface is sutured to the mucosal margin of the anterior pillar.

- Postoperative monitoring with a pulse oximeter.
- Otherwise as for tonsillectomy.

Alternatives

Laser Uvulopalatoplasty (LUPP)

Using the CO_2 or Nd:YAG laser, the procedure is basically the same as for a UPPP, yet the uvula is completely resected and the operation is on the whole more radical.

Laser-Assisted Uvulopalatoplasty (LAUP)

Using the CO_2 or Nd:YAG laser, parauvular vertical incision is through the mucosa of the anterior and posterior pillars with partial or total resection of the uvula. Here, the muscularis layer is also slightly incised to a varying extent. The operation may also be performed gradually in several stages and can usually be done under local anesthesia (**Fig. 9.39**).

Radiofrequency Ablation/Somnoplasty

Focusing radiofrequency energy on the soft palate tissue leads to a controlled thermal lesion and subsequently to a widening and stiffening of the velopharyngeal segment secondary to tissue shrinkage and scar formation, while preserving the intact mucosa. For this purpose, needle-shaped applicators are advanced into the soft palate in the direction of the uvula from median and paramedian locations under local anesthesia, introducing the energy in a temperature-controlled manner (**Fig. 9.40a, b**). The technique may be used in the region of the pharyngeal wall and, in particular, at the base of the tongue. Several sessions are usually required, depending on the outcome. Edema may occasionally occur.

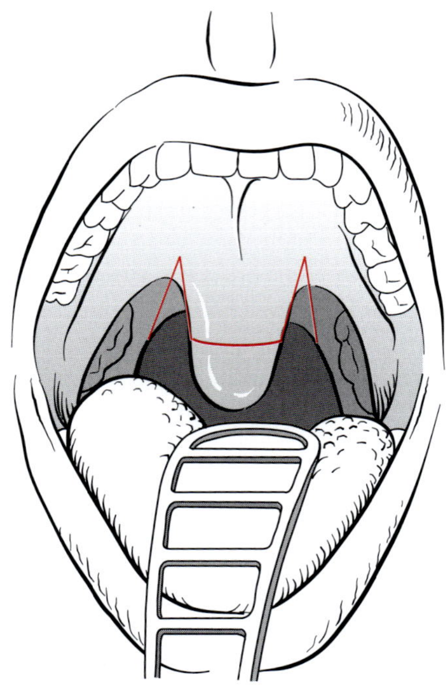

Fig. 9.39 Laser-assisted uvulopalatoplasty. Para-uvular incision and uvular reduction.

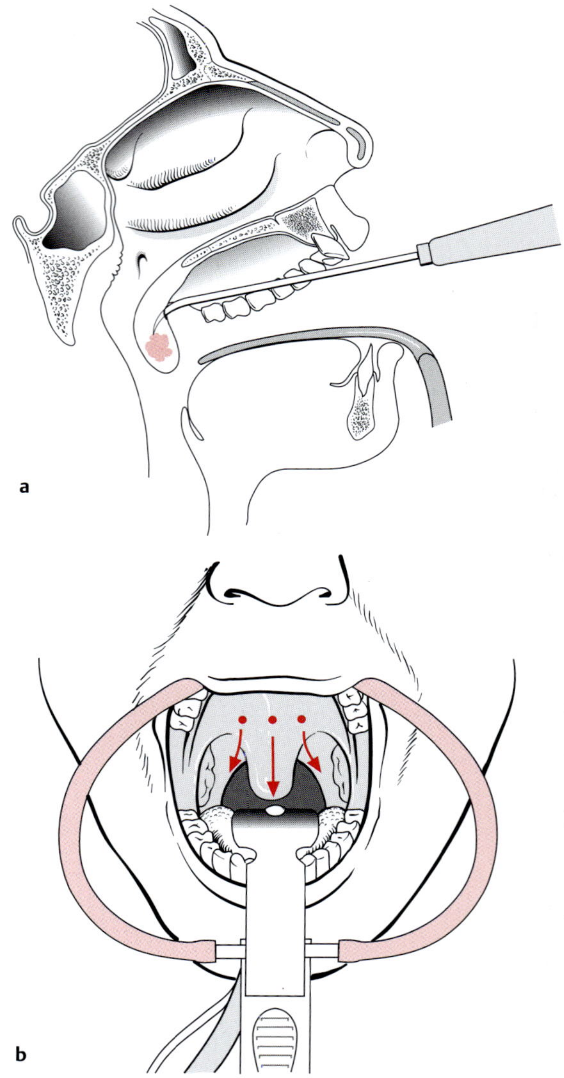

Fig. 9.40a, b Radiofrequency ablation/somnoplasty.
a Position of the needle electrode in the uvula.
b Puncture sites on the soft palate.

10 Surgery of the Larynx, Hypopharynx, and Trachea

Endolaryngeal Operations

Endolaryngeal operations may be performed under topical anesthesia using indirect laryngoscopy or—and this is virtually standard practice nowadays—under general anesthesia and under direct vision using the operating microscope. Direct microlaryngoscopy under general anesthesia has the additional option of using angled telescopes, which provide significantly better exposure for even poorly accessible areas.

Indirect Endolaryngeal Operations

Surgical Principle

Involves performing localized endolaryngeal operations under topical anesthesia using curved instruments, under mirror or angled endoscopic guidance (mirrored vision involves guiding the instruments in the opposite direction).

Indications

- Excisional biopsies.
- Excision of localized lesions of the vocal folds with the option of an intraoperative voice assessment.

Contraindications

- Hyperactive gag reflex, poor visualization due to the anatomical situation.
- Lesions situated in the anterior commissure; extensive lesions (e.g., extensive Reinke edema and leukoplakia).
- Children under the age of 14 years.
- Allergy to topical anesthetics.

Special Instruments and Implants

Curved cotton buds, Reichhardt epiglottis retractor, epiglottis double-cup grasping forceps and punches, or curved universal handpiece with various tools.

Binocular microscope with a 30-cm objective lens or magnifying laryngoscope.

Anesthesia

Premedication (atropine, administered IM 20 minutes before surgery, plus trifluopromazine or pethidine if required, although they are not obligatory for outpatient surgery.) The patient should be fasting.

Topical anesthesia with lidocaine. The oral cavity, pharynx, and laryngeal mucosa are sprayed successively, and the larynx is additionally brushed with anesthetic on a curved cotton bud under indirect laryngoscopic vision.

A hyperactive gag reflex will require a peripheral block of the superior laryngeal nerve from an external approach and infiltration of the glossopharyngeal nerve at the inferoposterior tonsillar pole, each with 2 mL 1 % lidocaine.

Surgical Technique

Positioning. The patient is positioned sitting upright, with slightly reclined head stabilized in the headrest in preparation for binocular microscopy. The assistant may stand just behind the patient's left shoulder.

Preparation. Appropriate instrument attachment piece (double-cup grasping forceps and punch); *the working direction of the attachment is parallel to the vocal fold and is verified using thumb and index finger of the left hand, which are spread apart in a V shape to simulate the position of the vocal folds.*

Insertion of the instruments. The tongue is held from the right by the patient or an assistant. The laryngoscope or magnifying laryngoscope is inserted with the left hand and the larynx visualized (if necessary, first adjust the microscope with the right hand). If necessary, ask the patient to phonate (**Fig. 10.1a**).

Technique for overhanging epiglottis. With an overhanging epiglottis, the Reichhardt retractor is positioned beneath the epiglottis and supported by the assistant.

Tissue removal. Using the right hand, the closed instrument is introduced laterally through the mouth into the larynx under vision. *The instrument is advanced with the position of the vocal folds during respiration and the tissue removed (optimal view and complete anesthesia are absolute prerequisites for precise positioning)* (**Fig. 10.1a–c**).

Hemostasis. The excision site is checked, a second sample is taken if necessary, the area is smoothed out, and hemostasis is achieved with a cotton bud soaked in a vasoconstrictive agent.

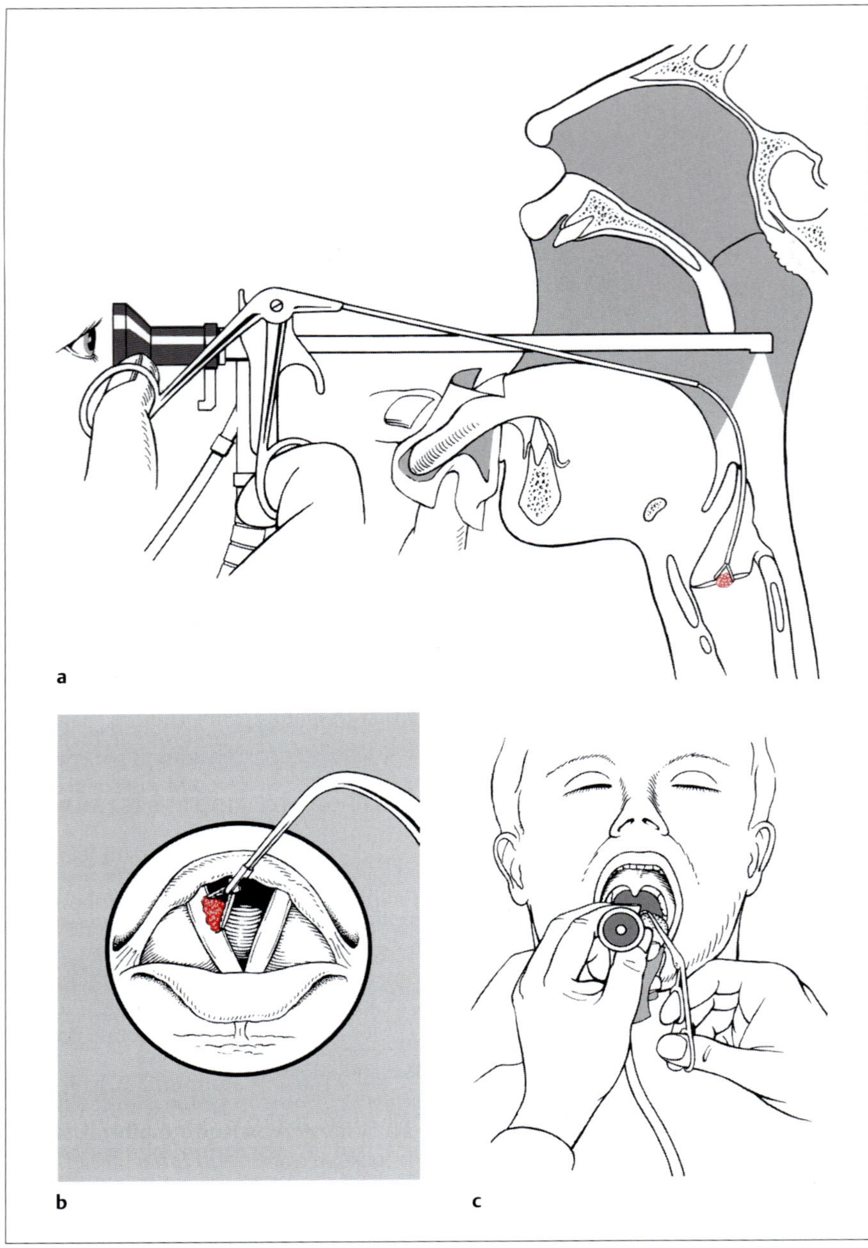

Fig. 10.1a–c Indirect biopsy from the larynx under the guidance of a magnifying laryngoscope.
a Cross-section. Head reclined. Tongue drawn far forward.
b Positioning the opened biopsy graspers with the position of the vocal folds during respiration.
c Directing the instrument from the angle of the mouth with the right hand, while guiding of the magnifying laryngoscope with the left hand.

! Risks and Complications

- Hoarseness secondary to tissue defects, injury to the vocal fold (which may be caused by wrongly chosen and wrongly placed instruments or inadequate anesthesia), scarring of the vocal fold, web formation.
- Swelling of the larynx with subsequent dyspnea; tracheotomy may become necessary if a stenosis (secondary to a tumor or similar lesion) is already present.
- Recurrence.

Postoperative Care

- Voice rest for 3–7 days, smoking and alcohol cessation.
- Oral intake 2 hours after completion of the operation at the earliest; inhalations; antitussive agents to suppress the urge to cough.
- If edema develops and/or a narrow glottis is present, observation under in-patient conditions; steroids if appropriate.

Alternatives

Direct laryngoscopy.

Direct Endolaryngeal Operations

Direct endolaryngeal operations are always performed under general anesthesia, usually as so-called "direct distending laryngoscopy."

Direct Distending Laryngoscopy Under General Endotracheal Anesthesia (Microlaryngoscopy after Kleinsasser)

Surgical Principle

After intubation using a relatively thin tube, a relatively wide, conical endoscope tube is introduced into the larynx and stabilized with a support placed on the chest. This allows fine manipulations to be performed bimanually under microscopic, stereoscopic vision and without time restrictions from pauses for breathing. The walls and the sinus of Morgagni are inspected using angled telescopes. The ventricle is held open with small retractors to allow inspection.

Indications

- Excisional biopsy, assessment of the extent of malignant lesions.
- Excision of benign alterations, such as leukoplakia, hyperkeratosis, polyps, fibromas, papillomas, Reinke edema.
- Scar revision, resections of web formations and diaphragms.
- Reduction of arytenoid cartilage dislocations.
- Endolaryngeal arytenoidectomy; augmentation or lateralization of the vocal folds, glottic expansion.
- Endolaryngeal resection of laryngeal and hypopharyngeal carcinomas.

Contraindications

- General disorders that preclude general anesthesia.
- Anatomical alterations of the cervical spine, which prevent a (sufficient) reclination of the head (ankylosing spondylitis, fractures, extensive spinal osteochondrosis) or disk herniation in the region of the cervical spine, mandibular prognathism, significantly protruding upper teeth.
- Trismus.
- Larynx too narrow, exposure impossible.

Specific Points Regarding Informed Consent

Microlaryngoscopy/hypopharyngoscopy, rigid tracheobronchoscopy:

- Dental damage or even loss of teeth.
- Mucosal injury.
- Disturbances of swallowing (dysphagia), nasogastric tube.
- Hoarseness or even loss of voice.
- Dyspnea, tracheotomy.
- Pneumonia, atelectasis.
- Mediastinitis.
- Pressure injury to the lingual, hypoglossal, or glossopharyngeal nerve, possibly causing loss of function.
- Recurrence.

Special Instruments and Implants

A set of operating laryngoscopes (e.g., Kleinsasser) with chest support and fiber-glass illuminator, distending laryngoscope (e.g., Weerda), the Lindholm self-retaining vocal fold retractor. A set of instruments for laryngeal microsurgery with double-cup grasping forceps and small scissors with various types of curved blades, needle holder, sickle blade, curette, suction tubes, and diathermy. Operating laryngoscopes and instruments should all have suction tubes for laser surgery.

Operating microscope with 400-mm lens, side-viewing endoscope.

Anesthesia

Intubation with a 24–28 Fr Woodbridge or single-use tube for adults, appropriately smaller tubes for children. Complete muscle relaxation should be achieved for inserting the laryngoscope. Alternatively, jet ventilation anesthesia or intermittent ventilation with the option of performing the operation during apnea.

Surgical Technique

Positioning. The patient should be positioned *absolutely flat* on the operating table, head dorsally flexed and stabilized in a small rubber ring. Remove dentures, if this has not already been done, and insert a mouth guard. After insertion of the laryngoscope, the whole operating table is inclined to approx. 30°.

Exposure. Recline the head with the left hand. Displace the lip to one side and introduce the laryngoscope from the right corner of the mouth—displacing the tongue to the left—and let it glide deeper down, using the intubation tube as a guide (**Fig. 10.2**). The tip of the blade elevates the epiglottis; it is introduced into the larynx under direct vision until the vocal folds are fully visible.

Fixation of the endoscope. Fix the endoscope in this position by placing the support onto the holding plate, which is positioned on the chest (**Figs. 10.3** and **10.4**). If insertion is difficult or there is inadequate visualization, the telescope may also lie obliquely in the corner of the mouth or in a gap in the teeth; in addition, a smaller-caliber tube may be resorted to.

Optimization of exposure. Tightening the adjusting screw on the side will improve the view of the anterior commissure as well as stabilizing the support; care should be taken here, however, because this increases pressure on the incisors. External counter-pressure on the larynx also improves the view into the anterior larynx (**Fig. 10.4**).

Exposure of the posterior commissure. The posterior commissure only comes into view after the tube has been elevated by the laryngoscope. The telescope should be advanced a little further if the vocal folds are obscured by the false cords; introducing the endoscope too deeply will excessively abduct and even occasionally injure the vocal folds.

Inspection of the subglottis and the sinus of Morgagni. The subglottic space and the sinus of Morgagni cannot be viewed completely, even with optimal visualization, and therefore need to be inspected with the aid of angled telescopes. It has proved helpful here to elevate the false cords with an angled blunt hook.

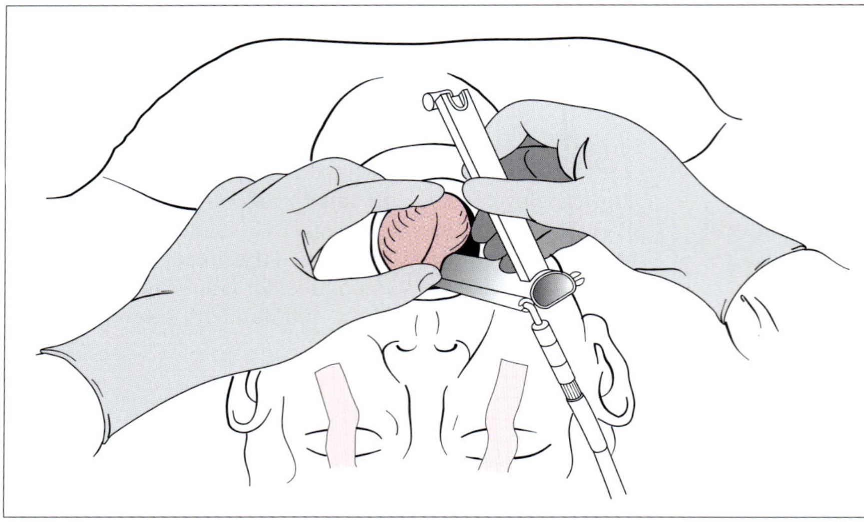

Fig. 10.2 Direct distending laryngoscopy: first step.
Insertion of the laryngoscope tube into the oral cavity and oropharynx.

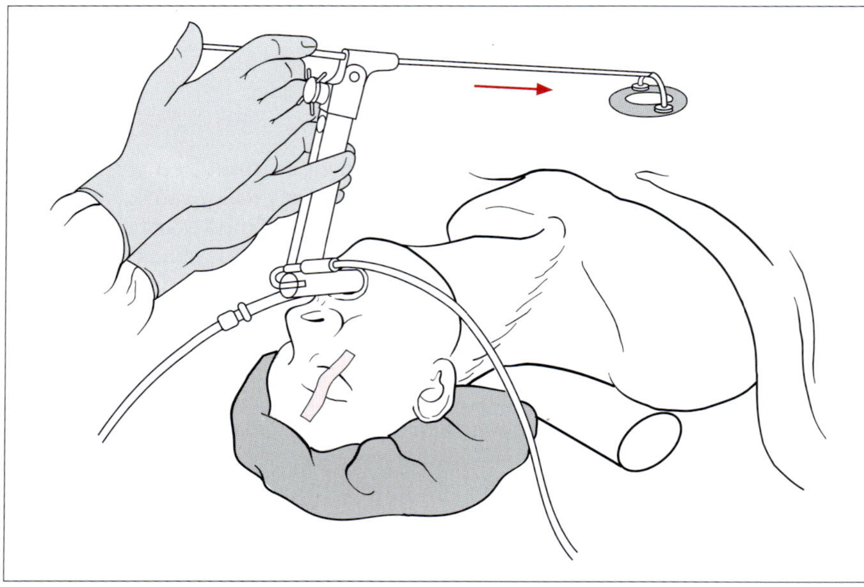

Fig. 10.3 Direct distending laryngoscopy: second step.
After the endolaryngeal space is exposed, the support is positioned on the chest.

Rules, Tips, and Tricks

Examination of the ventricles may be optimized by lateral pressure as well as by pressing the tip of the laryngoscope laterally against the false cord.

Risks and Complications

- Dental damage (chipping of tooth enamel, fractures of the tooth neck or loosening of teeth, tooth extractions); mandibular joint problems secondary to hyperextension.
- Hematomas and abrasions in the region of the palatal arches, tonsils, and base of the tongue.
- In extremely rare cases, dysfunction of the hypoglossal, lingual, or glossopharyngeal nerves secondary to pressure damage, resulting in disturbances of sensation, motion, and taste.
- Edema formation in the larynx, producing a risk of dyspnea in the presence of pre-existing stenosis.
- Hoarseness or increase of any pre-existing hoarseness, scar formation, and web formation with voice impairment.
- Jet ventilation carries the risk of bursting an emphysematous bleb.

Postoperative Care

- Voice rest, the duration of which depends on the endolaryngeal procedure being undertaken, consider voice therapy; daily inhalations may be indicated.
- Consider suppressing an irritated cough with antitussive agents and administering steroids to counteract the risk of edema.

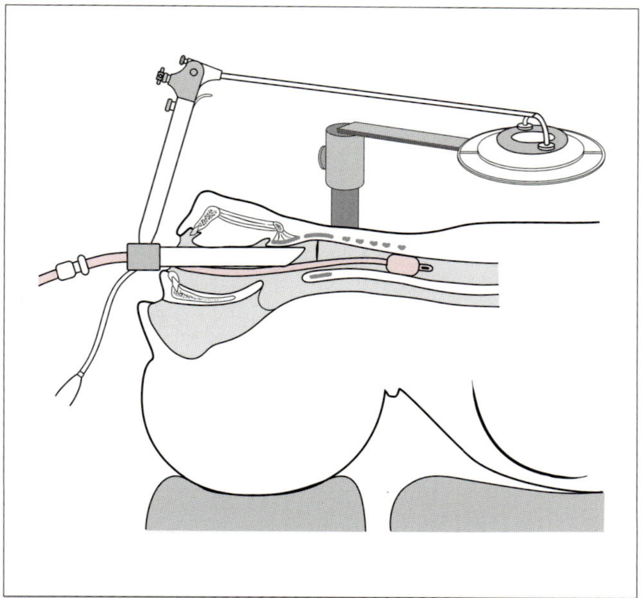

Fig. 10.4 Direct distending laryngoscopy: third step. The alignment of support and laryngoscope tube can be regulated by an adjusting screw.

Alternatives to Surgery Under Intubation

Jet ventilation allows an intubation-free general anesthesia with muscle relaxation when the larynx is narrow or where there are alterations in the most posterior part of the vocal folds or in the region of the posterior wall. Rapid insertion of the operating microscope is followed by connection of the injector cannula to the ventilator; the oxygen supply should be carefully monitored. If significant hemorrhage should occur, e. g., during carcinoma resection, then rapid intubation should be considered, followed by tracheobronchoscopy to aspirate blood, should hemostasis not be achieved immediately.

Direct Laryngotracheoscopy Using the Ventilation Laryngotracheoscope

Surgical Principle

Direct inspection of the larynx and trachea under general anesthesia using a thin tube (available also battery-operated for emergency cases) and ventilator connection, especially during emergency endoscopy or where intubation proves difficult.

Indications

- Direct laryngoscopy, incision biopsy, polypectomy, where narrow access or special anatomical conditions preclude intubation.
- Emergency endoscopy in the presence of intubation difficulties, laryngeal and tracheal tumors, laryngeal and tracheal injuries.

Contraindications

Severe general disorders precluding general anesthesia.

Specific Points Regarding Informed Consent

As for direct distending laryngotracheoscopy.

Special Instruments and Implants

Laryngoscope blades, emergency tracheoscope (various diameters and lengths), appropriate suction probes and double-cup grasping forceps which can be introduced through the tube.

Anesthesia

Before inducing muscle relaxation, it should be ensured that mask ventilation is possible or that insertion of the telescope through the glottis has been successful.

Surgical Technique

Positioning. Position the patient flat on the operating table, head slightly raised, neck maximally reclined. Remove dentures. Oxygenate well using mask ventilation before commencing the procedure. Ensure muscle relaxation (see above), consider insertion of a mouth guard.

Unfolding the pharynx. The laryngoscope blade (which should not be too large) is inserted with the left hand, past the right-hand corner of the mouth toward the midline, and the tip is slid as far as the vallecula. *Do not elevate the epiglottis.* The right hand maintains the head in reclination. *Lifting the blade in the direction of the laryngoscope handle* (do not lever it) will unfold the pharynx and raise the epiglottis until the arytenoid cartilage and posterior parts of the vocal folds come into view. Apply suction (**Fig. 10.5a, b**).

Introduction of the laryngoscope. With the right hand, pass the emergency laryngoscope tube (with tube size selected to suit the larynx or any stenosis present) from the corner of the mouth beneath the epiglottis—if possible, use any gap in the teeth—and then withdraw the laryngoscope blade.

Exposure of the larynx. The arytenoid cartilages with their mucosal coverage are now visible through the tube. Elevate the tip of the tube slightly and slide it under direct vision as far as the glottis. The tube is first rotated 90° just before the glottis and *the slender tip is introduced into the glottis; during the subsequent passage, the tube is rotated back again and the entire diameter of the tube is passed through the glottis.* During this maneuver, the tube is supported at the teeth with the thumb and index finger of the left hand, while the head is maintained in reclination (**Fig. 10.6**).

Inspection of the trachea. Carefully withdraw the tube past the level of the glottis to inspect the larynx and then advance it back into the trachea and ventilate. *Do not allow unduly long ventilation gaps. Check oxygen saturation.*

10

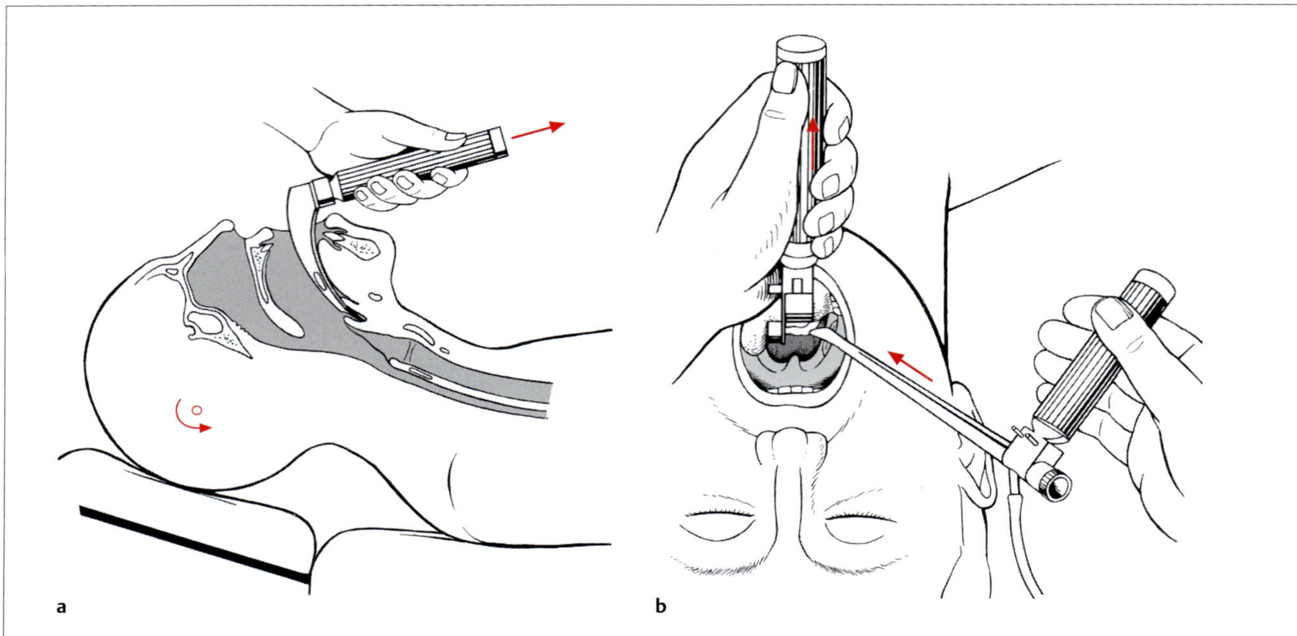

Fig. 10.5a, b Direct laryngotracheoscopy.
a Positioning with raised and reclined head. The laryngoscope blade is held with the left hand and drawn in the direction of the handle.
b The ventilation laryngotracheoscope is introduced with the right hand from the corner of the mouth. The tip of the tube slides over the epiglottis and is then raised slightly.

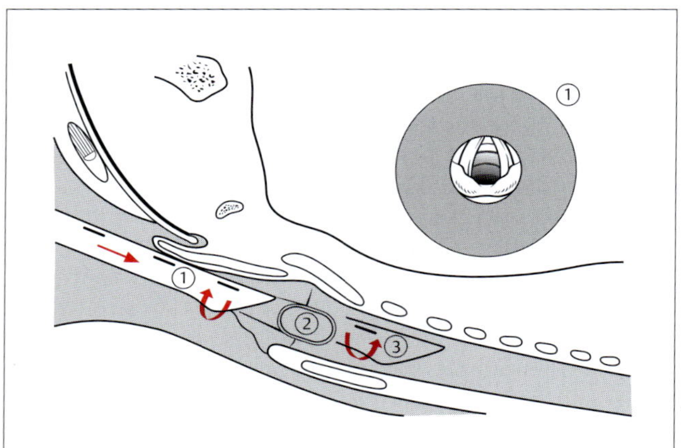

Fig. 10.6 Direct laryngotracheoscopy.
1 arytenoid cartilage, vocal folds, vestibular folds are visualized
2 for insertion into the trachea, the tip of the tube is positioned in the sagittal direction and then advanced through the glottis
3 rotating the tube 90° allows its entire circumference to pass the glottis when advanced further

Rules, Tips, and Tricks

- Excisional biopsies, polypectomies, and similar procedures are done with long double-cup grasping forceps. The instruments are guided with the right hand by right-handed surgeons, while the left hand stabilizes the tube, which is then advanced back past the glottis, and ventilation is re-commenced. Hemostasis is achieved with a cotton bud soaked in naphazoline.
- For difficult intubations: insert emergency tube into the trachea. Then advance a thin, well-lubricated bougie as far as the bifurcation and withdraw the tube. Then an intubation tube, which has been lubricated on its inner and outer surface, is threaded over the bougie and advanced into the larynx and trachea under digital guidance. The bougie is then withdrawn (**Fig. 10.7**).
- For cases where identification of the laryngeal aperture is difficult due to edema, tumor, or trauma: once the pharynx has been well visualized with the aid of the laryngoscope blade, have firm pressure applied to the chest; the escaping air stream indicates the way to the glottis.
- Always consider performing flexible fiberoptic intubation over a thin bronchoscope. This can be done via a transnasal route; however, the transoral route is preferable in an emergency situation. For this purpose, the tube is threaded over the flexible bronchoscope and secured with a tape at the transition to the handle, at that point where it can no longer be advanced further cranially. Then the intubation blade is inserted by an assistant, who pulls the right-hand corner of the mouth laterally. Now the person undertaking the intubation advances the bronchoscope over the tip of the intubation blade under direct vision as far as the epiglottis and then directs it under endoscopic guidance through the level of the glottis into the trachea as far as the bifurcation. Only now is the threaded tube advanced by the assistant, who maintains the position of the endoscope throughout the examination. After the tube has been placed, the endoscope is withdrawn.

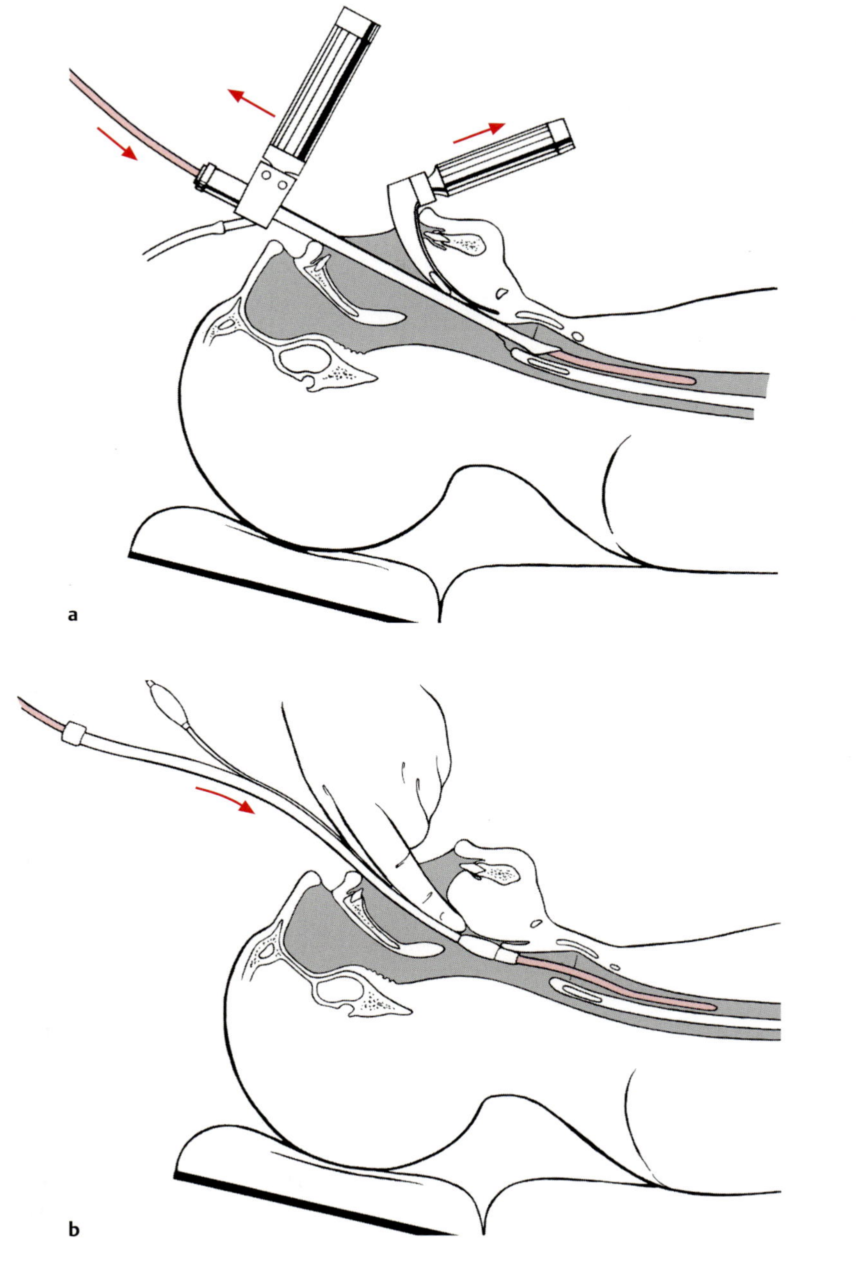

Fig. 10.7a, b Procedure for the difficult intubation.
a A thin bougie is introduced into the trachea via a ventilation tracheobronchoscope.
b Intubation via the bougie, under digital guidance.

! Risks and Complications

- Dental damage or tooth loss, especially in the presence of preexisting dental damage or crowns.
- Hoarseness or increase of any pre-existing hoarseness secondary to swelling, or even as a result of scar formation and web formation.
- Laryngeal swelling with dyspnea, consider tracheotomy or intubation in the presence of pre-existing stenosis.
- Slipping and simultaneous brusque advancement of the telescope can, in exceptional cases, even result in hypopharyngeal perforation.

Postoperative Care

- Antitussive agents against the urge to cough should already be given intraoperatively.
- With edema formation or in the presence of a narrow glottis: administer steroids before completion of the operation, postoperative observation.
- Voice rest, depending on the state of the larynx.

Transoral Cold-Steel Resection of Benign Lesions of the Larynx

Polyps of the Vocal Folds

Surgical Principle

Place the polyps on traction with grasping forceps and incise the mucosa around the base of the polyp with straight or curved scissors, without injuring the muscle or vocal ligament. If necessary, the incision margins can be carefully evened out with small scissors. *Avoid creating opposing mucosal defects in the anterior commissure.*

Hyperkeratoses

Surgical Principle

Hyperkeratoses are often indistinguishable macroscopically from carcinomas in situ. Therefore, always *excise completely leaving an adequate safety margin—but superficially*. One option is to inject a vasoconstricting agent into a lesion-free area of the vocal fold to elevate the superficial mucosal layer from its undersurface (hydrodissection). Incise the mucosa behind the hyperkeratosis transversally using scissors, a sickle blade, or a straight disk blade, then slit it anteriorly along the sinus of Morgagni and incise again using scissors anteriorly, in front of the anterior commissure as far as the free border of the vocal fold. Then elevate the mucosal flap thus created with a fine forceps and release it extensively with scissors or the disc blade before excising it behind the end of the lesion at the free border of the vocal fold. Hemostasis is achieved with a cotton bud soaked in epinephrine, for example.

Reinke Edema

Surgical Principle

In the presence of Reinke edema, it is recommended to open Reinke space along the ventricle, i.e., in the direction of vocal folds, and remove the thick liquid contents by suction (**Fig. 10.8**). The part of the mucosa covering the region of incision is reflected back. Then, any excess mucosa is carefully excised, avoiding removing too much. If bilateral treatment is required, an incision is made on one side transverse to the anterior commissure, which is not correspondingly denuded.

It should be emphasized that with Reinke edema, excision of the edema can be done bilaterally as long as the anterior commissure is not de-epithelialized. If the edema has extended as far as the anterior commissure, the contralateral side should not be approached during the same session, but completion of epithelialization should be awaited, 6–8 weeks later at the earliest.

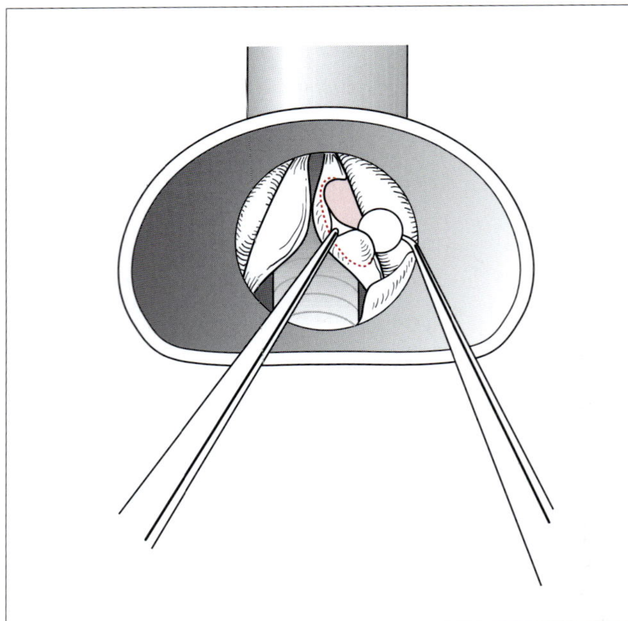

Fig. 10.8 Opening the Reinke space with the curved blade or the disc blade.

! Risks and Complications
Mucosal injuries in the region of the anterior commissure with an opposing wound surface in the region of the anterior vocal folds may become the origin of extensive web formations, which will then require treatment.

Postoperative Care

Postoperative voice therapy is advised for polyps of the vocal folds and occasionally also for Reinke edema.

Cysts

Surgical Principle

Surgical treatment of cysts may consist either of excision or, in many cases, enucleation. Cysts of the vocal folds are by no means always confined to the free margin, but may also occur on the subglottic wall.

Indications

More or less pronounced phonatory gap with subsequent hoarseness.

Contraindications

None, apart from medical aspects.

Surgical Technique

Mucosal incision. After exposing the lesion using microlaryngoscopic technique, the mucosal membrane covering the vocal folds is incised and drawn medially with fine forceps.

Excision of the cyst. The complete enucleation of the cyst then follows.

Laser Surgery

The real value of selective laser surgery undertaken with low performance parameters in the treatment of Reinke edema and vocal fold polyps has not yet been clarified. The question remains: Why should a thermal resection technique be used when the above-mentioned indications can be successfully treated with cold-steel surgery and complementary speech therapy?

Rules, Tips, and Tricks

Always use microscopic magnification. Use both hands: the left hand guides the forceps to grasp the tissue and puts it on stretch, while the right hand dissects. Flex the arms slightly and if necessary support the elbows.

Ensure optimal visualization, remove blood by suction, consider infiltration with a saline solution supplemented with epinephrine (1:10000). Ensure hemostasis by pressure of a cotton bud soaked in naphazoline, and also consider microsuction diathermy.

Laryngeal Web

Surgical Technique

Exposure. First, ensure optimal exposure of the anterior commissure.

Web release. The web is released on one vocal fold side as far as the anterior commissure, either using cold steel or by laser surgery; the epithelial tip thus formed is held up with a suture or tissue glue.

Insertion of the spacer. If recurrence of the web occurs, the web lamina is excised as a triangle and a narrow triangular dilator made of silicone is inserted into the anterior commissure for ca. 3–4 weeks. It is important to mention that the increased production of granulation tissue is occasionally observed after spacer insertion, and can considerably interfere with the healing process.

Positioning the spacer. A thin cannula is inserted into the larynx at the inferior edge of the thyroid cartilage; a nylon suture is passed through its lumen into the larynx, grasped with a fine grasping forceps, and withdrawn superiorly. The cannula is then withdrawn. The triangular silicone wedge is threaded onto the suture; the length of the dilator should not exceed 1.5–2 cm. The superior thread is now re-introduced into the larynx, a Reverdin needle is inserted slightly obliquely in an inferior direction through the thyroid notch, and the suture is threaded onto the needle and withdrawn. The thread is then knotted externally over a dental swab under mild traction, after checking the position of the dilator on the inside and, if necessary, correcting it. An instrument for advancing the needle, which was developed by Lichtenberger, has proven of assistance during this maneuver (Endo-extralaryngeal Needle Holder, 8267.50, Wolf, Knittlingen, Germany) and may also be used for the reversible endo-extralaryngeal expansion of the glottis (p. 200).

Postoperative Care

After completion of epithelialization, which usually takes about 4 weeks, the dilator is removed by repeat endoscopy. Tracheotomy is not usually required.

Alternatives

Even though long-term trials and controlled studies still remain to be undertaken, there are indications that topical application of mitomycin C after division of the anterior glottic stenosis demonstrates better long-term results than those after web release alone. Web release can be done with cold steel or using a CO_2 laser.

Incomplete Glottic Closure in the Presence of Unilateral Adductor Paralysis—Endolaryngeal Approach

Surgical Principle

An excavated vocal fold in the intermediate position can be medialized by injecting autologous fat or collagen; this is known as augmentation. The problem with autologous fat injection is that the absorption rate is unpredictable, requiring a repeat injection after months to years.

Indications

Unilateral incomplete glottic closure.

Contraindications

Severe general disorder that does not justify the risk of a general endotracheal anesthesia.

Specific Points Regarding Informed Consent

Complications as for microlaryngoscopy.

Special Instruments

Three-ring syringe (e.g., Ultra-Asept K. Storz, Tuttlingen, Germany), injection cannula (e.g., PV 27200S 18-cm injection cannula, K. Storz, Tuttlingen, Germany).

Surgical Technique

Augmentation

(Peri-)umbilical skin incision with harvesting of fat and transfer into the injection cannula. Abdominal wall fat is harvested surgically via a skin incision extending into the umbilicus and is then manually fragmented.

Alternative technique for autologous harvesting of abdominal wall fat. An 18 G needle is inserted into the subcutaneous abdominal fatty tissue. The plunger is retracted to create a vacuum. Material is harvested by moving the needle around in the subcutaneous tissue. The harvested material is rinsed with saline solution. When allowed to stand it settles out into three layers: (1) free fatty acids; (2) fat cells; (3) blood cells, saline solution, and cellular particles. The layer containing the fat cells is filtered out with a sieve (e.g., a tea strainer) to separate it from the other layers.

Endolaryngeal injection. The harvested fat is injected with a three-ring syringe using a long 19 G needle. The autologous fat can easily be injected through this long needle. Autologous fat injection can be used on the vocal folds, the false cords, the aryepiglottic folds of the larynx, and the medial wall of the piriform sinus.

Autologous fat can be injected at the vocal fold membrane into the thyroarytenoid muscle to improve atrophy of the vocal fold and incomplete glottic closure. The fat is also injected into the thyroarytenoid muscle at the part near the cartilage to produce rotation of the arytenoid cartilage.

Autologous fat may also be injected into the false cord and the aryepiglottic fold. Fat injections into the vocal fold, false cord, or aryepiglottic fold are intended to compensate atrophy of the laryngeal tissue and to facilitate glottic closure.

In addition, fat can also be injected into the medial wall of the piriform sinus of the hypopharynx to reduce its width.

Open Approach

Since the introduction of the basic technique of thyroplasty by Isshiki over 25 years ago, it has become a frequently used procedure in laryngeal surgery for the treatment of incomplete glottic closure. Various modifications of Isshiki type I thyroplasty have been suggested to improve operating time, placement of the implant, and implant material (e.g., autologous cartilage implants or alloplastic material such as hydroxylapatite, vitalium [miniplates], and polytetrafluoroethylene [Gore-Tex]). In 1999 Friedrich, from Graz, Austria, reported a surgical technique in which external vocal fold medialization is undertaken using an adjustable, pre-formed titanium implant for vocal fold medialization. It is the author's view that this procedure, which has since been increasingly used, may be regarded as a proven form of therapy for vocal fold medialization in cases that remain unsuccessful, or apparently so, after medialization by augmentation using autologous fat transfer. The reason is the titanium prosthesis developed by Friedrich, which allows an uncomplicated and time-saving operation with adequate fixation over the thyroid cartilage.

Surgical Principle

Inadequate medialization achieved by autologous fat injection (although fat injection is not necessarily a prerequisite).

Indications

Unilateral incomplete closure of the glottis.

Contraindications

Severe general disorder that does not justify the risk of a surgical intervention.

Specific Points Regarding Informed Consent

Complications as for microlaryngoscopy, skin incision at the level of the thyroid cartilage, titanium spacer, wound infection, wound breakdown, intolerability, dyspnea, tracheotomy.

Special Instruments

For example, the Friedrich prosthesis (K. Storz, Tuttlingen, Germany), microlaryngoscopy (MLS) tube, drill if needed.

Anesthesia

The operation should be performed under local anesthesia to be able to adjust the depth of the implant intraoperatively to the optimal voice quality achieved.

Surgical Technique

Friedrich Vocal Fold Medialization

Skin incision. After infiltration using 1% lidocaine with the addition of epinephrine, a skin incision is made at the level of the thyroid cartilage, which is then exposed while protecting the perichondrium.

Construction of a cartilaginous window. A reference line is drawn parallel to the inferior edge of the thyroid cartilage, beginning in the middle between the superior and inferior borders of the thyroid cartilage arch. The line divides the distance between the superior and inferior borders of the thyroid cartilage in a ratio of 2:1 and corresponds to the free border of the vocal folds in the endolarynx. A further important landmark for the fenestration is the oblique line. The cartilaginous window should be positioned caudal to the reference line and the inferoposterior corner of the window, close to the oblique line. For the 13-mm implant (which is normally used for female patients), the size of the window should be 6 × 11 mm, while for the 15-mm implant (normally used for male patients) it should be 6 × 13 mm.

After the window is marked, cartilage and bony material are drilled out with a steel drill until the internal perichondrium becomes visible (**Fig. 10.9a**). Once the internal perichondrium has been reached, the edges and corners of the window are smoothed with a small diamond drill. The internal perichondrium is incised along the dorsal margin and in part along the

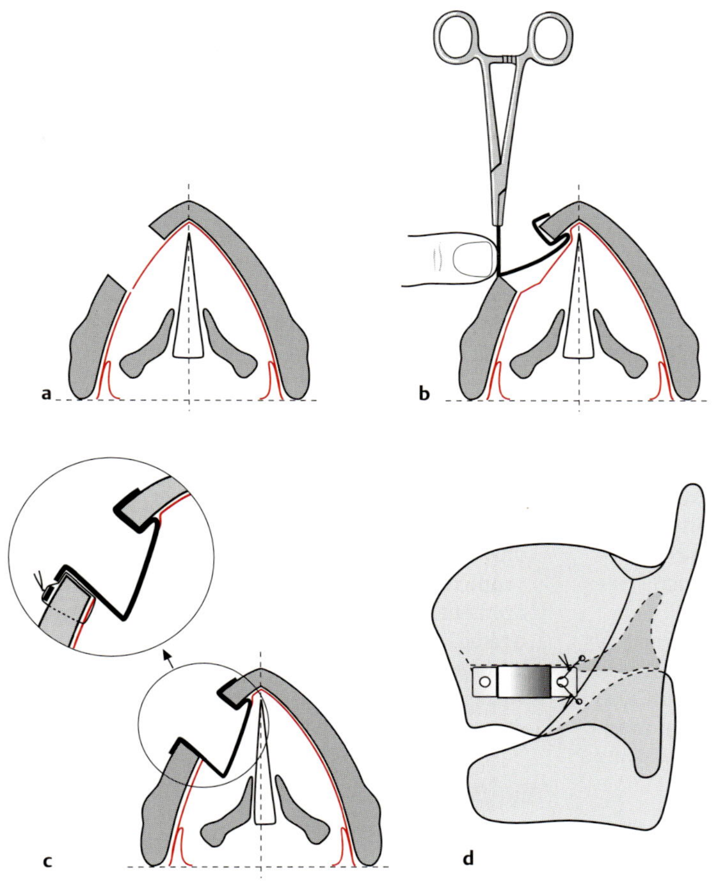

Fig. 10.9a–d Medialization of the vocal folds after Friedrich.

- **a** A cartilaginous window is drilled out down to the inner perichondrium.
- **b** Creation of subperichondrial pocket ventrally, insertion of the Friedrich prosthesis with the aid of a clamp—first ventrally, then dorsally.
- **c** Fixation of the Friedrich prosthesis in a dorsal direction using a monofilament suture.
- **d** Final appearance after dorsal placement of the Friedrich prosthesis and fixation with two sutures.

inferior and superior margin, using an electric knife. It is important that the paraglottic space is not encroached upon and the endolaryngeal vessels are not touched.

Placement of the implant. A subperichondrial pocket is created ventrally. The dorsal edge of the Friedrich prosthesis is held with a clamp and first inserted ventrally (**Fig. 10.9b**). The basal plate of the Friedrich prosthesis is 2 mm larger than the cartilaginous window. The implant must therefore be slightly bent between the clamp and index finger of the other hand. This allows the prosthesis to be inserted through the cartilaginous window into the endolarynx under mild tension. The optimal depth of medialization is determined by pressing the prosthesis in and marking the position with the clamp according to the optimal voice achieved. The dorsal edge is bent in a dorsal direction at the level of this mark and the prosthesis secured with two stitches of a monofilament, nonabsorbable suture (**Fig. 10.9c**). Due to the form of the prosthesis, no further fixation in the ventral region is usually required (**Fig. 10.9d**).

Rules, Tips, and Tricks

It is recommended to administer a single dose of 250 mg prednisolone and a one-off perioperative dose of a broad-spectrum antibiotic, which should be given 30–60 minutes before surgery.

Postoperative Care

Adjuvant speech therapy is beneficial.

Alternatives

Isshiki or Montgomery vocal fold medialization.

Transoral Laser Microsurgery

General Remarks

Laser surgery of benign and circumscribed malignant tumors of the larynx has become a common treatment concept in many institutes. The final assessment of this method in terms of reproducible long-term results has not yet reached a conclusion, especially as a therapeutic concept for advanced laryngeal carcinoma and in comparison to possible alternative treatments.

The use of laser surgery techniques is inextricably linked to the need for sound surgical training. It should in no way be understood as being "easier" than partial surgical resection using an open approach. This is all the more true when laser surgery is used for transoral treatment of advanced laryngeal carcinomas, although the required experience in this very demanding microsurgical technique may be lacking. Furthermore, situations will always arise, even with very experienced surgeons, where the difficulties of a tumor exposure that is "just about" acceptable or functional limitations during the postoperative course become apparent. These caveats indicate why endolaryngeal laser surgery has its detractors. There are some recognized laryngologists who regard laser surgery merely as a helpful alternative in certain indications, and a few who strictly rule out laser surgery of the larynx.

Modern laser technology allows surgery using a precisely aligned laser beam without producing any significant carbonization. A micromanipulator that produces a laser beam well below 0.5 mm in diameter should be used. The physical properties of the laser beam allow maximum use of both cutting qualities and coagulation.

Special Instruments

Laryngoscope tube and instruments with special suction units; protective eyewear.

Anesthesia

Operations may be carried out under general anesthesia, intermittent apnea, or jet ventilation. Various safety precautions must be observed during use of the laser in order to avoid serious complications, such as ignition of the endotracheal tube with its potentially fatal outcome. It is known that the endotracheal tube usually ignites if the laser beam accidentally penetrates unprotected components of the tube. The greatest risk potential lies in the cuff region and the tip of the endotracheal tube. Because the cuff region is particularly vulnerable, it is recommended to cover it with damp neurosurgical cotton padding. The risk can be further minimized by inflating the cuff with dyed physiological saline instead of air. The blue dye will immediately indicate that the cuff is damaged. If the tube ignites despite these precautions, then immediate disconnection of the ventilation tube from the ventilator is necessary, with removal of the laryngoscope, followed by re-intubation and interdisciplinary emergency management of the patient (depending on the severity—pulmonology, intensive care, visceral surgery, nephrology, etc). After extubation, laryngotracheal injection of Ringer solution may be initiated using a preprepared 50 mL syringe, provided the laryngoscope is still in its original position.

Benign Disorders

The introduction of the CO_2 laser into laryngology began with the treatment of benign disorders. The benign lesions of the larynx described in this chapter, such as cysts and granulomas, may also be resected using cold-steel instruments, with equivalent therapeutic results. For certain indications, such as laryngeal papillomatosis, however, laser surgical treatment is usually more advantageous than conventional surgery.

Granulomas

Indications

- The surgical removal of *contact granulomas* is indicated only in exceptional cases. Instead, speech therapy, in part supplemented by psychotherapy, forms the primary management modality. The possibility of reflux should be investigated.
- *Intubation granulomas* should not be excised earlier than 4 weeks after intubation. Exceptions are possible and include severe incidents of dyspnea or marked voice disorders.

Anesthesia

Intubation should be avoided. Excision of the intubation granuloma should be undertaken during an apnea phase or, if appropriate, using jet ventilation.

Surgical Technique

The glottis is exposed using a closed laryngoscope; the granuloma is grasped and excised at its base.

Rules, Tips, and Tricks

Unnecessarily excessive exposure of the arytenoid cartilage should be avoided.

! Risks and Complications

Because of the presence of persisting inflammation, recurrences in the region of the vocal process may originate from the perichondrium. This also applies after careful removal using the CO_2 laser.

Postoperative Care

Speech therapy.

Laryngocele

Surgical Principle

Excision or marsupialization of the soft, more or less spherical, bulge of mucosa protruding from the ventricle or the mucosa and extending into the supraglottic space.

Indications

Circumscribed external laryngoceles which are accessible by the open or endolaryngeal route.

Specific Points Regarding Informed Consent

As for microlaryngoscopy.

Surgical Technique

Exposure. Transoral surgery of laryngoceles requires exposure of the supraglottic region with the aid of a closed or open laryngoscope.

Identification of the laryngocele. The mucosa covering the laryngocele is incised in the region of the false cord or the aryepiglottic fold and the wall of the laryngocele is identified.

Opening the laryngocele. After the laryngocele is opened, it becomes apparent whether it contains air or thin or viscous mucus.

Transoral resection of the laryngocele. The secretion is removed by suction. After the subsequent collapse of the laryngocele, it may be dissected peripherally and completely excised, even in the case of smaller laryngoceles.

Marsupialization. Often wide marsupialization of the laryngocele in the direction of the internal larynx is also possible. This applies particularly to extensive laryngoceles.

Approach for external laryngoceles. Depending on their extent, external laryngoceles are removed using conventional surgical technique via an open approach (p. 282) or, in special cases, marsupialization is performed transorally using the CO_2 laser surgical technique as described above.

Papillomas

Surgical Principle

Vaporization of papillomas, which at the time may comprise multiple foci, may be repeated at short intervals, depending on the activity of the disorder, e.g., to avoid the necessity of a tracheotomy. Histological confirmation of the disorder is absolutely essential, however, even with more or less complete vaporization. In addition to endolaryngeal manifestations, patients with laryngeal papillomas must be assessed for possible extralaryngeal involvement of the tracheobronchial system as well as the region of the upper digestive tract.

Indications

Papillomatosis of the upper aerodigestive tract.

Specific Points Regarding Informed Consent

As for microlaryngoscopy.

Anesthesia

Surgery for laryngeal papillomas is performed on the intubated patient or with intermittent apnea or using jet ventilation to allow an optimal endolaryngeal view.

Surgical Technique

A slightly defocused laser beam is usually employed. Low laser power allows the controlled removal of the polyps, while ensuring that surgery is restricted to the mucosa. With bilateral involvement of the vocal folds it should be ensured that near the anterior commissure the laser is only used unilaterally to minimize the risk of postoperative web formation.

Rules, Tips, and Tricks

- Extubation is usually possible after surgery, even in very advanced cases.
- It has proved advantageous to maintain smaller areas of healthy mucosa between the individual papillomas to allow more rapid re-epithelialization of the endolarynx.

Postoperative Care

A single-dose application of a steroid (e.g., 3 mg/kg prednisolone) may be helpful to avoid postoperative dyspnea.

Alternatives

In addition to laser surgery, promising results have been achieved using photodynamic therapy. Further studies in the future will show to what extent long-term freedom from papillomas is possible with this type of treatment.

There is an increasing number of trials using systemic treatments for extensive forms of papillomatosis with involvement of the tracheobronchial tree. Isolated results with interferon-α2b or the intralesional injection of the antiviral drug cidofovir do not as yet allow a conclusive assessment of the value of this type of therapy.

Laryngomalacia

About 60–70% of stridor-associated laryngeal anomalies in childhood are attributed to laryngomalacia. The stridor associated with laryngomalacia is either congenital or manifests itself within the first weeks after birth. The symptoms of stridor will have reached their maximum by the age of 6 months, after which they usually recede by the end of the second year of life. Active surgical intervention is required in ca. 20% of cases of laryngomalacia.

Surgical Principle

An inward collapse of the supraglottic mucosa during inspiration is an indication for a so-called *supraglottoplasty*. This term includes all forms of surgical treatment that are aimed at reducing the hypermobile supraglottic tissue. In most cases this involves the mucosa of the aryepiglottic folds and the arytenoid cartilage regions.

If the symptoms of stridor result from *short aryepiglottic folds*, then bilateral laser surgical incision of these anatomical structures can usually be made.

On the other hand, if there is an *inward collapse of the epiglottis* during inspiration, then a so-called epiglottopexy should be performed.

These various treatment strategies for infants suffering from severe laryngomalacia underline the need for a careful preoperative diagnostic assessment, including an examination of the tracheobronchial system.

Indications

Swallowing problems (dysphagia), dyspnea, and life-threatening symptoms of apnea.

Anesthesia

Intermittent apnea or general endotracheal anesthesia (e.g., for epiglottopexy).

10

Surgical Technique

Intubation and general approach. All the following measures are preceded by flexible laryngo(tracheobroncho)scopy, with the infant held upright. To diagnostically assess the underlying cause of inspiratory stridor in infancy or childhood, the supraglottic region is viewed using an intubation blade. This is followed by rigid endoscopy and imaging via a monitor with the child sedated and breathing spontaneously. This will allow the diagnosis of laryngomalacia and the various forms of laryngeal and tracheal stenosis to be obtained. A tracheobronchoscopy may be regarded as obligatory.

If the condition is to be treated transorally using laser microsurgery, then the question arises as to whether to operate with the patient intubated or using intermittent apnea. If the latter technique is to be used, the endotracheal tube is inserted into the trachea via the operating microscope. Oxygen saturation is monitored by the anesthetist. Once 100% oxygen saturation is achieved, the tube is removed and laser surgery commenced. If oxygen saturation falls below 90% (which sometimes does not occur until after 5 minutes if the patient has been sufficiently pre-oxygenated), then the patient is re-intubated via the tube until 100% oxygen saturation has been regained.

Membranous Laryngotracheal Stenosis

If a short-segment stenosis is present, the membranes often have a web-like appearance; this is an excellent indication for laser surgery. Anesthesia is performed as described above and CO_2 lasering is commenced. It is not necessary to undertake a circular resection of the entire membranous web, as subsequently this carries the risk of creating a circumferential stenosis. Instead, a star-shaped incision should be made in the membrane, or a semi-circular portion excised.

Laser Surgical Epiglottopexy

Surgical Technique

Creation of opposing wound surfaces. This involves vaporizing or superficially resecting a circumscribed part of the tongue base using laser microsurgery, subsequently creating an opposing laser wound at the lingual epiglottic fold (laser power 1–2 W) (**Fig. 10.10a**).

Fixation of the epiglottis to the base of the tongue. Next, the epiglottis is fixed to the base of the tongue with the aid of two or three interrupted sutures using an absorbable suture material (e.g., Vicryl 4/0) (**Fig. 10.10b–d**).

Laser Surgical Division of Short Aryepiglottic Folds

Surgical Technique

Short aryepiglottic folds require incision using CO_2 laser (1 W, 0.25 mm). Tissue beneath the folds must be protected from injury during the procedure.

Hemangiomas and Vascular Malformations

Hemangiomas typically present as well-defined, reddish, space-occupying lesions in the posterior part of the subglottis, often at the subglottic undersurface of the vocal fold. Hemangiomas, which develop in the region of the posterior commissure and then extend along subglottic undersurfaces of both vocal folds, are less frequently seen than lesions in the region of the anterior commissure. The various therapeutic options for subglottic hemangiomas range from tracheotomy to a submucous surgical excision and systemic or intralesional steroid injections as well as the systemic administration of interferon-α2a. Circumscribed lesions can also be brought to involution using CO_2 laser and low laser energy (1–2 W). The use of a Nd:YAG laser is no longer recommended because of the often significant postoperative fibrin exudation. Following the adoption of propanolol for the treatment of problematic hemangiomas in infants, it is to be hoped that the excellent effect of this medication will also be extended to reduction of the volume of subglottic hemangiomas.

Unlike the biological behavior of the hemangiomas described above, vascular malformations of the larynx often only manifest themselves clinically in adulthood or are only discovered incidentally. Typical symptoms include foreign-body sensation, urge to clear the throat, or a slowly developing, usually mild stridor.

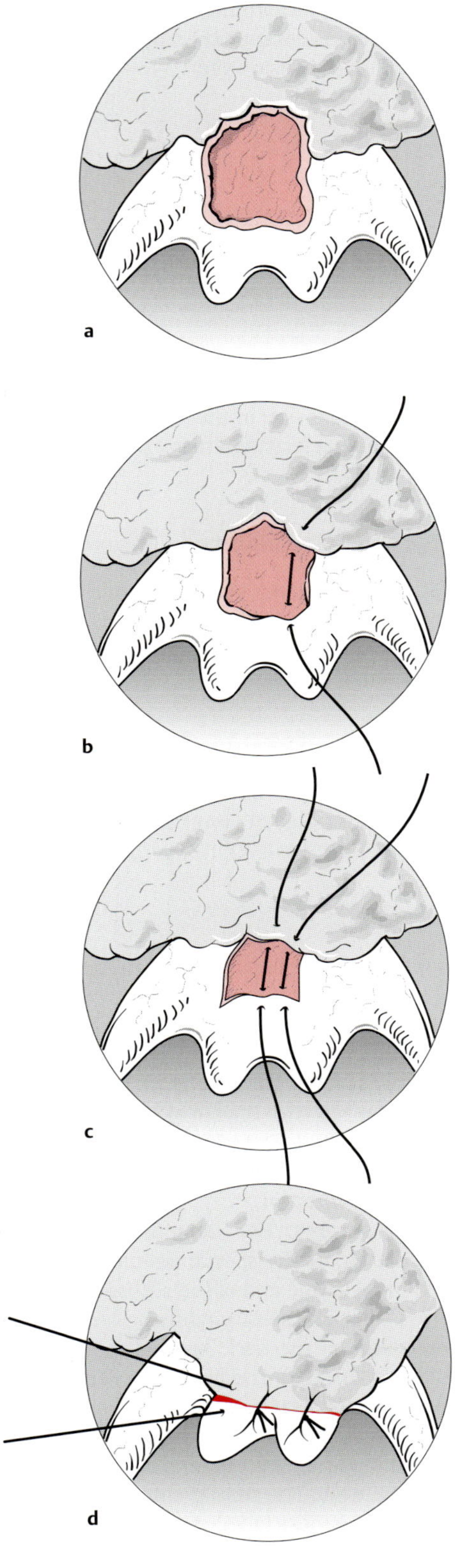

Fig. 10.10a–d Epiglottopexy
a Laser microsurgical vaporization of lingual epiglottal mucosa and the opposing mucosa of the base of the tongue.
b–d Stepwise fixation of the epiglottis to the base of the tongue using as many as three interrupted sutures.

Indications

- *Subglottic hemangioma*: progression in size with subsequent dyspnea and stridor.
- *Vascular malformations*: progression in size with swallowing difficulties (dysphagia), disturbances of articulation, recurrent bleeding, recurrent infections, or dyspnea.

Contraindications

There are no contraindications in the presence of an absolute indication with compromise of vital functions.

Anesthesia

General endotracheal anesthesia, surgery using intermittent apnea, jet ventilation.

Surgical Technique

Subglottic Hemangiomas

CO_2 laser treatment of subglottic hemangiomas is performed either with the aim of shrinking the lesion, which is achieved by single laser spots (2 W) placed at adequate distances apart, or via a mucosal incision followed by enucleation of the angioma. Postoperative edema formation can usually be avoided by the careful use of CO_2 laser treatment. A tracheotomy should be performed in uncertain cases. Cortisone administration is indicated. The possibility that the excellent efficacy of propanolol will be extended to subglottic hemangiomas has already been alluded to.

10

Vascular Malformations

Vascular malformations may be excised; this particularly applies to cases where the differential diagnosis is uncertain. If histological clarification is dispensed with, the vascular malformation may be brought to involution by using the Nd:YAG laser (e.g., 20 W, 0.5 seconds in single applications, bare fiber 0.6 mm).

Rules, Tips, and Tricks
Oral medication using prednisolone, 3–5 mg/kg body weight distributed over three doses per 24 hours, has proved successful in the management of subglottic hemangiomas (in addition to laser surgical vaporization). This should be undertaken in close cooperation with pediatricians to immediately diagnose and adequately treat any subsequent arterial hypertension or temporary diabetes mellitus.

! Risks and Complications
Hemorrhage, edema formation with the need for tracheotomy, infection with the subsequent risk of stenosis.

Postoperative Care

- Careful monitoring of the patient's respiratory condition in order to counteract immediately any postoperative edema formation by the administration of steroids.
- Inhalation with β-sympathomimetic agents and steroids.
- Oral and, if necessary, antibiotic therapy with a cephalosporin.

Surgery for Glottic Stenosis

Paralysis of the vocal folds is most often the result of thyroid gland surgery. Its incidence depends on the surgical technique, bearing in mind that injury to the recurrent laryngeal nerve can occur even in the hands of experienced surgeons. Unilateral injuries may initially remain undetected, only to become clinically manifest in the further course of the disorder. For this reason, pre- and postoperative assessment of vocal fold function should be standardized. In the presence of unilateral vocal fold paralysis, patients usually complain of isolated dysphonia. Bilateral paralysis, however, results in a paramedian position of the vocal folds, which produces a noticeable inspiratory stridor, usually associated with dyspnea at rest and in many cases quite well-preserved voice quality.

Some of those affected are capable of tolerating the associated dyspnea without any further surgical intervention, although additional infections of the upper respiratory tract can sometimes also lead to a life-threatening increase in dyspnea. Other patients, however, need immediate surgical intervention, which is usually undertaken in the form of a tracheotomy.

Currently four basic operative approaches are available for expanding the glottis:

- Endo-extralaryngeal expansion of the glottis (e.g., after Lichtenberger).
- Endolaryngeal microlaryngoscopic glottic expansion.
- Extralaryngeal laterofixation.
- Combined extra-endolaryngeal approach after thyrotomy.

Lichtenberger Endo-Extralaryngeal Expansion of the Glottis

Surgical Principle

This technique is based on the development of a special suture instrument with which, in the case of a bilateral paralysis of the vocal folds, a vocal fold can be temporarily lateralized. Lateralization is performed on the less mobile vocal fold.

The operation should be performed as early as possible to avoid injury to the vocal fold tissue secondary to intubation, while also sparing the patient symptoms of dyspnea, which considerably affect the quality of life and are associated with anxiety states.

Indications

- Fresh bilateral paralysis of the recurrent laryngeal nerve.

Contraindications

Given that restitution cannot be expected after more than 12 months, a definitive expansion of the glottis should be undertaken in cases of recurrent laryngeal nerve paralysis lasting longer than 1 year.

Specific Points Regarding Informed Consent

The same as for microlaryngoscopy, plus chondritis, soft-tissue infection, scar formation, sensory disturbances, injury to the hypoglossal nerve, wound infection, suture line breakdown, revision surgery for removal of sutures.

Special Instruments and Implants

Monofilament sutures (e.g., Prolene 2/0), special Endo-extralaryngeal Needle Holder, (8267.50, Wolf, Knittlingen, Germany), special needles (8267.951, Wolf, Knittlingen, Germany).

Anesthesia

Intermittent apnea, high-frequency jet anesthesia.

Surgical Technique

Visualization of the level of the glottis. Once the level of the glottis has been visualized with the aid of a distending laryngoscope (**Fig. 10.11a**), the endo-extralaryngeal sutures are positioned after temporarily removing the endotracheal tube (*ensure adequate pre-oxygenization*).

Positioning the sutures. Two monofilament sutures are positioned with the aid of the special needle holder, using a translaryngeal approach. One end of the suture attached to the needle is inserted through the laryngoscope and brought out through the soft tissue of the neck, below the posterior third of one vocal fold (**Fig. 10.11b**). The needle holder is then withdrawn, the remaining end again attached to a needle, which is inserted using the needle holder above the posterior third of the vocal fold to form a loop (**Fig. 10.11c**) and brought out through the soft tissue of the neck. The second suture inserted to perform the laterofixation is positioned in an appropriate fashion ca. 2–3 mm ventral to the first suture loop (**Fig. 10.11d**). If the first suture loop is sufficient, the second loop may be dispensed with.

Fixation of the sutures. After knotting the second suture loop subcutaneously, the orginal skin incision is closed.

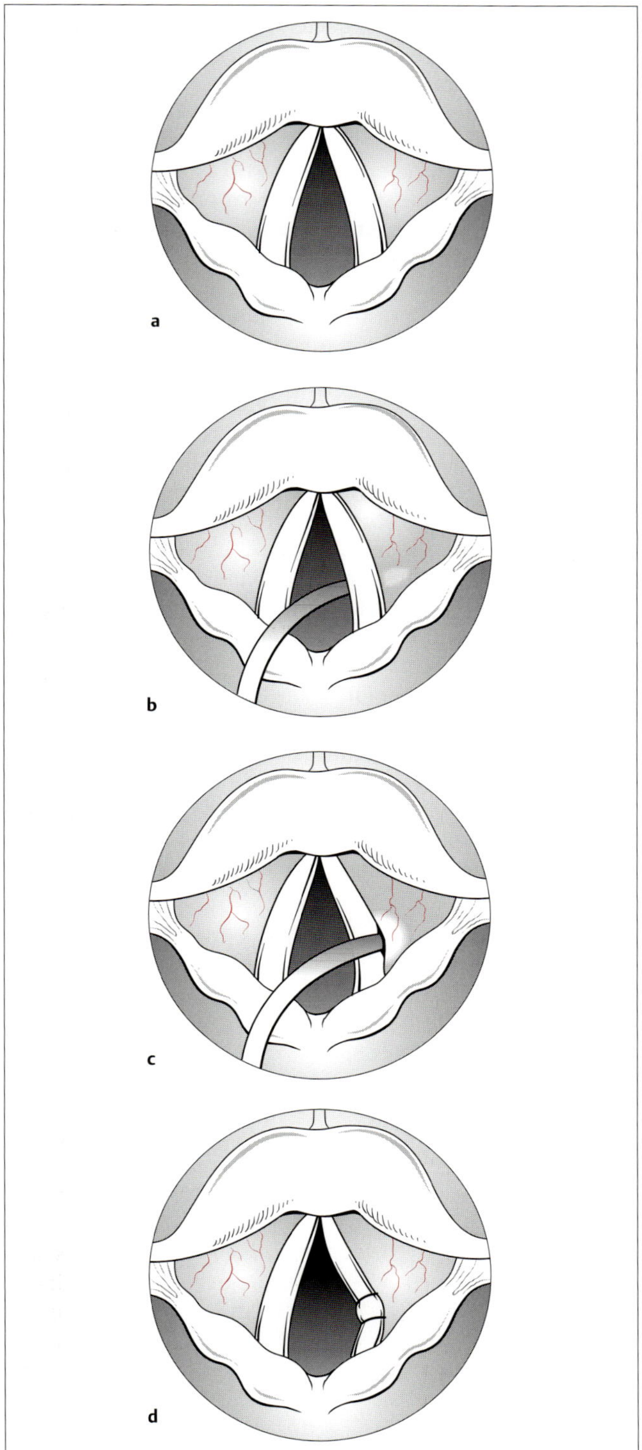

Fig. 10.11a–d Endo-extralaryngeal expansion of the glottis after Lichtenberger.
a View onto the glottic and supraglottic region using a distending laryngoscope.
b Subglottic positioning of the instrument for advancing the needle just in of front the vocal process with subsequent puncture through the soft tissue of the neck.
c The remaining endolaryngeal suture is once again passed through the needle and brought out via the ventricle.
d Final appearance with two suture loops.

Rules, Tips, and Tricks

To achieve an optimal surgical result using the endo-extralaryngeal suture technique, the guide suture should be placed as far dorsally as possible, close to the vocal process. Occasionally there is difficulty here because the adjacent part of the thyroid cartilage is often compacted or even ossified. If it is impossible to bring the suture out transcutaneously for this reason, the method may be modified to pierce the thyroid cartilage further ventrally.

! Risks and Complications

The sutures may create a superficial tear or even a deep tear in the vocal fold tissue, especially when operating under inflammatory conditions. The perioperative administration of a broad-band cephalosporin is initiated as infection prophylaxis, given that bacterial colonization of the soft tissues of the neck cannot be excluded after endo-extralaryngeal passage of the suture.

Postoperative Care

With regard to regaining the initially lost function of the vocal folds, the further outcome must be awaited with patience. Certainty as to whether or not physiological vocal fold function has been regained is not usually to be expected until at least 12 months after the operation. It should also be borne in mind that the prognosis of bilateral paralysis may differ for the two affected sides.

Endolaryngeal, Microlaryngoscopic Expansion of the Glottis

Surgical Principle

Unilateral arytenoidectomy (Thornell 1948) and attenuation of the posterior part of the vocal fold muscle with lateral retraction of the vocal fold (Kleinsasser 1976), or partial resection of the false cord and craniolateral fixation (Langnickel and Koburg 1970) of the posterior vocal fold under distending microscopic visualization of the larynx. Since the introduction of the CO_2 laser into otorhinolaryngology, laser surgical expansion of the glottis after Dennis and Kashima (1989) or a modification of this technique is increasingly being undertaken. The advantage of this procedure in comparison with the open approach is a better postoperative voice, on average; expansion of the glottis cannot, however, always be achieved to the same extent as with an open approach.

The dilemma of operations to expand the glottis is that they can only improve the voice at the cost of breathing, or vice versa. Surgery can only represent the *best possible compromise* between a reduction in voice quality and improvement of breathing.

Indications

Bilateral vocal fold paralysis in the paramedian position, associated with dyspnea.

Contraindications

Subglottic stenosis or tracheal stenosis.

Specific Points Regarding Informed Consent

- As for microlaryngoscopy.
- As for laser surgery of laryngeal tumors, the operation cannot reproduce normal findings; compromise between loss of voice and improvement in breathing; tracheotomy is often required with the conventional approach.

Special Instruments

CO_2 laser with its appropriate instruments.

Surgical Technique

The patient is positioned flat on the operating table. For special instruments see “Microlaryngoscopy.”

Transoral Arytenoidectomy

Identification of the level of the glottis. Exposure of the larynx using the largest possible distending laryngoscope. The arytenoid cartilage and the posterior region of the vocal folds and false cords must be completely visible. The arytenoid cartilage and the posterior third of the vocal folds are infiltrated with a vasoconstricting agent.

Incision. Under the microscope, a longitudinal incision is placed over the vocal fold, extending in an anterior-to-posterior direction over the vocal process, upward as far as the dome of the arytenoid cartilage. This incision was previously done with scissors or a sickle blade, but nowadays is usually done by CO_2 laser. A further incision is made from the end of this incision over the arytenoid cartilage in a lateral direction toward the aryepiglottic fold for a distance of approximately 8–10 mm; a third incision is made from this end point to the vocal process. The mucosal triangle incised in this fashion is later discarded.

Excision of the arytenoid cartilage. The cartilage is carefully taken up with grasping forceps and released from its surroundings (**Fig. 10.12a**). The cartilage must be removed *in toto.*

Thinning out the posterior third of the vocal fold. Excision of the vocal fold musculature. The previously placed incision is deepened and the vocal fold musculature is largely removed in its posterior and middle parts. *The conus elasticus is vertically incised posteriorly* (**Fig. 10.12b**).

Mucosal suture. The incision is repaired with two interrupted sutures (4/0 absorbable). The needle is passed first into the lower and then the upper fold using the special curved delicate needle holder. The surgical knot is tied in front of the tube and then the short end of the suture directed in an inferior direction using the grasping forceps, keeping the long end under tension. The second knot is tied as an instrument knot and drawn downward using a double hook or opened double-cup grasping forceps. Alternatively, the wound may be closed using fibrin glue (**Fig. 10.12c, d**).

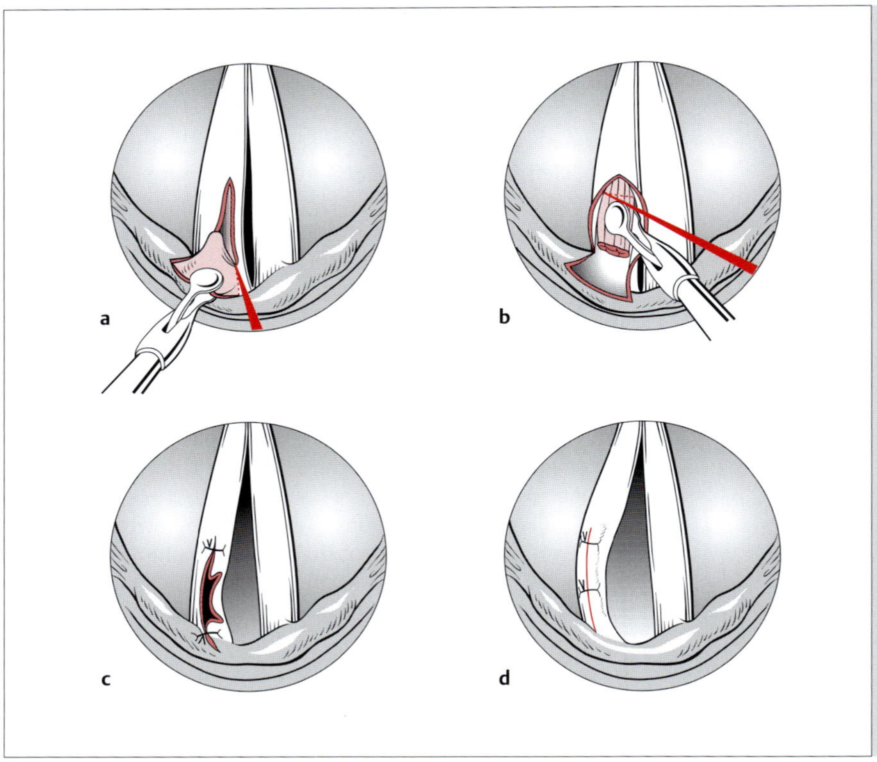

Fig. 10.12a–d Endolaryngeal microscopic expansion of the glottis after Kleinsasser.
a Longitudinal incision over the posterior vocal fold and triangular mucosal excision over the arytenoid cartilage using a CO_2 laser.
b Release of the arytenoid cartilage.
c Excision of the vocal fold muscles using scissors and grasping forceps, incision of the conus elasticus.
d Suture repair of the incision.

Endolaryngeal Laser Surgical Expansion of the Glottis After Dennis and Kashima (Posterior Cordectomy)

Surgical Principle

Incision of the dorsal vocal folds in the region of the vocal process while protecting the arytenoid cartilage. This approach allows an individually adapted compromise between adequate breathing and voice function.

Surgical Technique

Exposure of the posterior glottis. Surgical division of the vocal ligament and the musculature of the vocal muscle by CO_2 laser (usually low power) immediately in front of the arytenoid cartilage. The tissue is divided lateral to the vocal process, down to the level of the thyroid cartilage.

Modifications

Good respiratory results are achieved in the long term by an additional incision extending from the lateral tip of the excision area in the direction of the anterior commissure and resection of the lateral thyroarytenoid muscle. Without these measures, the initially wide glottis not infrequently becomes narrow again as a result of scar formation in the excision area. Steiner (of Göttingen, Germany) favors the bilateral posterior cordectomy to avoid injuring the ventral part of the vocal folds, which is so important for phonation. All the techniques described presuppose sound knowledge of the anatomy of each individual patient. This also allows a choice of treatment method, tailored to suit the patient.

For "Rules, Tips, and Tricks" and "Risks and Complications" see p. 201.

Postoperative Care

- Extubation after a single-dose administration of a steroid (e.g., 250 mg prednisolone IV); a tracheotomy is not necessary.
- Antibiotic coverage for 3 days.
- Revision surgery may be necessary to remove fibrin deposits and/or granulations, which can narrow the glottis.

Extralaryngeal Lateral Fixation

Surgical Principle

Open exposure of the laryngeal framework. Identification of the arytenoid cartilage via a window in the thyroid cartilage lamina, mobilization, and lateral displacement of the vocal process with a suture. As breathing is improved, the voice deteriorates. The procedure described here is based on the technique reported by McCall and Gardiner. This technique may be considered above all for the situation where a transoral exposure is not possible.

Preoperative diagnostic examinations, indications, and contraindications, as well as the choice of sides, are the same as for the endolaryngeal technique.

Anesthesia

Intubation, tracheotomy, re-intubation. The orotracheal tube is left in the glottis to displace the arytenoid into the operative field.

Surgical Technique

Positioning. A roll is placed beneath the shoulders; the head is turned to the contralateral side.

Incision. The skin incision runs obliquely from the anterior margin of the sternocleidomastoid muscle, in an antero-inferior direction over the lamina of the thyroid cartilage. The incision is deepened through the platysma; the omohyoid muscle and the prelaryngeal strap muscles are divided. If still present, the thyroid gland may need to be displaced caudally. Identification of the thyroid cartilage (**Fig. 10.13a**).

Creation of a window in the thyroid cartilage. A window is made in the thyroid cartilage. The perichondrium is incised above the planned window as an inferiorly based swing-door flap. The window is created in the cartilage with a scalpel or punch, leaving only a relatively narrow (ca. 0.5 cm) frame posteriorly and superiorly (**Fig. 10.13b**). The internal perichondrium is divided and a large blood vessel that regularly traverses the area is diathermied. The exposed musculature is bluntly spread apart posteroinferiorly until the arytenoid cartilage is encountered in the depths.

Arytenoidectomy. While holding the musculature aside with a retractor, the arytenoid cartilage is released down to the vocal process with small scissors and the disk blade. The articular cartilage and the cricoarytenoid ligament in particular must be safely divided (**Fig. 10.13c**).

A nonabsorbable polyester suture (e.g., Mersilene) is passed around the vocal process, which is exposed but still firmly attached to the vocal ligament, knotted initially over the cartilage, then drawn downward around the previously exposed thyroid cartilage and then knotted again. Before finally pulling this knot tight, the position of the vocal fold must be confirmed by endolaryngeal inspection with a laryngoscope and, if necessary, corrected (**Fig. 10.13d, e**).

Wound closure. Fixation of the elevated perichondrium using a retention suture, insertion of a suction drain, wound closure in a layered fashion.

Modifications

Mündnich approach. The superior and posterior frame of the thyroid cartilage as described above is also excised; this considerably facilitates dissection of the arytenoid cartilage and placement of the suture during this approach, which is otherwise practically similar to that described above. In addition, a notch is placed in the inferior part of the thyroid cartilage to guide the suture. However, a partial collapse of the corresponding half of the larynx later occasionally affects the inner stability of the larynx.

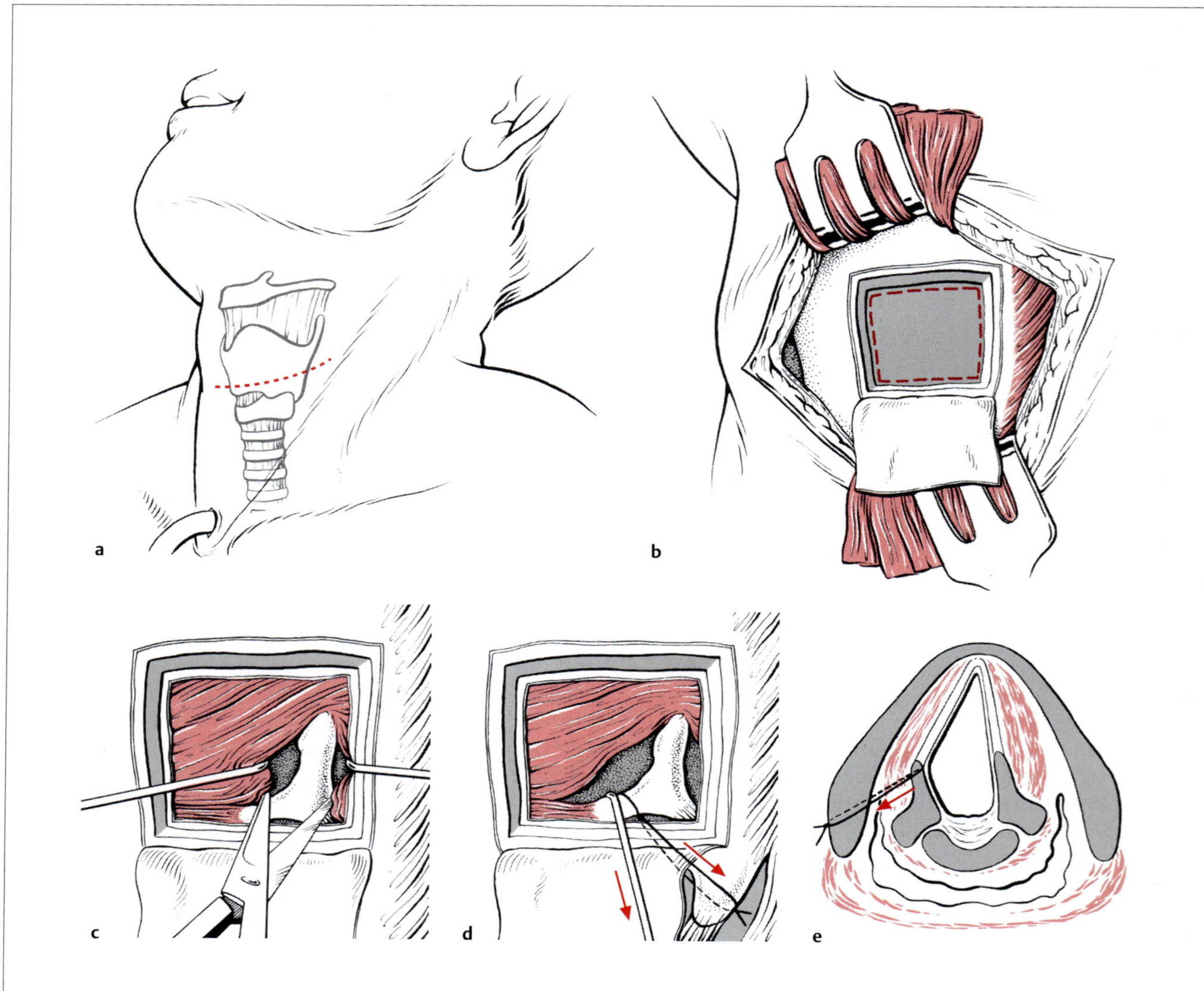

Fig. 10.13a–e Lateral fixation from an open approach.
a Oblique skin incision over the lamina of the thyroid cartilage.
b Creation of a window in the thyroid cartilage after elevation of overlaying cervical muscles.
c Identification of the arytenoid cartilage.
d Lateral fixation of the arytenoid cartilage with a suture passed around the vocal process and the inferior horn of the thyroid cartilage.
e Lateralization as shown in the cross-section.

10

! Risks and Complications

- Postoperative bleeding, formation of hematoma, or persisting edema with persistent glottic stenosis.
- Dehiscence of the vocalis suture, perichondritis of the laryngeal framework.
- Injury to the hypopharyngeal mucosa with fistula formation (surgical revision with coverage, release of the lower horizontal fibers of the inferior pharyngeal constrictor muscle).
- Hoarseness (inevitable), aphonia secondary to exaggerated lateral fixation.
- Tracheal stenosis secondary to tracheotomy.

Postoperative Care

Antibiotic, voice rest, antitussive agents, steroids for significant edema. Remove drain on the second or third day; phoniatric treatment may be indicated later. Decannulation after the endolaryngeal swelling has receded.

Combined Extra-Endolaryngeal Expansion of the Glottis

Surgical Principle

After thyrotomy or laryngofissure, all adductors (lateral, external and transverse muscles) are removed unilaterally or, if necessary, bilaterally in a submucous plane. Additionally the posterior wall of the cricoid lamina may also be split. Tracheotomy is always required.

Indications

- Recurrences following laterofixation.
- Narrow glottis secondary to bilateral paralysis of the recurrent laryngeal nerve in addition to a laryngeal stenosis secondary to scar tissue formation.
- Traumatic or postoperative laryngeal stenosis.

Contraindications

As with endolaryngeal lateral fixation.

Special Instruments and Implants

Dilator.

Anesthesia

General endotracheal anesthesia, re-intubation after preliminary tracheotomy.

Surgical Technique

Incision. Midline skin incision, extending from the hyoid bone to the suprasternal notch, tracheotomy.

Approach. Thyrotomy or, in the presence of a high-grade stenosis, laryngofissure with subsequent division of the cricoid lamina (laminotomy) (**Fig. 10.14a**).

Arytenoidectomy. Curved incision from the medial tip of the arytenoid cartilage downward, circumventing below the vocal fold to the anterior commissure. The arytenoid cartilage is elevated with a small hook. Division of the capsule of the arytenoid joint. Release of the mucosa from the posterior margin of the arytenoid. Division of the transverse muscle. The incision is deepened along the vocal fold and the adductors removed, if necessary under the microscope (**Fig. 10.14b**).

Wound closure. Mucosal suture; if appropriate, the same approach is repeated on the contralateral side.

Stenosis secondary to scar formation requires a mucosal incision and a submucous resection of the scar tissue, followed by splitting of the posterior wall across the entire cricoid lamina in the midline from top to bottom, followed by lateral displacement.

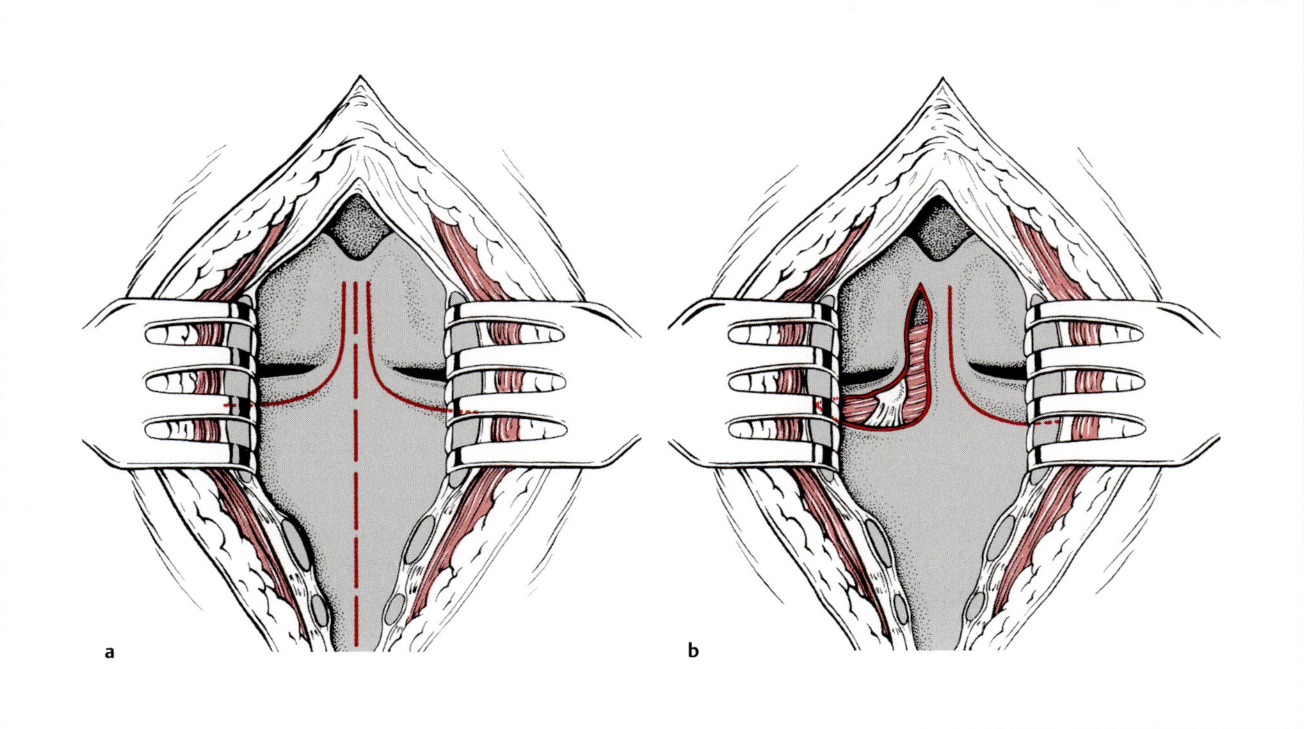

Fig. 10.14a, b Combined endo- and extralaryngeal lateral fixation after Rethi.

a Mucosal incisions to remove the adductors. Auxiliary incision in the middle of the posterior wall to enable laminotomy.
b The incision is spread open to remove the adductors.

Dilator implantation. In all cases, with or without laminotomy, a dilator is inserted to tamponade the mucosa and expand the interior of the larynx. The dilator lies on the cannula. Wound closure.

> **! Risks and Complications**
> - Risk of perichondritis, edema formation, pressure ulcers in the larynx or trachea, formation of granulation tissue, later scar formation with recurrent stenosis in the region of the larynx or trachea.
> - Massive deterioration in voice quality, often aphonic.

Postoperative Care

- Antibiotic coverage.
- Dilator must be left for several months.

Spasmodic Dysphonia

Spasmodic dysphonia, a form of pharyngeal dystonia, is a chronic neurological phenomenon characterized by action-induced spasms of the vocal folds. It usually presents as the adductor type, less often spasms of the abductor type are observed, and in some cases there is a combined adductor–abductor disturbance of function.

Surgical Principle

Spasmodic dysphonia is nowadays preferably treated by the injection of botulinum toxin type A (Botox), either transoral and endoscopically controlled or transcutaneous and electromyographically controlled. Various studies have shown that this should be done unilaterally. It is known that patients who have been treated long-term and at short intervals with a high cumulative total dose develop antibodies against neurotoxins. In this case, conversion to neurotoxin type B (e.g., Neuro-Bloc) is indicated.

Dose. Botox: 3.75 units/0.1 mL. For neurotoxin type B the equivalent dose must be verified individually by multiple injections. At the moment the literature recommends a dose between 250 MU and 1 250 MU of Neuro-Bloc. (An MU, or "mouse unit," corresponds to the LD_{50} using Swiss-Webster mice.)

Indications

Adductor spasmodic dysphonia.

Specific Points Regarding Informed Consent

- As for microlaryngoscopy.
- Anaphylactic shock.
- Multiple injections.

Operative Planning

Verification of spastic dysphonia by magnifying laryngoscopy, fiberoptic endoscopy and videolaryngostroboscopy with the assessment of vocal performance and voice quality, together with the auditory evaluation of voice quality using electroacoustic methods in the form of a hoarseness diagram.

Special Instruments

High-pressure syringe (Order Nr. 771 400, High Pressure Syringe, K. Storz, Tuttlingen, Germany), butterfly needle (needle diameter 0.6 mm, 23 G).

Anesthesia

Topical anesthesia of the mucosa of the mouth, pharynx, and larynx using lidocaine spray.

Surgical Technique

To reduce saliva flow and the urge to cough, an oral premedication of 0.5 mg atropine and 20 mg codeine is administered.

Positioning. The transoral intralaryngeal injection technique is performed with the patient placed in a seated position.

Transoral approach. First the level of the glottis is visualized endoscopically. After exposing the ventricularis and thyroarytenoid muscles, the injection is applied using a butterfly needle, causing only a small amount of tissue traumatization. The approach is usually unilateral.

Modification

The injection may be applied transcutaneously under electromyographic guidance. This approach is less effective because the muscles are targeted less accurately.

> **Rules, Tips, and Tricks**
> Current studies found in the literature indicate that unilateral injection is preferable to the bilateral approach.
> A single injection results in healing in 20 % of the patients; the remainder return for follow-up within the first 2 weeks postoperatively. If these patients have suffered no problems, an additional injection in the region of the contralateral side with 0.6–2.5 units/mL is indicated. About one-third of patients require the additional oral administration of clonazepam, trihexyphenidyl, or baclofen. A lateralization thyroplasty is indicated for recalcitrant cases.
> The time required to reach an optimal voice function is highly variable, both inter- and intra-individually.
> The onset of effect of the botulinum injection usually occurs after a latency of 2–8 days and the effect subsides after 3–6 months on average.

Risks and Complications
The development of antibodies against botulinum toxin, anaphylaxis. The bilateral injection of botulinum toxin into the cricoarytenoid muscle can result in stridor.

Postoperative Care

The combination of the botulinum toxin injection with postoperative voice therapy is strongly recommended.

Surgery for Stenosis of the Larynx and Trachea

Therapy of stenosis of the larynx and trachea is highly varied, given the different locations and forms as well as the heterogeneous pathogenetic mechanisms.

Approach for Laryngeal Stenosis

Congenital circumferential stenosis, especially if situated at a subglottic level, may initially be dilated with bougies. Repeated bougie dilation is possible.

Web-like membrane formations in the anterior commissure (congenital or post-intubation) are incised using a microlaryngoscopic technique.

Stenosis of the glottic aperture—post-traumatic, radiotherapeutic, or postoperative in origin—can often be managed with a supraglottic transverse laryngectomy.

Long-segment stenosis in the larynx secondary to trauma, surgery, or intubation usually requires a laminotomy.

Major plastic surgical measures are required for atresia or stenosis secondary to large defects.

Surgical Principle

Circumferential subglottic web-like stenosis. First, the extent of the subglottic stenosis is assessed by laryngotracheoscopy. The extent of the often circumferential button-hole stenosis may be palpated with a small curved hook. Web-like stenoses with a thickness of a few millimeters are released using laser surgery by making a stellate incision, e.g., at 2 o'clock, 6 o'clock, and 10 o'clock positions.

Rules, Tips, and Tricks
Full-thickness excision of the circumferential stenosis must be avoided at all costs. Such an approach will result in recurrent stenosis, leading in some cases to complete obstruction of the trachea.

Risks and Complications
A functionally irrelevant residual stenosis often remains and usually does not require any further management.

Postoperative Care

A laryngotracheoscopic follow-up examination should be performed, e.g., 6–8 weeks after the operation.

Web Formation in the Region of the Anterior Commissure

Postoperative management following the release of a web formation in the region of the anterior commissure is a problem that still has not been solved definitively. One option is for the surgeon to remove the fibrin deposits from the commissure under local anesthesia using a curved instrument and indirect laryngoscopy, with the patient holding out the tongue. The interval between removal sessions should be decided according to each individual case. Another possibility is applying mitomycin C intraoperatively onto the wound surface after web release to reduce postoperative fibrin exudate. But not only does the efficacy of mitomycin C on the anterior commissure remain unexplained, but the question of whether the fibrin deposits should be removed at all remains unanswered. More conservatively orientated surgeons dispense with removing fibrin from the anterior commissure altogether, because they do not believe it to be worthwhile. This difference of opinion illustrates the difficulty that still exists with regard to postoperative management.

Stenosis of the Proximal Larynx

See supraglottic transverse resection of the larynx, p. 248.

Stenosis of the Laryngotracheal Junction

Over the years stenosis in the region of the laryngotracheal junction has undergone a change in its varied ethiopathology. Thess stenoses used to be primarily congenital or of inflammatory origin, but nowadays they are usually iatrogenic, the result of complications secondary to long-term intubation or tracheotomy. The incidence of cicatricial stenosis of the laryngotracheal segment in newborns and infants has increased as a result of the growing number of intensive care measures performed in patients of this age group.

One-half of all cases stenoses caused by long-term intubation are found in the region of the cricoid cartilage. Surgical treatment of these poses a significant challenge. Here laminotomy, described for the first time by Rethi as early as 1956, and its modifications, as well as partial resection of the cricoid cartilage with subsequent thyrotracheal anastomosis as reported by Persson et al. in 1975, has proved effective in a large number of cases.

A clinically simple and commonly used grading system of subglottic stenosis originates from Myer. Grade I stenosis corresponds to an obstruction of 0–50% of the lumen, grade II to an obstruction of 51–70%, grade III to an obstruction of 71–99%, and grade IV to complete obstruction of the lumen.

Resection

Surgical Principle

Resection of the stenosis with division of the cricoid cartilage and insertion of a stent.

Indications

Subglottic stenosis of the cricoid secondary to perichondritis, supraglottic stenosis, complete stenosis of the glottis, combined stenosis or atresia of the cricoid and the upper trachea.

Specific Points Regarding Informed Consent

- Complications as for microlaryngoscopy, skin incision over the thyroid cartilage, stent placement, wound infection and wound breakdown, sensitivity, paralysis of the lingual nerve, dyspnea, tracheotomy.
- Placement of a stent for several months, repeated endoscopic follow-up examinations.

Operative Planning

Microlaryngoscopy and tracheobronchoscopy for the exact assessment of the indication for stenosis surgery, CT diagnostic examination.

Special Instruments and Implants

Cartilage graft (rib, also the auricle in children), stent (e.g., Aboulker stent, or a tailored transparent stent, e.g., made of Plexiglas).

Anesthesia

General endotracheal anesthesia.

Surgical Technique

Incision. The skin incision commences in the midline below the hyoid bone and continues to the upper border of the tracheostoma, where it proceeds in a semicircle around the upper border of the tracheostoma.

Laminotomy. Division of the cricoid cartilage, and also if necessary the thyroid cartilage, in the midline using a scalpel. If the thyroid cartilage is significantly ossified, it may be divided with Killian scissors.

> Scar tissue should not be removed from the inner lateral wall of the larynx, to prevent the recurrent formation of wound surfaces and subsequent scar formation.

Division of the posterior laryngeal wall. Corresponding to the approach for the anterior wall of the larynx, the posterior laryngeal wall is now opened, ensuring that the mucosa covering the external larynx wall, which already constitutes part of the hypopharynx, remains intact. The incision runs between the arytenoid cartilages, starting vertically in the midline and continuing downward past the level of the thyroid cartilage, 1–2 cm into the trachea. The lamina of the cricoid cartilage is now divided with a strong scalpel. If it is ossified, it should be carefully divided using primarily stab incisions.

A Freer elevator is then used to verify that the cartilaginous wall has been completely divided. After this, two single hooks or two Rethi hooks are inserted to separate the two halves of the larynx. The transverse muscle is identified and resected. An autologous cartilage graft is then sutured between the incision margins of the cricoid lamina, making the width of the posterior wall gap ca. 1 mm per year of the patient's age (rule of thumb for children). With regard to the use of this technique in children, it should be pointed out here that alternative procedures have increasingly won recognition, not least because of their long-term results.

To avoid an open laryngotracheal groove, the laminotomy is often supplemented by a "stepped incision" as described by Evans and Todd. For this purpose, two caudally or cranially based mucosal flaps are elevated using microsurgical ear instruments to almost completely cover the surface of the expanded lumen as a pedicled U-flap. Then the stent is inserted into the larynx, coming to rest on the tracheotomy cannula and projecting slightly over the level of the vocal folds.

> **Rules, Tips, and Tricks**
> - Retention time of the stent should not be less than 2 months, if possible, as otherwise shrinkage and subsequent narrowing of the lumen is to be expected.
> - It is imperative for the success of the operation to regularly check the position of the stent, initially every week.

> **! Risks and Complications**
> Residual stenosis, perichondritis.

Postoperative Care

Endoscopic follow-up of the stent: initially weekly, later 3- to 4-weekly.

Management of Tracheal Stenosis

Operations purely for support (lateropexy, augmentation) are indicated for compression and collapse stenoses. Resection procedures (transverse laryngectomy, longitudinal split, open groove) must be chosen for stenoses secondary to scar formation and associated with loss of substance. Diaphragms and short stomal stenoses, i.e., those in the region of a tracheostoma, may be managed using laser surgery. The option of a stent implantation should also be considered.

Lateropexy of the Trachea

Surgical Principle

Stabilization of the tracheal wall, softened by pressure, by creating a muscle loop using the sternocleidomastoid muscle after prior resection of the compressing parts of the goitre or after scar revision.

Indications

External compression of the trachea, in the region of the neck affecting breathing, by a goitre or scar with loss of cartilage elasticity but without scar formation involving tracheal cartilage or mucosa.

Contraindications

- Severe underlying general condition.
- Scarring of the mucosa or cartilage defects secondary to scar formation; intrathoracic development of a compression stenosis.

Specific Points Regarding Informed Consent

As for a transverse resection of the trachea (see p. 210).

Operative Planning

Laryngotracheoscopy, thyroid scintigraphy, lateral and anterior–posterior spot films of the trachea (sucking–pressing), CT if appropriate (including 3D reconstruction).

Anesthesia

General endotracheal anesthesia.

Surgical Technique

Incision with identification of the trachea. Kocher transverse collar incision, resection of compressing goitre nodes in typical fashion, resection of hypertrophic scars lateral to the trachea. Identification of the ventral tracheal cartilage.

Release of the trachea. A tunnel is created on either side of the stenosis beneath the scar tissue attached to the lateral tracheal wall (**Fig. 10.15a**).

Creation of the sternocleidomastoid muscle loops. Next, the sternal tendon of the sternocleidomastoid muscle is divided and the attachment released further proximally. The mobilized tendon is passed through and around the scar tunnel at the trachea and secured back to the clavicle or the clavicular head of the sternocleidomastoid. If it is not possible to draw the muscle through the scar tunnel, it may also be secured with several sutures to the lateral tracheal wall (**Fig. 10.15b**).

Wound closure. Wound closure over a suction drain.

Modification

Instead of stabilizing the trachea using a muscle sling, elastic material may be used for stabilization, placing it onto the trachea as a strut and securing it with a suture.

Rules, Tips, and Tricks

Beware of the recurrent laryngeal nerve: when dissecting lateral and posterior to the trachea, spread the tissue only in the direction of the course of the nerve. For remarks on the course of the recurrent laryngeal nerve see page 285 . If no tracheostoma is present, then tracheotomy as a rule is not essential.

! Risks and Complications

- Recurrent collapse of the trachea associated with stridor.
- Unilateral or bilateral injury to the recurrent nerve.

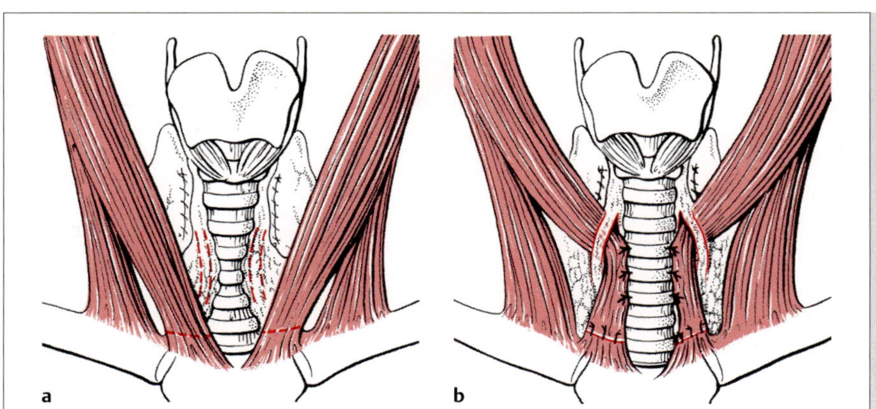

Fig. 10.15a, b Lateropexy.
The trachea is supported by loops created from the sternal bellies of the sternocleidomastoid muscles which are passed through the lateral tunnels created within the scar tissue.

- Postoperative bleeding with renewed compression of the trachea.
- Perichondritis of the tracheal cartilage.
- Mediastinitis, pneumothorax, injury to major intrathoracic vessels.

Postoperative Care

Postoperative observation for possible respiratory failure; antibiotic; remove drain depending on amount collected.

Transverse Tracheal Resection with End-to-End Anastomosis

Surgical Principle

The part of the trachea contracted by scar formation is resected; the resulting gap is bridged by mobilizing the distal and proximal stumps and repaired with sutures.

Indications

Cicatricial tracheal stenosis with a maximum length of 4–5 cm secondary to scar formation with loss of cartilaginous and mucosal coverage.

Contraindications

- Length of stenosis—usually more than 5 cm.
- Deep thoracic stenosis (not accessible via a collar incision).
- Stenosis at the cricotracheal junction (after resection of the cricoid there is a problematic difference of calibre between the lumen at the inferior border of the thyroid cartilage and that of the trachea, thus posing a relative contraindication).

Specific Points Regarding Informed Consent

- Long-term mechanical ventilation.
- Suture tear-out with dislocation or slippage of the trachea into the thorax.
- Poor healing of the skin margins.
- Cicatricial stenosis of the trachea, tracheitis.
- Hoarseness, loss of voice, paralysis of the vocal fold nerve.
- Difficulty with swallowing (dysphagia), insertion of a nasogastric tube.
- Possible tracheotomy with insertion of a tracheotomy tube.
- Possible extension of the operation, thoracotomy.
- Pneumonia.
- Pneumothorax, insertion of a chest drain.
- Hemorrhage/surgical emphysema of the mediastinum with mediastinitis.
- Chondritis.

Operative Planning

Endoscopy, spot films of the trachea, CT diagnostic investigation.

Anesthesia

General endotracheal anesthesia, usually initially via an already present tracheostomy, followed by intraoperative re-intubation.

Surgical Technique

Skin incision. Longitudinal midline incision, extending from the hyoid to the suprasternal notch, or large transverse Kocher collar incision. Exposure of the tracheal anterior wall of the larynx.

Identification of the trachea. Skeletonization of the trachea; dissection is strictly along the lateral wall, spreading the tissue only in the direction of the course of the recurrent nerve.

Resection of the stenosis. Transverse incision of the trachea at the caudal end of the stenosis, ensuring that the level of resection is free of scar tissue. The distal stump of the trachea is secured with two lateral stay sutures. The narrowed segment is then carefully released from the anterior wall of the esophagus under protection of the recurrent nerve and resected back to healthy tissue (**Fig. 10.16a**).

Mobilization of the trachea. To bridge longer defects, the trachea is mobilized in an inferior direction, down into the thoracic space (release is done only between sternum or esophagus and the trachea due to the lateral vascular supply). The straight prelaryngeal musculature and the thyrohyoid membrane are incised at the hyoid bone, allowing the larynx to be also moved downward.

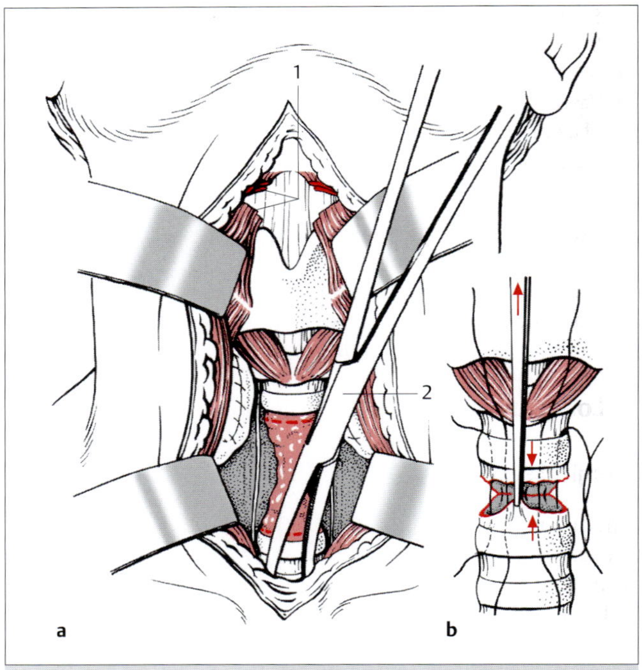

Fig. 10.16a, b Transverse tracheal resection with end-to-end anastomosis for cicatricial tracheal stenosis.
a After resection of all scar tissue, a transverse incision is made through the strap muscles at the level of the hyoid bone (1) and the trachea is released between sternum and anterior tracheal wall (2) and between posterior tracheal wall and esophagus.
b Suture repair of the tracheal stumps.

Tracheal suture repair. Suture repair using 2/0 absorbable sutures. The suture is inserted in the intercartilaginous space, passed inside in a submucosal plane, again inserted in the submucosal plane of the other tracheal segment, to be brought out again below the tracheal ring. All the sutures, including those of the posterior wall, are left untied until the end, when the knots are brought to lie on the outside.

Wound closure. In layers over a suction drain.

Rules, Tips, and Tricks

- Bring the head into anteflexion before tying the knots (**Fig. 10.16b**).
- The tracheostoma is included in the incision if there is a stenosis in the region of the tracheostoma. Intubation is performed via the tracheostoma; after the incision re-intubation is from a cranial approach by threading the tracheal stumps over the tube. Alternatively, a new tracheostoma may be created caudal to the anastomosis.
- Strict anteflexion of the head should be observed during the postoperative observation period. With very extensive segment resections, some surgeons recommend maintaining the head in anteflexion by applying a head–thorax cast or suturing the suprasternal notch to the tip of the chin to reduce tension on the suture line.

! Risks and Complications

- Suture-line dehiscence, residual stenosis associated with stridor.
- Injury to the recurrent nerve, pleural injury.
- Mediastinitis.
- Vascular injury, bleeding from vascular erosion in the presence of a deep tracheostoma.

Postoperative Care

Antibiotic, nasogastric tube, antitussive agent, 250 mg cortisone, anteflexion of the head.

Longitudinal Division of the Trachea

Surgical Principle

Longitudinal division of the anterior and posterior wall of the trachea with expansion (anteroposterior split widening), keeping it open with a stent or by insertion of a free spreading graft in the anterior and posterior wall.

Indications

- Extensive cicatricial stenosis of the cervical trachea (with an extent of >5 cm).
- Stenosis at the cricotracheal junction.

Contraindications

- Severe underlying general disorder.
- Inoperable coexisting laryngeal stenosis.
- Extension of the stenosis into the thorax.

Specific Points Regarding Informed Consent

As for transverse resection of the trachea.

Operative Planning

As for transverse resection of the trachea.

Special Instruments and Implants

Prosthesis for tracheal stenting (e.g., Montgomery T-tube or Aboulker prosthesis).

Surgical Technique

Skin incision and identification of the trachea. There is usually a tracheostoma already in place: if it is sited caudal to the stenosis, it is left untouched; if it is situated in the region of the stenosis, it is included in the incision. A midline skin incision is made over the narrowed tracheal segment, followed by skeletonization of the trachea beyond the stenosis. Compressing scars or a goitre are resected.

Tracheotomy. Longitudinal division of the anterior wall of the trachea along the entire narrowed segment until normal tracheal tissue is reached (**Fig. 10.17a**). After separating the trachea with thyroid retractors, the posterior wall of the trachea is divided to the same extent, down to the muscle layer of the esophagus. The narrowed region is held open to its normal calibre and a free mucosal graft, obtained from the oral mucosa, is inserted into the gaping posterior wall where it is glued (**Fig. 10.17b**).

Insertion of the stent. A stent (Montgomery T-tube or Aboulker prosthesis) is inserted to maintain tracheal patency. In addition, a lateropexy of the tracheal walls may be performed using the sternal head of the sternocleidomastoid muscle (**Fig. 10.17b, c**).

The incision margins of the anterior wall are epithelialized as an open groove with the aid of advancement flaps from the skin of the neck. The insertion of a Montgomery T-tube renders a tracheotomy unnecessary, whereas other prostheses require a tracheotomy below the stenosis.

Removal of the prosthesis and indication for tracheotomy. Subsequent to removal of the prosthesis after 4 weeks, the groove is closed using plastic surgical means by turning in the mobilized lateral skin and stabilizing with a free cartilage graft. The donor site is resurfaced with a transposition flap.

Modification

Insertion of a free costal cartilage graft to widen the anterior wall. The internal mucosal coverage is accomplished by mobilizing the mucosa of both lateral walls and advancing it medially as a bipedicled flap. The resulting larger defect on the posterior

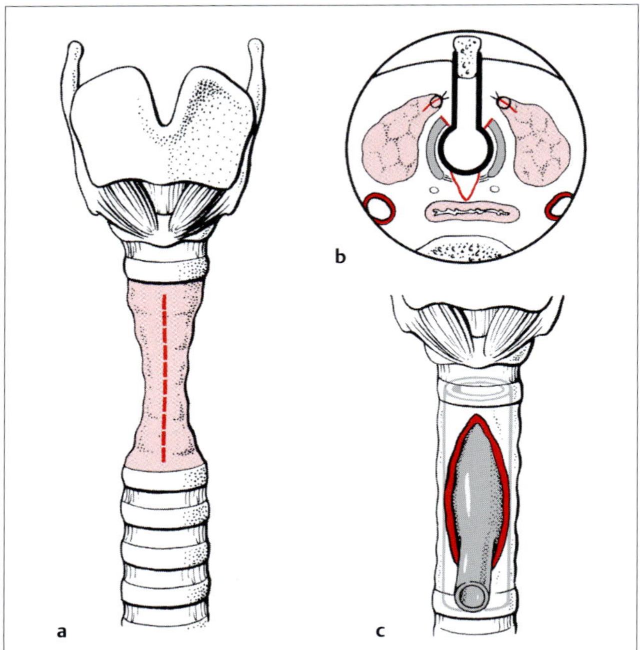

Fig. 10.17a–c Longitudinal division of the trachea for tracheal stenosis (after v. Ilberg).
a Longitudinal division of the entire segment of tracheal stenosis until healthy tracheal lumen is reached.
b Correspondingly, the posterior wall of the trachea is divided medially down to the esophageal musculature and kept open with a stent.
c Position of the stent.

wall is covered with a more extensive free mucosal graft. The external wound is closed with an advancement flap.

Postoperative Care

As for an end-to-end anastomosis after a transverse resection, except that fixation of the head in anteflexion is unnecessary.

Tracheal Stent Implantation

The surgical approach employing a transverse tracheal resection or operative tracheoplasty is the treatment of choice for symptomatic, proximal, benign tracheal stenosis. For several years, the use endoscopic procedures using various stents and laser surgical resections has been increasing.

Since the introduction of metal tracheal stents in the late 1980s, the use of tracheal stents has become an increasingly common procedure, mainly for the treatment of malignant stenosis of the tracheobronchial system. Metal stents are used particularly by pulmonologists and radiologists. Implantation of a tracheal stent is indicated for benign stenosis if a conventional surgical procedure would have no chance of success, or to avoid postoperative complications in high-risk patients suffering from additional severe comorbidities, such as cardiovascular compromise.

Important criteria for successful stent implantation are rapid and simple handling, optimal positioning of the stent against the tracheobronchial wall, high flexibility in the longitudinal direction without displacement, shear force adequate to expand even a marked tracheal stenosis, and the more or less extensive preservation of mucociliary clearance of the tracheal epithelium.

Surgical Technique

Stent implantations are usually performed under general anesthesia with intermittent apnea or with orotracheal intubation. Once satisfactory oxygen saturation has been achieved, the endotracheal tube or laryngeal mask is removed and intermittent ventilation commenced (depending on the oxygen saturation and the stenosis situation). Oxygen saturation should not fall below 90%. A Kleinsasser C-tube is positioned so that the endolarynx is well visualized. Laryngotracheobronchoscopy is performed by introducing rigid endoscopes of various sizes through the C-tube into the trachea. The trachea and the narrowed segment are meticulously examined. After the stenosis is located, metal markers can be placed on the skin using transillumination to achieve an adequate stent implantation in the further course of the procedure.

An stent appropriate to the length and diameter of the stenosis is selected. The diameter of the trachea proximal and distal to the stenosis is measured in advance by CT. In general, the diameter of the stent should correspond to the size of the proximal and distal tracheal lumina. The expanded stent diameter, however, must be 1–2 mm larger than the measured tracheal lumen to allow fixation of the stent wires to the tracheal wall.

A firm guide wire is introduced and passed across the stenosis. Under visual control, the catheter together with the stent is introduced into the narrowed segment via the wire and released under direct vision. During insertion, it is possible to reposition the stent until it is centered in the stenosis. Owing to the positioning mechanism from distal to proximal, however, the partially aligned stent can only be moved in a dorsal direction. The catheter is withdrawn directly after placement of the stent. Now an appropriate balloon catheter is advanced over the wire to expand the stent to the desired diameter. Complete self-expansion of the stent may be expected within the first 24 hours after implantation. The position of the stent is then checked using a rigid endoscope. In addition, a conventional chest radiograph or CT of the thorax is ordered 24 hours after the procedure to verify the position of the stent.

> **! Risks and Complications**
> Long-term complications include the formation of secretions, stent dislocation, and the development of granulomas.

Surgical Management of Tracheal Stenosis in Children

The majority of infants and children with pediatric laryngotracheal stenosis requiring treatment are tracheotomized while definitive management of a congenital stenosis is awaited, or because the initial treatment of damage secondary to intubation has been unsuccessful. The use of endoscopic techniques in the treatment of pediatric laryngotracheal stenosis is very limited. Open surgical techniques, laryngotracheal reconstruction with cartilage grafting, are undertaken for grade II and mild grade III stenosis with minimal morbidity and a high chance of decannulation. Partial cricotracheal resection may be more promising in more severe cases of stenosis, although this requires a more complex approach than laryngotracheoplasty with tracheal mobilization (including larynx release in some cases), with excision of a larger piece of trachea if a tracheotomy is included in the resection. Given that laryngotracheal reconstruction is less complicated, it is preferable when appropriately indicated. Experienced laryngologists choose a partial cricotracheal resection for severe grade III or grade IV stenosis, especially if the stenosis can be clearly delineated from the vocal folds.

It is rare for subglottic stenosis in childhood not to be associated with glottic stenosis and tracheal injuries secondary to tracheotomy. In addition, laryngeal, mediastinal, cardiologic malformations, or malformations associated with syndromes with or without neurological, cardiological, or pulmonary symptoms may make treatment difficult.

The most difficult situations observed in this group of pathologies result from:

- Failed reconstruction of the airways resulting in distortion of the larynx.
- Improper laser use.
- Incorrect placement of a tracheostoma, causing injury to the otherwise healthy trachea.

It is obvious that the patient has the greatest chance of success during the first operation. This means that the surgeon must be trained in pediatric tracheoscopy and laryngotracheal surgery, given that improper procedure can have irreversible consequences in pediatric laryngotracheal stenosis.

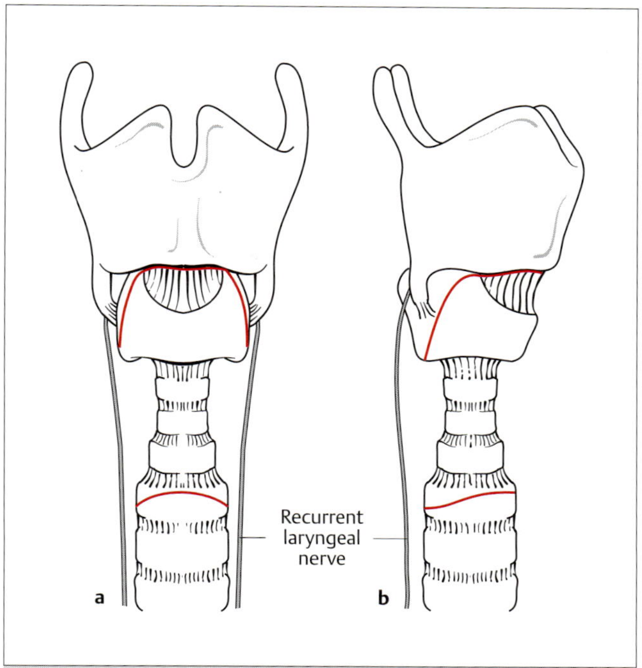

Fig. 10.18a, b Cricotracheal resection.
a Resection through the cricoid cartilage and the narrowed superior tracheal rings.
b Resection of the cricoid cartilage anterior to the cricothyroid joint. The posterior lamina of the cricoid cartilage is thus exposed.

Laryngotracheal Reconstruction Using Cartilage for Lumen Expansion

This operation involves enlargement of the laryngotracheal complex by splitting the cricoid cartilage in the anterior and/or posterior midline and inserting a cartilage graft to expand the tracheal lumen. Anteriorly, the incision is typically placed through the lower third of the thyroid cartilage, the thyrohyoid membrane, the cricoid cartilage, and the upper two or three tracheal rings (**Fig. 10.18a, b**). For the posterior cartilage graft, it is necessary to extend this incision into a complete median laryngotomy to divide interarytenoid scars accurately and position the graft exactly. Grade II stenosis is reconstructed with an anterior graft, generally without inserting a stent. Mild grade III stenosis usually requires an anterior graft together with a posterior cricoid split, supported by an endoluminal stent. Severe grade III stenosis ("eye-of-the-needle stenosis") requires both an anterior and a posterior graft with a long-term stent. Partial cricotracheal resection is an alternative technique for cases of severe grade III and grade IV stenosis.

If the operation is confined to an anterior graft, with or without posterior cricoid split, then a single-stage laryngotracheal reconstruction may be considered when the tracheostoma is closed. Tracheal reconstruction with costal cartilage grafting incorporates the tracheostoma. An endotracheal tube is used as a stent, usually for 5–7 days. It is necessary to prevent bacterial infections and any possible wound-healing problems. Tracheostomal collapse or stenosis is treated by extending the anterior graft into the stoma. This does not necessarily make subsequent decannulation necessary. If extubation fails, however, renewed tracheotomy may be required, which may possibly involve releasing the grafted material. Severe grade III stenosis may allow a single-stage reconstruction of the laryngotrachea with an anterior and a posterior graft, usually leaving the tracheotomy untouched and using a stent for 4–6 weeks to support the grafts. A one-stage technique is not indicated for grade IV stenosis; a stent is necessary for at least 6 weeks.

Partial Cricotracheal Resection

To improve the surgical outcome of severe (grade III/IV) laryngotracheal stenosis, the concept of partial cricotracheal resection was developed as an alternative to laryngotracheal reconstruction. It involves removal of the affected segment of the trachea and thus allows decannulation. The technique of partial cricotracheal resection with primary thyrotracheal anastomosis bypasses the glottis and reconstructs a rounded, "more normal" subglottic airway. If possible, the operation is undertaken as a single-stage procedure: the tracheostoma is removed as part of the resected segment and an endotracheal tube left for 7 days. If more than four or five tracheal rings need to be removed, the

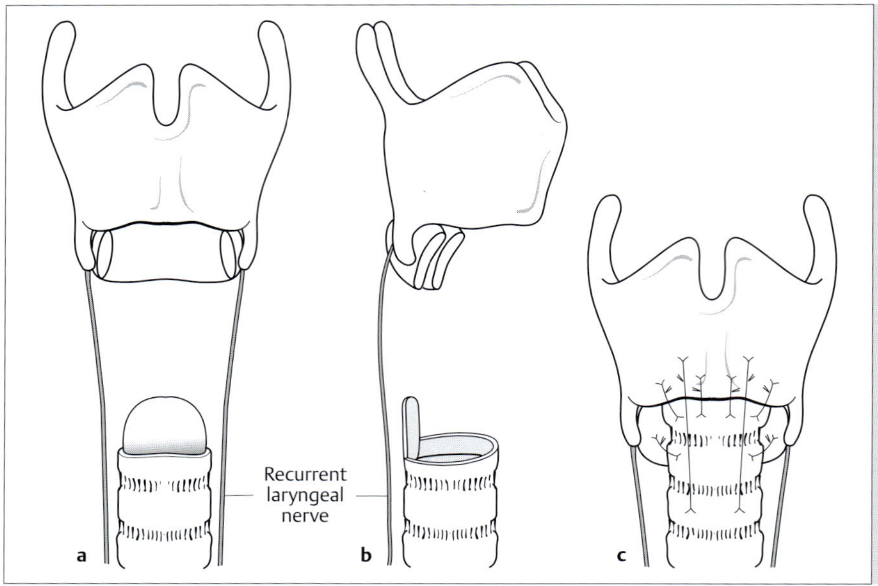

Fig. 10.19a–c Cricotracheal resection.
a, b After resection of the narrowed tracheal segment, the pedicled membranous posterior flap of the trachea is identified.
c Anterior thyrotracheal and lateral cricotracheal anastomosis.

trachea requires extensive mobilization to be able to achieve a tension-free anastomosis.

Extended Partial Cricotracheal Resection

This term refers to a partial cricotracheal resection with additional open surgery of the airway (**Figs. 10.19** and **10.20**). Typical indications include pediatric laryngotracheal stenosis with involvement of the glottis, either a posterior glottic stenosis with possible fixation of the cricoarytenoid joint, vocal fold fusion, or distortion of the larynx after failed laryngotracheal reconstruction. Alternatives are either laryngotracheal reconstruction with anterior and posterior cartilage graft, or a partial cricotracheal resection with posterior cricoid split and posterior cartilage graft and costal cartilage graft followed by stent insertion for 4–6 weeks. In this case, partial cricotracheal resection cannot be done as a single-stage procedure. The tracheotomy must be left until the trachea has completely healed and has become stable.

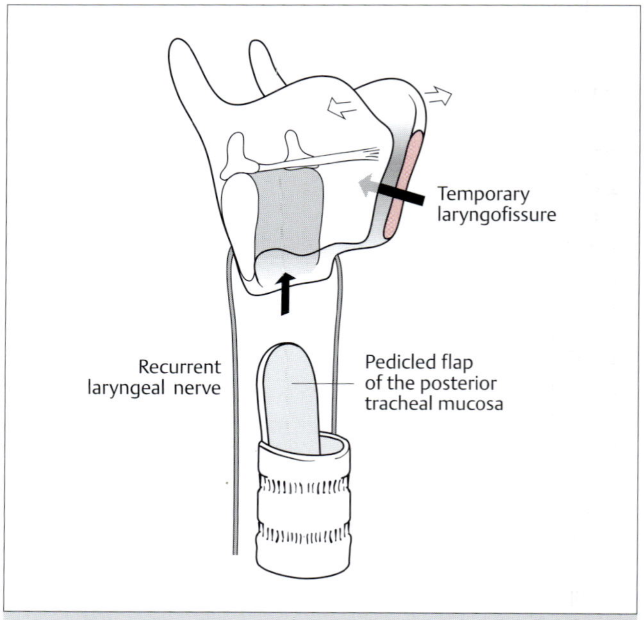

Fig. 10.20 Cricotracheal resection, combined with the excision of a posterior glottic stenosis.
The lamina of the cricoid cartilage is covered by the mucosa pedicled on the posterior tracheal wall. A temporary division of the thyroid cartilage in the midline is done to position the flap.

Postoperative Care

- Antibiotic administration is initiated during the operation and continued for a further 7 days.
- Antireflux medications are prescribed routinely for 6 weeks; children diagnosed with reflux are given these medications for at least 3 months.
- After the one-stage approach, intubated patients are maintained in a mildly sedated state, without muscle relaxation or ventilation. This reduces the risk of pulmonary atelectasis or infection.
- A nasotracheal tube must be securely fixed to prevent accidental extubation and dislocation of the tube. Nutrition via a nasogastric tube is initiated as soon as possible.
- The patient undergoes endoscopy after 5–7 days to assess the healing process and to check the calibre of the reconstructed trachea. If the result is good, the endotracheal tube is replaced with a smaller one. The child is extubated 24 hours later under the administration of steroids.
- After extubation, everything should be done to avoid renewed re-intubation, including the systemic administration of steroids and, if necessary, inhalation with nebulized epinephrine and steroids.
- Occasionally, granulation tissue will require removal during the healing process. For this reason, it is recommended to

examine the patient endoscopically 7–10 days after extubation.

- Any inserted stent is removed after 4–6 weeks. The patient must undergo repeat endoscopy 7–10 days later to remove any possible granulations. Endoscopy is once again performed 6 weeks later to confirm that the healing process has been completed and the trachea can be decannulated.
- Decannulation is done during an inpatient stay of a few days: the tracheotomy tube is reduced to 3 mm, closed for 24 hours and then removed if closure is well tolerated during waking and sleeping phases. If the stoma does not close spontaneously after removal of the tube, it is closed surgically.

Surgery for Fresh Injuries of the Larynx and Trachea

Laryngotracheal injuries occur as closed injuries following blunt trauma to the neck, or as open or penetrating injuries.

The patterns of injury are very varied; they range from a laryngeal contusion not requiring treatment, or nondislocated fractures of the thyroid or cricoid cartilages, to acute life-threatening rupture of larynx or trachea, or tracheal avulsion. Open laryngotracheal injuries are often complicated by an associated injury of the hypopharynx or esophagus.

Therapeutic and diagnostic measures depend on the presenting symptoms and in particular on the acute danger to life; in the presence of avulsion of the trachea they must be performed at dramatic speed.

Preoperative Diagnostic Investigations and Emergency Measures

Comminuted fracture of the larynx, laryngeal tear, or avulsion must be assumed in the presence of a contusion mark on the neck associated with hematoma and surgical emphysema, severe dyspnea, and hemoptysis.

First and foremost, the airways must be secured: do not intubate, but after visualizing the larynx using a laryngoscope blade, insert a long, thin emergency tracheoscope into the trachea. An intubation tube could result in the complete avulsion of the trachea by catching on tracheal tears; the posterior wall of the trachea often remains intact, despite considerable separation of the cartilage rings, and can serve as a guide for the emergency tracheoscope to locate the distal stump.

If an emergency tracheotomy is unsuccessful, then the distal stump must be located without delay via an external incision and retrieved.

Cases of blunt neck trauma with less severe dyspnea require diagnostic examination using a magnifying laryngoscopy, imaging (anterior–posterior and lateral soft-tissue radiographs of the neck, CT) and tracheoscopy with assessment of the tracheal wall using a 90° telescope.

Penetrating injuries to the larynx and trachea are usually easily recognized. They can be easily explored with a probe and confirmed by the exit of air or surrounding surgical emphysema.

Fractures without dislocation or contusion of the larynx usually only result in hematomas. If breathing is adequate and no major mucosal lesions are present, a conservative expectant approach may be adopted.

Management of Dislocated Laryngeal Fractures and Injuries

Surgical Principle

Meticulous early management with reconstruction or reduction of the laryngeal framework, either endoscopically or by exposing the laryngeal framework from an open approach, with or without medial laryngotomy, and with resurfacing of the mucosal defects to prevent scar formation and cartilage infection. Usually a tracheotomy is necessary.

Indications

Injury to the larynx with considerable dislocation, significant mucosal injury, and associated disturbance of breathing and voice.

Contraindications

Severe shock; patient with multiple injuries requiring management of the associated injuries after securing the airway.

Specific Points Regarding Informed Consent

- Tracheal stenosis.
- Hoarseness.
- Loss of voice.
- Paralysis of the vocal fold nerves.
- Difficulty with swallowing (dysphagia).
- Possible insertion of a nasogastric tube.
- Chondritis.
- Cartilage necrosis.
- Hypertrophic scar formation.
- Necessity for further surgery (revisions).

Anesthesia

General endotracheal anesthesia, if necessary over the inserted tracheoscope or via the tracheostoma after prior tracheotomy.

Surgical Technique

Positioning. Flat, supine, shoulders slightly raised, head reclined.

Secure airways, tracheoscopy, tracheotomy.

Laryngoscopy. Inspection of the larynx using the laryngoscope and angled telescopes; consider retrograde laryngoscopy using an angled telescope via the tracheostoma. The subsequent procedure will depend on the presenting findings.

Simple fracture. *With simple dislocation of the laryngeal framework*, attempt to straighten the larynx by levering with the laryngoscope or the emergency tube with simultaneous counter-pressure or guiding the larynx externally to interlock the fragments. Additional straightening may be achieved using a narrow Langenbeck retractor introduced through the stoma.

Dislocated fracture. *With considerable dislocation of the laryngeal framework, use an open approach.* A midline skin incision is made, extending from the hyoid bone to the suprasternal notch and incorporating any wounds. It is deepened down through the midline between the strap muscles to the larynx, followed by division of the thyroid isthmus. Unless already done, a tracheotomy through the second and third tracheal rings is often necessary.

If there is not already a full-thickness opening in the larynx, and if the mucosa is not significantly torn, the cartilage fragments may be reduced directly, followed by an endoscopic assessment of the success of the reconstruction, which may if necessary be corrected by a combination of internal pressure and external alignment. The fragments are secured either with titanium screws and plates or with absorbable plates. This avoids creating additional scars in the anterior commissure (**Fig. 10.21**).

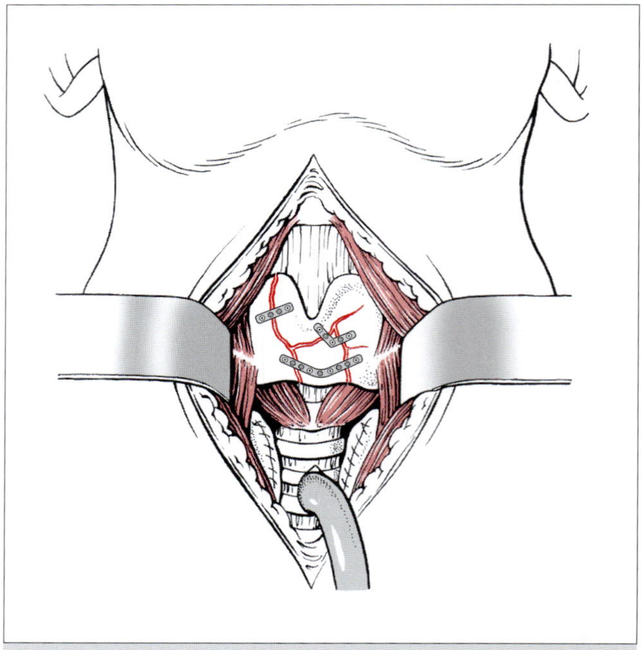

Fig. 10.21 Management of a fresh laryngeal injury.
Large midline incision extending from the hyoid bone to the suprasternal notch. Reduction of the borders of the thyroid cartilage followed by fixation of the osteo(chondral) fracture(s).

Mucosal suture. After open reduction and fixation of the fragments—do not sacrifice any cartilage, also reduce the arytenoid cartilage—repair the mucosa by suturing. Loss of substance is covered using pedicled flaps from the ventricle of Morgagni, the posterior laryngeal wall, or the tracheal region. If there is not enough tissue, then a free graft harvested from oral, septal, or turbinate mucosa is used and secured with retention sutures and fibrin glue.

Hypopharyngo-esophagoscopy. Injuries to the hypopharyngeal and esophageal mucosa are looked for using endoscopy and under direct vision, and then repaired by primarily suture.

Endolaryngeal stenting. If the larynx is stable enough after completion of reduction and closure of the medial laryngotomy with a perichondrial suture and the lumen is adequate as verified by endoscopy, an endoluminal stent may be dispensed with. If the larynx collapses, a sponge pack with a triangular cross-section (silicone tube, silicone block) placed in a rubber finger-stall is inserted as an endoluminal stent. A suture is placed through the inferior part for fixation and brought out through the stoma, while a further suture is passed out through the larynx (**Fig. 10.22**).

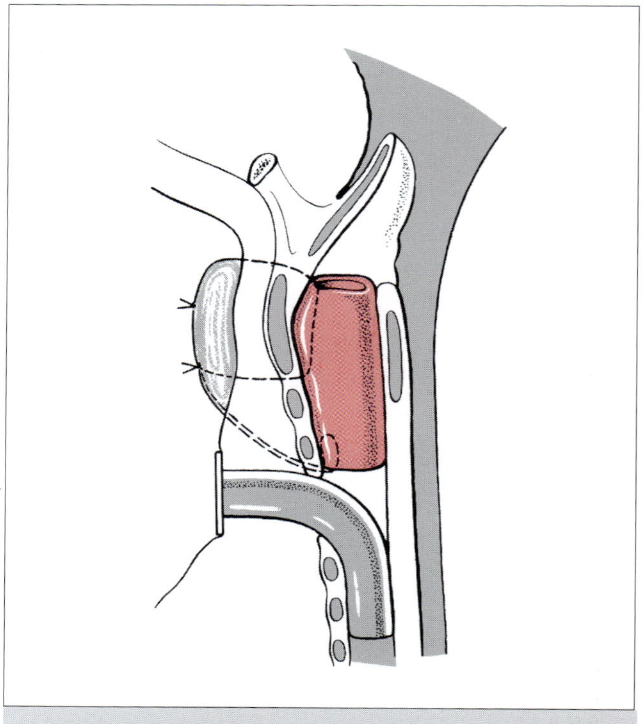

Fig. 10.22 Laryngeal fracture.
Support of the larynx with a stent, which is secured with a translaryngeal suture and a stomal suture.

Wound closure. Wound closure in layers. Suction of the tracheobronchial system.

Hemostasis. Meticulous hemostasis: superior laryngeal or cricothyroid arteries may be torn; thyroid arteries may also be injured.

Risks and Complications

- Postoperative bleeding from vessels that have been injured and not ligated, (surgical revision), aspiration of blood into the lungs, pneumonia.
- Laryngeal perichondritis, mediastinitis.
- Late sequelae: laryngeal stenosis, hoarseness, bilateral paralysis of the recurrent nerve, disturbances of swallowing (dysphagia).

Postoperative Care

- Antibiotic, nasogastric tube.
- Endoscopic removal of an endoluminal prosthesis after approximately 10 days, endoscopic follow-up.

Management of Tracheal Avulsion

Surgical Principle

Securing the airways, either by endoscopic bridging with an emergency tube or by directly locating the peripheral tracheal stump from the neck. End-to-end anastomosis of the tracheal stumps, if necessary with a tracheotomy placed caudal to the anastomosis.

Specific Points Regarding Informed Consent

- Long-term mechanical ventilation.
- The suture may tear out, allowing the trachea to slide back into the thorax.
- Cicatricial stenosis of the trachea, tracheitis.
- Hoarseness, loss of voice, paralysis of the vocal cord nerve (also bilateral).
- Difficulty with swallowing (dysphagia), insertion of a nasogastric tube.
- Possible tracheotomy with the insertion of a cannula.
- If necessary, extension of the wound, thoracotomy.
- Pneumonia.
- Pneumothorax, insertion of a chest drain.
- Bleeding into / emphysema of the mediastinum with mediastinitis.
- Chondritis.

Even in an emergency situation informed consent should be obtained if at all possible.

Anesthesia

General anesthesia as soon as the airways have been secured; if the trachea has to be bridged with an emergency tube, muscle relaxation and induction of anesthesia will need to be done in one stage together with emergency endoscopy.

Surgical Technique

Incision. Long midline skin incision, extending from the hyoid bone to the suprasternal notch. The strap muscles are retracted; if necessary the thyroid isthmus is held aside or divided.

Access. Provided a transoral insertion of a tracheoscope is possible, the tube is palpated and the peripheral tracheal stump located by blunt release of the overlying tissue. *The position of the stump is palpated using the index finger*; the stump is grasped with a clamp and retrieved from the thoracic cavity. Even without tracheoscopic guidance, it is necessary to palpate and locate the distal end of the trachea with the index finger to grasp the stump with a clamp and retrieve it. An emergency tube may then be initially inserted into the stump along the finger to allow suction and ventilation (**Fig. 10.23**).

This is then followed by oral translaryngeal intubation (the tube is threaded through the tracheal stumps) using a thin tube, or a tracheostoma is created caudal to the site of the tear.

Tracheal suture. End-to-end suture repair of the tracheal stumps. *The thyrohyoid muscles and the thyrohyoid membrane are released from the hyoid* to relieve tension on the suture line. First, the mucosa of the posterior wall is approximated exactly with 3/0 absorbable sutures. Then the tracheal rings are drawn together with 2/0 sutures, which encircle the rings. Each of these sutures is initially only placed; they are not knotted until the last suture is in place. The sutures are then tied so that the knots come to lie externally (**Fig. 10.24**).

10

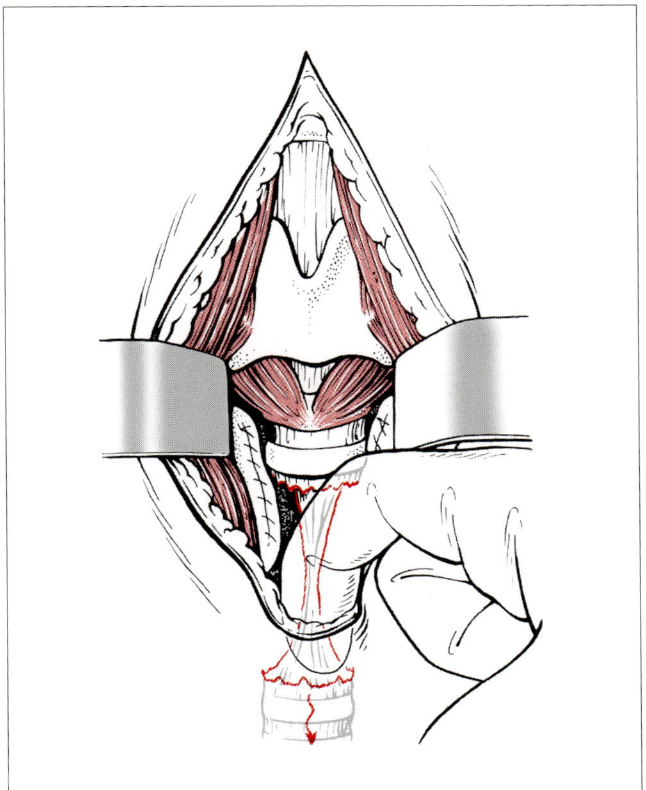

Fig. 10.23 Management of a tracheal avulsion.
The tracheal stump is located using the palpating finger.

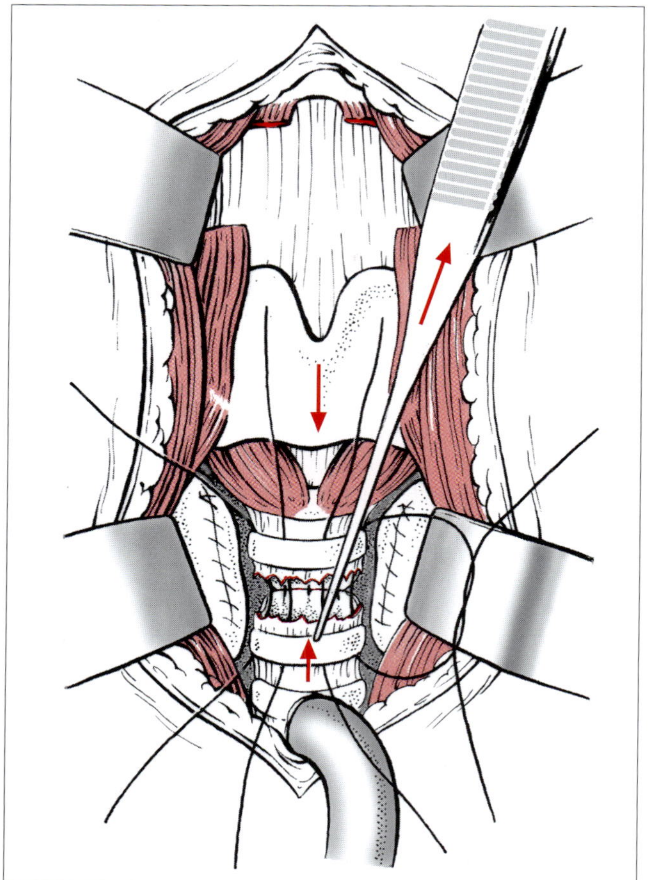

Fig. 10.24 End-to-end anastomosis for tracheal avulsion. After adaptation of the posterior wall, sutures are placed around the tracheal rings. Tension is taken off the suture line by releasing the strap muscles between larynx and hyoid bone.

Laryngoscopy at the end of the operation. After knotting the sutures, *do an endoscopic examination using a thin tube*. If the tracheal lumen is wide enough and there is no more bleeding, then—if not already done—a tracheotomy is dispensed with and the operation concluded with meticulous hemostasis and closure in layers over a suction drain.

! Risks and Complications

- Suture-line dehiscence, postoperative bleeding, pneumonia, perichondritis, mediastinitis, injury to the recurrent laryngeal nerve (in some cases as a direct result of the trauma).
- Pneumothorax.
- Injury to major intrathoracic vessels.
- Mild stenosis, which has no functional effect, is not uncommon.
- Cicatricial stenosis with dyspnea (damage to cartilage, loss of blood supply), possible tracheotomy later.

Postoperative Care

It used to be customary to secure the head in anteflexion by suturing the chin down in the direction of the sternum. Nowadays there is the tendency is just to have the head positioned in anteflexion. Antibiotics, feeding tube, voice rest, suppression of the cough reflex, endoscopic and, if appropriate, radiological assessment of the anastomosis, exact monitoring of breathing (risk of suture-line breakdown with renewed obstruction of the airways). If the tube has been left in situ, it should be removed, if at all possible, after 2 days.

Laryngotomy and Tracheotomy

Coniotomy

Indications

Life-threatening dyspnea that is no longer manageable by any other means (emergency intubation, emergency tracheoscopy).

Surgical Technique

Hyperextend the neck, palpate the cricoid cartilage, make a small vertical incision over the inferior thyroid and superior cricoid cartilages, spread the tissue bluntly in the midline, palpate the superior border of the cricoid cartilage, make a stab incision in the cricothyroid membrane, insert a cannula (e.g., split cannula with dilator). In an emergency situation, a full-thickness horizontal incision between the cricoid and thyroid cartilage is equally possible and fulfils the same purpose, although the risk of inadvertently damaging the cartilage is higher than with the dissection technique described above.

Modification

Alternatively, the larynx may be entered with a coniotome, which is inserted directly through the skin into the larynx under palpation of the cricoid and thyroid cartilage. After withdrawing the trocar, the guide sheath is left as a cannula (**Fig. 10.25**).

Rules, Tips, and Tricks

Classic tracheotomy once the airways have been secured.

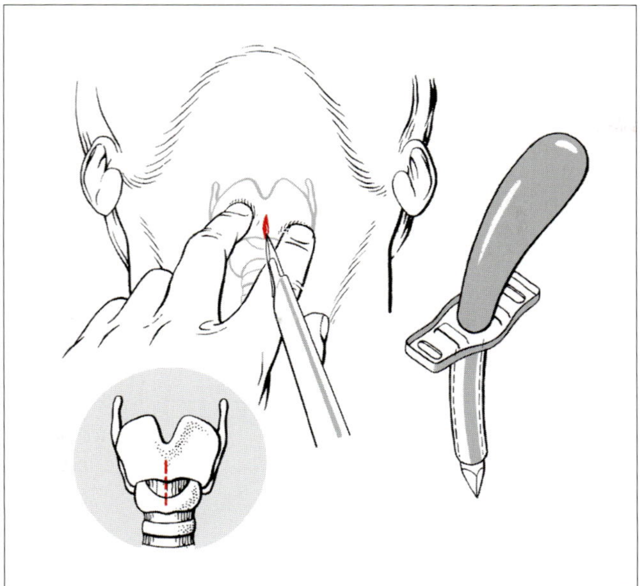

Fig. 10.25 Coniotomy.
Palpation of cricoid and thyroid cartilages. Incision using scalpel. Coniotome with attached cannula.

Tracheotomy

Surgical Principle

Exposure and opening of the cervical trachea, insertion of a tracheotomy cannula.

The distinction between superior, middle, and inferior tracheotomy, which is determined by the position of the tracheostoma in relation to the thyroid isthmus, is practically irrelevant, as the position usually arises inevitably out of the situation. In adults a middle tracheotomy is usually performed, i.e., with dissection or sometimes resection of the thyroid isthmus, unless a low entry into the trachea is necessary because of trauma, stenosis, or tumor. A superior tracheotomy is only possible in adults when the isthmus is narrow and low-lying. In children an inferior tracheotomy is usually appropriate because of the position of the thyroid isthmus.

Indications

- Obstruction of the airways by tumors in the pharynx, larynx, trachea, or esophagus, as well as for obstructing laryngeal carcinomas, where debulking of the tumor using laser surgery may alternatively be considered.
- Injuries to airways secondary to laryngeal or tracheal carcinoma.
- Bilateral recurrent nerve paralysis with stridor. Alternatively: the Lichtenberger reversible endo-extralaryngeal lateralization (p. 200).
- Dyspnea secondary to scalding or chemical burn in the pharynx and laryngeal aperture.
- Relevant congenital laryngeal or tracheal stenosis.
- Craniofacial and mandibular injuries with obstruction of the airways.
- Prolonged mechanical ventilation in intensive care.
- Conversion of a needle tracheotomy with the complications associated with this procedure.
- Aspiration secondary to dysphagia, especially in neurological disorders.
- Dead space reduction secondary to respiratory failure (not without controversy).
- Stenosis of the larynx and trachea secondary to scar formation.
- Inflammatory and edematous swelling at the laryngeal aperture, meso-, and hypopharynx, if not enough patency is obtained with steroids and intubation is not possible.
- As a preliminary tracheotomy for operations of the oropharynx and hypopharynx as well as the larynx.

Contraindications

- As a rule, there are no contraindications in life-threatening situations.
- But in an emergency, always assess whether intubation or emergency tracheoscopy is impossible (especially in the presence of edema, inflammation).

Specific Points Regarding Informed Consent

- Nonhealing of the wound margins.
- Stenosis of the trachea secondary to scar formation, tracheitis.
- Hoarseness, voice loss, paralysis of the vocal fold nerve.
- Problems with swallowing (dysphagia), insertion of a nasogastric tube.
- Insertion of a tracheotomy cannula.
- Possible extension of the skin incision.
- Mucosal injury, mediastinitis.
- Chondritis.

Operative Planning

- Indirect or direct laryngotracheoscopy.
- Posterior–anterior and lateral soft-tissue radiographs of the trachea (stenosis or tracheal deviation) are now rarely required. When imaging is requested nowadays, it is usually CT.

Special Instruments and Implants

Soft-tissue instruments, thyroid retractors, a set of tracheostomy cannulas, Killian speculum, bougies of various sizes as a guide for the tracheotomy cannulas. Emergency tracheoscope. If required, bone punch for the tracheal window in the presence of ossification of the trachea.

Anesthesia

If at all possible, general anesthesia after intubation or insertion of an emergency tracheoscope (tracheotomy over the inserted tube).

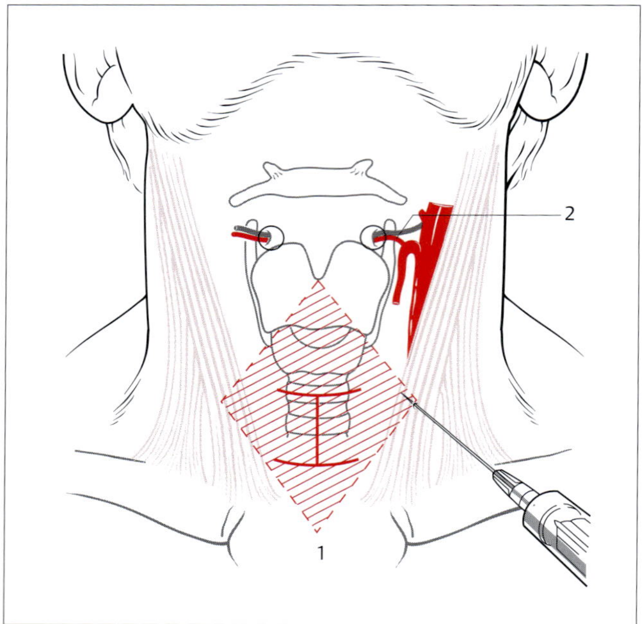

Fig. 10.26 Local anesthetic for tracheotomy.
Diamond-shaped infiltration of the surgical site from the thyroid notch to the suprasternal notch (1). If an additional thyrotomy is planned, the superior laryngeal nerve (2) is also anesthetized.

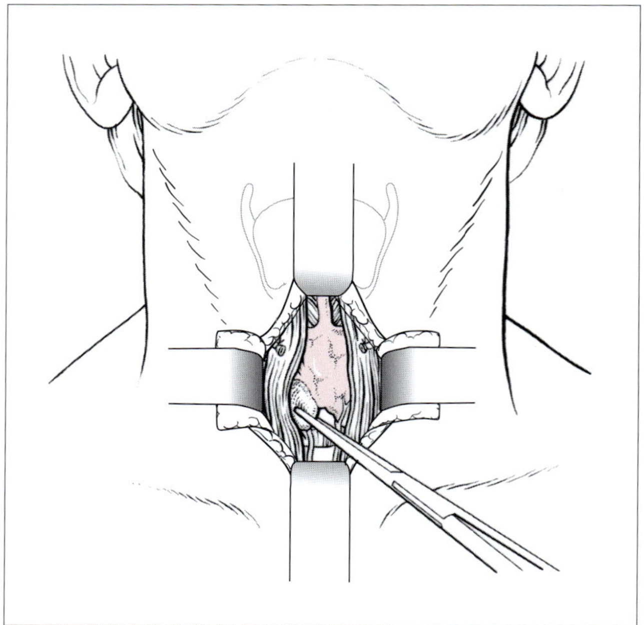

Fig. 10.27 Tracheotomy.
Midline skin incision. Ligation of the superficial neck veins, followed by exposure of the strap muscles and the thyroid gland by blunt dissection.

Local anesthesia: premedication if time allows, otherwise venous access, IV administration of atropine.

Diamond-shaped infiltration of the operation site between the thyroid cartilage and suprasternal notch via a lateral puncture site over the sternocleidomastoid muscle. Midline infiltration in the region of the skin incision as well as in the deeper layers. The incision area should also be infiltrated with a vasoconstricting agent when using general anesthesia (**Fig. 10.26**) to reduce the intensity of intraoperative bleeding.

Surgical Technique

Tracheotomy in Adults

Positioning. Supine, neck hyperextended by placing a roll beneath the shoulders and reclining the head. This position is usually not achievable under local anesthesia because of dyspnea; the upper body usually needs to be elevated.

Incision. Midline skin incision from the cricoid cartilage down to the suprasternal notch. Alternatively, an H-shaped skin incision may be made to prepare the skin flaps required to line the tracheotomy canal. The subcutaneous fatty tissue is spread apart in the midline and any traversing veins are ligated. The skin flaps are firmly retracted laterally with broad retractors and the strap muscles swept aside with a large dissection swab.

Dissection of the prelaryngeal soft tissues. The middle (pretracheal) layer of the cervical fascia is incised between the two muscle bellies using the dissecting scissors. The capsule of the thyroid gland is identified by splitting apart and sweeping aside the overlying connective tissue using the dissector swab. The strap muscles are taken up by retractors (**Fig. 10.27**).

Release of the thyroid isthmus. The cricoid cartilage is identified by palpation. A pyramid lobe is isolated by parallel separation of the overlying tissue on either side of the cricoid cartilage; a clamp is passed beneath it before the lobe is clamped off and resected. The thyroid isthmus is released by placing a transverse incision along the inferior border of the cricoid cartilage. The thyroid gland is elevated further from the anterior tracheal wall bluntly using a dissecting clamp or dissector swab (**Fig. 10.28**).

A thyroid gland with a low-lying isthmus and large inferior veins is displaced superiorly with dissector swabs and the soft tissue overlying the trachea is retracted downward with blunt hooks. The veins are isolated with the dissector swab by spreading apart and displacing the tissue before ligating them.

Division of the thyroid isthmus. The thyroid isthmus is released and a long clamp is passed beneath it; two large clamps are placed on either side of the midline to clamp off this lobe of the thyroid gland. The isthmus is then sharply divided in the middle. Both stumps are oversewn with a continuous suture and carefully released from the lateral wall of the trachea, until the anterior wall is completely exposed. When dividing the isthmus, it may be necessary to undertake resection of a troublesome goitre (**Fig. 10.29**).

Tracheotomy and creation of an epithelialized tracheostoma. A longitudinal incision of the trachea is made over the second and third tracheal rings before excision of a window corresponding to the size of the cannula to be inserted later. This is accomplished by excising the lateral parts or, in the presence of ossification, a punch is used. Alternatively, an increasingly fa-

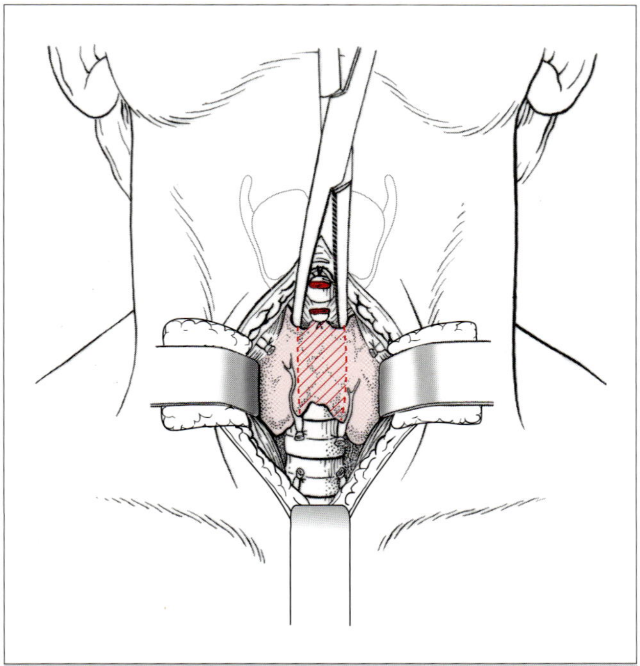

Fig. 10.28 Tracheotomy.
Release of the isthmus of the thyroid gland from the trachea after resection of any pyramidal lobe.

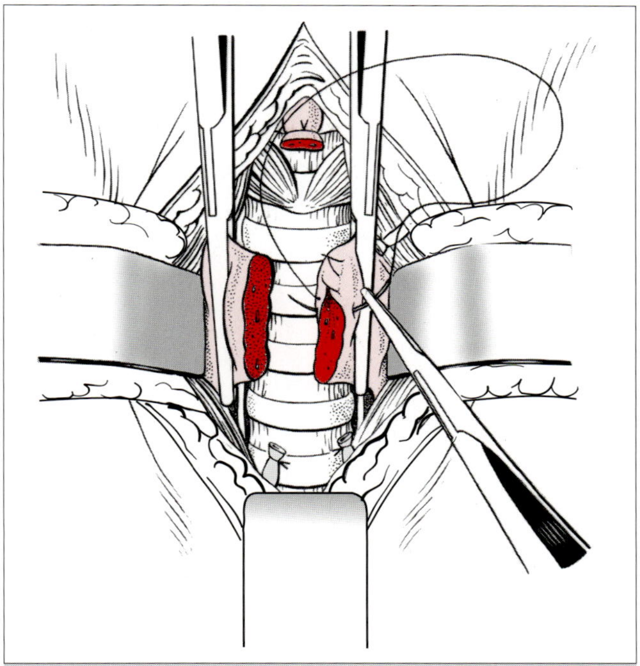

Fig. 10.29 Tracheotomy.
Division and management of the thyroid isthmus.

vored approach is to create an inferiorly based U-shaped flap by placing a transverse incision in the anterior wall of the trachea: A transverse incision is made between the first and second (alternatively second and third) tracheal rings, after which the second and third (third and fourth) rings are divided on either side down to the space between the third and fourth (fourth and fifth) tracheal rings, corresponding to the intended anterior-wall window. The resulting cartilaginous flap is sutured to the corresponding external skin to form the inferior border of the stomal epithelialization (**Fig. 10.30**). Opening the trachea in the space between the second and third tracheal rings provides the greatest protection against damage to the cricoid cartilage. The final level of the tracheotomy, however, must always be determined on the merits of each individual case.

The mobilized external skin is sutured to the incision margins. If the tracheostoma does not need to be left open just for a short time over a few days, the tracheotomy canal is epithelialized by mobilizing the surrounding wound edges of the external skin and suturing them without tension to the tracheal margin.

Denecke flap. If there is too much tension, a flap is elevated below the suprasternal notch at right angles on either side in continuation with the tracheotomy incision. After elevation, the skin flap is sutured without tension to the tracheostoma. The resulting defect is closed by mobilizing the surrounding skin.

Re-intubation. After creation of a window or epithelialization of the tracheostoma, the patient is re-intubated or a tracheostomy cannula is inserted (**Fig. 10.31**). A cannula such as a Rügheimer TracheoFlex is inserted if mechanical ventilation is required, or a silver or plastic cannula if the patient is breathing spontaneously.

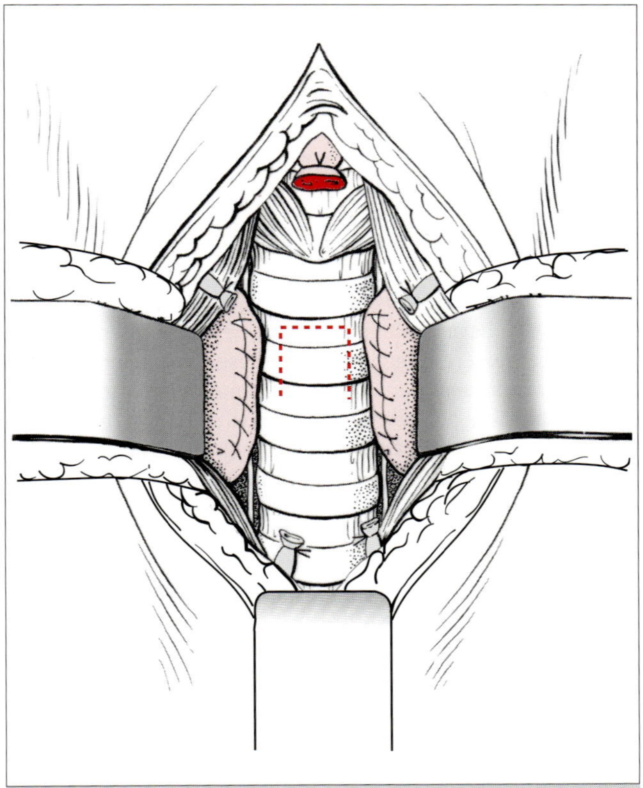

Fig. 10.30 Tracheotomy.
Creation of a window in the trachea by elevating a pedicled U-shaped flap in the anterior tracheal wall.

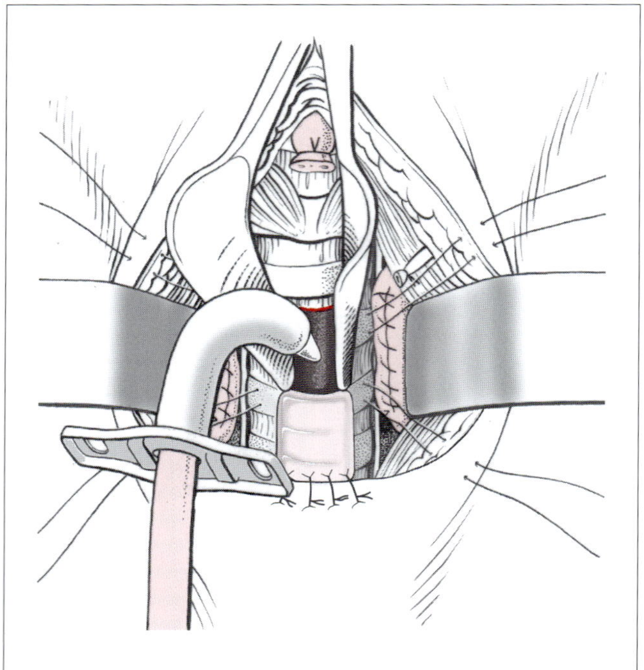

Fig. 10.31 Tracheotomy.
Epithelialization of the tracheostoma with U-shaped flaps and the external skin of the neck. Insertion of a tracheostomy cannula using an obdurator and Killian speculum.

After removal of the orotracheal tube, the tracheostoma is held open with a speculum or two fine hooks and the cannula is introduced into the trachea, using a bougie as a guide if necessary.

Tracheotomy in Children

In the past, tracheotomies were created more often in children, mainly for acute obstruction of the airways secondary to infection. The development of special pediatric intensive care facilities has now resulted in most of these children undergoing endotracheal intubation. Although antibiotics and vaccinations ensure that there are now fewer serious infections, tracheotomy of infants and children has nevertheless once again become a focus of interest, due above all to the success achieved in the treatment of premature babies and children with chronic, often neurological, disorders.

The classic method of tracheotomy in infants is to incise between two tracheal rings and cannulate the trachea via this window. The skin is approximated to the cranial and caudal borders of the window. In the following paragraphs an alternative technique (after Koltai) is described which lends itself to the longer-term management of tracheotomy in infants and children.

Incision. An X-shaped incision is made halfway between the suprasternal notch and the cricoid cartilage (**Fig. 10.32a, b**). The limbs of the X form the diagonals of a 1 cm × 1 cm square. This X-shaped incision may need to be proportionally larger in children older than 1 year, so that for an adolescent the square will be ca. 2 cm × 2 cm in size.

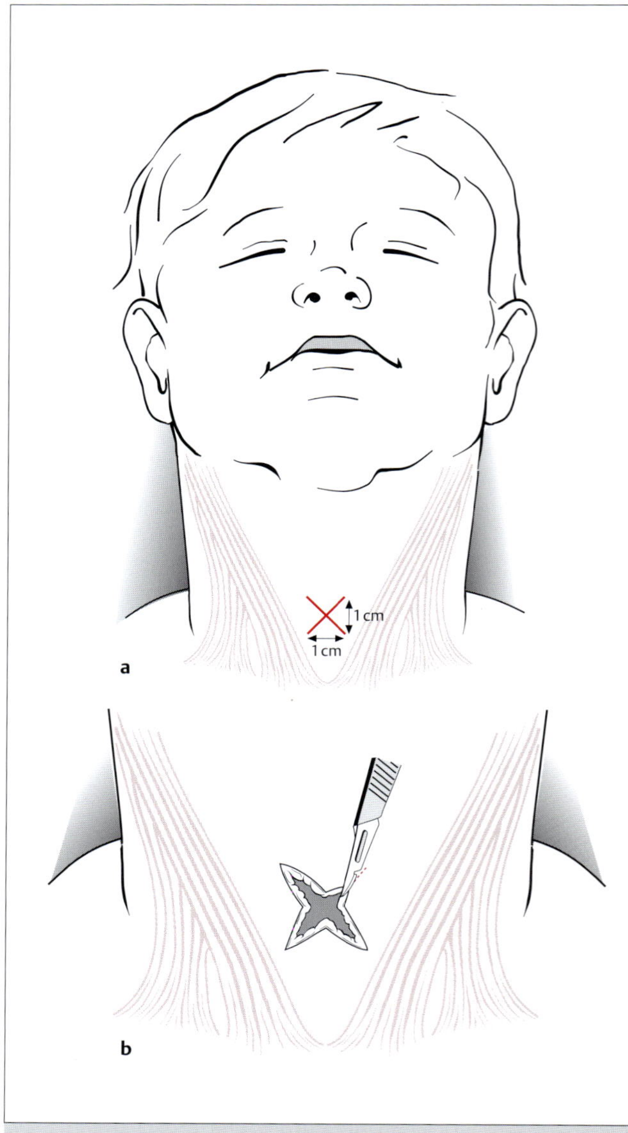

Fig. 10.32a, b Tracheotomy in a child.
a Marking the x-shaped incision.
b Skin incision followed by dissection and elevation of the skin flaps.

Identification of the thyroid and tracheotomy. After elevating the skin flaps and releasing the pretracheal fascia off the anterior trachea, an x-shaped incision is made in the anterior tracheal wall (**Fig. 10.33a–e**). The horizontal limb extends from one side of the tracheal wall to the other. The vertical midline limb of the incision is through two tracheal rings above and two tracheal rings below the horizontal limb.

Creation of a tracheostomy canal using plastic-surgical technique. Because the skin and tracheal incisions are offset by 45°, the tips of the skin flaps align with the troughs of the tracheal flaps and vice versa. The tip of the right upper tracheal flap is approximated to the right upper skin trough using 5/0

Vicryl. The needle is mattressed through the skin, 4 mm from the notch of the trough, then passed through the distal tip of the tracheal flap, taken back through the skin again 2 mm from the notch, and then tied. The other flaps are similarly sutured in place (**Figs. 10.33f–l** and **10.34**) and the tracheostomy cannula is introduced into the funnel-shaped stoma.

Subcutaneous and skin sutures. Wound closure is achieved using subcutaneous and skin sutures.

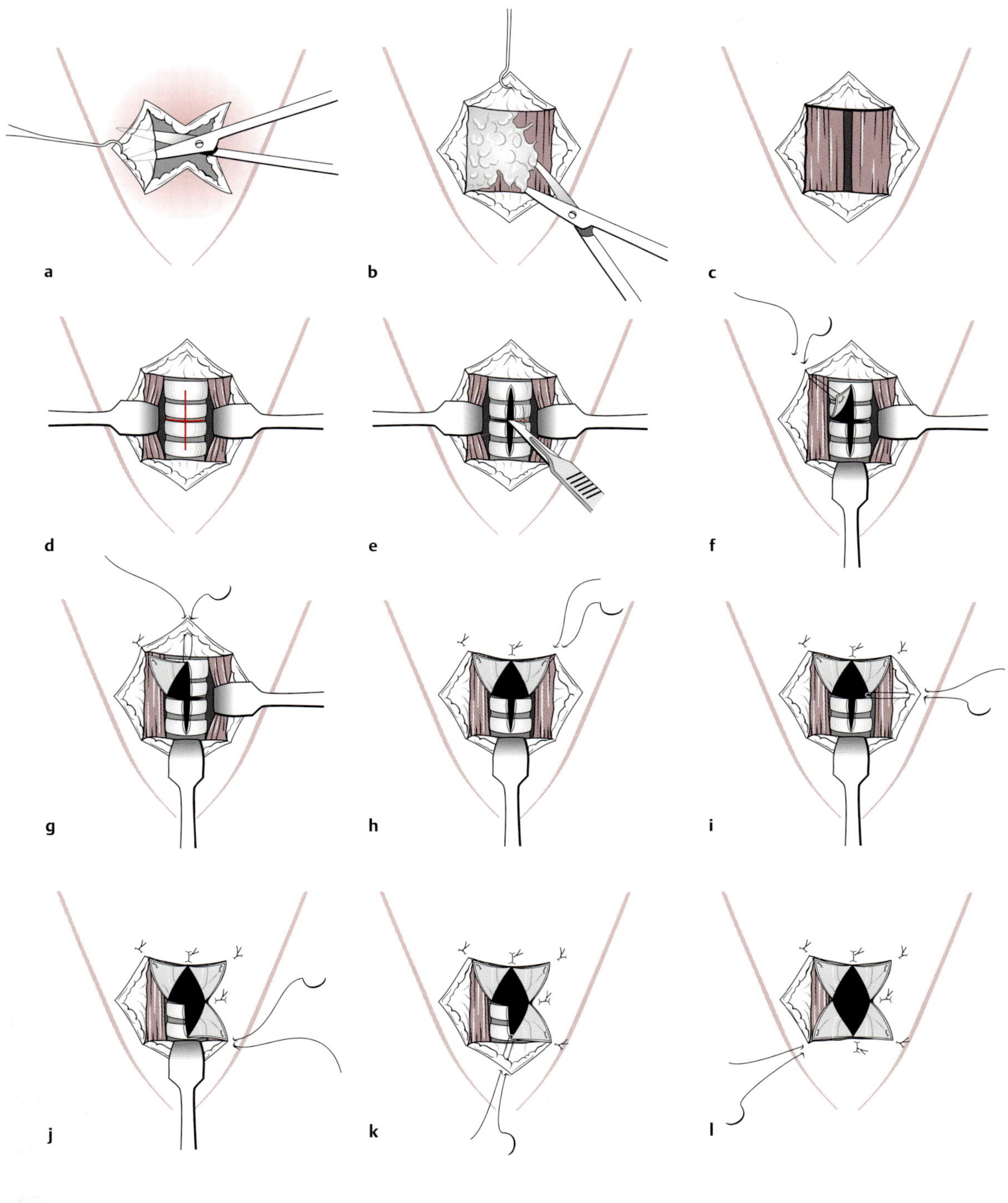

Fig. 10.33a–l Tracheotomy in a child: stages of dissection. After elevation of the skin flaps, a plus-shaped incision is made in the tracheal wall. Since the skin and tracheal incisions are offset by 45°, the tips of the skin flaps come to lie over the troughs between the tracheal flaps and vice versa.

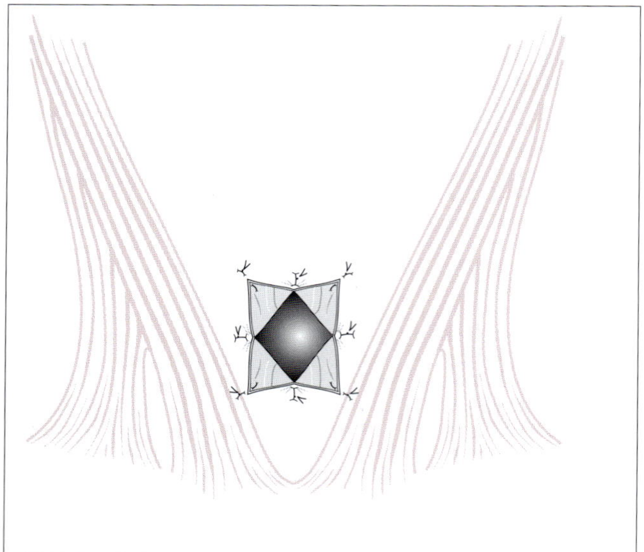

Fig. 10.34 Tracheotomy in a child.
Final appearance showing the funnel-shaped tracheostoma.

Rules, Tips, and Tricks

- Excise the cartilaginous window as sparingly as possible and select an appropriately sized cannula to ensure adequate ventilation.
- The length and curve of the tracheostomy cannula should correspond to the anatomical circumstances, i.e., allow for the distance between the external neck and the depth of the trachea. The cannula should extend ca. 2 cm below the lower border of the internal tracheostoma. Cannulas with too strong a curve or which are too long will injure the anterior wall and can result in erosion of the brachiocephalic trunk.
- Stenosis situated deep in the thorax: consider first undertaking tracheoscopy with an emergency tracheoscope and dilating the stenosis with bougies, then insert a lobster-tail tube.
- Displacement of the trachea by an external mass: orientation is always according to the larynx; identify the cricoid arch, from where the trachea is located by palpation. The trachea can also be identified over the emergency tube by having an assistant raise the tip of the tube. If identification is still difficult, puncture the trachea with a long needle attached to a syringe half-filled with water: if the trachea has been punctured, aspiration will cause air bubbles to rise in the syringe.
- The dressing consists of an incised dressing gauze for tracheostomy cannulas placed beneath the cannula plate. The cannula tapes are tied tight enough to prevent the cannula from slipping back too far.
- Do not excise cartilage in infants and small children.

! Risks and Complications

- Intraoperative and postoperative bleeding (from the thyroid and brachiocephalic vein).
- Surgical emphysema, air embolus, pneumothorax.
- Deep neck infection, mediastinitis, pneumonia, lung abscess, oesophagotracheal fistula.
- Tracheal stenosis with difficult decannulation.
- Problems with swallowing (dysphagia).
- Incorrect placement of the cannula with subsequent stridor.
- Formation of granulation tissue at the end of the cannula (removal of the granulation, change the length of the cannula).
- Crusted tracheitis (inhalation, consider corticosteroids, secretolytic agents).

! Risks and Complications

Especially in children:

- Pneumothorax.
- Dislodged cannula.
- Tracheal stenosis. It has been shown that the formation of a clinically relevant stenosis does not depend on the operative technique, but is more like to originate from an infection of the tracheal cartilage around the tracheostoma.
- Slight collapse of the anterior tracheal wall resulting in a mild flattening of the tracheostoma occurs in most children and is normally not clinically relevant. Nevertheless, this stenosis may have severe consequences in some children and result in difficulties during decannulation. Pressure of the tracheostomy cannula on the superior part of the anterior tracheal wall and infections of the involved cartilage may result.

Postoperative Care

- Postoperative observation (breathing, hemorrhage, surgical emphysema).
- Antibiotic, antitussive agent, secretolytic agents.
- Regular suctioning, moisturization of inspired air (inhalation, heat and moisture exchanger).
- Cannula care, cleansing of the internal cannula.
- First cannula change on the second or third day (bougie, speculum, lubricating agent required). During insertion, the opening of cannula is first introduced transversely and then advanced to its final position while rotating it 90°.
- Tracheostomy dressing change, skin protection against dermatitis using moisturizing cream.

Tracheostoma Reversal

Surgical Principle

A tracheostoma that is not epithelialized will tend to close spontaneously. If closure does not take place, or the stoma epithelializes, it is closed using plastic surgical technique.

Indications

- Sufficient patency of the natural trachea.
- Plastic surgical closure of an epithelialized stoma or residual stoma after removal of the cannula.

Contraindications

- Marked dermatitis of the skin around the stoma.
- Insufficient airway patency.
- Uncertain prognosis of an underlying condition.

Specific Points Regarding Informed Consent

- Unsatisfactory cosmetic result/hypertrophic scar formation.
- Poor healing of the wound margins.
- Tracheal stenosis, tracheitis.
- Hoarseness, loss of voice, paralysis of the vocal fold nerve.
- Dysphagia, insertion of a nasogastric tube.
- Insertion of a tracheotomy cannula.
- Possible extension of the skin incision.
- Mucosal alterations, mediastinitis.
- Chondritis.

Operative Planning

Laryngoscopy, tracheoscopy, retrograde approach through the stoma is also an option.

Surgical Technique

Spontaneous closure of the tracheostoma. After removal of the cannula, the stoma margins are approximated using adhesive tape. Usually the nonepithelialized tracheostoma canal will contract rapidly and close spontaneously. If a residual lumen is left, closure may be effected using an adaptation suture.

Plastic surgical closure. Make an incision around the stoma, at least 1 cm from the mucosal margin. The superior and inferior corners of the skin are excised. The skin margins are then sufficiently mobilized to allow the skin flaps to be approximated from either side over the middle of the trachea without tension. Suturing is accomplished with absorbable 4/0 material. The incision margin of the epithelium must be folded toward the tracheal lumen. The surrounding skin is undermined from the incision surfaces, mobilized, and the wound closed (**Fig. 10.35a–c**).

Modification

If the skin around the tracheostoma is in a poor condition, a transposition flap is elevated, based beyond the sternocleidomastoid muscle and incised over the suprasternal notch and clavicle, to close the defect. The donor site can be closed directly after undermining the skin.

Rules, Tips, and Tricks
Recannulation

If stridor recurs shortly after decannulation—tracheal collapse, scar stricture—then the cannula will need to be re-inserted. The tracheostoma may be re-opened by inserting and opening out a Killian speculum or by dilating with hard rubber bougies. The cannula is then introduced over the bougie.

If a longer period of time has passed since decannulation, it may be quicker to insert an emergency tracheoscope and to re-tracheotomize over the existing tube, or to re-open the tracheostoma canal using bougies.

! Risks and Complications

- Wound infection with subsequent healing by secondary intention, re-opening of the stoma.
- Stenosis.
- Deposition of hair and epithelium in the trachea.

Postoperative Care

Consider administering an antibiotic, monitor breathing.

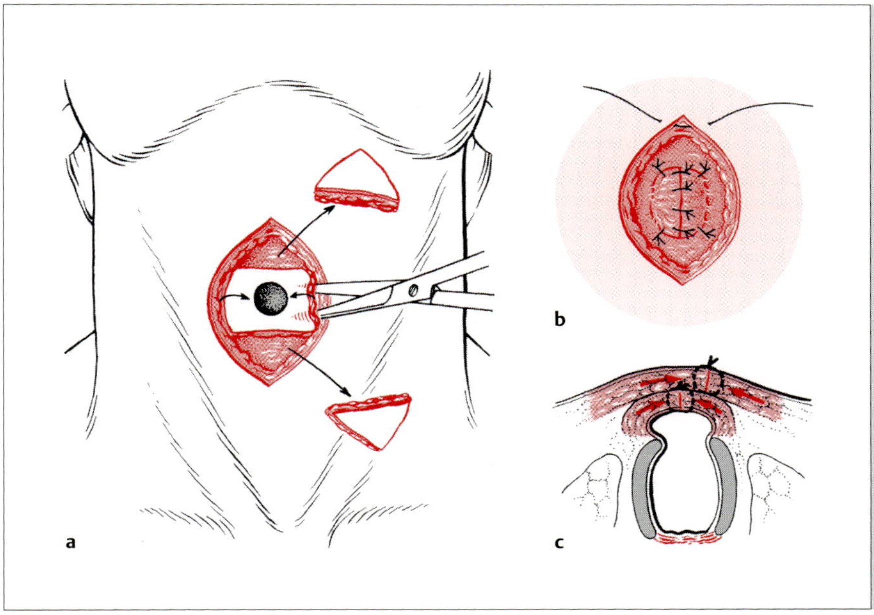

Fig. 10.35a–c Closure of an epithelialized tracheostoma.
a Elliptical incision, the superior and inferior tips are discarded, the skin surrounding the stoma is mobilized and inverted.
b Approximation of the mobilized external skin to come to lie over the buried tracheostomal epithelium.
c Cross-section. External and internal sutures are offset.

Surgery for Inflammatory Diseases of the Hypopharynx and Larynx

Surgery of an Epiglottic Abscess

Circumscribed abscesses are visible during laryngoscopy, especially at the margin of the epiglottis or toward the vallecula, and are incised transorally using cold steel or possibly CO_2 laser via an endolaryngeal or endopharyngeal route. Depending on the extent of the pathology, a simultaneous temporary tracheotomy may be indicated as sudden inflammatory edema not infrequently results in dyspnea.

Specific Points Regarding Informed Consent

As for microlaryngoscopy and laser surgical treatment of supraglottic tumors; tracheotomy, nasogastric tube if appropriate.

Operative Planning

CT or MRI examinations to assess the extent of the abscess.

Special Instruments

Consider CO_2 laser with appropriate instruments.

Anesthesia

General endotracheal anesthesia.

Surgical Technique

If the abscess cannot be exposed via a transoral route, or if transoral surgery is not an option for other reasons, the following procedure is followed via an open approach: a small longitudinal midline incision is made between the upper margin of the hyoid and thyroid notch; the underlying spaces are spread apart bluntly with dressing forceps until the abscess empties itself (**Fig. 10.36**). Alternatively: transoral (laser) incision (CO_2 laser, e.g., 10 W) until the abscess has been widely opened.

! Risks and Complications
- Laryngeal edema associated with stridor.
- Deep infection of the soft tissues of the neck.
- Mediastinitis.

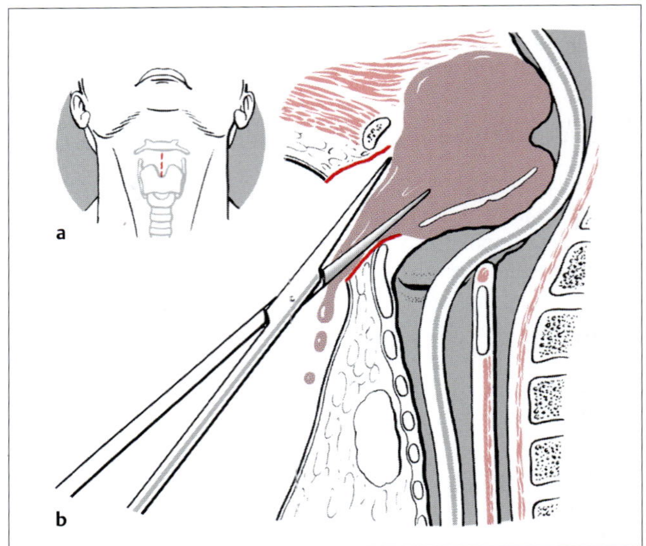

Fig. 10.36a, b Incision and drainage of a deep epiglottic abscess.
a Longitudinal incision between hyoid and thyroid cartilage.
b The abscess cavity is entered inferior to the hyoid and spread open.

Postoperative Care

Insertion of a soft drain if incised from an open approach, antibiotic, consider steroids. Monitor breathing, with stridor initially consider intubation; if the swelling is prolonged, consider tracheotomy.

Management of Laryngeal Perichondritis

Cases of perichondritis of the larynx are initially treated with high doses of antibiotics. Steroids are given for severe edema formation. The presence of stridor requires tracheotomy. If necrolysis occurs in the laryngeal framework, then the larynx must be exposed from an open route, abscesses drained, and necrotic areas of cartilage resected. Plastic surgical measures may be necessary after the inflammatory changes have settled, but complete resolution of the inflammatory process is the prerequisite for this.

Surgery for a Hypopharyngeal Diverticulum

Transoral Surgery

In recent years, transoral division has increasingly come into use. Unlike the transcutaneous operative technique, transoral cricopharyngeal myotomy may be performed repeatedly without any significantly increased risk. Patients recover more quickly and hospital stay is shortened as a result of the short operating time. Because the functional outcome is usually very good and the complication rate lower in comparison with the transcervical approach, especially with regard to the occurrence of accidental recurrent pharyngeal nerve injury, transoral cricopharyngeal myotomy has meanwhile become the preferred management for Zenker's diverculum, using either laser surgery or a stapler.

Surgical Principle

Transoral division of the diverticular pouch developing through the pharyngeal constrictor muscles using the CO_2 laser or a stapler.

Indications

A symptomatic hypopharyngeal (Zenker) diverticulum.

Contraindications

Because increase in size and associated inflammatory symptoms with the increased risk of mediastinitis, cachexia, and dyspnea are to be expected, practically the only contraindications are the inability to tolerate general anesthesia, severe cervical kyphosis or ankylosis, cervical disk prolapse, nonidentifiable diverticulum, or nonexposable diverticular pouch (e.g., due to irregularities of the maxillary teeth).

Specific Points Regarding Informed Consent

- Dental damage, loss of teeth.
- Dysphagia, nasogastric tube.
- Hoarseness, even voice loss.
- Dyspnea, tracheotomy with the insertion of a tracheotomy cannula.
- Pneumonia, atelectasis.
- Mucosal injury, perforation of the esophageal wall.
- Mediastinitis, pneumomediastinum.
- Paralysis of the lingual nerve.
- Paralysis of the hypoglossal nerve (pressure neuropathy).
- paralysis of the glossopharyngeal nerve (pressure neuropathy).

Special Instruments and Implants

The Weerda distending diverticuloscope, CO_2 laser or stapler.

The Anesthesia

General endotracheal anesthesia.

Surgical Technique

To facilitate delineation of the diverticular pouch from the esophagus, some days preoperatively the patient is asked to swallow a small perforated lead weight tied to the end of a 6–7-m-long silk thread, facilitating the process by drinking fluid if necessary. A radiological assessment after 2–3 days confirms the migration of the lead weight into the stomach. Inadvertent slippage of the lead weight into the diverticular pouch may already be clinically verified by the premature curtailment of the thread's passage into the stomach. In these cases, a new lead weight may be swallowed. This technique is in no way obligatory, but time and again it has helped even experienced surgeons to identify the diverticulum, especially in revision cases and with very large diverticula.

Insertion of the diverticuloscope. The patient is positioned with the head slightly elevated and reclined. First, a mouth guard is inserted, and then the Weerda distending diverticuloscope is introduced as for a rigid esophagoscopy. Following the previously introduced thread as a guide, the epiglottis is elevated and the arytenoid cartilages are identified. Saliva, which is usually present, is removed by suction. After the Weerda distending diverticuloscope has been inserted behind the arytenoid cartilage, the piriform sinus is passed while carefully observing through the endoscope. Elevating the diverticuloscope slightly will place the cricopharyngeal bar under tension and render it recognizable. The lower blade places the diverticular pouch under tension, the upper blade passes the esophageal aperture and allows identification of the direction of the esophagus (**Fig. 10.37a**). After identification of the cricopharyngeal bar, undigested food particles can occasionally be removed from the diverticular pouch by suction. To avoid accidental damage to the esophageal mucosa during myotomy when using laser surgery, a damp cotton pledget attached to a thread may be placed in the part of the esophagus behind the cricopharyngeal bar.

Laser surgical cricopharyngeus myotomy. This begins with an incision in the middle of the cricopharyngeal bar (1–2 W, CW mode, diameter of the beam e.g., 0.25–0.5 mm). After the mucosal incision (**Fig. 10.37b**), separation of the muscle fiber bundles is visible under the operating microscope. Separation is continued until the lower horizontal fiber bundles of the inferior pharyngeal constrictor muscle are completely divided. The resulting wedge-shaped defect allows free visualization into the esophagus. By the end of the operation a wide passage has been created into the esophagus. The feeding tube is inserted transnasally under direct vision, i.e., with the distending diverticuloscope still in place (**Fig. 10.37d**).

Cricopharyngeus myotomy using the stapler. After identifying the cricopharyngeal bar, the stapling device (e.g., Multifiber Endo Gia 30 3.5 mm, REF 303813, Tyco Healthcare, Norwalk, USA) is introduced, the two blades are opened in front of the bar and placed in the midline above and below the bar. The stapling device is activated, simultaneously dividing and closing the cricopharyngeus muscle with a multilayer staple line. The incision margin should then be inspected once again, as the author has on occasion observed bleeding from the tip of the resulting V-shaped incision.

Rules, Tips, and Tricks

Complete division of the muscle is essential.

! Risks and Complications

- Severe intraoperative hemorrhage is extremely rare. Laser surgery considerably reduces the risk of bleeding. Even the pulsation of small vessels can be easily recognized under microscopical vision. If they are too large in calibre for adequate coagulation by the CO_2 laser, then bilateral monopolar vascular coagulation or bilateral placement of titanium clips on the vessels is undertaken before division of the cricopharyngeal bar.

10

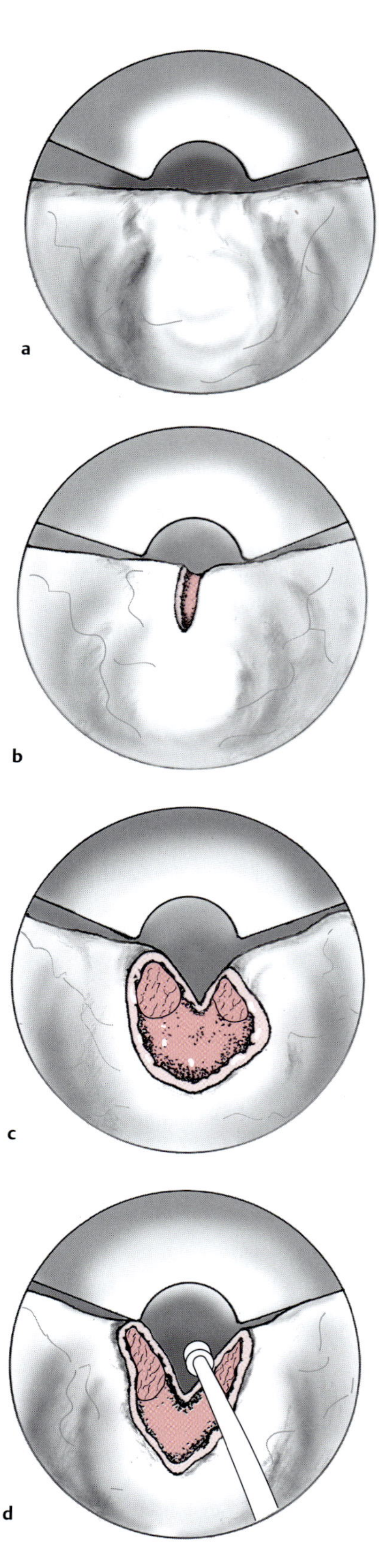

- Unlike cricopharyngeus myotomy using the stapler, the laser surgical approach often results in opening the mediastinum. This results in a usually irrelevant associated mild mediastinitis, which is closely monitored by checking C-reactive protein (CRP; see Postoperative Care, below).
- Esophageal perforation, pulmonary embolus, bronchopneumonia.

Postoperative Care

Postoperative monitoring appears to be less problematic after stapler use than after laser surgery, for which the authors, based on their wide experience, have developed their own strict protocol to be able to recognize complications in good time. This protocol comprises the following points:

- Liquid food is given on the first postoperative day. If healing develops uneventfully, the transnasal feeding tube may be removed on the second postoperative day.
- To manage the above-mentioned initial associated mediastinitis, which is regarded as an inflammatory irritation, for laser surgical cricopharyngeus myotomy we administer
  - on the evening *before* the operation:
    - 150 mg H_2 receptor antagonist (e.g., ondansetron [Zofran]), 1.5 g cefuroxime, and 0.5 g nitroimidazole (e.g. Clont), administered intravenously
  - *intraoperatively*:
    - 4 mg ondansetron
    - 1.5 g cefuroxime and 0.5 g nitroimidazole IV.
  - *postoperatively*:
    - 4 mg ondansetron (2 and 6 hours postoperatively)
    - Novaminsulfone 6-hourly (40 drops)
    - 1.5 g cefuroxime and 0.5 g nitroimidazole IV for a further 5 days
    - Estimation of CRP 6 hours and 24 hours postoperative, then daily. (A CRP rise of 50 during the first 36 hours is regarded to be little cause for concern in the absence of any severe concomitant symptoms. A CRP rise clearly above this level should prompt the ordering of a chest radiograph check (even CT) and, if appropriate, the additional administration of netilmicin sulfate (e.g. Netromycin) 400 mg b.d. and consideration regarding a mediastinotomy via a collar incision.

This protocol is the result of many years of intensive analysis of all laser surgical diverticulotomies that the authors have undertaken. Of course, the protocol is only to be regarded as a recommendation. However, it must be pointed out that this treatment procedure must always be accompanied by a high level of alert-

Fig. 10.37a–d Transoral laser microsurgical cricopharyngeus myotomy of a Zenker diverticulum.
a Exposure of the diverticular pouch and cricopharyngeal bar using the distending diverticuloscope.
b Laser microsurgical division of mucosa and submucosa under vision using the operating microscope.
c Laser microsurgical division of the lower horizontal fibers of the cricopharyngeal muscle.
d Insertion of the nasogastric tube into the esophagus with the distending diverticuloscope still in place.

ness during the postoperative phase. Laser cricopharyngeus myotomy is certainly not an operation to be underestimated in terms of its risk potential.

Choice of Endoscopic Approach

After introduction of transoral laser cricopharyngeus myotomy, this technique was for a long time the therapy of choice. Cricopharyngeus myotomy using the stapler appears to be associated with fewer complications owing to an absent or less extensive mediastinotomy. This procedure has its complications too, however, e.g., hemorrhage, which is why the treatment of a Zenker diverticulum is to be undertaken with special care. Laser cricopharyngeus myotomy has therefore in no way been replaced by the stapler technique. Time and again there are situations where the stapler cannot be adequately positioned over the diverticular pouch. Knowledge of both endoscopic techniques is required, as well as of diverticulectomy from an open approach, to adequately treat this disorder.

Resection of a Zenker Diverticulum from an Open Approach

Indications

Diverticular pouch that cannot be visualized transorally.

Contraindications

Inability to tolerate general anesthesia.

Specific Points Regarding Informed Consent

- Sensory disturbances in the region of the neck and/or ears.
- Poor healing of the skin flap.
- Paralysis of the suprascapular, vagus, phrenic, lingual, hypoglossal, recurrent, or facial nerve.
- Hoarseness, even loss of voice.
- Dyspnea, tracheotomy with insertion of a tracheotomy cannula.
- Unsatisfactory cosmetic result, hypertrophic scar formation.
- Possible extension of the skin incision.
- Mucosal injury, mediastinitis.
- Persistent secretion of lymph fluid (lymphatic fistula).

Surgical Technique

Positioning. Supine, head turned to the right, reclined, slight padding under the shoulders.

Incision and dissection down to the prevertebral fascia. A skin incision is made over the anterior margin of the left sternocleidomastoid muscle, extending from the suprasternal notch to the level of the hyoid bone. Identification of the anterior margin of the sternocleidomastoid muscle and location of the carotid sheath from where it is crossed by the omohyoid muscle, which is divided. Medial to the carotid sheath, which is retracted laterally with Langenbeck hooks, blunt dissection is used down to the prevertebral fascia. Transverse thyroid veins are ligated, if necessary also the superior thyroid artery and the inferior thyroid artery as far laterally as possible if they are obstructing.

Identification and exposure of the diverticular pouch. Palpation of the cricoid lamina allows identification of the diverticular neck, from where the entire diverticular pouch is delivered by spreading apart and carefully sweeping off the surrounding fibrous tissue (**Fig. 10.38a**). Dissection stays strictly

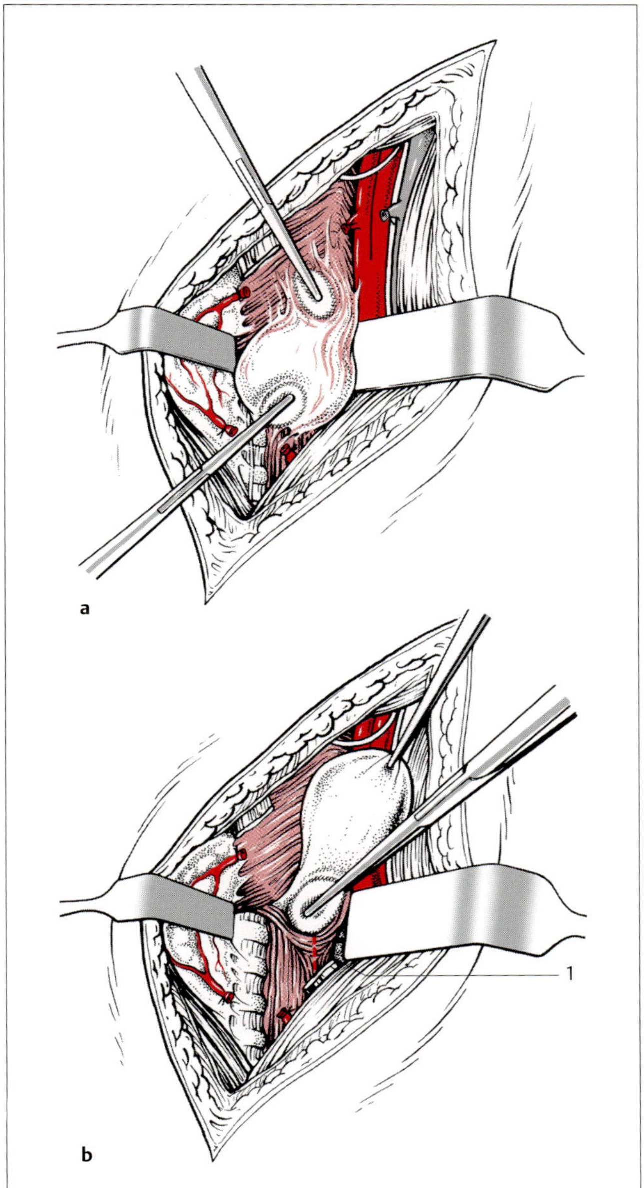

Fig. 10.38a, b Surgery of a hypopharyngeal diverticulum using an open approach.
a Identification of the diverticular pouch. The vascular sheath is retracted laterally, with larynx and thyroid gland rotated medially. Superior and inferior thyroid vessels have been ligated. Dissection of the diverticulum off the prevertebral fascia.
b The diverticular pouch is put on stretch, still pedicled on the esophagus. The horizontal pharyngeal constrictor muscle (1) is divided vertically in the midline.

close to the posterior wall of the hypopharynx and esophagus in order not to endanger the recurrent laryngeal nerve. Once the tip of the diverticular pouch has been reached, it is grasped with a blunt clamp and elevated. The pouch may then be completely released from the muscular and fibrous tissue, until the diverticulum has been exposed in its entirety (**Fig. 10.38b**).

Myotomy. The transverse muscle fibers of the cricopharyngeal muscle are divided in the midline, ca. 2 cm distal to the diverticular neck, after carefully spreading it apart without breaching the mucosa. This step is absolutely essential. The diverticular pouch is held up to allow (transnasal) insertion of the feeding tube.

Resection of small diverticula. Smaller diverticula may be invaginated. The diverticular neck is first encircled with a purse-string suture and the pouch then buried through this narrow opening, the suture tied and once again oversewn. The author, however, favors diverticulectomy.

Resection of larger diverticula. Two sutures are placed at the junction between hypopharynx and diverticulum for orientation. About 2 cm above this junction a noncrushing bowel clamp is placed on the diverticular neck and the diverticulum divided above it. The resection margins are secured with interrupted sutures or a continuous suture, which must securely invert the mucosa, and once again covered with a second suture line. In either case, an additional myotomy of the horizontal part of the cricopharyngeal muscle is obligatory.

Wound closure. Insertion of a small suction drain, wound closure in layers.

Rules, Tips, and Tricks

At the beginning of the operation the diverticular pouch may be packed with a ribbon-gauze tamponade to facilitate its identification.

! Risks and Complications

- Perforation of the diverticular fundus or of the esophagus requires immediate oversewing.
- Suture-line dehiscence with subsequent esophago-cutaneous fistula or mediastinitis: surgical revision.
- Bleeding from the inferior thyroid artery.
- Paralysis of the recurrent nerve.
- Stenosis resulting from too generous excision of the diverticular pouch: dilation treatment or esophagoplasty.

Postoperative Care

- Enteral nutrition for at least 1 week, then careful advancement of the postoperative diet.
- Antibiotic, remove drain once secretion stops.

Tracheobronchoscopy

Two preferred techniques, using a *rigid bronchoscope* or a *flexible fiberoptic bronchoscope* for different indications, are available for tracheobronchoscopy.

The advantages of the rigid bronchoscope is its large working channel, through which it is possible to manipulate and suction better, especially with large foreign bodies, and the better optical image of the respective angled telescopes.

Flexible bronchoscopy may be performed under topical anesthesia, can be used for difficult intubations, and allows a clearer peripheral view than the angled telescopes of the rigid tube.

Tracheobronchoscopy with a Rigid Bronchoscope

Surgical Principle

Under general anesthesia, a rigid telescope is advanced into the trachea and the main and secondary bronchi, the bronchial origins are visualized with angled telescopes, and diagnostic and therapeutic measures performed.

Indications

- Diagnostic investigation for suspected foreign body and suspected tumor, for hemoptysis of unknown origin.
- Acute and chronic inflammatory diseases.
- Stenosis in the tracheobronchial system.
- Clarification of operability of tumorous lesions.
- Bronchial toilet, intensive care.

Contraindications

- Severe general disease or cardiovascular disease (consider flexible bronchoscopy), obstacle to intubation secondary to alterations of the cervical spine.
- There are no contraindications for foreign-body aspiration with dyspnea.

Specific Points Regarding Informed Consent

- Dental damage, loss of teeth.
- Dysphagia, nasogastric tube.
- Hoarseness, even voice loss.
- Dyspnea, tracheotomy with the insertion of a tracheotomy cannula.

- Pneumonia, pneumothorax.
- Mucosal injury, perforation of the esophageal wall.
- Mediastinitis, pneumomediastinum.
- Paralysis of the lingual nerve.

Special Instruments and Implants

Ventilation bronchoscopes of all sizes (pediatric bronchoscopes with proximal illumination, adult bronchoscopes with distal illumination), suction catheter, biopsy and foreign-body forceps (alligator forceps), peanut forceps, 30° and 90° angled telescopes, optical forceps; *optical peanut forceps for infants have proved particularly useful.*

Anesthesia

Always general anesthesia with muscle relaxation and mechanical ventilation via the bronchoscope, if appropriate, jet ventilation via a bronchoscope with injector channel.

Surgical Technique

Positioning. *The head should be slightly raised by elevating the head rest to allow insertion of the bronchoscope.*

Insertion of the bronchoscope. Head slightly elevated, maximally reclined. Mouth guard. Insertion of laryngoscope blade, visualization of the larynx (**Fig. 10.39a**).

The bronchoscope tube is inserted under vision into the larynx with the right hand from the oral commissure. If only the arytenoid cartilages are initially visible, then the base of the tongue and the epiglottis are elevated. With the opening vertical, the tip of the tube is then advanced between the vocal folds and completely passes the glottis while rotating the tube by 90°. The laryngoscope blade is then removed. The tube is attached to the ventilator (**Fig. 10.39b**).

The tube is advanced under vision as far as the carina, while simultaneously slightly lowering the head. While advancing the bronchoscope, it is slid between thumb and index finger of the left hand to protect the maxillary teeth and the upper lip (**Fig. 10.39c**).

Tracheobronchoscopy. Slight rotation of the patient's head to the left allows the tip of the tube to be advanced into the right bronchial system. Immediately laterally on the left the origin of the upper lobe bronchus is recognized tangentially, while ventrally the origin of the middle lobe and at about the same level, again tangentially, the apical bronchus of the lower lobe become visible after further advancement. The other lower lobe origins are visualized further ahead in the depths. For further diagnostic assessment, a 30° telescope is passed through the tube and slightly rotated to demonstrate the entrances to the lower and middle lobes. Then the tube is partially withdrawn past the origin of the upper lobe to allow inspection of the upper lobe with the 90° telescope. By rotating the 90° telescope by 180° and simultaneous slight withdrawal of the bronchoscope, the origin of the upper lobe on the left side can be exactly visualized (**Fig. 10.39d**).

The left bronchial system is visualized after withdrawing the bronchoscope tube over the carina, turning the head to the right, and renewing advancement of the tube. Again the upper lobe origin can be visualized with the 90° telescope, while the apical, posterior, and anterior origins can only be seen with the 120° telescope. The lower-lobe segmental bronchi may be visualized with the 30° telescope (**Fig. 10.39e**).

The tube is finally withdrawn under vision and anesthesia reversed using mask ventilation.

Rules, Tips, and Tricks

- Unless jet ventilation is used, always allow repeated breaks for ventilation when inspecting or working on the bronchial system; withdraw the tube into the trachea in the presence of unfavorable anatomical conditions to ventilate the contralateral side better.
- Bronchial secretion is removed by suction and retrieved (for cytology and bacteriology); perform lavage with saline irrigation and subsequent suction in the bronchial origins.
- Biopsies are taken with rigid optical forceps connected to the forward-oblique telescope or the flexible forceps combined with the angled telescope or the double-cup grasping forceps.
- Foreign-body extraction is done using the alligator forceps or peanut forceps. Use the optical peanut forceps for infants because of its decisive handling advantages.

! Risks and Complications

- Dental damage, loss of teeth.
- Injury to the vocal folds, hoarseness.
- Laryngeal edema, dyspnea.
- Pneumomediastinum, pneumothorax (when performing therapeutical measures).
- Hemorrhage secondary to biopsies or puncturing.

Postoperative Care

- Monitor breathing, suppress the urge to cough.
- Adminster steroids against laryngeal edema during long operations, especially in children.

Tracheobronchoscopy with a Flexible Bronchoscope

Surgical Principle

Endoscopy of the tracheobronchial system with a flexible fiberoptic bronchoscope.

Indications

Basically the same as for bronchoscopy with a rigid telescope, especially:

- Endotracheal suctioning, bronchial lavage.
- Assessment of airway dynamics, assessment of the very peripheral bronchial segments.

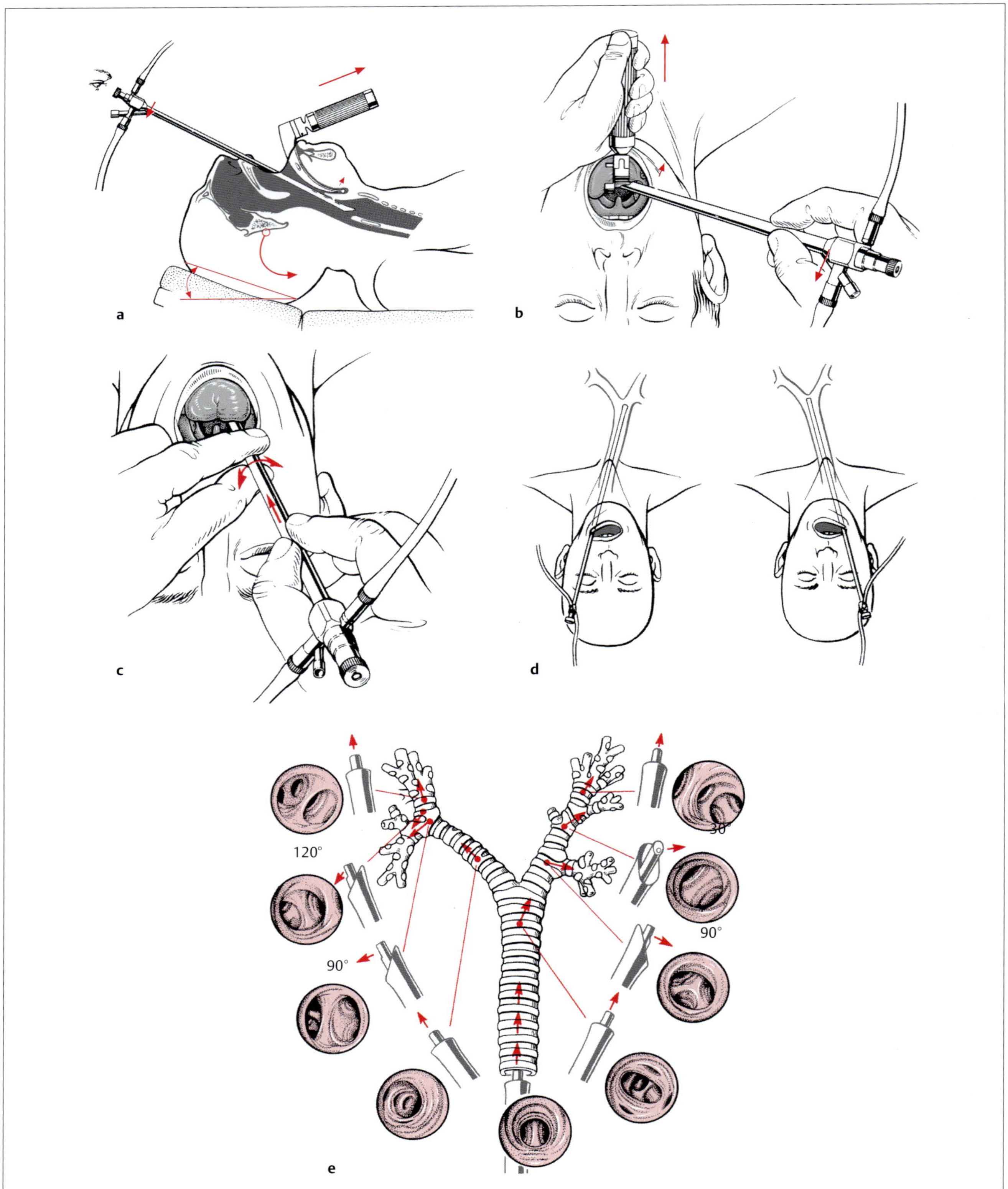

Fig. 10.39a–e Tracheoscopy using a rigid telescope.

a Positioning: head slightly elevated and reclined. Visualization of the larynx is achieved by traction in the direction of the handle of the laryngoscope. The tip of the bronchoscope is raised after passing beneath the epiglottis.

b The bronchoscope is introduced from the right corner of the mouth. The epiglottis is elevated.

c The bronchoscope glides over the thumb of the left hand (which at the same time protects the teeth).

d The left main bronchus is inspected from the right corner of the mouth. The bronchoscope is moved to the left side of the mouth to enter the right main bronchus.

e Schematic illustration of the bronchial divisions with the corresponding telescope angles.

- Therapeutic follow-up of conservative management of malignancies.
- Bronchoscopy for patients who are not fit for general anesthesia.

Contraindications

- Massive pulmonary hemorrhage, biopsies from highly vascularized tumors.
- Relative contraindication: removal of a large foreign body in a child.

Specific Points Regarding Informed Consent

As for rigid tracheobronchoscopy.

Special Instruments

Fiber-optic endoscope with additional instruments (forceps, brushes, puncture needles, catheter).

Anesthesia

General endotracheal anesthesia or topical anesthesia.

Topical Anesthesia

Mucosal anesthesia of the nose (for transnasal approach) or oral cavity (for transoral approach), pharynx and larynx by spraying and brushing with lidocaine spray or 4% lidocaine (maximum dose without vasoconstricting agent = 200 mg = 5 mL). Lubricate the intubation component of the fiberoptic bronchoscope with 2% lidocaine gel.

After introducing the fiberoptic bronchoscope and visualizing the glottis, 1 mL 4% lidocaine is sprayed through the instrument channel around the region of the vocal folds during phonation (5-mL syringe with 1 mL anesthetic and 4 mL air); the air blows the anesthetic through the instrument channel. The deeper tracheobronchial system can be anesthetized in the same manner (use diluted 2% lidocaine solution). Alternative technique: inhalation of 5 mL 4% lidocaine with an ultrasonic nebulizer.

Surgical Technique

Positioning. The patient is placed in a recumbent position with the upper body elevated by 30°; the examiner stands beside the patient, or at the head end of a supine patient (**Fig. 10.40**).

Insertion of the bronchoscope. With the left hand, the endoscope is carefully inserted at the floor of the decongested and anesthetized nose, angled downward in the nasopharynx by pulling the lever (right hand) and advanced under optical guidance as far as the glottis by reversing the angulation (left hand).

Tracheobronchoscopy. After repeating anesthesia and allowing the urge to cough to settle, the endoscope is advanced into the trachea. On reaching the carina, the tip of the endoscope is directed under visual guidance into the main bronchi and further into the periphery. *When further advancing the instrument, the tip must always be kept in the middle of the lumen by careful angulation and must not press against the wall. Light rotation of the endoscope about its axis allows the direction to be adapted to the instrument tip (small arrow on the edge of the field of vision)* (**Fig. 10.41**).

Inspection of the entire bronchial system is accomplished by advancement and angulation of the telescope; repeat anes-

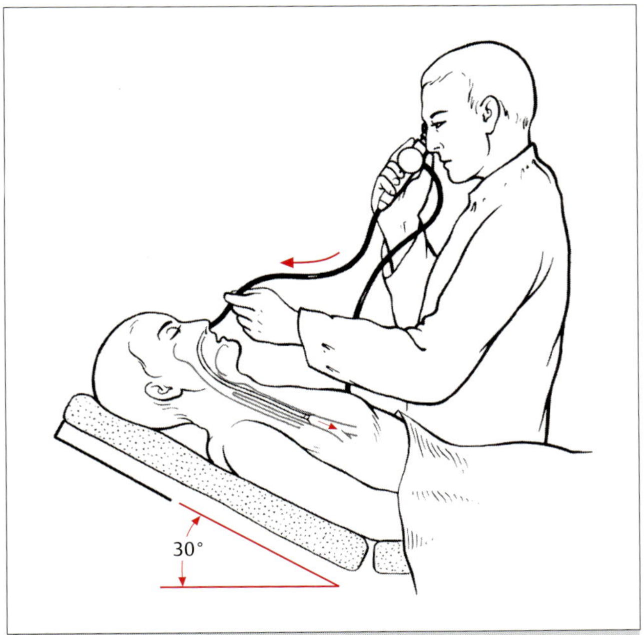

Fig. 10.40 Bronchoscopy using a flexible endoscope. The examiner stands next to the patient, whose upper body is raised to 30°.

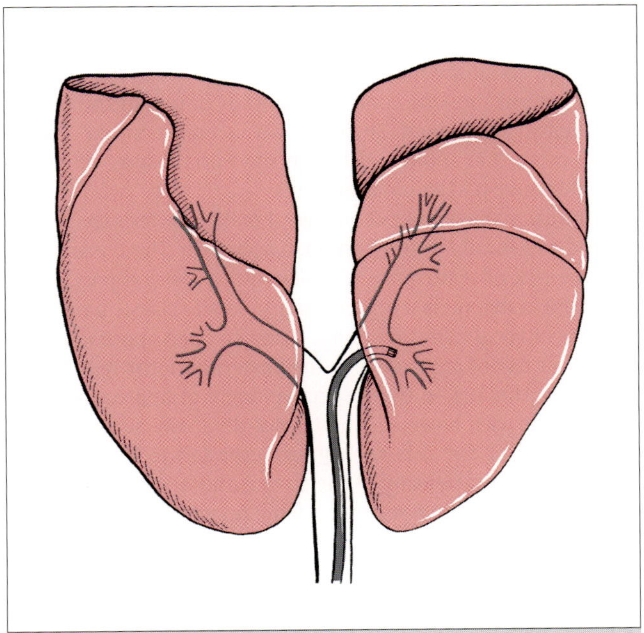

Fig. 10.41 Bronchoscopy using a flexible endoscope. Angling the tip of the endoscope allows access to the bronchial divisions.

10

thesia via the instrument channel may be required. Mucus is removed by suction via the instrument channel.

Biopsy. A grasping forceps is advanced via the instrument channel after temporarily straightening up the tip of the instrument. *To maintain good visualization, do not advance the telescope too close to the lesion.* The inserted forceps is advanced in the open position toward the lesion, into which it is then pressed. The instrument is then closed on cue by an assistant and withdrawn again by the surgeon. It is recommended to apply drops of a vasoconstricting agent beforehand. As many as four biopsy samples should be taken to increase the accuracy of the histology. When using a catheter or brush, it is passed several times over the suspicious area and the harvested material quickly processed. For fine-needle aspiration biopsies, the cannula is advanced through the instrument channel and inserted into the tissue. After removing the mandrin, suction is achieved with a 20-mL syringe, while at the same time moving the spiral tube to and fro. After withdrawing the needle, the entire instrument is removed.

Rules, Tips, and Tricks

- Always ensure optimal visualization; occasionally the fiber endoscope has to be withdrawn, cleaned, and re-inserted. However, visualization can often be regained by mere suctioning.
- It may be necessary to administer oxygen via a nasal tube in patients with dyspnea.

! Risks and Complications

As with the approach using a rigid bronchoscope.

Modifications

The endoscope must be protected by a mouth guard during transoral insertion of the bronchoscope.

If endoscopy is done under general anesthesia, then a so-called T-adapter (e.g., from Portex) is used, which has a lateral connection for delivery of the anesthetic gas and a sealable duct above for the endoscope. The endoscope is sprayed with a lubricant.

For endoscopy via a tracheotomy cannula or a tracheostoma, the trachea is anesthetized with a few sprays of lidocaine before the lubricated endoscope is inserted.

Malignant Diseases of the Larynx

When considering the management of laryngeal carcinoma, any discussion about the most suitable form of therapy for the individual patient must be conducted in the context of the overall oncological background. The more advanced the tumor disease is, the more this applies, although the initial stages of cancer should receive particular attention.

Surgical management of laryngeal malignancies may be performed transorally or from an open approach. The basic rule is that the risk of recurrence is higher in the ventral part of the larynx for transoral laser microsurgery, while classic partial resections of vocal fold carcinomas using an open approach carry the higher risk of recurrence in the posterior glottic region. The reason for this lies in the respective angle of approach. These general remarks, however, should not deter the surgeon from one method or the other; they are intended to draw certain problems to the attention of the novice and as a reminder that neither laser surgery nor conventional open surgery is suitable for resecting every single carcinoma with the highest degree of safety. Sound training in both surgical procedures will allow the indication to be made responsibly and provide individually tailored surgical management of laryngeal carcinoma.

In what follows, it will be repeatedly stated that transoral resection of carcinomas of the larynx—and the same applies for carcinomas of the oral cavity, oro- and hypopharynx—may be performed either in one step or piecemeal, as originally described by Steiner (of Göttingen, Germany). However, it should be mentioned that as a rule the fragmentation technique contradicts the principle of classic block resections (no-touch method). The prevalence of the fragmentation technique is based on the experience so far gained on a large number of treated patients and on the observation that the laser beam seals off the lymph ducts of healthy tissue. There is currently no clinical evidence that tumor fragmentation is associated with an increased incidence of lymphogenic metastatic spread. Critics of this technique counter with the argument that a not insignificant number of these patients undergo postoperative radio(chemo) therapy, particularly for carcinomas of the larynx, which in any case metastasize more often. There are also indications based on animal studies that fragmentation of very aggressively growing carcinomas is followed by a higher rate of lymph node metastasis than classic block resection. This discussion is intended to make it clear that it is currently not possible to judge whether the principle of classic en bloc tumor resection can be abandoned in favor of the strategy of fragmentation by laser surgery, without increasing the risk of lymphogenic metastatic spread. This issue may in future be fundamental in choosing the most suitable moment for neck dissection after tumor fragmentation by laser surgery. Steiner carries out neck dissection in two stages, which may have the result that detached clusters of tumor cells are removed with more certainty during the subsequent lymph node resection than during simultaneous laser resection of the primary tumor.

Transoral Partial Laryngectomy—Laser Surgery

Indications

Decision-making about individual treatment strategies for laryngeal carcinomas goes hand in hand with a meticulous preoperative diagnostic examination. The larger the tumor, the more this applies. If preoperative CT examinations reveal that there is deep infiltration of the laryngeal framework or extralaryngeal spread, only a few laryngologists will take this as an indication for laser surgery. Laser surgical treatment of advanced laryngeal carcinomas demands particularly great expertise on the part of the surgeon.

Specific Points Regarding Informed Consent

- Dental damage, loss of teeth.
- Dysphagia, nasogastric tube.
- Hoarseness, even voice loss.
- Dyspnea, tracheotomy with the insertion of a tracheotomy cannula.
- Pneumonia, pneumothorax.
- Mucosal injury, perforation of the pharyngeal wall.
- Mediastinitis.
- Paralysis of the lingual, hypoglossal, and glossopharyngeal nerves.
- Choking, with aspiration of gastric contents.
- Ignition of the endotracheal tube with subsequent severe damage to the trachea, bronchi, and lung.
- Inflammation of the thyroid and cricoid cartilages with the risk of late development of severe laryngeal stenosis.

Special Instruments and Implants

- Laryngoscope tube and instruments with special suction appliances; laser safety eye wear.
- Special laryngoscope tubes for transoral laser microsurgery of the larynx have been reported by various surgeons. Deciding which of these tubes is most suitable in a given situation is ultimately a question of individual preferences and techniques. Particularly for laser surgery of advanced carcinomas, it is not an infrequent occurrence for several laryngoscopes to be used to resect a tumor. A carcinoma can only be resected responsibly if the tumor margins can be clearly identified. In rare cases, whether one- or two-staged, conversion to an open procedure will have to be considered if the transoral approach does not allow complete resection.
- A CO_2 laser may be used for vaporization and also as a cutting instrument. The vaporization technique is contraindicated for malignant neoplasms, as this approach does not allow the histopathological assessment of the tissue and the resection margins. The only exception is to achieve a rapid reduction in tumor volume, as may be indicated in a palliative approach. The incision technique is indicated for all curative laser surgical tumor resections. This is done in a focused or lightly defocused manner, which allows an almost bloodless resection.

Carcinoma of the Vocal Folds

Carcinoma in Situ, Circumscribed Microinvasive Carcinomas

Surgical Technique

Small lesions of the vocal folds, which have only developed superficially, are typically removed as an excisional biopsy with a narrow safety margin and submitted for histopathological evaluation. This excision may be done with cold steel or by laser microsurgery (**Fig. 10.42**). Both techniques may be preceded by the injection of a mixture of physiological saline and epinephrine into the superficial layer of the lamina propria of the vocal fold (hydrodissection). This facilitates the distinction between a superficially circumscribed carcinoma and a tumor infiltrating into deeper tissue layers. If the lesion appears to be infiltrating the deeper layers and no histological result has yet been obtained, the histology should be verified first and no deeper resection attempted, given that confusion with benign lesions can happen, even with experienced surgeons.

If the indication for laser surgical resection has been established, the procedure begins with determining the peritumoral incision line (**Fig. 10.43**). The experienced surgeon will often undertake the resection in one continuous stage. It is, however, equally possible, and no less efficient, to first mark the imaginary excision line with individual laser spots. Once the laser incision has been completed behind or in front of the lesion, the incision margin facing the tumor is grasped with fine forceps and dissection then completed in the apparently tumor-free tissue layer. The excised sample is then placed on a cork, marked with differently colored needles to indicate which margin should be tumor-free, and sent to the pathologist.

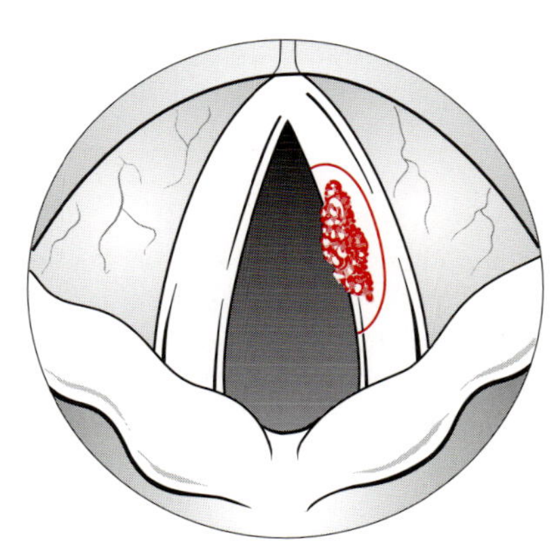

Fig. 10.42 Excisonal biopsy of a superficial hyperkeratotic lesion of the right vocal fold, confined to the mucosa.

10

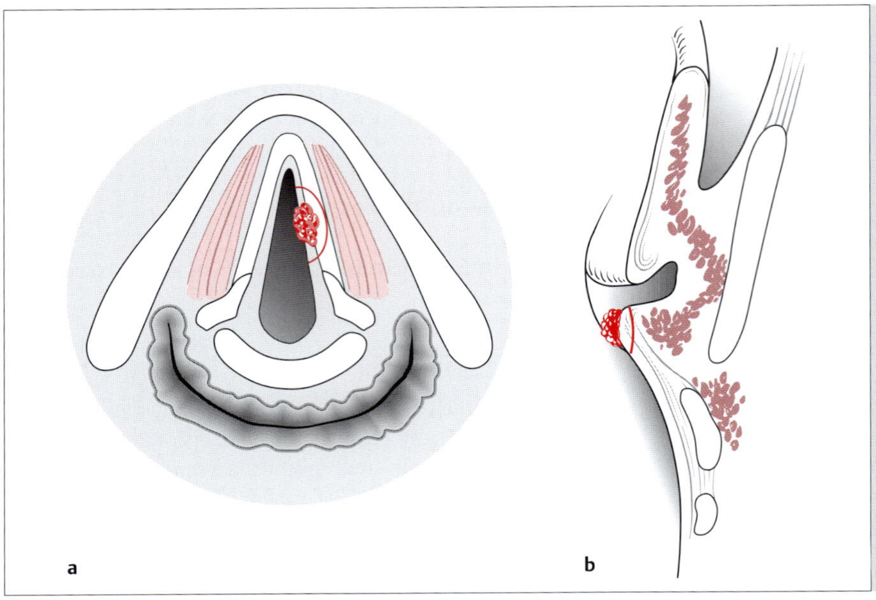

Fig. 10.43a, b Laser microsurgical resection lines for a right-sided carcinoma of the vocal fold.
Using an operating microscope, resection is done under direct vision, keeping close to the lesion and respecting the laser microsurgical behaviour of the tissue.
a Frontal view.
b Lateral view.

T1b Carcinomas of the Vocal Folds

Surgical Technique

The indication for transoral surgery of a T1b carcinoma of the vocal folds presupposes its reliable exposure. Compromises during tumor resection are associated with an increased risk of recurrence. Laser surgical treatment of T1b carcinomas of the vocal folds may be done in at least three ways:

- Histologically confirmed carcinoma is excised in one piece (**Fig. 10.44**).
- The carcinoma is divided in or near the midline and removed in two or more portions. This applies above all for deeper infiltrating carcinomas and those extending far ventrally (**Figs. 10.45** and **10.46**).
- A carcinoma that has developed superficially, and has been confirmed histologically as being highly differentiated, can be removed in two stages: first the more affected side, then the residual tumor after 6–8 weeks. Here the aim is to avoid postoperative web formation in the region of the anterior commissure and thus to achieve a good functional result. Deeper carcinoma infiltration and moderate grade differentiation militate against this two-stage form of treatment.

! Risks and Complications

Involvement of the anterior commissure bears the risk of postoperative web formation. Similarly, the danger of recurrence is based around this problem zone. There are several explanations for this. On the one hand, the transoral approach itself makes adequate exposure of the anterior commissure difficult; this applies particularly for patients with a narrow or prominent larynx, which is not infrequently also associated with a prominent maxilla. A further difficulty lies in the potential tangential growth of the tumor into ossified areas of the thyroid cartilage along the Broyle tendon or along the blood vessels that enter the ossified part of the cartilage. In the case of a deep invasion of the anterior commissure

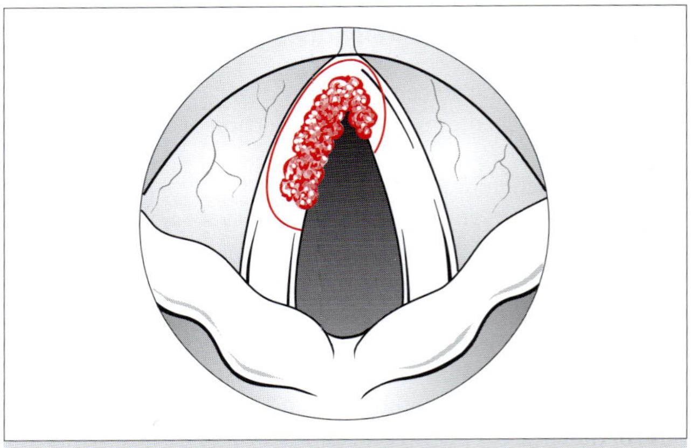

Fig. 10.44 T1b carcinoma of the vocal fold, predominantly on the right.
The laser microsurgical resection can be done in one piece.

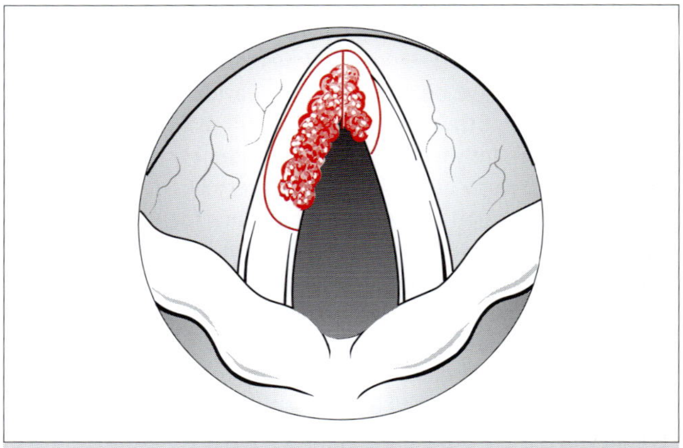

Fig. 10.45 T1b carcinoma of the vocal fold, predominantly on the right.
The laser microsurgical resection is done in two portions, with a vertical incision in the midline.

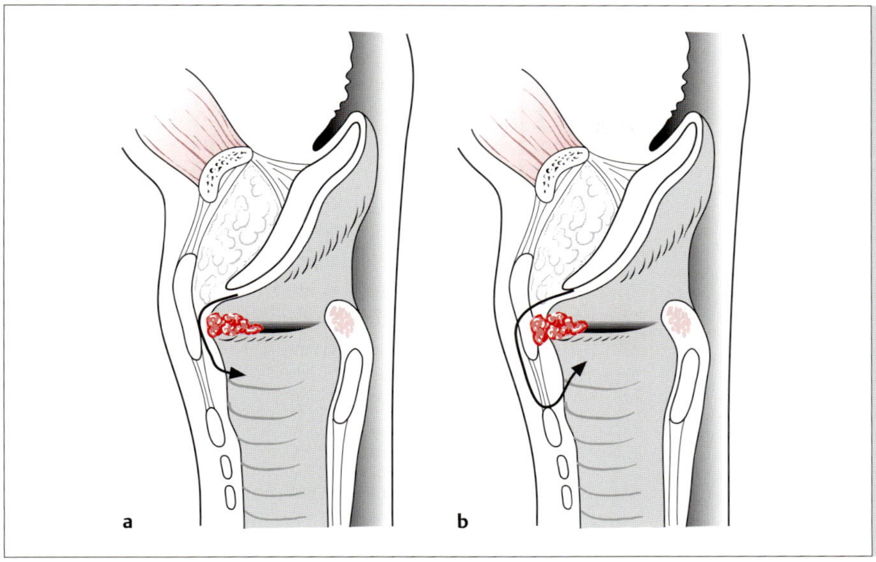

Fig. 10.46a, b Transoral laser microsurgical resection of a ventrally located carcinoma of the vocal fold.

a If the perichondrium of the thyroid cartilage is recognized to be uninvolved, resection is done along the cartilage and includes the perichondrium.

b If the perichondrium is involved, with invasion of the ossified thyroid cartilage, the involved part of the thyroid cartilage can also be resected transorally using laser microsurgical technique. A prerequisite for this is the adequate exposure of the aforementioned region.

these arguments demand particularly careful weighing up of the choice between the indication for transoral laser surgery and that for partial laryngectomy using an open approach.

T2 and T3 Carcinomas of the Vocal Folds

Surgical Principle

Transoral laser microsurgical resection of extensive carcinomas is done in one stage or piecemeal. If the latter technique is used, particular attention must be paid to the exact marking of the incision margins in order to be able to confirm histologically the complete resection of the tumor, which of course must be the aim of these treatment measures. When planning the operation, the approach to the tumor must be determined. Sometimes it is appropriate—and this applies particularly for advanced glottic carcinomas—to begin dissection from above the tumor, i.e., from the supraglottic region, e.g., along the thyroid cartilage, in a caudal direction. In this context, the question regarding the necessity as well as the extent of any possible false-cord resection is important and should be considered during operative planning. This is important above all during the postoperative phase, when the question arises regarding the possibility of learning a new voice at the level of the false cords. An uncritical complete resection of the false cords is not indicated.

Given all the above arguments relating to the technique of tumor resection, the question of postoperative function must not be disregarded when drawing up the surgical plan for treating laryngeal carcinoma. From a purely technical surgical point of view, the majority of advanced laryngeal carcinomas are resectable by the experienced laser surgeon. The remaining functional limitations are, however, highly significant, especially for laryngeal carcinomas. Thus, the absence of one arytenoid cartilage can often be compensated for by adequate swallowing training, but the removal of both arytenoid cartilages is unacceptable from a functional point of view.

Surgical Technique

Tumor fragmentation. If the carcinoma can be removed completely in one piece, the technique does not principally differ from that already described for circumscribed vocal fold carcinomas. The fragmentation technique usually involves incisions that are directed laterally toward the thyroid cartilage and caudally toward the superior border of the cricoid. They follow the extent of the tumor down into the depths of the musculature, until finally tissue is reached that has the laser absorption characteristics of healthy tissue, as observed under high amplification of the operating microscope (**Fig. 10.47**). If the

10

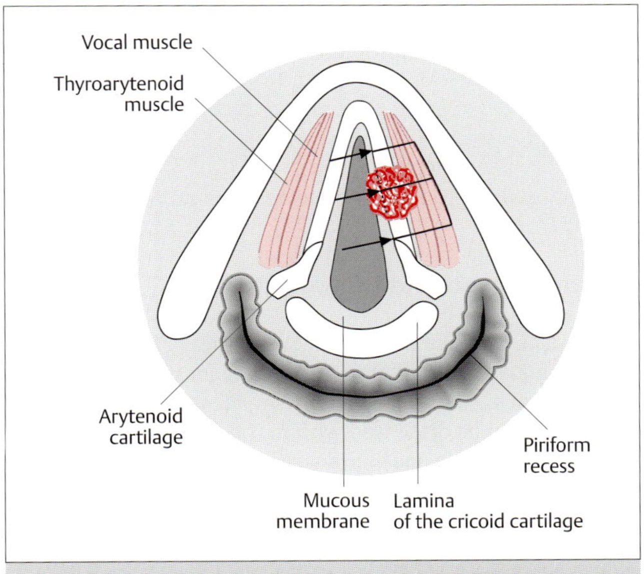

Fig. 10.47 Carcinoma of the right vocal fold with invasion of the muscles.
Laser microsurgical resection of the carcinoma under the view of the operating microscope allows adequate differentiation between healthy tissue and tissue affected by the tumor.

musculature is infiltrated as far as the perichondrium, then the carcinoma may also be resected along the inner surface of the thyroid cartilage. Of course, the thyroid cartilage may also be included in the resection, but this technique necessitates adequate experience on the part of the surgeon. One prerequisite for the laser surgical indication, as put forward by practically all laryngologists, is that the tumor has not grown in a paralaryngeal direction in a cranial and/or caudal direction.

Rules, Tips, and Tricks

- Functional reasons, such as the inevitable dysphagia following resection of the arytenoid joint, limit the technical possibilities of resectability.
- Unilateral removal of the arytenoid cartilage can usually be functionally compensated, but functional reasons forbid a bilateral resection.

! Risks and Complications

- Local infections.
- Surgical emphysema.
- Fistula formations.
- Hemorrhage.
- Dyspnea secondary to web formation.
- Stenosis or edema.
- Difficulties with swallowing (dysphagia) or aspiration pneumonia.
- Severe postoperative bleeding, hoarseness and even loss of voice.

Postoperative Care

Voice therapy and, if appropriate, swallowing training; bedside inhalator.

Alternatives

Conventional surgical resection techniques, radiotherapy.

Carcinoma of the Supraglottis

Transoral CO_2 laser resection of malignancies of the supraglottis is a technique that is not unduly stressful for the patient and is usually associated with little morbidity. Since a temporary tracheostomy can be dispensed with in the vast majority of cases and, unlike with the open approach, nutrition via a nasogastric tube is often restricted to only a few days, the quality of life after partial endoscopic resection is to some extent clearly superior to the conventional open approach, at least during the first postoperative weeks. Furthermore, most surgeons set no age limit for partial supraglottic resection using an open approach. The superiority of the functional results characterizes endoscopic laser surgical resection as an excellent treatment method for supraglottic carcinomas.

Surgical Principle

Transoral exposure of the supraglottic carcinoma after prior diagnostic imaging examinations. Decision regarding the approach (e.g., via epiglottis splitting, division of the glossoepiglottic fold) and the question of any possible infiltration of the pre-epiglottic space, the question of performing a neck dissection, one- or two-stage operation.

A particular advantage of laser microsurgical forms of treatment of the supraglottic region lies in the fact that, unlike with the vocal folds, wider safety margins to the carcinoma can be often maintained without noticeably increasing the extent of functional problems.

Indications

Carcinomas of the free epiglottic margin, central suprahyoid carcinomas, and carcinomas of the lingual surface of the epiglottis, the margin of the false cords, or the region of the aryepiglottic folds are all particularly suited for endoscopic laser surgical resection.

Surgical Technique

Circumscribed carcinomas of the suprahyoid epiglottis. Resection in one piece, similar to the technique for resecting early carcinomas of the vocal folds (**Fig. 10.48**).

Carcinomas of the infrahyoid epiglottis. The actual extent of the depth of the carcinoma is often difficult to identify preoperatively, and this particularly applies to the region of the epiglottic petiole. In addition, differentiation between T1 and T3 carcinomas can also prove difficult.

Clinical experience has shown that with carcinomas of the infrahyoid region, infiltration of the pre-epiglottic space must always be considered. Such an infiltration does not represent a contraindication to laser surgical resection. The precondition for this type of resection, however, is the complete identification of the tumor after division of the pre-epiglottic fat pad. A laser surgical approach through the vallecula is recommended to achieve this objective.

Identification of the pre-epiglottic fat pad. Conventional electrocautery of the vascular bundle in the pharyngo-epiglottic folds is followed by a midline division of the glosso-epiglottic fold. Bleeding usually occurs and if it proves uncontrollable, the use of special titanium clips (Ligating Clip Cartridge, Ethicon Endo-Surgery, Cincinnati, USA; Endolaryngeal Clip Forceps, 8665 L, Karl Storz, Tuttlingen, Germany) has proven effective. Furthermore, division of the suprahyoid epiglottis may then be undertaken, in a sagittal (**Figs. 10.49, 10.50, 10.51**) or parasagittal direction. After identification of the pre-epiglottic fat pad and the laryngeal aspect of the infrahyoid epiglottis bearing the tumor, the carcinoma is usually divided sagittally by an incision running in a caudal direction. In some cases the extent of the tumor also requires a horizontal incision through the lesion (**Figs. 10.52, 10.53, 10.54, 10.55**). If the tumor has infiltrated the thyroid cartilage or one of the arytenoid cartilages, these structures may be included in the resection.

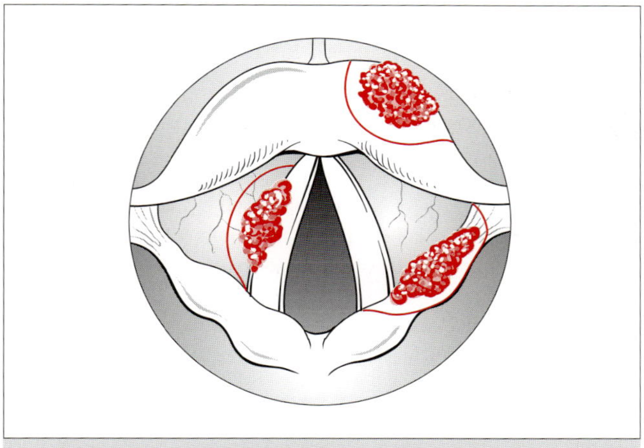

Fig. 10.48 Small supraglottic carcinomas are excised using laser microsurgical technique, adapted according to the individual extent of the tumor.

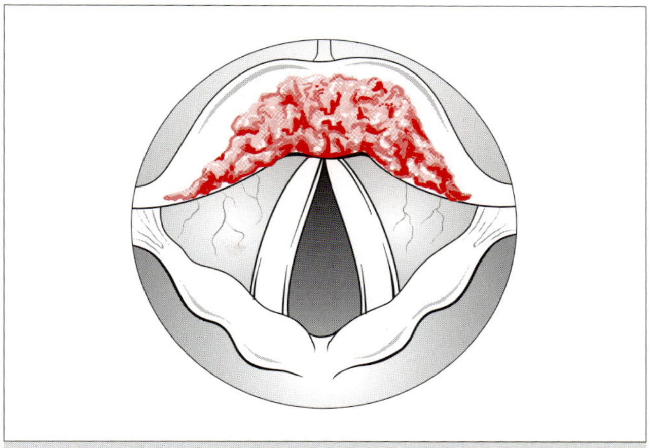

Fig. 10.49 Extensive carcinoma of the laryngo-epiglottic fold.

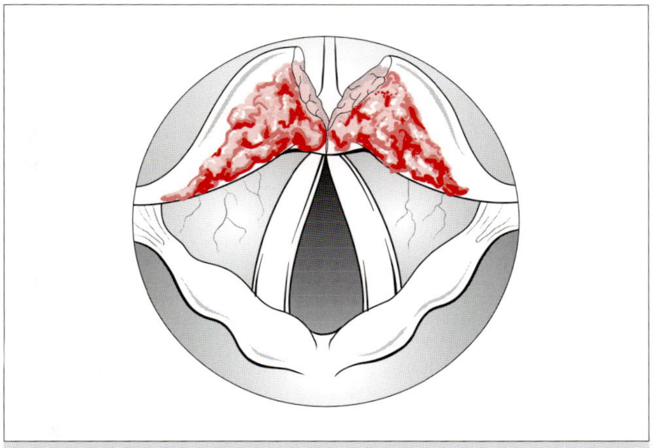

Fig. 10.50 Laser microsurgical division of the epiglottis in the midline, giving the opportunity of determining exactly the extent of the supraglottic carcinoma.

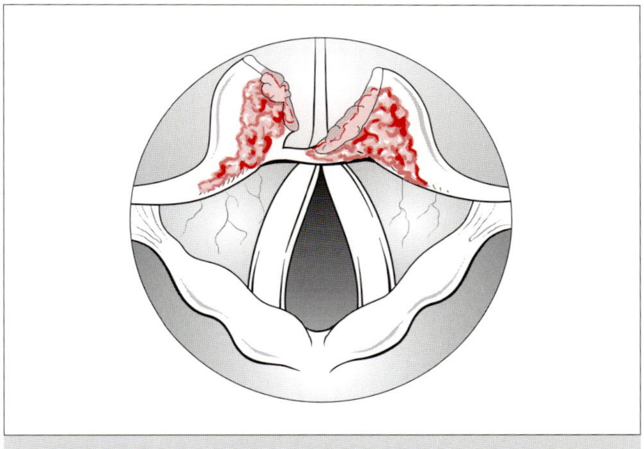

Fig. 10.51 The affected supraglottic area is resected piecemeal, corresponding to the exact location of the tumor.

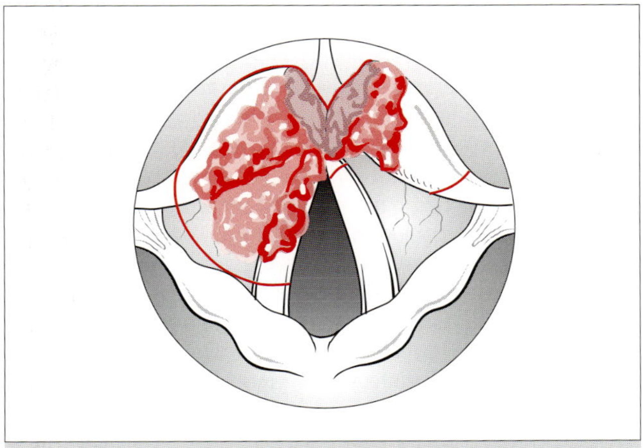

Fig. 10.52 Extensive supraglottic carcinoma with implied line of resection.

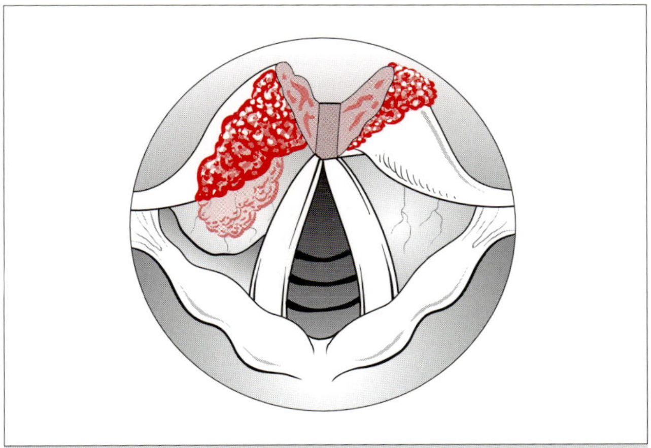

Fig. 10.53 Midline laser microsurgical division of the epiglottis with recognizable extent of the carcinoma, which also extends to the lingual aspect of the epiglottis.

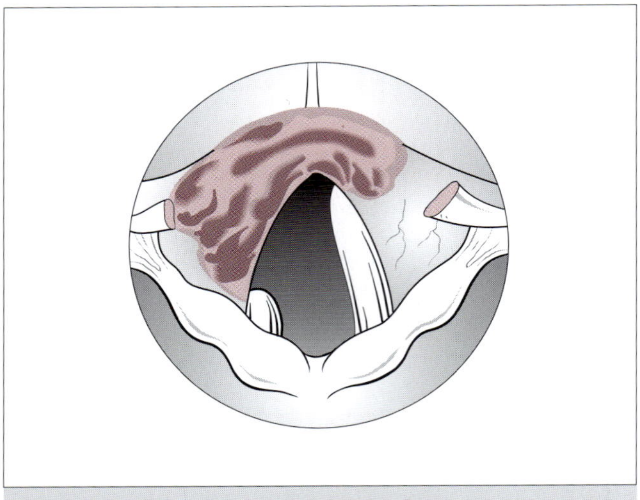

Fig. 10.54 Extensive supraglottic carcinoma.
Parts of the false cord and the true vocal fold as well as the base of the tongue are included in the resection.

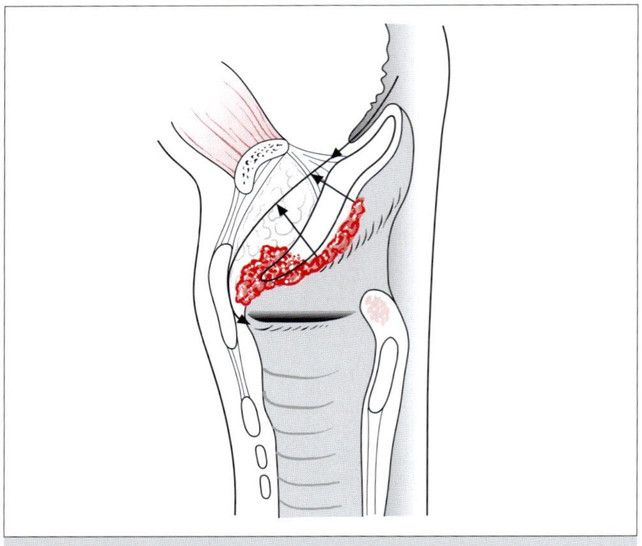

Fig. 10.55 Supraglottic carcinoma with invasion of the pre-epiglottic space.
Transoral laser microsurgery allows a supraglottic resection along the thyroid cartilage with inclusion of the pre-epiglottic tissue and, with it, inclusion of the part of the tumor that is located here.

Rules, Tips, and Tricks

As already mentioned above, a more or less significant degree of postoperative dysphagia should be expected, depending on the extent of the unilateral resection in the arytenoid region. Both arytenoid cartilages should not be resected, as this will result in the most severe postoperative dysphagia.

! Risks and Complications

- Local infections.
- Surgical emphysema.
- Fistula formations.
- Hemorrhage.
- Dyspnea secondary to stenosis or edema.
- Difficulties with swallowing (dysphagia) or aspiration pneumonia.
- Severe postoperative bleeding, hoarseness and even loss of voice.

Postoperative Care

Voice therapy and, if appropriate, swallowing training; bedside inhalator.

Carcinoma of the Hypopharynx

Surgical Principle

Transoral resection along the individual extent of the tumor; no comprehensive block resections of the tumor and neck dissection specimen. Tumor and healthy tissue in the hypopharynx can often be very easily distinguished from each other under the operating microscope.

Indications

T1 and T2 hypopharynx carcinomas, which can be exposed in their entirety from a transoral approach.

Contraindications

Carcinomas infiltrating deep into the soft tissue of the neck.

Operative Planning

The preoperative diagnostic work-up includes an endoscopic examination and CT. The results of these examinations help in reaching a decision about the possibility of partial transoral resection. Of course, the experience of the surgeon also has an influence on the final decision, and it goes without saying that oncological safety must be considered. Occasionally the extent of the tumor as reflected by the mucosal surface is not an indication of the actual size of the lesion. Carcinomas of the piriform sinus can invade the paraglottic space and the pre-epiglottic space, the arytenoid cartilage region, the thyroid cartilage, or the soft tissue of the neck without any pathology being evident at endoscopy. Only in cases of extensive infiltration, e.g., of the cricoarytenoid joint, does the extent of the tumor become clinically evident as a result of the limited mobility or fixation of the arytenoid cartilage.

Surgical Technique

It is generally recommended to resect the tumor step-by-step in a craniocaudal direction. For this purpose, the distending laryngoscope is positioned so that a margin of healthy tissue of ca. 10–12 mm remains between the blade of the speculum and the edge of the visible tumor. The mucosal incision should be made under higher magnification using the microscope.

The tumor is removed by block excision and excision in layers. The tumor may be divided into small segments by placing horizontal and vertical incisions in a criss-cross fashion. The junction between healthy tissue and tumor is usually identifiable under the operating microscope.

Modifications

If the tumor is not resectable by laser surgery because of its poor exposure or location, a partial laryngectomy from an open approach or even laryngectomy with partial pharyngectomy is usually indicated. In such cases the option of radiochemotherapy should be considered.

Rules, Tips, and Tricks
A relatively wide resection margin (≥10 mm) may be maintained in this region without entailing major functional consequences, which could otherwise result from further loss of tissue. This means increased safety during tumor resection.

Postoperative Care

In transoral laser surgical removal of hypopharyngeal carcinomas, it may be assumed that the wound will heal spontaneously with complete epithelialization. Wound healing is usually accomplished within 8 weeks, giving good functional results.

! Limitations and Complications of Laser Surgery
Following on the remarks made in this section, the limitations and complications of transoral laser surgery of laryngeal carcinoma should once again be pointed out. As with any other surgical procedure, the experience of the surgeon has an important influence on the complication rate. Transoral resection of large tumors is possible provided exposure is good and the surgeon has sufficient experience. The limitations of laser surgery are determined less by the technical possibilities than by the postoperative functional results.
Apart from acute dyspnea, postoperative hemorrhage is the most dangerous complication. This is preventable by meticulous intraoperative hemostasis, partly with the use of the titanium clips mentioned above. Nevertheless, even after an uneventful intraoperative course, severe postoperative bleeding can occasionally occur, demanding immediate action. In such a situation, centres experienced in the use of laser surgery for advanced laryngeal carcinomas will concentrate on rapid hemostasis by coagulation or vascular clips, followed immediately by tracheobronchoscopy. If justifiable, a tracheotomy should be avoided; controlled postoperative mechanical ventilation, e. g., for a day, should be considered.

With regard to resection of T1b glottic carcinomas, it should be emphasized that one functional aspect is the potential danger of web formation, sometimes extensive, secondary to the development of opposing wound surfaces in the region of the anterior commissure. Depending on the extent, this may result not only in considerable dysphonia, but also in stridor which will require treatment. The resection of both arytenoid cartilages is also contraindicated, due to unavoidable aspiration, and may be associated with more or less severe postoperative dysphagia, depending on the extent of the unilateral resection in the arytenoid region.
Although these serious events are rare, they must be considered when planning treatment and also, of course, when obtaining informed consent.

Partial Laryngectomy—Transcutaneous or Open Approaches

Cordectomy after Thyrotomy

Surgical Principle

After temporary division of the thyroid cartilage, excision of that part of the vocal fold affected by tumor.

Indications

Carcinoma of the vocal fold with maintained vocal fold mobility without extension into the anterior commissure or arytenoid region or sinus of Morgagni.

Operative Planning

- Clarification of general operability.
- Confirmation of the histological diagnosis by biopsy.
- Magnifying laryngoscopy to gain an impression of the tumor site and mobility of the vocal folds.
- Distending microlaryngoscopy with exact assessment of the tumor site and extent, view of the sinus of Morgagni and subglottic space using the angled telescope.

Special Instruments and Implants

Sagittal microsaw or oscillating saw. Long, slender scissors; if appropriate, ear micro-instruments. If appropriate, microscope with 30 mm object lens for endolaryngeal resection.

Anesthesia

Local anesthesia or general endotracheal anesthesia. Even when operating under general endotracheal anesthesia, tracheotomy is only necessary in exceptional cases.

Local anesthesia. Infiltration is made in a diamond-shaped fashion in the midline from the hyoid bone to the suprasternal notch, extending in a lateral direction as far as the anterior margin of the sternocleidomastoid. Additional depots are placed at both superior laryngeal nerves over the superior horn of the thyroid cartilage. Later the larynx is punctured with a needle through the exposed conical ligament and lidocaine is instilled with the syringe after prior aspiration of air.

Topical anesthesia of the opened larynx with pantocaine; infiltration of the vocal fold with lidocaine plus epinephrine.

General endotracheal anesthesia. Thin Woodbridge tube (24–28 Fr), positive–negative pressure ventilation.

Surgical Technique

Positioning. The patient is positioned flat on the operating table, shoulder elevated with a roll, head reclined. The surgeon stands on the healthy side (good view of the lesion).

Skin incision. Midline skin incision, extending from the hyoid bone to the inferior border of the cricoid cartilage (and further on to the suprasternal notch if a tracheotomy is planned). The incision is deepened exactly in the midline, down to the perichondrium of the thyroid cartilage. Traversing neck veins are ligated and the strap muscles are drawn laterally with retractors. Alternatively, an incision in a natural horizontal skin crease at the level of the cricoid cartilage is a possible option.

Thyroid cartilage dissection and division. The open thyroid cartilage perichondrium is swept aside with a dissector sponge and incised at a distance of 1 cm on the healthy side as well as on the upper and lower margin. The perichondrial flaps are swept back off the angle of the thyroid cartilage to be used later for coverage (**Fig. 10.56a**)

In the middle of the lower border of the thyroid cartilage, from the incision site of the perichondrium, the internal perichondrium is sparingly released with a Freer elevator. The sagittal saw with a rounded saw blade is placed exactly in the midline and the cartilage is divided (**Fig. 10.56b**).

Laryngotomy. The divided halves of the cartilage are drawn apart with hooks; the larynx is opened with a transverse incision at the inferior border of the thyroid cartilage, the soft tissues are divided from bottom to top either with scissors or, after inserting a hollow probe which is pushed into the anterior commissure, with the scalpel. With one stroke of the scissors the incision is extended upward into the pedicle of the epiglottis to achieve a wider opening (**Fig. 10.56c**).

The laryngeal framework is held apart with a retractor, the tube is elevated with a Langenbeck retractor, and the microscope is brought in.

The vocal fold region is infiltrated with a vasoconstricting agent without touching the tumor.

Tumor resection. An incision is made around the tumor with the sickle blade, initially superficially from posterior to anterior with a sufficient safety margin, i.e., ca. 0.5 cm. The incisions are deepened and the tumor released with fine scissors and a rasp from anterior to posterior. The incision is made through the muscle, again maintaining a safety margin to the tumor; if necessary the excision is extended as far as the internal perichondrium. The tumor is resected just before the vocal process; if the safety margin demands it, then the vocal process is also removed. Frozen-section confirmation is possible (**Fig. 10.57**).

Hemostasis and defect coverage. Meticulous hemostasis (microcoagulation). Coverage of the cordectomy area can be dispensed with (spontaneous epithelialization; a replacement vocal fold later develops from scar tissue). If resection of the vocal process was necessary, then the cartilaginous resection surface is resurfaced by elevating a small advancement flap from the region of the false cord.

Wound closure. To close the larynx, the previously incised perichondrium is returned to its position and sutured with 4/0 absorbable material (**Fig. 10.58**). If elevation of an external perichondrial flap was not possible, the soft tissue is sutured at the level of the upper and lower border of the thyroid cartilage. The musculature is approximated in layers over a half-tube rubber drain, which is brought out through the inferior wound pole to prevent the development of subcutaneous emphysema. Subcutaneous sutures and skin sutures are placed, followed by dressing gauze and adhesive tape.

Modifications

If during the operation the tumor is found to have extended beyond the cordectomy resection margins, then the operation will need to be extended.

Extended Cordectomy after St. Clair-Thompson

If the inner perichondrium has become involved from the body of the vocal fold, the external perichondrium is elevated and an incision is made from the thyrotomy site widely around the affected area of cartilage, which is then resected completely together with the attached area of vocal fold and false cord. Here too, defect coverage is not necessary, although it is possible to elevate a fascial flap from the middle (pretracheal) layer of the cervical fascia, which is turned into the wound bed and secured with fibrin glue (**Fig. 10.59**).

Frontolateral Partial Laryngectomy

If the tumor has reached the anterior commissure, then the operation must be altered to take the form of a frontolateral laryngectomy, with the result that the subsequent resection divides the tumor specimen into two parts.

! Risks and Complications

- Subcutaneous emphysema of the neck: remove some sutures, re-approximate the soft tissues to the larynx with a mild compression dressing. Surgical revision with additional waterproofing measures is necessary only in exceptional cases, when fibrin glue may be considered.
- Postoperative bleeding in the region of the neck from the cricothyroid artery: surgical revision and suture ligature; internal bleeding will require re-opening of the larynx followed by diathermy.
- Perichondritis: give antibiotics, consider wound revision.
- Mediastinitis, deep neck infection, and sepsis are virtually no longer a threat as a result of the administration of antibiotics.
- Postoperative laryngeal stenosis secondary to web formation or polyp formation: microlaryngoscopic resection.
- Tracheal stenosis following tracheotomy.
- Voice deterioration, which does however usually improve subsequently as a result of the formation of a scarred substitute vocal fold.

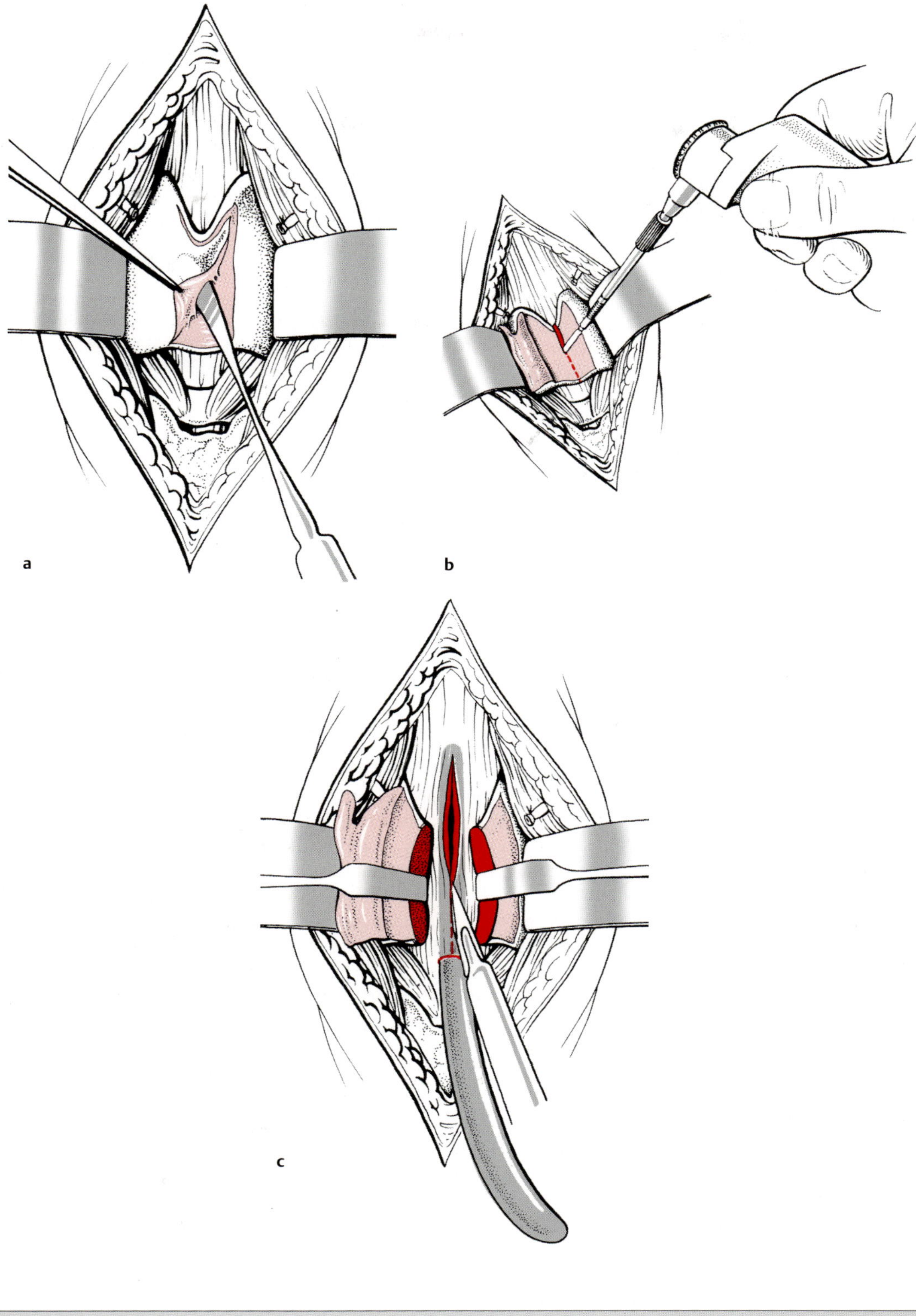

Fig. 10.56a–c Thyrotomy
a Elevation of a paramedian perichondrial flap 1 cm wide, reflecting it over to the contralateral side.
b Midline division of the thyroid cartilage using the sagittal saw.
c The inside of the larynx is opened strictly in the midline over a hollow probe inserted from below.

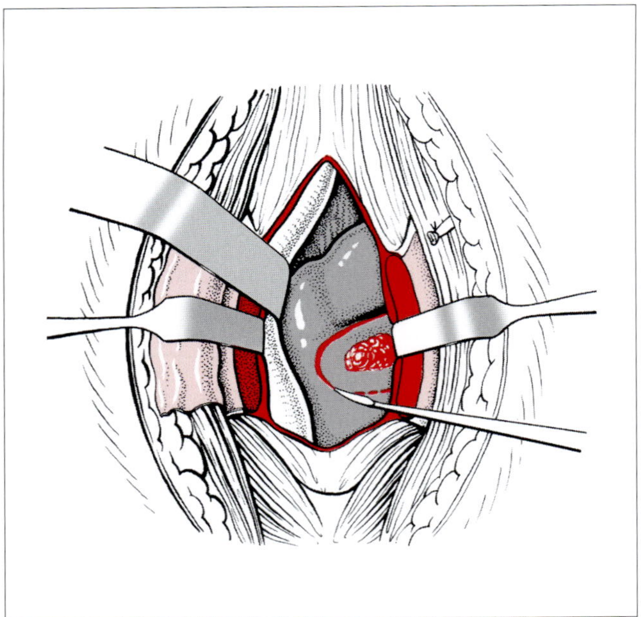

Fig. 10.57 Cordectomy.
Excision of the vocal fold using the sickle blade. The thin tube is retracted with the Langenbeck hook to allow visualization of the posterior parts of the larynx.

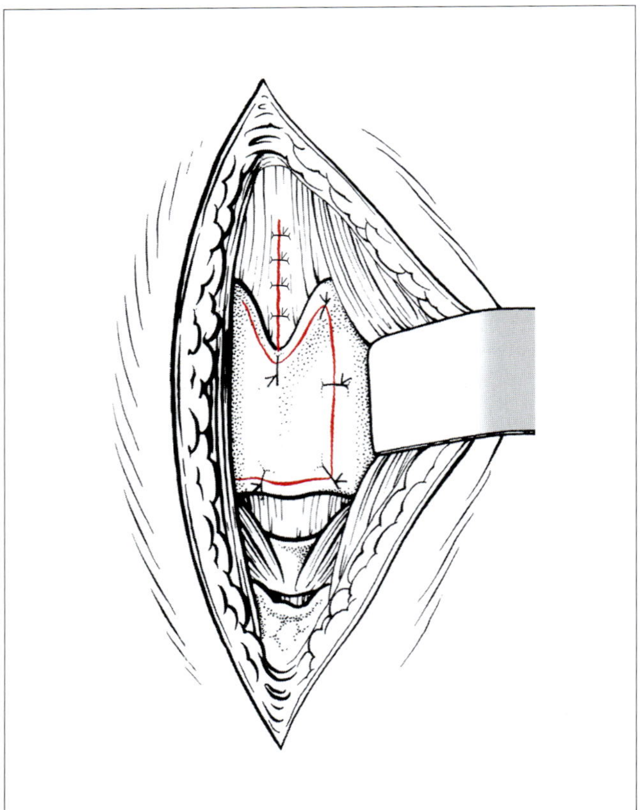

Fig. 10.58 Thyrotomy.
Closure of the larynx by suture repair of the perichondrium.

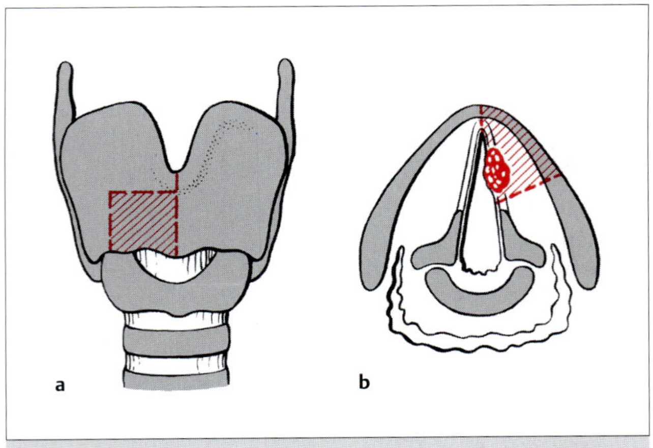

Fig. 10.59a, b Extended cordectomy after St. Clair-Thompson.
a Cartilage resection in the region of the thyroid cartilage.
b Encompassed area at the level of the vocal folds.

Postoperative Care

- Monitor breathing, inhalations, voice rest.
- Remove the rubber drain on the second postoperative day; if a tracheotomy has been done, decannulate around the seventh day.
- Antibiotics for 5 days, cough suppressants.
- Feeding tube if difficulties with swallowing (dysphagia) arise, otherwise soft diet.
- Subsequent regular follow-ups.

Alternatives

Given the excellent results that can be achieved with laser surgery, the procedure using an open approach as described above is increasingly becoming reserved only for special situations. This applies primarily to T1b vocal fold carcinomas with components in the region of the anterior commissure, which are not resectable with adequate safety margins using laser surgical technique, and cases where transoral exposure is not possible.

Frontolateral Pharyngectomy according to Leroux–Robert

Surgical Principle

Glottis carcinomas that extend into the anterior commissure or slightly onto the contralateral side may be excised, together with subglottic regions, by a triangular resection of the frontal cartilaginous component in the region of the angle of the thyroid cartilage.

Indications

Carcinomas of the vocal folds with retrograde extension as far as the vocal process, with anterior progression as far as the anterior commissure or those extending to the most anterior part of the contralateral vocal fold, laterally to the beginning of the sinus of Morgagni, but not onto its lateral wall or onto the false cord. Mobility of the vocal fold may be restricted, but not absent.

Contraindicationss

- Extension of the tumor beyond the described limits of indication, especially with involvement of the arytenoid cartilage or the cricoid.
- Severe general condition or ill-health which essentially does not allow a surgical approach.

Specific Points Regarding Informed Consent

- Sensory disturbances in the region of the neck/ear.
- Paralysis of the vocal folds and facial nerve.
- Hoarseness, even voice loss.
- Disturbances of swallowing (dysphagia), insertion of nasogastric tube.
- Dyspnea, tracheotomy with the insertion of a tracheotomy cannula.
- Unsatisfactory cosmetic result, hypertrophic scar formation.
- Possible extension of the skin incision.
- Mucosal injury, mediastinitis.

Special Instruments and Implants

Sagittal microsaw or oscillating saw, microscope, ear microinstruments.

Anesthesia

The operation is predominantly done under general endotracheal anesthesia. If a tracheotomy can be dispensed with—large larynx, a tumor that is well visualized and not too extensive—intubation is done with a thin tube (28 Fr) and positive–negative pressure ventilation.

Local anesthesia is also possible. The technique is as for cordectomy.

Surgical Technique

Positioning. The patient is positioned flat on the operating table; shoulder region elevated with a roll, the head is hyperextended backward. The surgeon stands on the healthy or less affected side.

U-shaped flap incision or midline skin incision. *U-shaped flap incision* (with the option of extension for laryngectomy if a simultaneous neck dissection is planned or there is a borderline indication): a transverse incision is made along the inferior border of the cricoid cartilage, with lateral incisions extending along the anterior margin of the sternocleidomastoid muscle to the level of the hyoid bone. The incision may also be extended upward to the mastoid with an auxiliary incision or downward and laterally to the clavicle (**Fig. 10.60**). Alternatively, *midline skin incision*: extending from the hyoid bone to below the cricoid cartilage and as far as the suprasternal notch if a tracheotomy is intended.

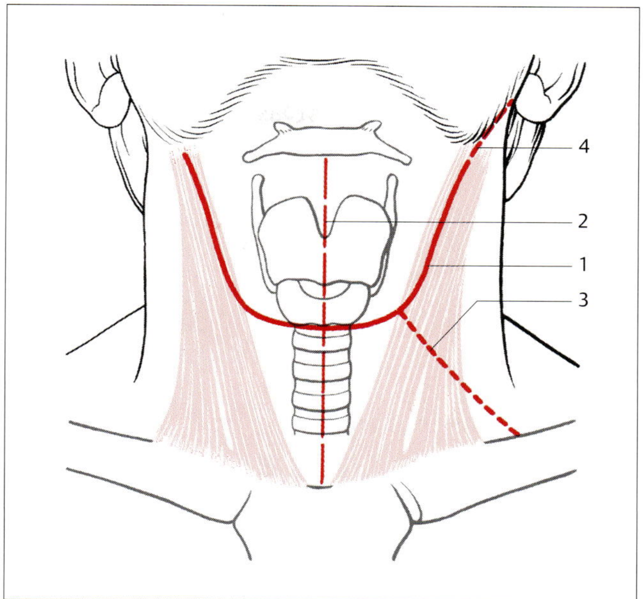

Fig. 10.60 External incision lines for laryngectomy, horizontal and vertical partial resections.
1 U-shaped flap elevation
2 midline skin incision extending from the hyoid to the suprasternal notch
3 auxiliary incision extending to the clavicle
4 extension for neck dissection

10

Dissection of the thyroid cartilage. The superficial cervical fascia is divided in the midline. The strap muscles are separated and the angle of the thyroid cartilage is identified. A pyramidal lobe or a high-riding thyroid isthmus is resected in typical fashion. If necessary, a tracheotomy is now done, followed by re-intubation.

The external perichondrium is incised in the midline and then carefully swept off beyond the intended line of cartilage excision. The perichondrium and the insertion of the conical ligament are divided at the lower border of the thyroid cartilage with a scalpel and the internal perichondrium is elevated from this position in the region of the cartilage incisions with an elevator (unnecessary if a sagittal microsaw is used).

Cartilage incision using the saw. A narrow equilateral triangle is resected if the tumor is located purely in the commissure; otherwise, if involvement is predominantly unilateral, an asymmetrical resection is done toward the more affected side. The apex of the resected cartilage triangle lies just below the laryngeal prominence; division of the two cartilage halves is accomplished by an auxiliary incision in the midline, extending downward from the thyroid notch (**Fig. 10.61**).

Opening the inside of the larynx. The conical ligament is divided along the base of the excised triangle with a scalpel. Any bleeding points encountered are coagulated. The internal laryngeal soft tissues are divided with slender scissors on the side less involved by the tumor, corresponding to the cartilage incision. For this purpose, the margins of the thyroid cartilage are held apart with small thyroid retractors. The incision may extended upward in the midline as far as the epiglottic petiole (**Fig. 10.62a**).

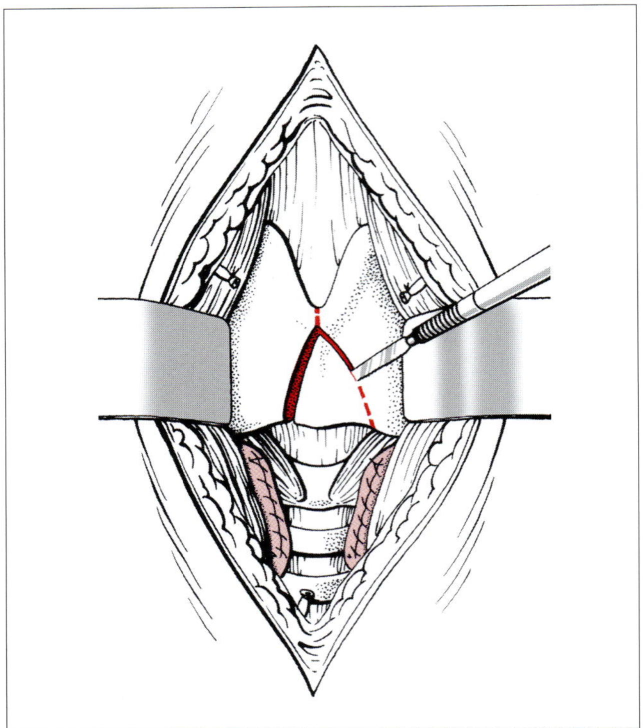

Fig. 10.61 Frontolateral partial laryngectomy.
Cartilaginous incisions. The tip of the triangle intended for resection lies beneath thyroid notch.

Tumor resection. The larynx is held open with a self-retaining retractor and the microscope adjusted. At the level of the tumor, the soft tissues are released off the thyroid cartilage perichondrium with an elevator. If a tracheotomy has not been made previously, the tube is held aside with a Langenbeck retractor. An incision is made under vision around the tumor within healthy tissue using fine scissors or ear instruments. The posterior level of excision usually ends in front of the vocal process. If the tumor has reached the vocal process it is resected, if necessary with larger parts of the arytenoid cartilage itself. Usually the superior resection margin runs within the sinus of Morgagni, with the inferior margin running along the lower border of the thyroid cartilage; these margins must, however, be adapted to the extent of the tumor. Meticulous hemostasis is achieved by immediate microcoagulation. Frozen-section confirmation is possible (**Figs. 10.62b** and **10.63**).

Defect coverage. The resulting defect is left to epithelialize spontaneously. Larger defects may require a mucosal transposition flap from the subglottic space or the region of the false cords.

Wound closure. The larynx is closed by suturing the elevated perichondrium in the thyroid notch and over the cartilage defect. If the retained vocal fold is to be released anteriorly, then it is also sutured to the perichondrium. This is covered by repair of the musculature in layers. A half-tube rubber drain is inserted and brought out through the inferior wound pole to prevent the development of subcutaneous emphysema. Subcutaneous sutures and skin sutures are placed, followed by dressing gauze and adhesive tape.

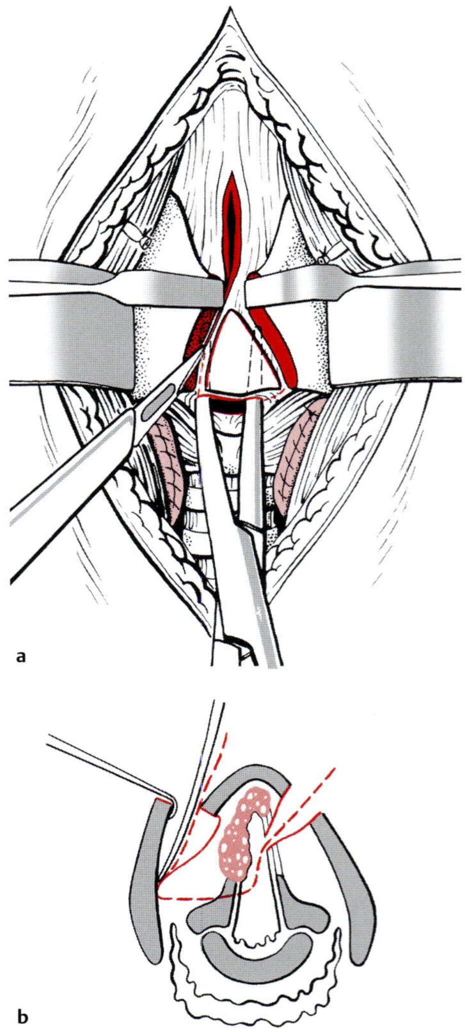

Fig. 10.62a, b Frontolateral partial laryngectomy.
a Opening of the internal larynx. Incision of the soft tissues via the conical ligament on the side less involved by tumor.
b Release is accomplished around the tumor along the cartilage.

Modification

If the tumor is situated only in the anterior commissure, an anterior partial resection is performed. This involves ipsilateral resection of the most anterior corner of the thyroid cartilage, followed by excision into the laryngeal soft tissues as already described.

! Risks and Complications

- As for cordectomy.
- The voice usually deteriorates (voice therapy).
- In rare cases, stridor secondary to scarring and web formation.

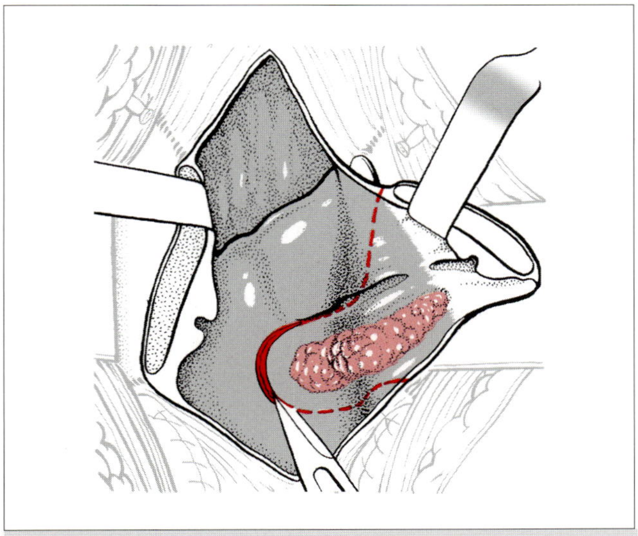

Fig. 10.63 Frontolateral partial laryngectomy.
Incision around the margins of the tumor along the mucosal aspect.

Postoperative Care

As for cordectomy. Granulation polyps often form in the anterior commissure and require excision.

Partial Laryngectomy according to Hautant

Surgical Principle

Hautant's original hemilaryngectomy—for tumors with a predominantly subglottic extension—involves the hemiresection of a vertical segment from the cricoid and thyroid cartilage. Since the posterior components of the laryngeal framework are preserved, it is not a complete hemiresection: the procedure offers the advantage, however, of a primary wound closure. The modification described here avoids any possible stenosis of the laryngeal aperture by preserving an upper arch of the thyroid cartilage. A tracheotomy is required.

Indications

Unilateral carcinoma of the vocal fold, extending anteriorly as far as the anterior commissure and reaching posteriorly onto the arytenoid cartilage, but without involving the cricoarytenoid joint and without supraglottic extension. Mobility of the vocal folds may be restricted and the tumor may extend caudally into the subglottic space.

Contraindications

- Complete involvement of the arytenoid cartilage, extension beyond the anterior or posterior commissure, encroachment of the supraglottic space.
- General disorders that do not allow major surgery.

Anesthesia

General endotracheal anesthesia. Temporary tracheotomy. Afterward, re-intubate via the tracheostoma.

Surgical Technique

Skin incision. Choice of skin incision and exposure of the larynx as for the frontolateral partial laryngectomy. This is followed by division of the thyroid isthmus and tracheotomy; if required, a neck dissection is performed first.

Elevation of a musculo-perichondrial flap. Exposure of the short strap muscles on the affected side. A flap is elevated from these muscles and the laryngeal perichondrium. An incision is placed over the thyroid cartilage, 0.5 cm lateral to the midline on the healthy side, beginning a few millimeters below the thyroid notch and extending caudally to the conical ligament. Here the flap is divided on the affected side and at the upper border of the thyroid cartilage and then released laterally from the thyroid cartilage. The base of the pedicled flap lies anterior to the posterior border of the thyroid cartilage.

Cartilage incisions. The following cartilage incisions are made with the electric saw: paramedian incision on the healthy side, extending cranially adjacent to the angle of the thyroid cartilage to ca. 0.5 cm below the thyroid notch, from where a transverse incision is made on the affected side to ca. 0.75 cm anterior to the posterior border of the thyroid cartilage, proceeding caudally parallel to the posterior border as far as the inferior border of the thyroid cartilage. The internal perichondrium is carefully released from the margin before each vertical incision. Corresponding, but slightly staggered, cartilage incisions are made through the cricoid cartilage (midline and junction between the arch and the lamina of the cricoid cartilage) (**Fig. 10.64a, b**).

Opening the inside of the larynx. The internal soft tissues are mobilized as far as the midline of the lamina of the cricoid cartilage, beginning at the posterior cartilage incision; it is important to stay close to the posterior surface of the cartilage. The arytenoid cartilage is released from its connection with the

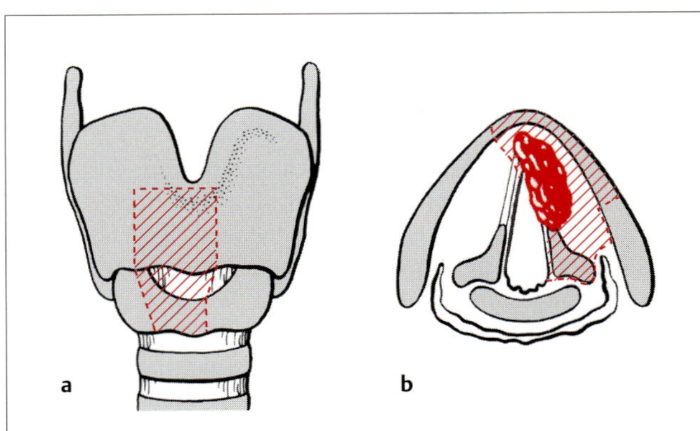

Fig. 10.64a, b Partial laryngectomy after Hautant (modified).
a Cartilage resection in the region of the thyroid and cricoid cartilages.
b Resection region at the level of the glottis.

10

lamina of the cricoid cartilage with a few strokes of the scissors. The fibrous bands attached to the conical ligament between cricoid and thyroid cartilages are also divided sharply.

The larynx is opened along the cartilage incision of the cricoid with a paramedian stepped incision through the soft tissues until beneath the thyroid notch, where the incision curves posteriorly. The specimen is taken inferiorly at the first tracheal ring. The larynx is then opened up and a longitudinal incision is made along the posterior wall in the midline. Superiorly, depending on the tumor, the specimen is taken either including the arytenoid cartilage, or preserving it, which is more favorable for the act of swallowing. Caudally the incision extends as far as the inferior border of the cricoid cartilage. The tissue that is to be removed can be released by separating and dividing the fibrous bands with scissors and excised by connecting the lateral incisions with the posterior longitudinal incision.

Defect coverage. The wound surface is covered with a large split-skin graft harvested from the thigh and secured with fibrin glue. A few additional safety sutures are also placed. The anterior part of the split-skin graft comes to lie on the replaced musculoperichondrial flap, which is secured to the preserved side of the larynx and the upper framework. The fibrin glue allows a Mikulicz tamponade to be dispensed with.

Wound closure. The wound is closed in layers as for a cordectomy.

10

! Risks and Complications

Marked hoarseness, even to the extent of aphonia. Disturbance of swallowing (dysphagia), which is often longer lasting. Risk of laryngeal stenosis secondary to scarring.

Postoperative Care

As for the frontolateral partial laryngectomy. A nasogastric tube is generally required.

Classic Hemilaryngectomy according to Gluck–Soerensen

Surgical Principle

Midline division of the larynx (medial laryngotomy), together with laminotomy and complete removal of the affected half of the larynx. The resulting defect is epithelialized with a skin flap from the neck after pulling together the pharyngeal defect. The pharyngolaryngostoma is later closed in two stages by plastic surgical technique.

The operation is technically demanding, may cause postoperative problems with swallowing and breathing, and is stressful for the patient because of the long phase of open treatment and the multistage approach.

Indications

Strictly unilateral carcinoma of the vocal fold, confined exclusively to the internal larynx without extending to the midline either anteriorly or posteriorly. Extension caudally as far as the lower border of the cricoid cartilage, cranially only as far as the laryngeal aspect of the epiglottis at most or to the aryepiglottic fold. This approach is used only in exceptional cases nowadays, given the many alternatives.

Contraindications

- Extension beyond the limits described above.
- Severe underlying general disorder, especially cardiac or pulmonary disorder.
- Distant metastases, or fixed regional metastases that cannot be completely resected within healthy tissue.
- Relative contraindication in elderly patients because of the special problems they encounter when re-learning how to swallow.

Anesthesia

General endotracheal anesthesia.

Surgical Technique

Depending on the lymph-node status, the operation may be combined with a neck dissection.

Skin incision. Laterally based, unilateral swing-door flap incision in the midline, extending from the hyoid bone to below the cricoid cartilage. Horizontal incisions as far as the sternocleidomastoid, extended if appropriate from there cranially and caudally for neck dissection. Unilateral skeletonization of the larynx (as for a total laryngectomy). Semicircular incision below the arch of the cricoid cartilage. Division of the thyroid cartilage and the cricoid cartilage from an open approach. The larynx is opened in the midline. Division of the lamina of the cricoid cartilage from an internal approach. The interarytenoid notch is divided, from where an incision is made along the aryepiglottic fold; the mucosa of the piriform sinus and that of the posterior wall of half of the larynx are elevated. Dissection of that half of the larynx. The pharyngeal mucosa is pulled together by suturing the thyroid membrane to the anterior pharyngeal wall. The swing-door flap is sutured to the mucosal margins of the posterior wall, the midline skin margins to the mucosa of the anterior commissure. Tracheostomy cannula and nasogastric tube are inserted. The laryngopharyngostoma is later closed by plastic surgical means after the healed swing-door flap is divided at its base (**Fig. 10.65a, b**).

! Risks and Complications

The operation is performed in two stages, which consequently involves a long postoperative management phase. Possible complications are:

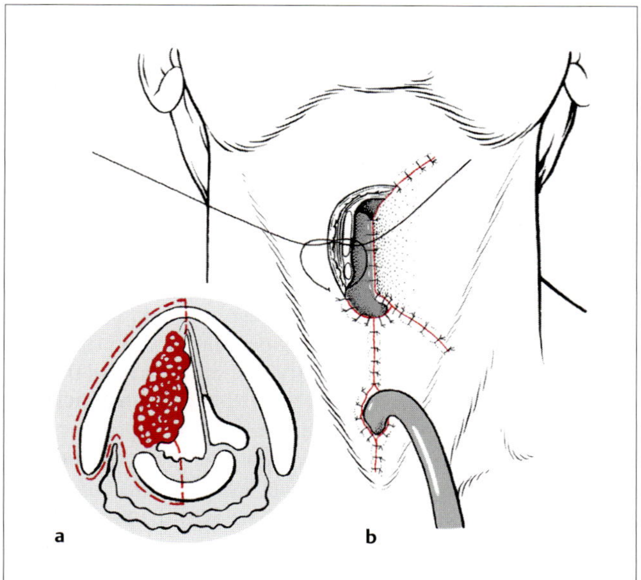

Fig. 10.65a, b Lateral hemilaryngectomy after Gluck–Soerensen.
a Resection region.
b Epithelialization of the wound surfaces, suture approximation of a swing-door flap created from external skin to the posterior mucosal incision margins. The midline skin surface is sutured to the anterior mucosal margin.

- Salivary fistula initially—obturator, frequent change of dressing.
- Sometimes considerable dysphagia—improved by using a Gollmitz suture: the swing-door flap is displaced cranially in the midline, displacing the act of swallowing to the contralateral side.
- Considerable dysphonia, possible laryngeal stenosis with the impossibility of decannulation.
- Wound infection, wound breakdown, necrosis of the swing-door flap, typical sequelae of a neck dissection and tracheotomy problems.

Horizontal Partial Laryngectomy

Surgical Principle

Excision of the supraglottic components of the larynx together with the epiglottis and the pre-epiglottic space. A tracheotomy is necessary. A selective or modified radical neck dissection is usually performed, depending on the state of the cervical lymph nodes.

The classic procedure of a transverse supraglottic resection as described by Alonso has meanwhile undergone several modifications. A modification according to Leroux-Robert, and Gosepath is now described.

Indications

- Tumors of the laryngeal aperture extending as far as the false cords.
- Carcinoma of the epiglottis, including the lingual epiglottic surface, even involving of the aryepiglottic fold and slight extension into the vallecula.

Contraindicationss

- Invasion of the piriform sinus or the cricoarytenoid joint; tumor involvement of the floor of the sinus of Morgagni, or invasion of the base of the tongue.
- Severe underlying general disorder, distant metastases, untreatable regional metastases.
- Old age (difficulties with re-learning how to swallow).
- Severely restricted pulmonary ventilation.

Special Instruments and Implants

Sagittal microsaw.

Anesthesia

General endotracheal anesthesia. Tracheotomy. Re-intubation.

Surgical Technique

Incision. U-shaped skin incision, extended upward on the neck-dissection side as far as the mastoid, with a corresponding incision on the contralateral side (for bilateral neck dissection) or reaching just above the hyoid bone. A transverse incision is placed at the level of the inferior cricoid border. An auxiliary incision down to the clavicle may be required for the neck dissection. Platysma and cutaneous veins are divided and the skin flap elevated (see **Fig. 10.60**). First, the neck dissection is performed, followed by exposure of the trachea, tracheotomy and re-intubation.

Skeletonization of the larynx. Using the electric saw, the strap muscles and the muscles of the floor of the mouth are released from the hyoid bone, which is later removed. The thyrohyoid, sternohyoid, and omohyoid muscles are then reflected inferiorly. The tissue over the exposed superior border of the thyroid cartilage, medial to the superior horn, is bluntly spread apart with dissecting pledgets to allow the superior laryngeal blood vessels to be isolated, ligated, and divided. *At the same time the superior laryngeal nerve, which runs parallel to the vessels, must be identified and protected as far as possible* (**Fig. 10.66**).

Laryngotomy. The perichondrium is incised along the superior border of the thyroid cartilage, the superior horn, and the most superior quarter of the posterior border, while the external lamina is elevated for a distance of 1 cm with the Freer elevator. From the incision margin, the internal soft tissues together with the internal perichondrial membrane are released on either side from the superior thyroid cartilage down to below the thyroid notch.

Resection of the thyroid cartilage. Resection of both upper parts of the thyroid cartilage with the saw or cartilage scissors, obliquely from the insertion of the horn anteriorly until just below the notch (consider further resection after opening the larynx).

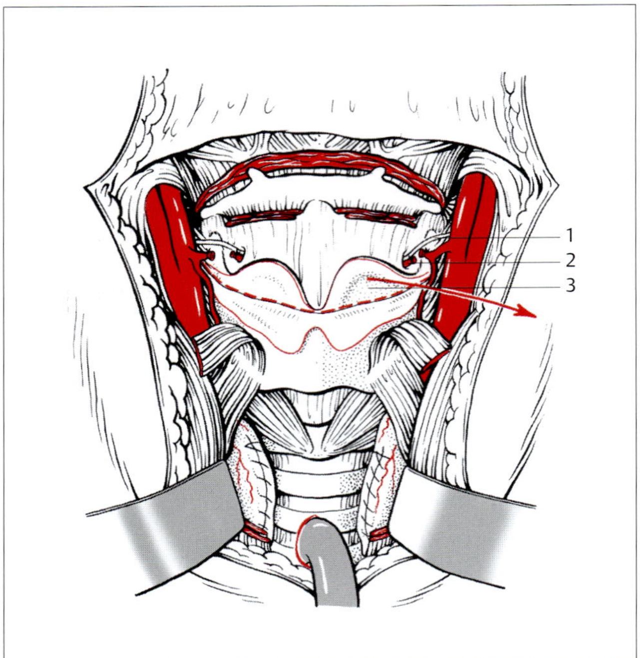

Fig. 10.66 Supraglottic partial laryngectomy.
Skeletonization of the superior larynx: the superior laryngeal vessels are ligated (2), the superior laryngeal nerve (1) is preserved, cartilage resection (3), perichondrium is released.

Pharyngotomy and resection of the tumor. The pharynx is opened using scissors laterally on the less involved side, anterior and superior to the dissected superior laryngeal nerve; superiorly the incision curves medially to the hyoid bone (**Fig. 10.67a**). Inserting a Langenbeck retractor into the gap will expose the epiglottis, allowing it to be drawn forward. The incision is now extended transversely along the hyoid bone to the contralateral side under direct vision using the electric saw and is then curved back again lateral to the epiglottis down toward the piriform sinus. Drawing the epiglottis in a caudal direction will offer the surgeon, who now changes position to the head end, a view of the entire tumor region. The incision then proceeds from the beginning of the piriform sinus through the soft tissues, which have been released from their attachments to the internal perichondrium, to just before the arytenoid cartilage. On the more affected side, this incision may be carried into the mucosa of the superior piriform sinus, while on the contralateral side it extends along the superior border of the aryepiglottic fold (**Fig. 10.67b**). The superior laryngeal nerve must be bluntly held aside by the assistant during this resection stage, as well as during the following stage in the region of the ventricle of Morgagni, to preserve it at least on the side less involved by tumor. From both sides of the arytenoid cartilage, the incision is made in the supraglottis in an anterior direction, keeping the supraglottic part containing the tumor continuously under tension; both incisions meet superior to the anterior commissure of the vocal folds, thus completing the resection (**Fig. 10.67c**).

10

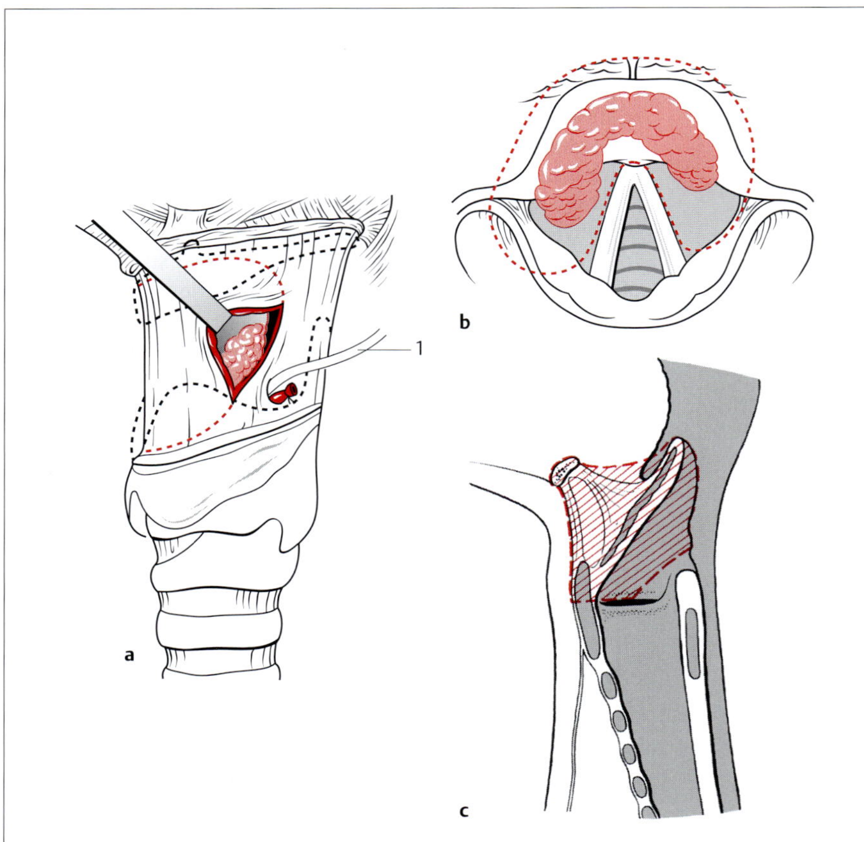

Fig. 10.67a–c Supraglottic partial laryngectomy.
- **a** Lateral opening of the larynx on the side less affected by the tumor. The incision is extended in a superior direction.
  1 superior laryngeal nerve
- **b** Incision line.
- **c** Lateral view of the resection area with inclusion of the epiglottis and the preepiglottic space.

If the tumor extends to the vallecula, its extent is assessed by palpation before making the transverse incision into the base of the tongue, in order to place the incision far enough within healthy tissue. The lamina of the thyroid cartilage can be resected, at least unilaterally and if necessary to just above the level of the vocal fold, to provide a better view into the inside of the larynx. *The anterior commissure, however, must not be released.*

Wound closure. The incision margins of the sinus of Morgagni/vocal fold and piriform sinus are approximated posteriorly with 4/0 absorbable suture material.

Coverage of the border of the thyroid cartilage. Anteriorly this is accomplished by turning over the released external perichondrium and suturing it with the incision margin of the vocal fold/sinus of Morgagni (**Fig. 10.68a**). *These sutures must be tight.* On the side not bearing the tumor, resection of the thyroid cartilage lamina should therefore not be too extensive *because a certain degree of tension of the external perichondrium, which is draped over the border of the thyroid cartilage, will later widen the glottis*; some authors dispense with all mucosal sutures and still achieve good results.

Pharynx suture. Closure of the pharyngostoma is achieved with strong absorbable sutures inserted through the prelaryngeal musculature and the thyroid cartilage and superiorly into the base of the tongue, immediately next to the mucosal margin. Three strong sutures are required on either side; the posterior part of the pharyngostoma is closed with inverting sutures. *The firm sutures from the larynx to the base of the tongue are all placed first, and then knotted after raising the previously reclined head.* This brings the base of the tongue to lie over the laryngeal aperture and later also serves to protect the larynx during the act of swallowing (**Fig. 10.68b**).

The divided strap muscles are also secured to the muscles of the base of the tongue. The U-shaped flap is folded back into place and suction drains are inserted on either side of the neck to also come to lie over the larynx. This is followed by closure of the wound in layers.

> **!** **Risks and Complications**
> - Stenosis of the laryngeal aperture due to chronic edema formation, ankylosis of the arytenoid cartilage, scar formation,
> - Wound breakdown, in rare cases pharyngeal fistulas.
> - Aspiration, aspiration pneumonia.
> - Permanent dysphagia, possibly dysphonia secondary to persisting edema or severe scar formation in the arytenoid region.

Postoperative Care

- Enteral nutrition, usually for 10–15 days. *To practise the act of swallowing: incline the head forward and sideways to the less involved side before swallowing.*
- Antibiotic coverage. Monitoring of the tracheostoma, frequent suctioning, consider administering atropine if there is a strong propensity to aspiration.
- Decannulate depending on the width of the glottis; consider administering a steroid in the presence of significant edema.

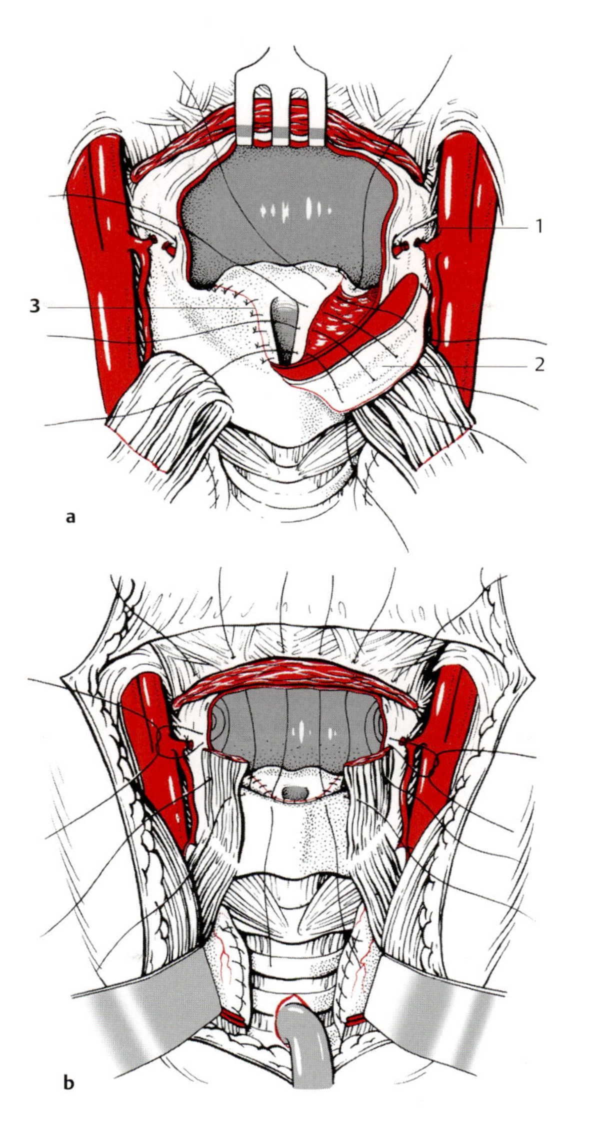

Fig. 10.68a, b Supraglottic partial laryngectomy.
a Mucosal sutures. Superior laryngeal nerve (1). Coverage of the cartilage by approximating the perichondrium (2) with the mucosal margin (3).
b Closure of the pharyngostoma using deep sutures through the prelaryngeal muscles, thyroid cartilage, and base of the tongue.

Supracricoid Partial Laryngectomy with Cricohyoidopexy Reconstruction

Subtotal partial laryngectomy with cricohyoido(epiglotto)pexy reconstruction was first reported by the Austrian surgeons Maier and Reider in 1959. Both of these procedures are widely employed in France, Italy, and North America for the management of T1 to T3 laryngeal carcinomas. In contrast, the good functional oncological results of partial endolaryngeal laser surgical laryngectomy achieved in Germany have resulted in a clear decrease in the number of so-called conventional extralaryngeal partial laryngectomies. Nevertheless, not all laryngeal carcinomas can be optimally resected via an endolaryngeal approach. The indication for cricohyoido(epiglotto)pexy may be justified in patients with carcinoma of the anterior commissure, carcinoma of the epiglottic petiole, or extensive supra- or transglottic laryngeal carcinomas, because these tumors may have unsatisfactorily high local recurrence rates after endolaryngeal partial laryngectomy or after primary radiochemotherapy alone. Depending on the extent of the tumor, the epiglottis can also be resected during resection of the tumor (so-called cricohyoidopexy), or preserved in its cranial part (cricohyoidoepiglottopexy).

Indications

Transglottic and supraglottic carcinomas:

- with involvement of the infrahyoid epiglottis or the ventricle;
- or with vocal fold fixation;
- and/or limited invasion of the pre-epiglottic space, but without fixation of the arytenoid cartilage;
- or with limited invasion of the thyroid ala without extension through the external perichondrium.

Contraindications

- Fixation of the arytenoid cartilage. Unlike vocal fold fixation, fixation of the arytenoid cartilage demonstrates involvement of the cricoarytenoid musculature or the cricoarytenoid joint. The cricoid cartilage cannot therefore be excluded from any oncologically based therapeutic approach.
- Infraglottic extension of the tumor more than either 10 mm anteriorly or 5 mm posterolaterally. Extension into these areas indicates possible involvement of the cricoid cartilage.
- Extensive invasion of the pre-epiglottic space. This is clinically evident by the presence of a bulge below the vallecula and/or expansion through the thyrohyoid membrane.
- Tumor extension superior to the hyoid bone or below the cricoid cartilage. Resection of these structures renders any reconstruction impossible.
- External perichondrial invasion of the thyroid cartilage. An extralaryngeal expansion of the tumor is a contraindication for organ-preserving surgery of the larynx.
- The operation cannot be performed adequately if the patient has been provided with a tracheostoma preoperatively.
- Poor general condition, especially with regard to pulmonary function, is a relative contraindication. A rule of thumb is that the patient should be able to climb two flights of stairs without becoming short of breath. Poor cognitive function is another relative contraindication because postoperative rehabilitation requires close cooperation with the patient.

Surgical Technique

- A bimastoid apron flap is elevated, extending inferiorly no further than two finger-breadths above the sternum. The tracheotomy is placed in line with the skin incision. A smaller incision is possible if no neck dissection is planned. A superior subplatysmal flap should be raised to a level of 2 cm superior to the hyoid bone. No inferior flap should be raised, to allow the tracheotomy to be more easily isolated and thus avoid the postoperative penetration of air into the neck.
- Superior laryngeal neurovascular structures must be identified bilaterally and protected. Preservation of laryngeal innervation is vital for a successful postoperative course.
- Division of the cervical fascia to expose the strap muscles in the midline from the superior border of the laryngeal cartilage to the level of the first tracheal rings (**Fig. 10.69**). These muscles are then divided, together with the sternohyoid and thyrohyoid muscles at the level of the superior border of the thyroid cartilage but not at the hyoid bone. These muscle flaps are retracted laterally and secured in this position bilaterally with sutures. In addition, the sternohyoid muscles are again divided at the inferior border of the thyroid cartilage, without injuring the underlying thyroid gland. The inferior constrictor muscles are transected at the posterolateral border of the thyroid cartilage. Next, the internal thyroid perichondrium and the piriform sinus are elevated and the latter is now opened. How far the perichondrium on the side involved by the tumor is elevated

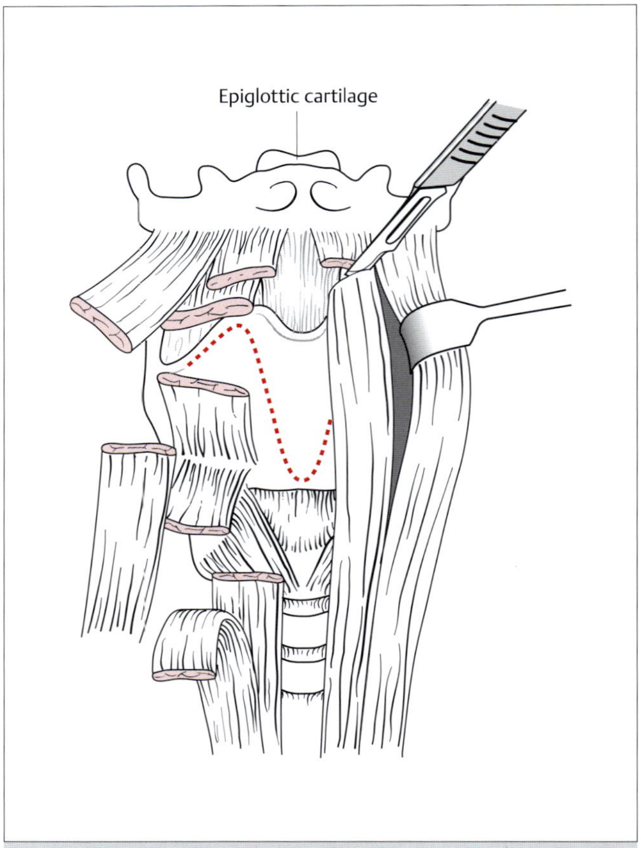

Fig. 10.69 Supracricoid partial laryngectomy with cricohyoidopexy (CHP).
Division of the strap muscles from the superior border of the thyroid cartilage and extending to the level of the first tracheal rings.

depends on the location of the tumor; elevation of the first third of the cartilage is often sufficient. On the contralateral side, the entire piriform sinus should be opened as far as the midline.

- Now follows the disarticulation of the cricothyroid joint (**Fig. 10.70**). A Freer elevator is placed on the inferior horn of the thyroid cartilage to disarticulate the joint. It is imperative here not to injure the recurrent laryngeal nerve. The region posterior and lateral to the inferior horn of the thyroid cartilage is avoided in order not to injure the nerve in this area. Both cricothyroid joints are disarticulated, before the isthmus of the thyroid gland is transected and sutured. Blunt dissection is used along the anterior wall of the trachea to divide adhesions, which can impair mobility of the trachea during reconstruction.
- Incision of the cricothyroid membrane along the superior border of the cricoid cartilage. Incision of the periosteum of the inferior hyoid bone. The larynx is entered via a small transvallecular pharyngeal incision. Now the epiglottis is drawn out (**Fig. 10.71**) and entire pre-epiglottic space is removed. The incisions are made medial to the main trunk of the internal branch of the superior laryngeal nerve. The false cord is transected where it adjoins the arytenoid. The vocal process and the true cords are divided directly posterior to the ventricle. It is essential here that the arytenoid cartilage is preserved on the side of the larynx not involved by the tumor. The cricoarytenoid joint must also be protected, to avoid the development of postoperative ankylosis. The pre-arytenoid incisions are connected with the cricothyroidotomy (**Fig. 10.72**). The cricothyroid and the lateral cricoarytenoid musculature are divided along the superior border of the cricoid cartilage. The surgeon takes hold of both thyroid alae, one in each hand, and cracks open the cartilage in the middle (like opening a book). Resection of the tumor is continued under direct vision. It is essential to preserve the posterior arytenoid mucosa to maintain adequate postoperative swallowing function. The subsequent resection is continued as described previously. Complete resection therefore includes the tumor, the epiglottis, the thyroid cartilage, the true vocal cords, the false cords, and possibly one arytenoid, completely or partially resected.
- Reconstruction begins after the pathology results are received. The arytenoid cartilage (or the posterior arytenoid mucosa) must be drawn forward to ensure that it remains in the correct position postoperatively. This is achieved with a 3/0 or 4/0 Vicryl suture placed directly above the vocal process (or in the arytenoid mucosa), fixing the cartilage at the superior end of the cricoid with an air knot. The

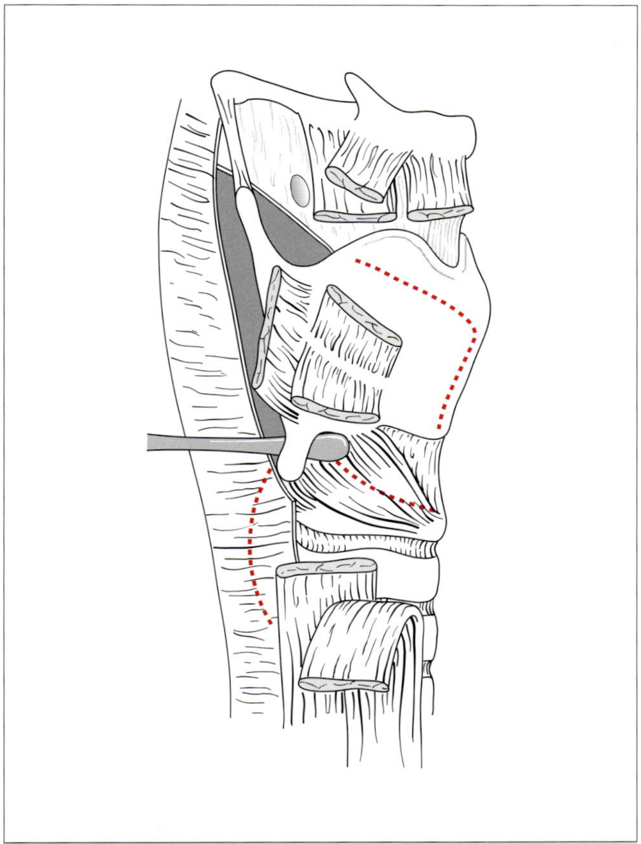

Fig. 10.70 Cricohyoidopexy.
Bilateral dislocation of the cricothyroid joint. The region posterior and lateral to the inferior horn of the thyroid cartilage is avoided in order not to injure the recurrent nerve.

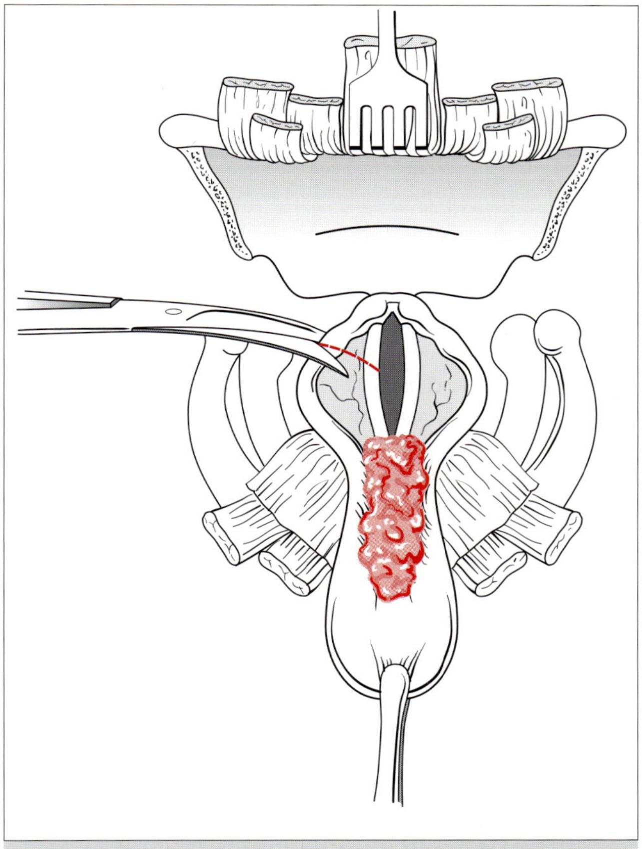

Fig. 10.71 Cricohyoidopexy.
After entering the larynx via a small transvallecular pharyngotomy, the epiglottis is drawn outward, after which the entire pre-epiglottic space is removed.

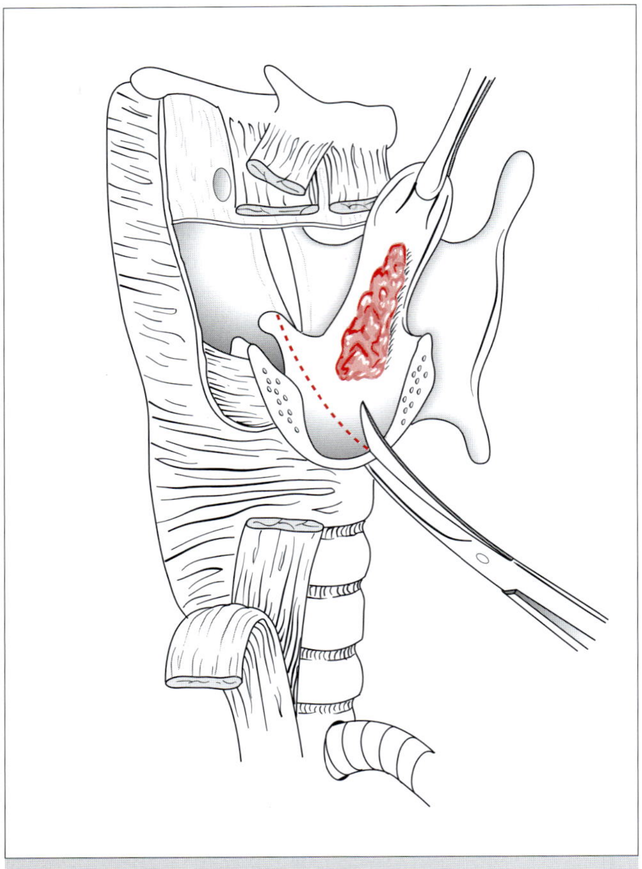

Fig. 10.72 Cricohyoidopexy.
Particular attention should be paid to ensure protection of the posterior arytenoid mucosa to allow a sufficient postoperative swallowing function.

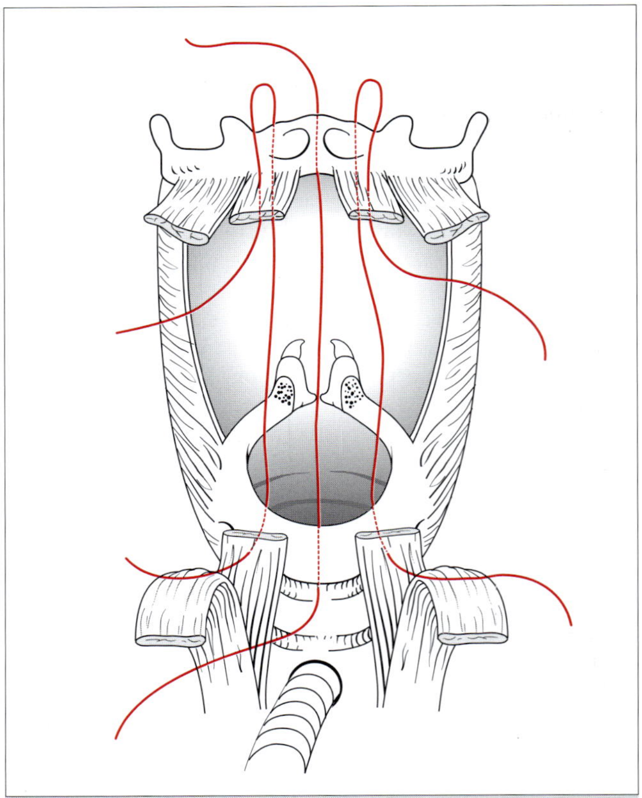

Fig. 10.73 Cricohyoidopexy.
Positioning the sutures.

arytenoids therefore do not remain at the posterior pharyngeal wall.

- A suture is placed on either side in the incision margin of the pharyngeal constrictor muscle, but not tied. This is followed by the cricohyoidopexy (**Figs. 10.73** and **10.74**). A 1/0 Vicryl suture with a 65-mm needle is used to place a submucosal stitch around the cricoid cartilage, exactly in the midline. The needle is then passed around the hyoid and deep into the musculature of the tongue base. This suture must be placed exactly in the midline and in the submucosal layer. Finally the needle is brought out at the base of the tongue and around the hyoid. This suture is not pulled tight until two further similar stitches have been placed exactly 1 cm either side of the midline. Any more stitches would fix the base of the tongue in place and the neolarynx would not be sufficiently covered. The cricohyoidotomy tube is removed before pulling the sutures tight; the trachea is lifted by pulling tight the two lateral cricohyoidopexy sutures. A tracheotomy is created in line with the skin incision. The tracheotomy tube is inserted into the tracheal opening. Now the cricohyoidopexy sutures may be securely tied—first the middle one, then the two lateral sutures.

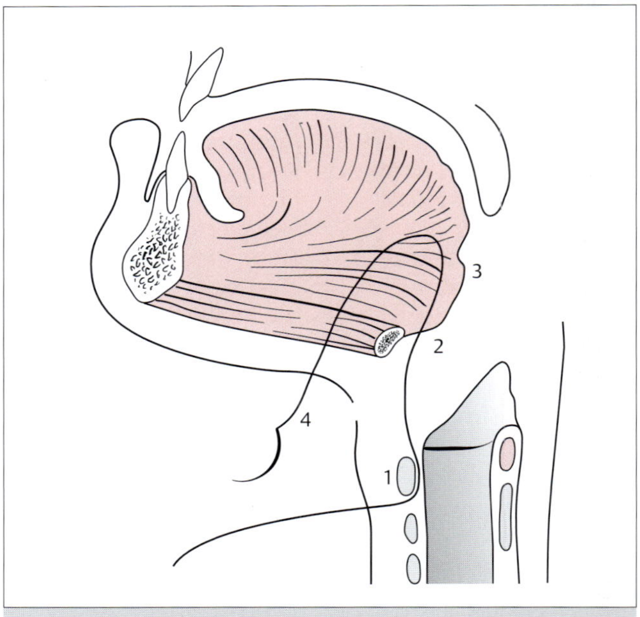

Fig. 10.74 Cricohyoidopexy.
Lateral view showing placement of the suture.
1 cricoid cartilage
2 hyoid bone
3 base of the tongue
4 suture

- During wound closure, it should be ensured that the region around the tracheotomy is separated from the rest of the wound with subcutaneous sutures. Wound closure is accomplished in two layers over a drain.

! Complications

The most frequent complication is pneumonia secondary to aspiration, with a frequency reported to be between 1.5% and >35%. These cases of pneumonia are typically not chronic and do not recur, as demonstrated in the literature by the low rate of permanent gastrostomies (1–4%) and the low frequency of laryngectomies due to untreatable aspiration (6%). Pneumonia is usually treated conservatively with antibiotics. Other complications such as wound dehiscence and laryngeal stenosis occur only very rarely. There is a slightly higher incidence of local complications in post-radiotherapy patients.

Rules, Tips, and Tricks

If fracture of the cricoid membrane occurs during closure, the cricohyoidopexy sutures are placed around the first two tracheal rings.

Supracricoid Partial Laryngectomy with Cricohyoidoepiglottopexy Reconstruction

Surgical Principle

Supracricoid partial laryngectomy with cricohyoidoepiglottopexy reconstruction is an effective surgical procedure for treating glottic carcinomas. Excellent follow-up results have been achieved and the functionality of speech and swallowing obtained without a permanent tracheostoma.

Indications

- Bilateral vocal cord involvement, with or without anterior commissure involvement (horseshoe lesion).
- Unilateral glottic carcinoma with anterior commissure involvement.
- Impaired true vocal fold mobility with limited subglottic (<1 cm) and ventricular extension.
- T3 glottic lesions with fixation of the true vocal fold and either impaired or mobile arytenoid.
- T4 glottic carcinomas with limited thyroid cartilage invasion.

Contraindications

The most important contraindication for supracricoid partial laryngectomy with cricohyoidoepiglottopexy is the preoperative evidence of poor respiratory function. Supracricoid partial laryngectomy alters the sphincter function of the larynx and so respiratory reserves are necessary to respond to the increased postoperative risk of aspiration with the simultaneous risk of atelectasis and pneumonia. *Patients who are unable to climb two flights of stairs without becoming short of breath should not undergo this type of procedure.*

Oncological contraindications:

- Tumors originating in the anterior commissure or ventricle. Such tumors have a propensity for early invasion of the pre-epiglottic space. They may be resected by supracricoid partial laryngectomy with cricohyoidopexy.
- Tumors of the glottis with ipsilateral fixation of the arytenoid cartilage.
- Tumors of the glottis with extension to the subglottis, reaching to the upper border of the cricoid cartilage or invading the cricoid cartilage.
- Tumors of the glottis invading the posterior commissure.
- Tumors of the glottis invading the outer perichondrium of the thyroid cartilage or with extralaryngeal spread of the tumor.

Surgical Technique

The initial operative steps are the same as for Cricohyoidopexy (CHP) (p. 251) as far as the incision of the cricothyroid membrane.

After completed transverse cricothyroidotomy, access to the larynx is gained superior to the false cords. This essentially avoids the entire epiglottis and the pre-epiglottic space. An Allis clamp is placed on the epiglottic petiole and drawn through the incision to facilitate direct visualization of the endolarynx. Resection is continued along the side with less tumor invasion. Curved Mayo incisions are used for the vertical part of the resection. One blade of the scissors is inside the laryngeal lumen, while the other lies between thyroid cartilage and elevated internal perichondrium of the thyroid cartilage. The incision begins anterior to the arytenoid cartilage, protecting the vocal process and the cricoarytenoid musculature. The incision allows resection of the entire false cord, posterior to the ventricle. The entire vocal fold is resected before an incision is placed below the level of the cricothyroid musculature and the subglottic mucosa to connect the operation to the horizontal cricothyrotomy. The larynx is opened like a book, allowing the resection on the side bearing the tumor to be performed under direct vision. Resection is continued from the cricoid cartilage in a cranial direction. If necessary, the arytenoid cartilage is removed, but the posterior arytenoid musculature on the affected side must be protected. T3 glottic carcinomas always require resection of the ipsilateral arytenoid cartilage and the ipsilateral cricoarytenoid muscle to leave adequate margins around the posterior and inferior paraglottic space. Specimens are taken from the inferior and posterior margins of the surgical site and analyzed to confirm that the extent of resection has been adequate. The further operative course again corresponds to the technique described for CHP, except for wound closure (**Fig. 10.75**).

Comment

The invasive nature of the conventional surgical transcervical laryngectomy described above, possible delayed wound healing, and the sometimes considerable functional deficits substantiate the superiority, confirmed by various surgeons, of the

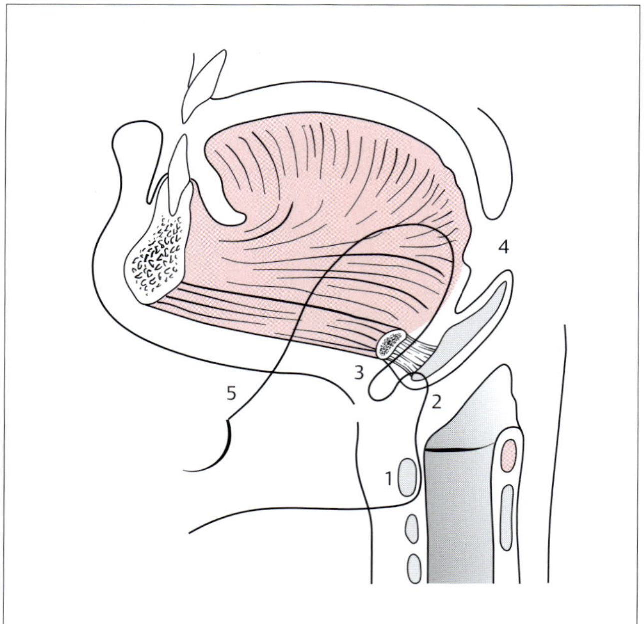

Fig. 10.75 Supracricoid partial laryngectomy with cricohyoidoepiglottopexy (CHEP).
Lateral view showing placement of the suture.
1 cricoid cartilage
2 base of the epiglottis
3 hyoid bone
4 base of the tongue
5 suture

endolaryngeal laser surgical technique of tumor resection. The clearly reduced hospitalization times often achieved with this technique, and especially the often better quality of life immediately postoperatively, must not, however, be achieved at the cost of oncologically poorer outcomes. Again, it is not a question here of a one-sided endorsement of only one operative technique. Knowledge of alternative surgical procedures contributes to making the decision best suited for each individual patient. Only once it is accepted that the choice of a surgical and/or radiochemotherapeutic treatment that is adapted to the individual situation can attain consensus only when founded on broad expertise will it be possible to comprehensively guarantee the adequate care of cancer patients in future.

Total Laryngectomy

Surgical Principle

Removal of the entire larynx from the base of the tongue to the trachea, if necessary with the resection of adjacent parts of the tongue, pharynx, trachea, or thyroid gland. Trachea and esophagus are separated by primary closure of the pharynx and suturing the trachea to the suprasternal notch.

Indications

Defining the indication for laryngectomy is proving to be more difficult today than it was in the 1990s. The reason for this current doubt is that treatment procedures sometimes compete with each other and their effectiveness has not been definitively and conclusively assessed. Mention is made here both of the further developments of transoral laser surgery and also of organ-preserving protocols, in part combined with chemo-induction therapy or radiochemotherapy. Both techniques harbour various possibilities, as well as risks, with organ preservation in principle only being achievable with difficulty in the presence of deep infiltration of the laryngeal framework. Apart from this, still classic, indication for laryngectomy (provided a partial resection is not adequate), there are several other indications that merit consideration in individual cases:

- Laryngeal carcinomas that exceed the indication limitations for laser surgical resection or conventional surgical horizontal or vertical partial resection.
- Supraglottic carcinomas with extension to the glottis or relevant invasion of the base of the tongue.
- Glottic carcinomas with bilateral involvement of the arytenoid cartilage.
- Extensive bilateral tumor involvement with immobility or restricted mobility of the vocal folds.
- Carcinomas with penetration through the cartilage and tumor invasion of the surrounding tissue.
- Carcinomas that have penetrated into the piriform sinus from the inside out or carcinomas of the piriform sinus or hypopharynx with invasion of the laryngeal framework and involvement of the arytenoid cartilage.
- Tumor recurrences after previous partial resection or unsuccessful radiotherapy or radio(chemo)therapy, e.g., also for processes that have followed organ-preserving protocols.
- Severe traumatic destruction of the larynx with failed attempt at plastic reconstruction.
- Extension of the operation in cases where the limitations of the indication have been exceeded during partial resection or after persistent dysphagia following partial resection.

Contraindicationss

- Severe general disorders or poor general condition precluding operability.
- Incurable distant metastases or synchronous tumors.
- Undissectable encasement of the common or internal carotid artery by metastases or continuous growth of a tumor.
- Extensive tumor invasion into the deep parts of the tongue or breaching of the prevertebral fascia.

Specific Points Regarding Informed Consent

- Sensory disturbances in the region of the neck/ears.
- Paralysis of the levator scapulae, vagus, phrenic, lingual, hypoglossal, and facial nerves.
- Disturbances of swallowing (dysphagia), insertion of a nasogastric tube.
- Dribbling of saliva/food from the wound.

- Voice loss, inability to learn esophageal speech, and malfunction of the voice prosthesis.
- Dyspnea, insertion of a tracheostomy cannula.
- Tracheitis, tracheal stenosis, tracheostomal stenosis.
- Poor healing of the skin flap or the tracheostoma.
- Possible extension of the skin incision.
- Mucosal injury, mediastinitis.
- Possible elevation of a musculocutaneous flap from the chest with extension to the neck.
- Musculocutaneous flap failure.

Operative Planning

- Clarification of the patient's general operability.
- Confirmation of the histological diagnosis by biopsy.
- Verification of the extent of the tumor by magnifying laryngoscopy and microlaryngoscopy, also with the aid of angled telescopes.
- Hypopharyngo-esophagoscopy (extent of the tumor, synchronous tumors).
- Ultrasonography of the cervicofacial lymph nodes.
- CT of the neck and thorax to determine the extent of the tumor and to exclude distant metastases.

Anesthesia

General endotracheal anesthesia. Transoral intubation, with reintubation into the tracheal stump after removal of the larynx. If the tumor renders intubation difficult, use a thin tube and consider emergency endoscopy.

Surgical Technique

Skin incision. U-shaped flap incision, with the transverse incision usually lying below the cricoid cartilage (**Fig. 10.60**); if the resection of tracheal rings is intended, the incision is placed lower, corresponding to the planned resection. The incision extends laterally to the sternocleidomastoid muscle and on the neck dissection side as far as the tip of the mastoid, away from the inferior wound pole to the middle of the clavicle. It ends on the contralateral side, above the hyoid bone, provided a bilateral neck dissection is not intended. The incision is deepened, while ligating the superficial neck veins, the flap is incised with inclusion of the platysma and beyond the hyoid bone, elevated and secured. Neck dissection then follows.

Neck dissection. Depending on the involvement of the lymph nodes as assessed on ultrasound, a selective or modified radical, unilateral, or bilateral neck dissection is undertaken. The corresponding indications are discussed in detail in Chapter 11.

Skeletonization of the larynx. The muscles are detached from the hyoid bone with the electric knife and the omohyoid and sternohyoid muscles are reflected downward. The muscle insertions at the oblique line of the thyroid cartilage are resected, again with the electric knife, and the insertions to the sternum reflected downward (**Fig. 10.76**).

If the thyroid gland is high-riding or enlarged, the isthmus is tunnelled and resected and the stumps suture ligated, allowing them to be dissected bluntly off the laryngeal framework. This brings the cricothyroid artery into view as it comes more under tension when the larynx is retracted sideward, allowing it to be ligated exactly. The laryngeal artery and vein, which traverse over the superior horn of the thyroid cartilage, are then ligated and divided after spreading apart the overlying tissues (**Fig. 10.77**).

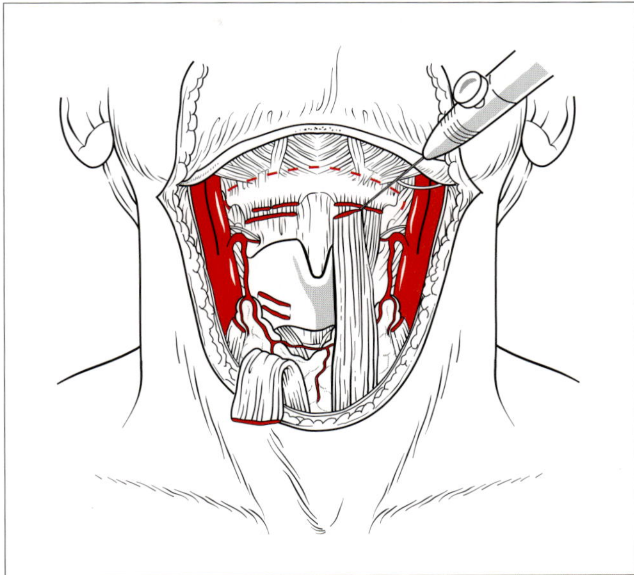

Fig. 10.76 Laryngectomy.
Division of the prelaryngeal muscles.

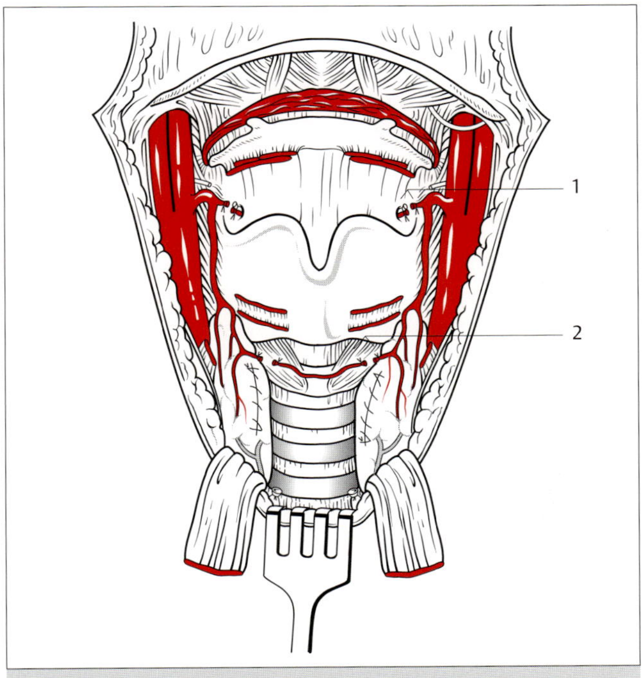

Fig. 10.77 Laryngectomy.
Ligation of the laryngeal vessels.
1 inferior laryngeal artery
2 cricothyroid artery

Detachment of the pharyngeal constrictor muscle. The larynx is retracted to the contralateral side with a single hook, while the thyroid gland is held aside with a Langenbeck retractor. The pharyngeal constrictor muscle is divided sharply at its insertion anterior to the posterior border of the thyroid cartilage with an incision extending from the superior to the interior horn of the thyroid cartilage and also dividing the perichondrium. Both muscle and perichondrium are swept back with a Freer elevator along the length of the incision to the posterior border of the thyroid cartilage. From here, the piriform sinus is released in a subperichondral plane from the internal surface of the thyroid cartilage using a dissecting swab (**Fig. 10.78**).

Release of the larynx. The larynx is drawn downward with single hooks and the base of the tongue is elevated with a wide Langenbeck retractor. The entire musculature of the floor of the mouth and tongue is removed above the hyoid bone with an electric knife, and the hyoid is released. Any bleeding is immediately coagulated.

Pharyngotomy. Pre-epiglottic tissue is grasped with a clamp and drawn downward. The pharynx is opened transversely at the level of the hyoid bone with an electric knife, allowing a clamp to be passed through the opening to grasp the epiglottis and draw it forward and downward (**Fig. 10.79a, b**). The mucosa on either side of the epiglottis is incised through the opening under direct vision and by palpation (the line of incision is adapted to the requirements of the tumor). The incision runs along the aryepiglottic fold at the superior border of the piriform sinus to behind the arytenoid cartilage. The incisions extend on either side and are connected with a transverse incision behind and beneath the arytenoid cartilages. To avoid injury to the piriform sinus, it is unfolded with a finger. Bleeding from the mucosa is controlled by bipolar diathermy (**Fig. 10.79c**).

Removal. While drawing the larynx further forward, the postcricoid mucosa is swept off the posterior cricoarytenoid (posticus) muscle below the transverse arytenoid incision (**Fig. 10.80a**). The larynx is now connected only to the trachea. To remove the larynx, an incision is made beneath the cricoid cartilage or, depending on the demands of the tumor, between the superior tracheal cartilages. This incision is gradually deepened down to the posterior wall; the larynx is drawn upward and completely released from the mucosa of the hypopharynx and the esophagus. Re-intubation is performed and a nasogastric tube inserted (**Fig. 10.80b**).

Pharyngeal suture. The patient's head is elevated forward to relieve tension along the suture line. The base of the tongue is unfolded with a wide retractor. Absorbable suture material is used. The wound margins of the pharyngostoma are stretched to achieve a straight suture line; a T-shaped wound closure is created only in exceptional cases where there is a corresponding loss of substance. A continuous inverting suture as described by Conley is placed using two threads (alternatively, an interrupted inverting suture or continuous inverting suture with one thread). The needle is inserted from the outside through the mucosa, immediately at the edge, brought out again from the mucosal aspect a few millimeters further on, then inserted again on the contralateral side through the full thickness of the wall, brought out again a few millimeters downward, and continued until reaching the middle. A suture line is placed in a similar fashion from the opposite wound pole, *carefully pulled tight* (clearly shortening the suture line) and then knotted with the upper suture (**Fig. 10.81a**).

A second layer of interrupted sutures is placed over the entire length of the first layer. For this purpose, the first suture line is once again tightened carefully by pulling on the sutures left long

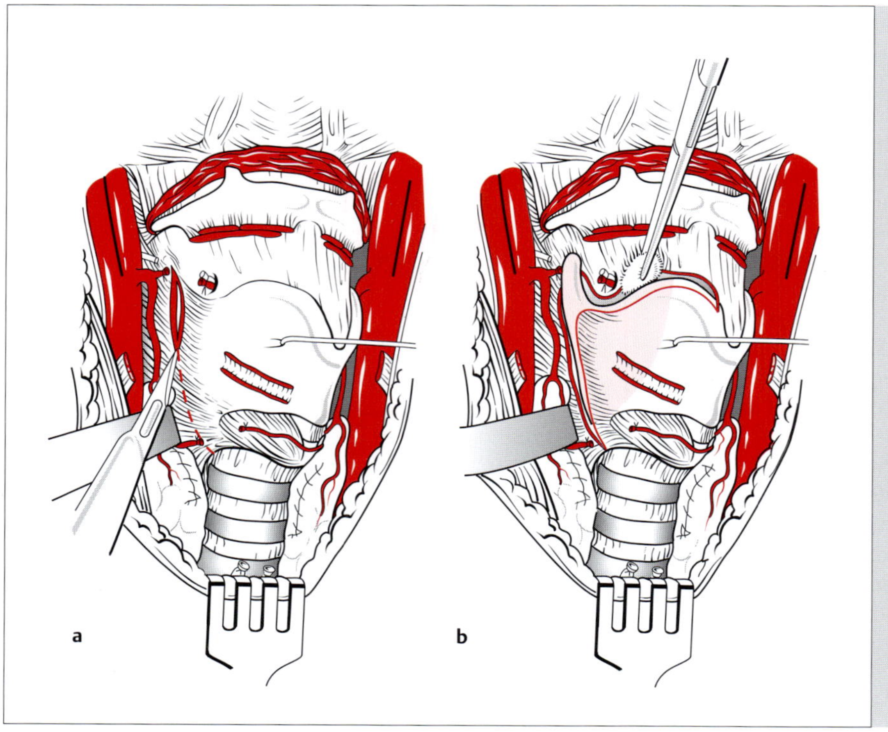

Fig. 10.78a, b Laryngectomy.
a Division of the pharyngeal constrictor muscle at the posterior border of the thyroid cartilage.
b Dissection of the piriform sinus after division of the perichondrium over the lamella of the thyroid cartilage.

at the superior and inferior wound poles, before the tissue lying directly next to the first suture line is taken up by the needle, without penetrating the mucosa, and brought over to cover the first suture line. The third suture layer includes the pharyngeal constrictor muscle and, if preserved, the sternohyoid muscle to cover the second line, taking care not to create any cavities, especially at the inferior wound pole (**Fig. 10.81b**).

Suture of the trachea. Strong size 0 skin suture material is used. The suture is inserted below the most superior tracheal ring and exits externally in the dermis. *All the sutures are placed first, and then knotted.* When knotting, the skin is placed by the assistant exactly on the cartilage incision margin. The lateral parts of the tracheal rings are sutured with a certain degree of traction in a lateral direction. When excising the larynx, a tongue-shaped flap may be elevated superiorly from the posterior membrane of the trachea and sutured to the lightly taught U-shaped skin flap (this tightens the posterior tracheal wall flap) (**Fig. 10.82a**).

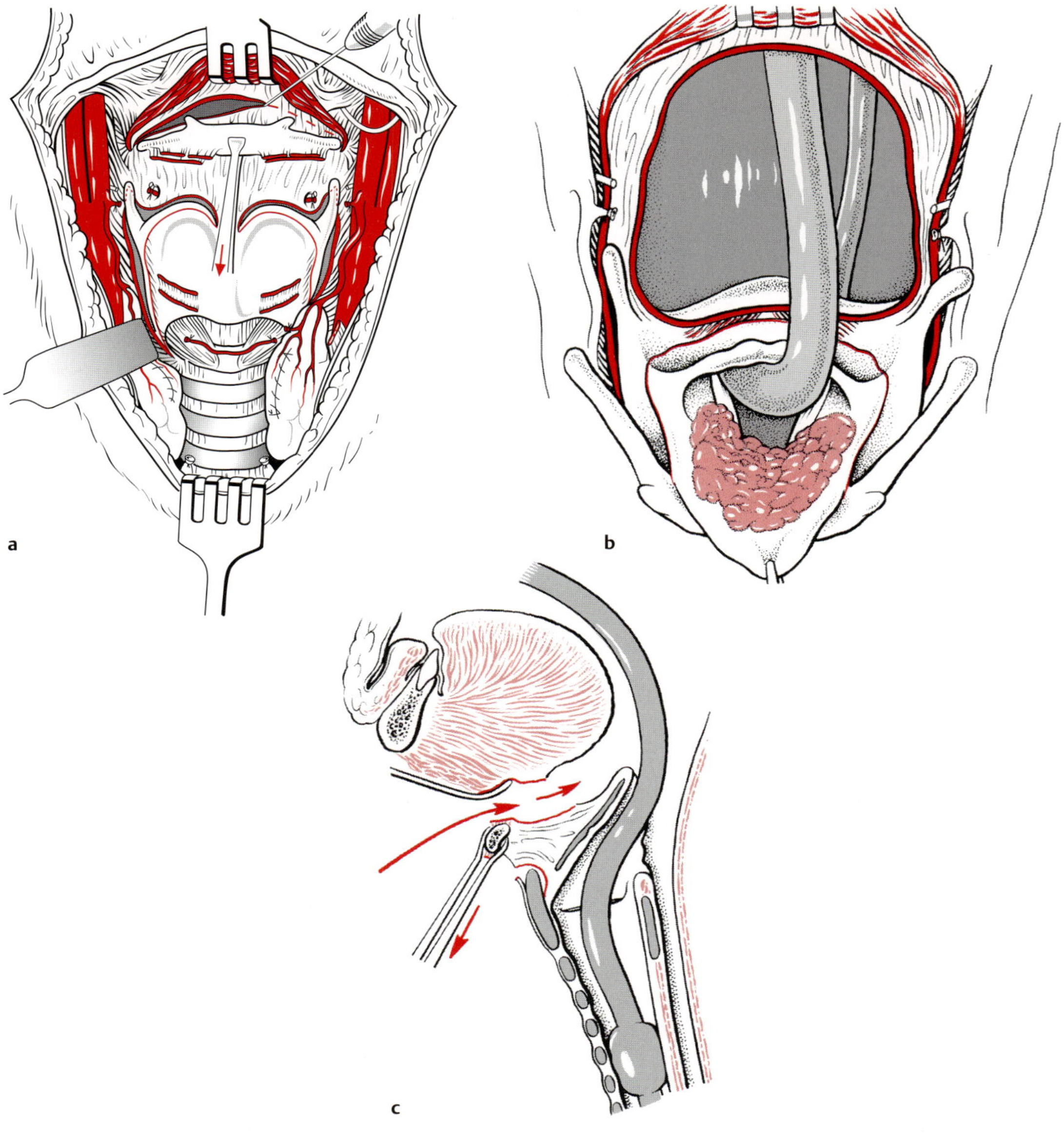

Fig. 10.79a–c Laryngectomy.
a The pharynx is opened via a transverse incision above the hyoid bone, which is drawn downward.
b Pharyngotomy in cross-section.
c Incision along the epiglottis, which is drawn forward, the aryepiglottic fold and the arytenoid cartilage.

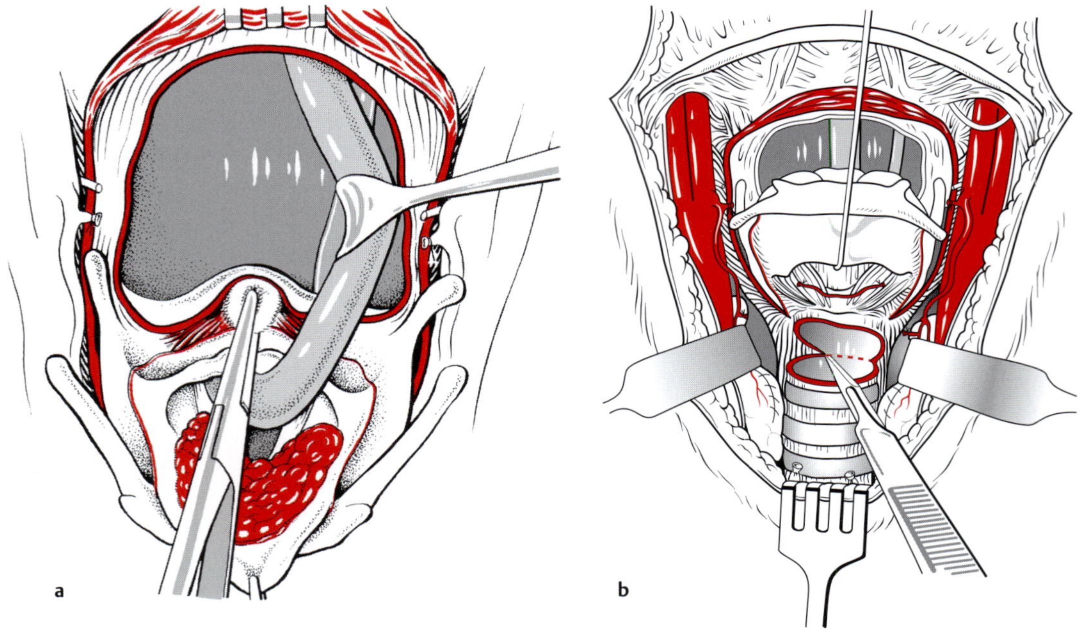

Fig. 10.80a, b Laryngectomy.
a The incised mucosa is elevated off the posterior aspect of the larynx.
b Division of the larynx below the cricoid cartilage by transverse transsection of the posterior wall.

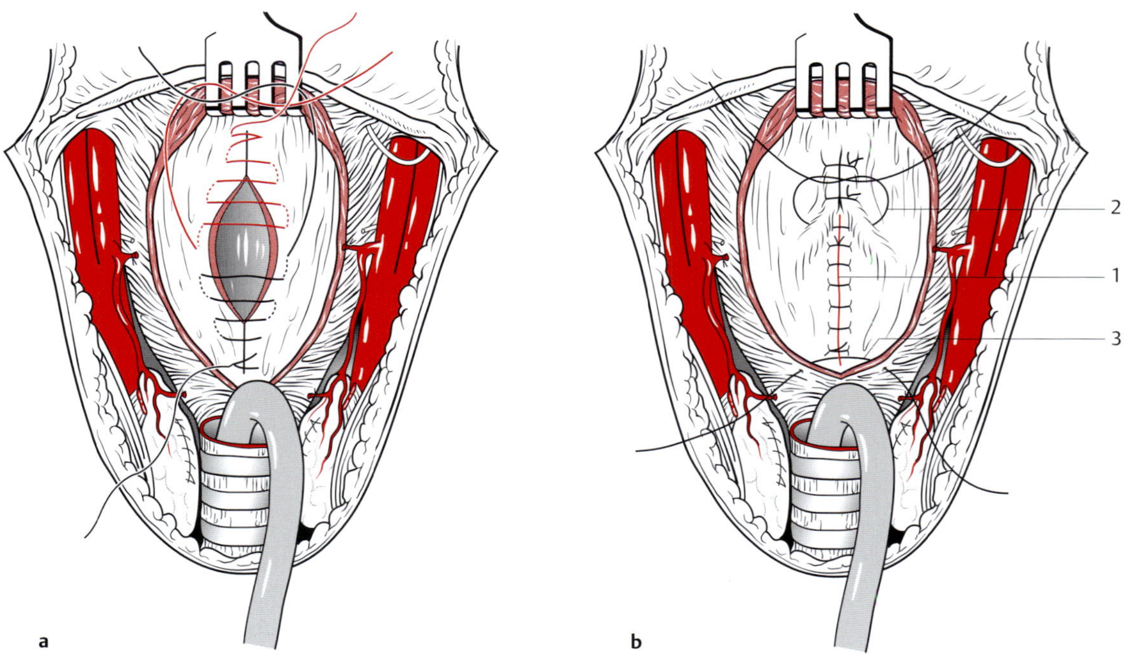

Fig. 10.81a, b Laryngectomy.
a Suture of the pharynx using a continuous inverting suture as described by Conley.
b Coverage in three layers after inverting the Conley suture (1), covered by interrupted sutures (2) and muscle suture of the pharyngeal constrictor muscle (3).

A suction drain is inserted from either side of the neck and placed next to the pharynx suture, followed by closure in layers (**Fig. 10.82b**). Mild compression dressing. A metal tracheostomy cannula is inserted.

Modification

The larynx may also be removed in the opposite direction, from below upward, but the operative steps basically remain the same. If the tumor has invaded the prelaryngeal soft tissues or the thyroid gland, then the involved tissue must be left attached to the larynx and removed with it en bloc. Even with larger expansions invading the piriform sinus or the pharyngeal mucosa, the whole tumorous region must be excised.

Instead of U-shaped flaps, a bilateral swing-door flap may be elevated, based laterally beyond the posterior margin of the sternocleidomastoid muscle. Tumor involvement of the skin or significant skin alterations secondary to radiotherapy will require a local or distant flap to be used for resurfacing.

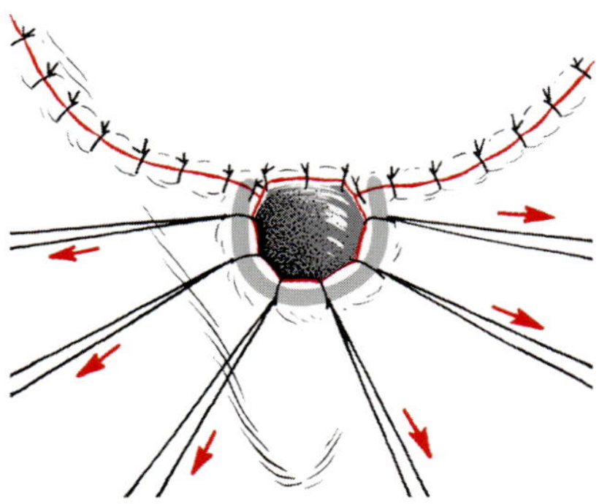
a

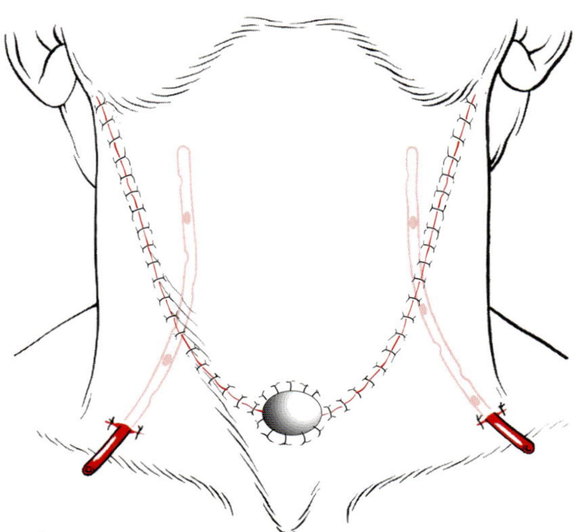
b

Fig. 10.82a, b Laryngectomy.
a Lateral fixation of the tracheal stump using the suture as described by Dietzel.
b Wound closure after the insertion of suction drains.

Rules, Tips, and Tricks

The mattress sutures for closure of the pharynx inevitably invert the mucosal edges (absolute requirement) and press outer surface against outer surface. The tracheostomy cannula must not rub against the anterior wall of the trachea; avoid too narrow a radius and ensure that the cannula is not too long, but has a wide lumen.

Risks and Complications

- Postoperative bleeding from the arterial vessels (superior and inferior laryngeal arteries): wound revision.
- Pharyngeal fistula, secondary to suture-line dehiscence or unrecognized perforation: insertion of a probe or leave the probe in situ and irrigate the fistula; if the fistula exits into the tracheostoma, try draining it obliquely in a lateral direction, encourage granulation formation and apply a pressure dressing; revise the wound if the fistula persists, place a new pharyngeal suture or perform a secondary plastic-surgical wound closure.
- Aspiration, aspiration pneumonia: antibiotic, packing of the fistula, suction the tracheobronchial system and administer a secretolytic agent.
- Wound infection, deep neck infection, mediastinitis.
- Loss of both voice and ability to speak.

Postoperative Care

- Antibiotic; consider secretolytic agents and possibly antitussive agents.
- Ultrasonic nebulizer, suction of secretions, cleansing of the internal cannula, cannula change on the second or third postoperative day, sooner if crusts develop.
- Monitoring of blood pressure and pulse, consider intensive care observation, Hb checks.
- Mobilization of the patient, compression stockings to prevent formation of emboli, consider heparinization.
- Depending on the amount of secretion produced, the drains are removed between the second and fourth days; change of dressing on the seventh day if the course is uneventful, wound check earlier if congestion, tendency to bleed or fever occurs. Remove sutures on the seventh day. Leave the tracheostoma sutures until the tenth day.
- After approximately 10 days attempt a trial of swallowing, e.g., with methylene blue; if no fistula is detected, remove the nasogastric tube.
- Postoperative radiotherapy, if appropriate, after 2–3 weeks,
- Tracheostoma: plastic cannulas are usually more suitable as indwelling cannulas than metal ones. To avoid pressure necrosis on the anterior tracheal wall, a flatter angle than with tracheostomy cannulas is required. If the stoma shows no tendency to shrink, then a cannula may be dispensed with entirely after an appropriate length of time. As a rule, problems basically arise with stomas when showering,

swimming, or taking a bath. Suitable appliances are available from specialist retail outlets. Depending on the amount of secretion produced or the tendency for desiccation, a suction appliance and the possibility of inhalations at home must be also arranged after discharge.
- Training in esophageal speech after 2–3 weeks at the earliest. It is advisable to arrange a meeting with the speech therapist during the initial preparations for surgery to facilitate comprehension and provide the opportunity to answer any questions. A small chalkboard or notebook should be available directly after surgery for communication.

Comment

After complete removal of the larynx, communication is initially considerably impaired but this impairment may be reduced by a well-directed approach to rehabilitation. The almost complete loss of the sense of smell and the reduction of the sense of taste are, on the other hand, irreversible. The missing olfactory and gustatory stimuli can only be marginally compensated for by fanning air into the oral and nasal cavities. As already mentioned, voice rehabilitation is basically possible in the form of the body's own capabilities of voice replacement (so-called esophageal voice), by the implantation of a voice prosthesis, by surgical reconstructive procedures, or by the use of electronic devices. All these rehabilitation measures must not conceal the fact that the total removal of the larynx is an extremely stressful, and unfortunately usually inevitable, destructive operation. Furthermore, there is often the additional loss of work, which is associated with sometimes considerable financial and thus social repercussions. Stigmatization and the patient's subsequent withdrawal from their social environment can find expression in depressive disorders and a general loss of activity.

Even after preservation of the larynx has been achieved by surgical or radio-oncological means, severe sequelae are possible. These include severe lymphedema secondary to permanent damage to the cervical lymphatic drainage system. The damage may be caused by surgery as well as by radiotherapy. A combination of both treatment procedures results in the most damage to lymph drainage. This is particularly relevant as treatment of advanced laryngeal carcinomas requires inclusion of the lymph drainage area in the therapeutic planning. Lymphedema is often associated with considerable functional restrictions and often involves long-term treatment applications of manual lymph drainage, funding for which may be difficult to secure. A proactive and early inclusion of follow-up care possibilities and the involvement of representatives of related specialties (speech therapy, physiotherapy, psychology) are essential.

Voice Rehabilitation after Laryngectomy—Functional Principle

Esophageal Voice

The oesophageal voice involves injecting air into the esophagus and then expelling it in a controlled fashion.
- Over time mucosal bulges form (pseudoglottis).
- The controlled release of air causes these mucosal bulges to vibrate.
- This produces perceptible sounds, which can be formed into speech sounds.

Voice Prosthesis

- The voice prosthesis is a valve, which is inserted surgically between trachea and esophagus.
- When the wearer of a voice prosthesis device closes the tracheostoma, the expiratory air enters the esophagus via the trachea and valve.
- It then flows on through the esophageal aperture into the oral cavity.
- The mucosal folds in the esophagus vibrate and so allow voice formation.

Electrolarynx

- The electrolarynx has a membrane that is held against the neck and transfers external vibrations into the pharynx.
- The sounds produced can be modulated in the mouth.
- For this purpose, lips and tongue are moved, as previously with a natural voice.

Surgical Rehabilitation of the Voice after Laryngectomy

The problem of surgical rehabilitation of the voice after laryngectomy has gained momentum over the years, yet a standard procedure has not yet emerged. It is basically possible to create the fistula while performing the laryngectomy, or to do it later with a simple puncture from the trachea into the esophagus.

Many centers have meanwhile abandoned Staffier's procedure and the method described by Asai. The former operation involves suturing the posterior hypopharyngeal wall onto the tracheal stump and creating a fistula 6–8 mm long in the middle or slightly laterally and achieving epithelialization by everting the mucosal margins; breathing is possible via a lower-placed tracheostoma. The Asai method creates a fistulous tract from the skin between the most superior part of the trachea and the base of the tongue.

The Herrmann glottoplasty procedure involves the insertion of a valve prosthesis during laryngectomy. To achieve good vocal function, several precautionary measures are necessary during the laryngectomy procedure to avoid scar formation.

There is also the alternative of first performing a laryngectomy in a conventional fashion and then awaiting the development of an esophageal voice. If this does not happen, then it is recommended to perform a puncture of the hypopharynx from the posterior tracheal wall and to insert, e. g., a Provox II prosthesis. As with all other methods, closure of the stoma with a finger is then necessary for the patient to speak. The quality of the voice produced depends decisively on the scar formation of the hypopharynx region and the expiratory air pressure required to open the hypopharynx. Of course, the voice prosthesis may also be inserted directly during laryngectomy, a technique which is undertaken in many centers.

External Approach for Malignant Tumors of the Hypopharynx

The same is true for hypopharyngeal carcinomas as for supraglottic and glottic carcinomas; namely that a laser surgical procedure may be considered for cases with complete transoral exposure of the tumor if the surgeon is adequately experienced, especially as the later postoperative and sometimes technically demanding flap elevation becomes unnecessary. The extent of the tumor and its exposure, however, does not always allow this, rendering a conventional approach necessary.

Partial Hypopharyngolaryngectomy with Preservation of the Larynx

Surgical Principle

Resection of the superior level of larynx, including the lateral pharyngeal wall together with the piriform sinus.

Indications

Smaller tumors in the piriform sinus without extension into its tip and without invasion into the inside of larynx, mobility of the vocal folds must be present; the tumor margins may at most lie on the mucosa lateral to the arytenoid.

Contraindications

Distant metastases, poor general condition, tumor invasion of the laryngeal framework, involvement of tip of the piriform sinus.

Specific Points Regarding Informed Consent

Unlike the transoral approach, a tracheotomy is the general rule and at least a selective neck dissection (levels II–IV) is necessary to gain access to the hypopharynx.

Anesthesia

General endotracheal anesthesia.

Surgical Technique

- Commence with a neck dissection, as explained in detail in Chapter 11.
- Tracheotomy.
- Resection of the upper level of the larynx as for the supraglottic transverse resection. The upper level of the larynx is excised from the healthy side, while from the affected side the piriform sinus and the adjacent lateral and posterior laryngeal walls are also excised. Depending on the area of resection, closure is achieved either primarily by drawing the defect together, or by gluing or suturing a split-skin graft.

Total Laryngectomy with Partial Pharyngectomy

Surgical Principle

Laryngectomy with resection of larger areas of the pharynx and reconstruction of the esophagus using residual pharyngeal mucosa.

Indications

Extensive tumor involvement in the hypopharynx and tumor invasion of the larynx, provided a bridge of mucosa at least 2 cm wide is preserved in the posterior hypopharyngeal wall while observing the margins of safety for tumor surgery.

Contraindications

- Severe general disorders precluding operability.
- Incurable distant metastases or synchronous tumors.
- Undissectable encasement of the common or internal carotid artery by metastases or continuous growth of a tumor.
- Penetration of the tumor into the prevertebral fascia.
- Tumor which is too extensive and only controllable by performing a transverse pharyngolaryngectomy.

Surgical Technique

Classic total laryngectomy with neck dissection. In modification of the standard procedure, the tumor region in the hypopharyngeal wall is also excised under direct vision, together with an appropriate safety margin. The hypopharynx is closed in typical fashion over an inserted nasogastric tube.

> **! Risks and Complications**
> As for a total laryngectomy. Pharyngeal fistulas are clearly more frequent. Stenosis within the esophagus.

11 Surgery of the Neck

Perioperative Antibiotics for Soft-Tissue Surgery of the Head and Neck

Distinction between Septic and Aseptic Surgery

The nature of the surgical procedure determines the risk of postoperative wound infection. A general distinction is made between aseptic and septic wounds. Examples of *aseptic* procedures are the excision of a simple neck cyst or lymph node. The term "clean-contaminated wounds" is used when an incision is made in the neck and connects with the salivary system. *Septic* wounds include traumatically or preoperatively infected wounds as well as surgically inflicted wounds in which the pharyngeal mucosa has been opened at operation.

Spectrum of Infectious Organisms

The organisms most commonly identified in the neck are *Staphylococcus aureus* and *S. epidermidis*, α-hemolytic streptococci, and especially Gram-negative organisms such as *Klebsiella* species, *Proteus mirabilis*, *Pseudomonas aeroginosa*, *Escherichia coli*, enterococci, and *Enterobacter* species. Second-generation cephalosporins have proven useful in the prevention of infection, but because their efficacy against some members of the Enterobacteriaceae family (*Klebsiella*, *Proteus*, *E. coli*) is not complete, a cephalosporin should be combined with metronidazole in any operation that opens the pharynx.

Timing and Duration of Antibiotic Therapy

The standard practice in noninflammatory surgery is to administer a single dose of perioperative antibiotic. A cephalosporin and/or metronidazole should be administered intravenously 30–60 minutes before the start of the operation to achieve active serum and tissue levels. An adequate level of efficacy is maintained for approximately 3 hours, and longer operations will require an additional dose. In procedures that open the pharynx, the large wound surfaces require a 3- to 5-day course of second-generation cephalosporin plus metronidazole.

Treatment of Wound Infections

Fever, leukocytosis, an elevated C-reactive protein (CRP), and/or cervical redness in the wound area may be the earliest signs of a postoperative wound infection. In patients with a frank postoperative wound infection, a specimen should be taken from the infected site for microbial analysis. Specific antibiotic therapy can then be administered on the basis of sensitivity results. Purulent soft-tissue infections should be evacuated and, if necessary, irrigated with an antiseptic solution (e.g., povidone iodine, Betaisodona) several times daily for several days.

A postoperative infection in the neck is occasionally associated with a defect in the cervical soft tissues as a result of thrombophlebitis. If the infection persists, this may lead to the formation of extensive pharyngocutaneous fistulas. With proper treatment, however, the wound will usually undergo secondary healing by granulation.

Surgery of the Lymph Nodes

Lymph Node Abscesses

Inflammatory swellings in the neck are managed by a staged therapeutic approach. In the absence of liquefaction, cellulitis, sepsis and laryngeal edema, treatment is conservative and consists of antibiotic therapy. It may also be necessary to locate and eradicate an inflammatory focus in the tonsils, tongue, oral floor, teeth, or salivary glands.

An abscess, on the other hand, requires immediate surgical drainage.

Surgical Principle

The abscess is opened and drained with respect for skin cleavage lines while preserving nerves and vessels that cross the operative field.

Indications

The indications are abscess formation and liquefaction (e.g., nonspecific inflammations, specific inflammations, actinomycosis, secondary inflammation of neck cysts).

Contraindications

There are almost no contraindications, because of the risk of sepsis.

Specific Points Regarding Informed Consent

- Sensory disturbances involving the neck or ear.
- Paralysis of the nerves supplying the trapezius, visceral muscles, diaphragm, lingual muscles, sublingual muscles, vocal cords, and facial muscles.
- Hoarseness or voice loss.
- Poor cosmetic result, excessive scarring.
- Possible need to extend the skin incision.
- Need for a second operation.
- Mucosal injury, mediastinitis.

Operative Planning

The pathogenesis of the abscess should be investigated at the time of diagnosis. Possibilities includes inflammatory skin diseases and diseases of the Waldeyer ring. Dentogenic abscesses are also common.

Special Instruments

Dressing forceps, drainage material (e.g., Easy-Flow-Drainage).

Anesthesia

General or local anesthesia (Dermajet may be used for intracutaneous injection). One has to wait longer for local anesthesia to take effect in infected case due to change of pH in the tissues.

Surgical Technique

Incision. The abscess is drained through a skin incision placed along RSTL over the mass. Generally the incision is 1–2-cm long.

Introducing the dressing forceps and opening the abscess. The dressing forceps is introduced through the incision, parallel to the course of the major neck vessels. Guided by external palpation, the abscess is located with the forceps, spread open, and drained. Entry into the abscess is usually indicated by the immediate drainage of purulent material (a sample is taken for analysis).

Draining the abscess. The dressing forceps is brought out below the abscess through an incision made over the forceps tip and opened wide enough to grasp the end of a drain (e.g., Easy-Flow-Drainage) and pull it upward through the abscess cavity.

Securing the drain. The drain sutured to the skin above and below with simple interrupted sutures.

Irrigation. At the end of the procedure, the drain is used to irrigate the abscess cavity with an antiseptic solution (e.g., povidone iodine, 11 % Betaisodona solution).

Rules, Tips, and Tricks

A sample is taken so that specific antibiotics can be administered at operation. Because the organisms identified in an abscess smear will generally include anaerobes, a combination of agents (e.g., a cephalosporin plus metronidazole) should be used for initial therapy. Additionally, tissue should be taken from the abscess membrane for histological or molecular diagnostic analysis to check for an underlying classic or atypical tuberculosis. Sterilized safety pins can also be used to secure the drain.
Easy-Flow-Drainage. Before insertion, elliptical openings ca. 1 cm long are cut in the lateral edges of the drain to allow for drainage of the antiseptic irrigating solution during the next few days.

! Risks and Complications

Septic complications; cellulitis; injuries to the marginal mandibular branch of the facial nerve, accessory nerve, recurrent laryngeal nerve, jugular vein, or other major vessels; postoperative bleeding; mediastinitis; laryngeal edema; keloid formation.

Postoperative Care

Antibiotic therapy. The abscess may have to be reopened and drained. The drain is shortened and may be removed as the drainage volume declines. The wound heals secondarily, and scar revision may be elected at a later date. If an underlying cyst is present, it should be extirpated after inflammation has resolved. A 6-month course of penicillin is indicated for patients with actinomycosis.

Cervicofacial Lymphadenectomy

Surgical Principle

Removal of one lymph node or several conglomerated lymph nodes for histological examination.

Indications

Persistent, noninflammatory lymph node swelling that requires benign–malignant differentiation.

Specific Points Regarding Informed Consent

- Sensory disturbance involving the neck or ear.
- Growth lag of the skin flap.
- Paralysis of the nerves supplying the trapezius, visceral muscles, diaphragm, lingual muscles, sublingual muscles, vocalis, and facial muscles.
- Hoarseness or voice loss.
- Dyspnea, which may necessitate a tracheostomy tube.
- Poor cosmetic result, excessive scarring.
- Possible need to extend the skin incision.
- Mucosal injury, mediastinitis.

- Persistent drainage of lymphatic fluid.

Operative Planning

B-mode ultrasonography. Fine-needle aspiration cytology may be necessary in some cases. Sectional imaging modalities (CT, MRI) are rarely necessary.

Anesthesia

General endotracheal anesthesia, which may be supplemented by local anesthesia with a vasoconstrictor to reduce bleeding. Local anesthesia alone is an option in some patients.

Surgical Technique

Skin incision. The skin incision of choice depends on the location of the lymph node and should follow the RSTL (**Fig. 11.1**).

Dissection of subcutaneous fat. After division of the skin, the subcutaneous fat is spread open and secured with a retractor. The tissue planes are successively spread open to enter the lymph node-bearing compartments.

Dissection at level I (submental and submandibular nodes). Particular attention is given to the marginal mandibular branch of the facial nerve in dissections of the submandibular nodes. The external incision is deepened through the platysma, and the posterior part of the wound is spread open to expose the *facial vein*, which is *ligated and reflected upward*. Localization of the lymph nodes is aided by manual or bimanual palpation while the oral floor is pushed forward (after first rinsing the oral cavity with antiseptic solution).

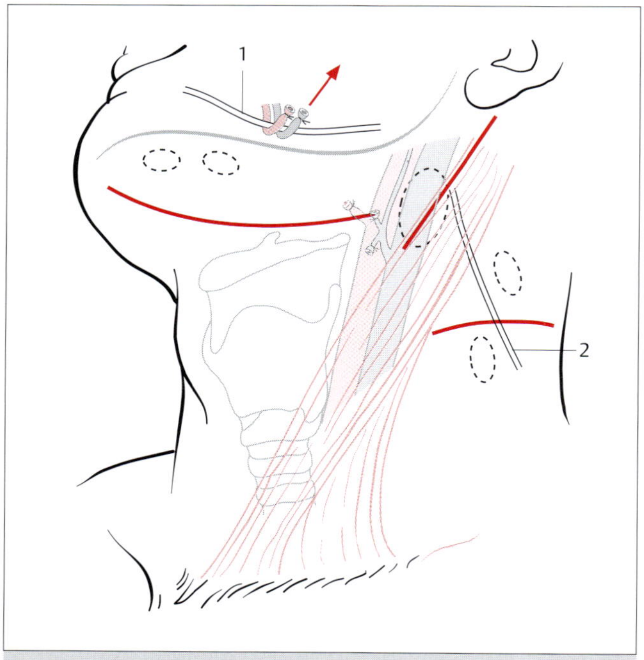

Fig. 11.1 Cervical lymphadenectomy.
External incisions along the RSTLs. Note the nerve locations: the marginal mandibular branch of the facial nerve (1) in the submandibular region (the facial artery and vein are ligated and reflected upward) and the accessory nerve (2) behind the sternocleidomastoid muscle.

Dissection at levels II–IV. Excisional biopsies are taken in proximity to the vascular sheath. Identification of the vascular sheath may be aided by locating the point where the omohyoid muscle crosses over the sheath.

Dissection at level V. *The accessory nerve occupies a very superficial location in the posterolateral triangle of the neck. Blunt dissection always proceeds parallel to the nerve, alternately pushing the connective tissue and fat aside with a dissecting sponge.* Small vessels are coagulated with bipolar cautery. The accessory nerve is carefully identified.

Exposing and freeing the lymph nodes. The lymph nodes are freed by blunt retraction and incision of the surrounding connective tissue bands. *The lymph nodes themselves should not be grasped with a forceps or clamp*, as this would hamper histological evaluation. Surrounding structures are held aside with retractors while the node is shelled out, aided if necessary by packing a gauze strip beneath it (the end should be left protruding).

Hemostasis. Hemostasis must be meticulous. A large wound cavity should be closed in layers over a small suction drain.

Management of Injury to Large Venous Vessels
If a large venous vessel is opened but cannot be grasped directly, it should be immediately packed off to prevent air embolism (unless endotracheal anesthesia is being used).

Management of Injury to Large Arterial Vessels
Arterial bleeding that cannot be immediately controlled should be packed off and the incision extended. Surrounding anatomical structures are identified, and the vessel is located and secured proximal to the site of the injury. The vessel is compressed proximal to the bleeding site with a mounted sponge. With injury to the common or internal carotid artery, consultation with a vascular surgeon may be necessary. Otherwise the head and neck surgeon may apply gentle, local compression with a small sponge, moving the compression site progressively closer to the tear. Pressure is applied caudal to the exposed vascular segment, and the tear in the vessel wall is repaired with sutures (e. g., 5–0 Prolene; note the compression time).

Management of Significant Nerve Injury
With an accessory nerve lesion, identify the stumps. If a primary nerve repair cannot be done, the nerve ends should be tagged for a secondary repair, but this is rarely necessary.

! Risks and Complications

- Various structures may be at risk, depending on the location of the lymph node:
  - the accessory nerve in the lateral cervical triangle
  - the marginal mandibular branch of the facial nerve in the submandibular region; the lingual nerve may also be at risk in very deep lymphadenectomies
  - in the vascular compartment: the vagus nerve, recurrent laryngeal nerve, hypoglossal nerve, carotid artery, and jugular vein (caution: air embolism)
  - at the supraclavicular level: the pleura, subclavian artery and vein, brachial plexus, and thoracic duct.

- Secondary infections, fistula formation due to incomplete removal of tuberculous lymph nodes. Postoperative bleeding, keloid formation.
- An extremely rare but potentially severe complication is to misidentify a carotid body tumor as a lymph node (differentiating signs: pulsations, transverse mobility on palpation with little or no vertical mobility). Careless dissection may result in massive bleeding with risk of carotid injury.

Postoperative Care

Drains are removed when the drainage volume falls to 30 mL or less. Sutures are removed on day 7.

Scalene Node Biopsy

Surgical Principle

The entire prescalene fat pad is removed along with the palpable and nonpalpable lymph nodes that it contains.

Indications

- Histological identification of inaccessible tumors, thoracic tumors, or tumors that have undergone intra-abdominal metastasis
- Exclusion of suspected sarcoidosis or tuberculosis, even in the absence of palpable lymphadenopathy
- Suspected Hodgkin or non-Hodgkin lymphoma
- Unexplained lymph node enlargement in the omoclavicular triangle

Contraindication

Severe debilitation.

Anesthesia

General endotracheal anesthesia is usually preferred. Local anesthesia is induced by infiltrating the area around the operative site. Caution: air embolism.

Surgical Technique

Skin incision and exposure of the prescalene fat pad. A 4- to 5-cm skin incision is made parallel to and just above the clavicle, starting over the medial head of the sternocleidomastoid muscle. The platysma is divided, and the crossing external jugular vein is ligated. The posterior border of the clavicular head of the sternocleidomastoid is isolated, and the muscle is retracted. The jugular vein is isolated by blunt dissection with a mounted sponge or dissecting forceps. The inferior belly of the omohyoid muscle is identified at the level of the vascular sheath and retracted upward (**Fig. 11.2**).

Mobilization of the prescalene fat pad. At this point the prescalene fat has been exposed between the jugular vein, clavicular margin, and omohyoid muscle. The deep cervical fascia is approached from the omohyoid by blunt dissection with two mounted sponges, and the fat–lymph node tissue is carefully dissected downward on the cervical fascia as far as the junction of the subclavian and jugular veins. The thyrocervical trunk is preserved. The deep cervical fascia should also be preserved to avoid injury to the phrenic nerve and brachial plexus (**Fig. 11.3**).

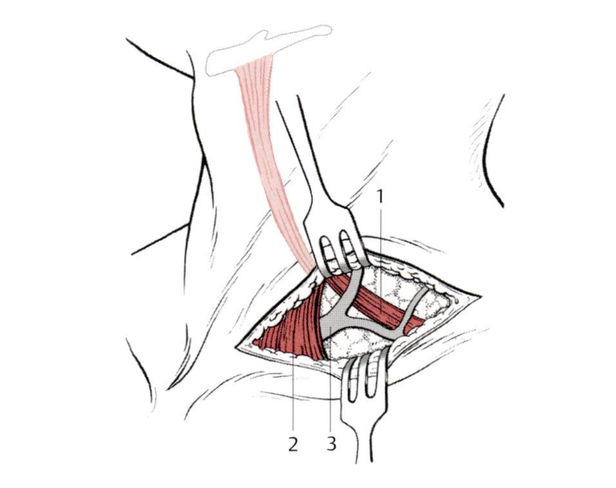

Fig. 11.2 Scalene node biopsy, step 1.
The skin is incised parallel to the clavicle. The external jugular vein (3) is ligated, and the clavicular head of the sternocleidomastoid muscle (2) and the inferior belly of the omohyoid muscle (1) are exposed.

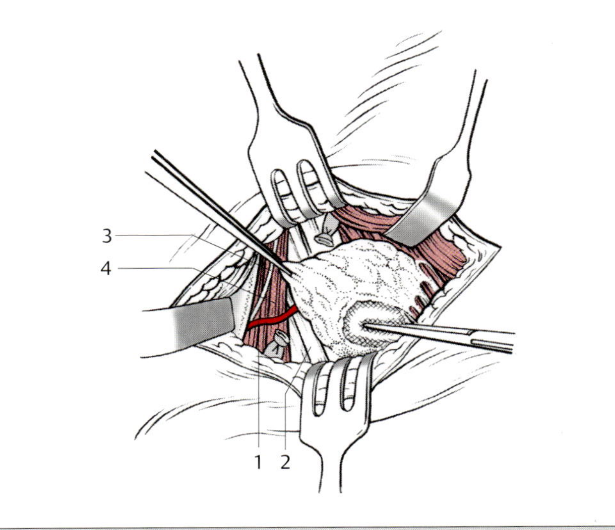

Fig. 11.3 Scalene node biopsy, step 2.
The sternocleidomastoid and internal jugular vein are retracted medially, and the inferior belly of the omohyoid muscle is retracted upward. The prescalene fat is exposed into the angle of the jugular and subclavian veins. The phrenic nerve (3) and brachial plexus (2) must be preserved. (1) Transverse cervical artery, (4) scalene muscle.

Wound closure. After the specimen has been removed, the wound is closed in layers over a small suction drain. A light pressure dressing is applied.

! Risks and Complications

- With injury to the thoracic duct, immediately locate and ligate the duct using the microscope. A chyle fistula that is detected after surgery can be managed conservatively in most cases by closely monitoring the chyle volume and obtaining a blood count, chest radiographs, urinary status, liver function, electrolytes, and serum protein assays including serum albumin. Most low-output fistulas can be successfully managed by a diet of medium-chain triglycerides to reduce chyle production. Parenteral nutrition alone is no longer considered a cost-effective approach. Conservative treatment measures for chyle fistula should be limited to 30 days so that planned postoperative radiotherapy can be instituted within a reasonable time frame. Chyle fistulas should be surgically repaired in patients with refractory hypoalbuminemia or if the fistula output is greater than 600 mL/24 hour.
- If the pleura has been opened, the wound edges should be carefully reapproximated and secured with sutures. A suction drain is inserted if necessary, and surgical consultation should be sought.
- Injuries to the subclavian artery and vein are surgically repaired.
- Injuries to the phrenic nerve or brachial plexus are referred for neurosurgical repair.
- Other risks are keloid formation and secondary infection.

Postoperative Care

The drain is removed when the drainage volume falls to 30 mL or less.

Neck Dissection

General

The Committee for Neck Dissection Classification of the American Head and Neck Society has issued a revised version of the cervical lymph node classification based on various discussions on regional definitions and the nomenclature of neck dissections. The lymph node groups are classified as follows:

- Submental group (level IA).
- Submandibular group (level IB).
- Upper jugular group (level II), which is subdivided by the oblique accessory nerve into level IIA (lymph node-bearing fat above the accessory nerve) and level IIB (lymph node-bearing fat below the accessory nerve).
- Middle jugular group (level III).
- Lower jugular group (level IV).
- Posterior triangle group (level V). An imaginary horizontal line at the level of the cricoid cartilage subdivides this group into level VA (lymph node-bearing fat above the imaginary line) and level VB (lymph node-bearing fat below the imaginary line).
- Anterior compartment group (level VI).

Lymph nodes omitted in this classification include:

- The retroauricular lymph nodes.
- The suboccipital lymph nodes.
- The parotid lymph nodes.
- The retropharyngeal lymph nodes.

The current neck dissection classification published by Robbins (2002) still distinguishes among a radical neck dissection, extended radical neck dissection, modified radical neck dissection, and selective neck dissection.

Radical neck dissection. A radical neck dissection involves the complete removal of levels I–V lymph nodes including all three major nonlymphatic structures—the accessory nerve, internal jugular vein, and sternocleidomastoid muscle. The resection does not include the suboccipital lymph nodes, periparotid lymph nodes, retropharyngeal lymph nodes, or anterior compartment lymph nodes (level VI).

Extended radical neck dissection. An extended radical neck dissection consists of a radical neck dissection plus the removal of one or more additional lymph node groups and/or nonlymphatic structures such as the external carotid artery, hypoglossal nerve, vagus nerve, or paravertebral muscles.

Modified radical neck dissection. This operation removes the level I–V lymph nodes in addition to one or more nonlymphatic structures (accessory nerve and/or internal jugular vein and/or sternocleidomastoid muscle).

Selective neck dissection. This operation removes the lymph node levels that principally drain a malignant tumor of the upper aerodigestive tract while sparing all three major nonlymphatic structures. The classic types of selective neck dissection are designated I–III, I–IV, II–IV, and II–V. If only two levels are removed, the selective neck dissection is named accordingly (e.g., SND II–III).

Indications for Neck Dissection in the Treatment of Head and Neck Malignancies

Radical neck dissection. In Europe and at most institutions, a radical neck dissection is reserved for the treatment of N3 metastasis or metastases that involve nonlymphatic structures.

Modified radical neck dissection. Most head and neck surgeons currently perform a modified radical neck dissection in all patients with clinically detectable lymph node metastasis. There is a definite trend, however, toward sparing certain levels such as level IIB in hypopharyngeal carcinoma or level I for the same tumor entity. A bilateral modified radical neck dissection is performed in patients with an N2c neck, or bilateral lymphogenous metastasis. Every effort consistent with oncologic requirements should be made to preserve the internal jugular vein on at least one side of the neck to prevent potentially severe lymphedema. A selective neck dissection should be considered in patients with a contralateral N0 neck in consideration of the overall prognosis. Thus, an ipsilateral metastasis at level IV would be more detrimental to survival than a metastasis at level II. Some authors would advocate a selective neck dissection even in patients with an N+ status, but the validity of this policy has yet to be established.

Selective neck dissection. The indication for an elective neck dissection is more controversial in patients with a clinical N0 neck than in patients with clinically apparent cervical lymph node involvement. Two different goals can be addressed. On the one hand, the dissection of a clinical N0 neck can be performed as a staging procedure. Selective neck dissections are increasingly used for this purpose and are followed by radiotherapy in cases where lymphogenous metastasis is found. In rare cases the staging procedure may be followed by the secondary removal of lymph node regions that were left intact in the initial operation. In other cases an elective neck dissection may be performed for curative intent in a clinical N0 neck. The goal of selective neck dissection in these cases is to provide definitive treatment of cervical lymphatic drainage. Further details on the pros and cons of these issues may be found in the literature.

At this point we wish to provide the surgeon in training with some principles that may be followed for the oncologically sound surgical management of the clinical N0 neck. **Table 11.1** lists types of selective neck dissection that are recommended for specific primary tumor sites in the upper aerodigestive tract. It is important to consider selection criteria for a bilateral selective neck dissection in the clinical N0 neck. The policy at many centers is to recommend this operation in cases where the primary tumor is located in the midline or has transgressed the midline. Of course, the table presents only one of several possible surgical strategies whose application will depend on the overall oncologic policy of the particular institution.

Radical Neck Dissection

Surgical Principle

En bloc resection of all cervical lymphatic tissue and fat at levels I–V in continuity with major nonlymphatic structures—the sternocleidomastoid muscle, internal jugular vein, and accessory nerve. By definition, this operation includes removal of the submandibular gland.

Indications

Fixed cervical lymph node metastases, N3 metastases.

Contraindications

Debilitated patient who is a poor candidate for surgery. Incurable primary tumor, incurable distant metastases, invasion of the carotid artery (relative contraindication, may be avoided by vascular grafting). Metastasis with contiguous invasion of prevertebral and nuchal soft tissues. Clinical N0 neck.

Specific Points Regarding Informed Consent

- Sensory disturbances involving the neck or ear.
- Growth lag of the skin flap.
- Paralysis of the nerves supplying the trapezius, visceral muscles, diaphragm, lingual muscles, sublingual muscles, vocal and facial muscles.
- Hoarseness or voice loss.
- Dyspnea, which may necessitate a tracheostomy tube.
- Poor cosmetic result, excessive scarring.
- Possible need to extend the skin incision.
- Mucosal injury, mediastinitis.
- Persistent discharge of lymphatic fluid.
- Lymphedema.
- Shoulder–arm syndrome.
- Limitation of motion by scar adhesions.

Operative Planning

B-mode ultrasonography and CT of the cervical soft tissues, plus thoracic CT to exclude distant metastases.

Table 11.1 Types of selective neck dissection recommended for the clinical N0 neck

Primary tumor site	Levels removed	
	Classic SND	More limited approach
Upper lip	I–III + parotid lymph nodes	IB–II + parotid lymph nodes
Lower lip	I–III	I–II
Floor of mouth	I–III	I, II
Mobile tongue	I–IV	I–II
Soft palate	II–IV	II–III
Tonsil	II–IV	II–III
Tongue base	II–IV	II–III
Supraglottis	II–IV	IIA–III
Glottis	II–IV	IIA–III
Piriform sinus	II–IV	IIA–IV
Posterior wall of pharynx	II–V	II–IV

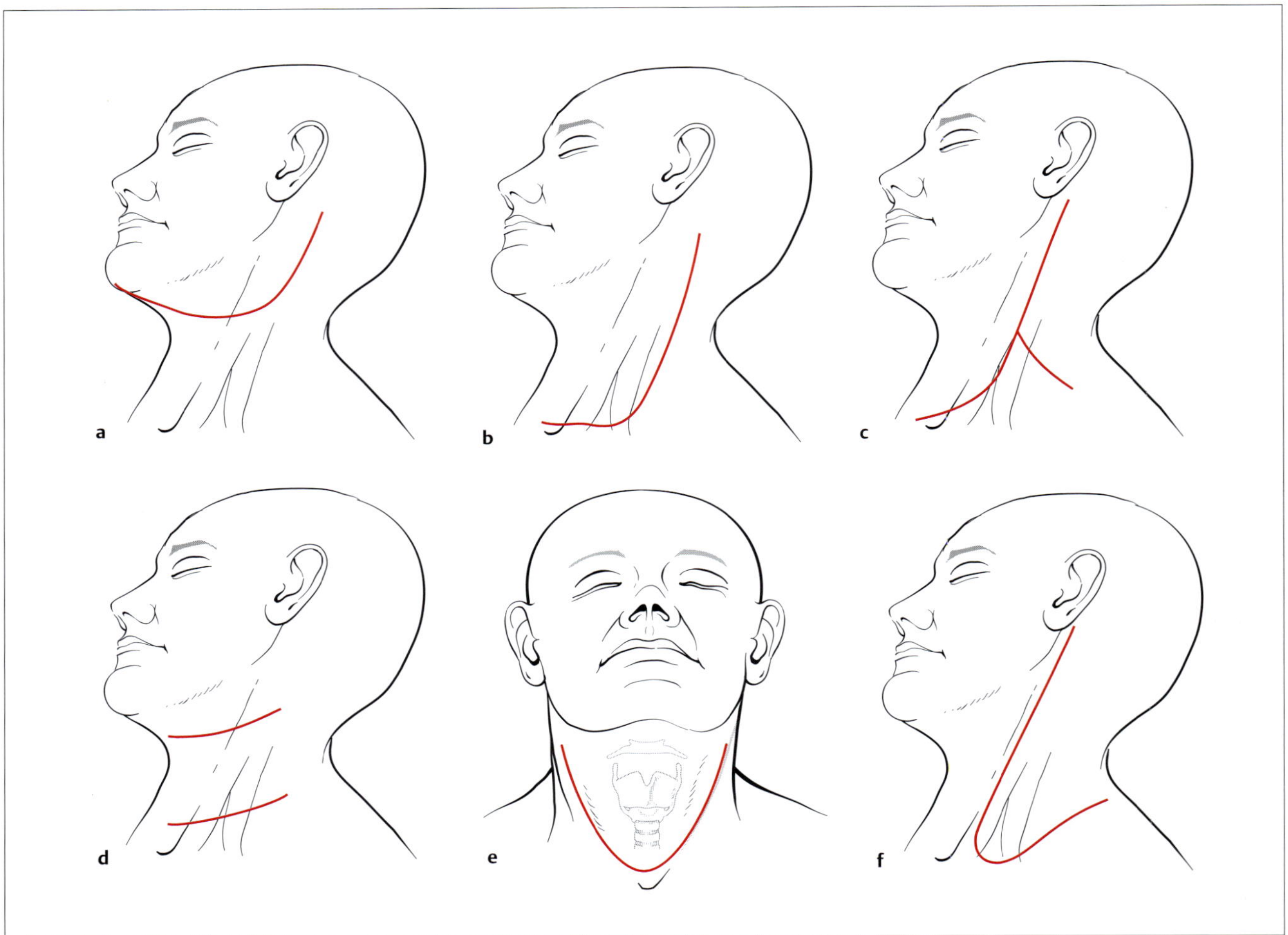

Fig. 11.4a–f Skin incisions for neck dissection.
a, e U-shaped incisions.
b, c Modified "hockey stick" incisions.
d MacFee incision.
f De Quervain incision.

Anesthesia

General endotracheal anesthesia.

Surgical Technique

Skin incision. Key anatomic landmarks—the mandibular angle, the tip of the mastoid process, and the sternum—are first marked on the skin. The skin incision (**Fig. 11.4**) starts at the tip of the mastoid process and curves along the anterior border of the trapezius, passing two finger-widths above the clavicle and curving toward the sternum to terminate at the cervical midline.

Dissection of the skin flap. The first step after the skin incision is to elevate the skin flap. This is aided by constant tension applied by an assistant. The platysma is integrated into the skin flap to maintain an adequate blood supply to the flap. The flap can be developed with a scissors, scalpel, or electrocautery. A radical neck dissection will include resection of the external jugular vein, which may be ligated with absorbable suture material (2–0 Vicryl) or nonabsorbable material. By contrast, the

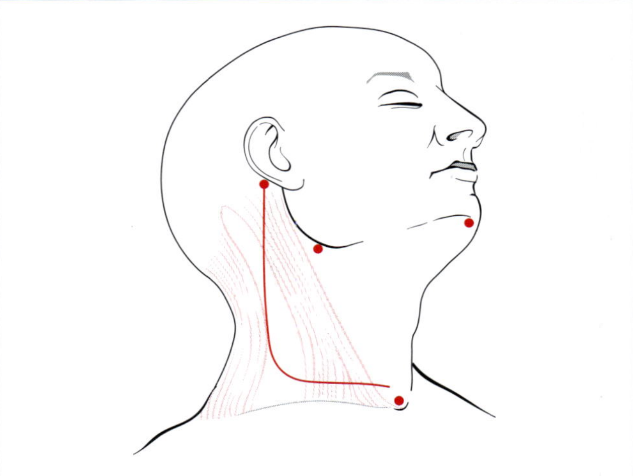

Fig. 11.5 Possible incision for radical neck dissection.
Key anatomic landmarks are marked on the skin before the incision is made.

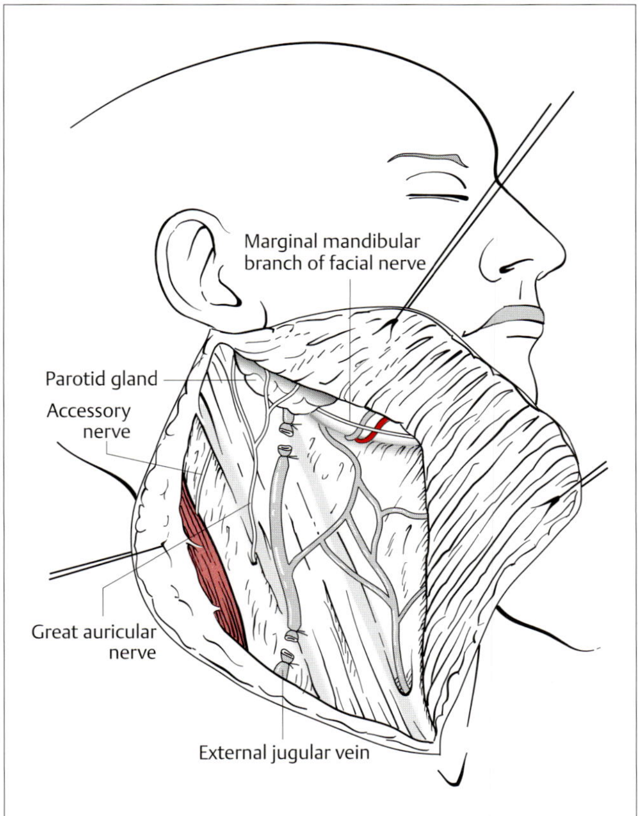

Fig. 11.6 Radical neck dissection.
The external jugular vein and its branches are incorporated into the surgical dissection.

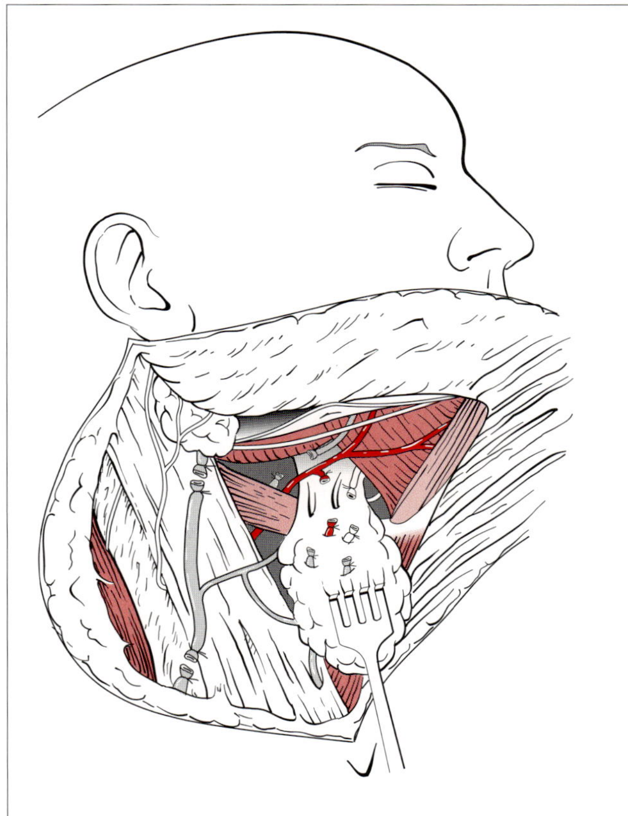

Fig. 11.7 Radical neck dissection.
The level I dissection includes removal of the submandibular gland. Nerves in that region are preserved.

internal jugular vein is always ligated with nonabsorbable suture material (e.g., 2–0 or 0 Mersilene) (**Figs. 11.5** and **11.6**).

Division of the great auricular nerve. The great auricular nerve is divided and the stumps cauterized with bipolar current to prevent neuroma formation. Dissection of the skin flap now continues toward the inferior pole of the parotid gland and the vertical ramus of the mandible, taking care to preserve the marginal branch of the facial nerve and the facial artery.

Fixation of the skin flap. The skin flap is retained by sutures to the surgical drapes.

Development of the inferior skin flap. The superficial fascia of the posterior triangle is incised and carefully spread open to expose the fatty tissue bearing the level V lymph nodes. The superficial fibers of the accessory nerve will enter the operative field during this part of the dissection. Because the accessory nerve may be sacrificed in a radical neck dissection, no special care is taken to preserve its superficial fibers. The inferior skin flap should be dissected to the anterior border of the trapezius muscle.

Dissection of level I nodes and the submandibular gland. The marginal branch of the facial nerve is at risk during resection of the level I nodes and submandibular gland. Generally this nerve branch crosses over the facial vein and artery at the approximate level of the inferior mandibular border (**Fig. 11.7**). The nerve branch should be identified at that location and traced a short distance posteriorly so that it can be safely mobilized upward from the field. Generally the facial vein is ligated. The hypoglossal nerve is exposed by elevating the intermediate tendon of the digastric muscle, whose course is traced cephalad. The hypoglossal nerve branch passing to the ansa cervicalis is ligated at the level where it crosses both carotid arteries. The dissection proceeds along the mandible to the submental attachment of the anterior belly of the digastric. The soft tissue between the anterior belly of the digastric and the mandible is mobilized. The dissection proceeds from the submental area across the anterior belly of the digastric to the midline raphe of the mylohyoid muscle, then continues on the mylohyoid to the free posterior border of that muscle. This requires a progressive posterior mobilization of the submandibular gland while identifying the excretory duct of the submandibular gland and the lingual nerve. Next, the submandibular (Wharton) duct is ligated with nonabsorbable 2–0 suture material (e.g., Mersilene). Care is taken to preserve the lingual nerve and the hypoglossal nerve, which runs from anterior to posterior in the adjacent fat. The hypoglossal nerve runs across the hyoglossus muscle, deep to the intermediate tendon of the digastric and behind the submandibular duct. When mobilization is completed, the submandibular gland can be separated from the facial artery in continuity with the surrounding lymph node-bearing soft tissue and reflected downward into the neck dissection specimen.

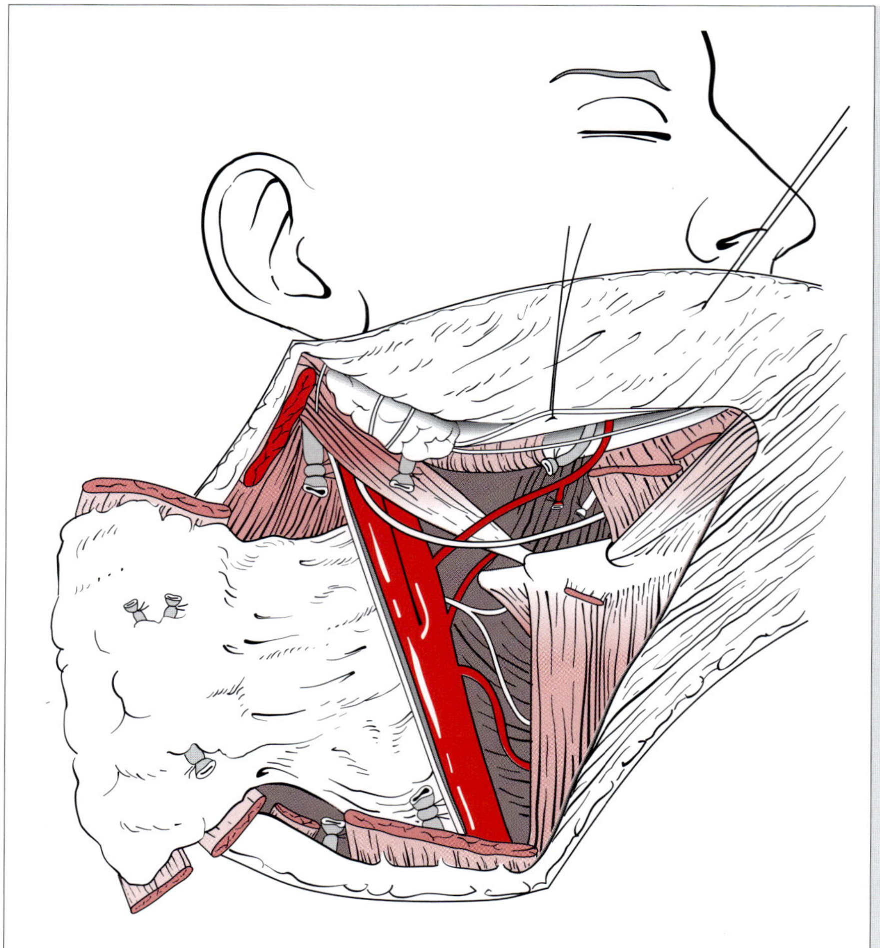

Fig. 11.8 Radical neck dissection. Levels I–IV have been removed.

Dissection of levels II–IV. The sternocleidomastoid muscle is progressively detached in a lateral-to-medial direction (e.g., with an electrocautery) until all its fiber bundles have been released (**Fig. 11.8**). The detached sternocleidomastoid is reflected downward to expose level II. The digastric muscle is the landmark that defines the superior limit of the field. The jugular vein is exposed by elevation of the digastric muscle. The accessory nerve and vagus nerve are identified at their site of emergence from the jugular foramen. Next, the jugular vein is carefully freed from surrounding soft tissue and doubly ligated with nonabsorbable sutures. The vessel is suture-ligated to prevent slippage, and the ligatures can be tied together. The upper vascular stump is additionally fixed to the deep cervical fascia or the posterior belly of the digastric. The accessory nerve is ligated and its proximal end coagulated as a precaution against neuroma formation. The lymph node-bearing fat at levels II–IV is dissected downward from the carotid artery. The sternocleidomastoid and omohyoid muscles are released from their sternal and clavicular attachments. The jugular vein is divided between ligatures and fixed ca. 1 cm above the clavicle, taking special care to preserve the vagus nerve. The opening of the thoracic duct into the internal jugular vein should be identified, especially on the left side, and the vein completely ligated at that site. Any aberrant lymphatic trunks should also be identified and ligated. Next, the inferior portion of the internal jugular vein is ligated and divided. This is done by positioning two clamps parallel to the clavicle and one cranially directed clamp at its lower end. The internal jugular vein is divided with scissors between the upper and middle clamps. It is then ligated with nonabsorbable suture material between the middle and lower clamp placed parallel to the clavicle. When the ligatures are tied, the middle clamp is slowly opened to confirm that the ligatures are secure. The vascular stump is then grasped and suture-ligated to prevent slippage.

Dissection of level V. The usual practice is to perform an en bloc resection of levels II–IV and V, the dissection of region V paralleling the dissection of levels II–IV. The plane of the dissection is on the deep cervical fascia. The cutaneous branches of the cervical plexus are divided and coagulated. The deep cervical fascia should not be opened, as the phrenic nerve runs unprotected on the scalene muscle deep to the fascia. Meticulous care should be taken to preserve the phrenic nerve (**Fig. 11.9**). The tissue to be removed is clamped and detached along the anterior border of the trapezius to prevent the development of a chyle fistula and prevent bleeding from branches of the transverse cervical artery. The accessory nerve is additionally coagulated and divided at the posteroinferior resection margin.

Wound closure. The wound is irrigated with warm Ringer solution following the en bloc resection. A suction drain is inserted and fixed at skin level with a 3–0 Vicryl suture. The

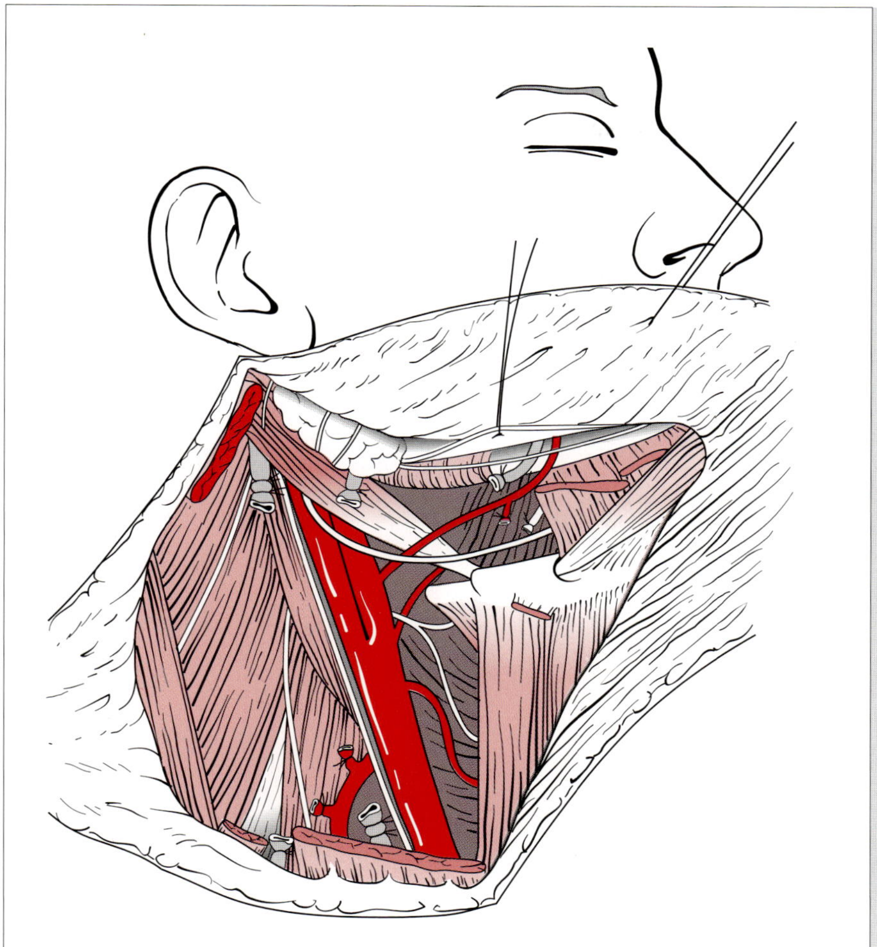

Fig. 11.9 Appearance of the operative field on completion of the radical neck dissection.

wound is closed at the level of the platysma with subcutaneous absorbable sutures (2–0 or 3–0 Vicryl). The skin margins are approximated with 3–0 or 4–0 sutures (e.g., Seralon).

! Risks and Complications

- Wound infection with secondary healing.
- Arterial or venous postoperative bleeding (immediate wound exploration).
- Bleeding from the common or internal carotid artery or subclavian artery (vascular surgical repair).
- Chyle fistula (milky discharge): first, try to close the fistula with pressure. If the discharge persists, repair by ligation or suture–ligation under the operating microscope (treatment details on p. 267).
- Vagal nerve injury (recurrent laryngeal nerve palsy), division of the marginal mandibular branch of the facial nerve, phrenic nerve division, brachial plexus injury. (If the prognosis is good, proceed with [neurosurgical] nerve repair.)
- Transient pharyngeal or laryngeal edema with hoarseness, dysphagia, and occasional dyspnea.
- Severe edema may develop after bilateral radical neck dissection and radiotherapy. Check vision in patients with severe eyelid edema.
- Sensory disturbances in the distribution of the brachial plexus.
- Motor disturbances and dropped shoulder due to accessory nerve injury.
- Motor disturbances in the neck and cervical spine due to loss of the sternocleidomastoid muscle and scarring.
- Apical pleural injury with pneumothorax and pneumomediastinum.
- Horner syndrome.

Postoperative Care

Postoperative care includes intravenous antibiotics (if the pharynx has been opened), hemoglobin checks, and suction drainage. The drain is removed between days 2 and 4 when the drainage volume has fallen to 30 mL or less. Low-molecular embolism prophylaxis (e.g., enoxaparin) is given. The patient is closely monitored for possible development of laryngeal edema. If both internal jugular veins were resected in one sitting, potentially severe edema may develop. If this prevents voluntary eye opening, regular ophthalmologic examinations should be done to reduce the risk of undetected blindness due to venous congestion. Postoperative Horner syndrome is managed with high-dose vitamin B therapy and artificial tears to protect the cornea. Ophthalmologic consultation is strongly advised.

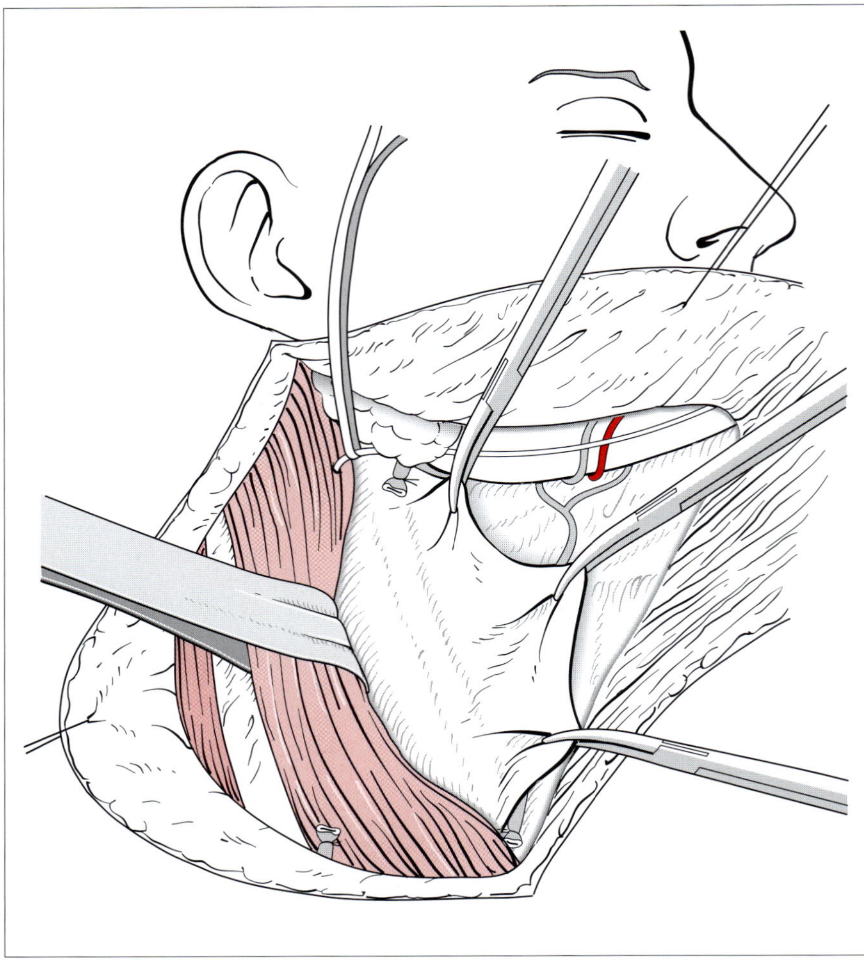

Fig. 11.10 Modified radical neck dissection. The sternocleidomastoid muscle is separated from its fascia, which is included in the surgical dissection.

Modified Radical Neck Dissection

Surgical Principle

Resection of lymph node-bearing fat at levels I–V while preserving at least one of the nonlymphatic structures (accessory nerve and/or internal jugular vein and/or sternocleidomastoid muscle). This operation is more time-consuming than a radical neck dissection.

Indications

Clinical suspicion of unilateral and/or bilateral metastasis. May be appropriate for refractory cervical lymph node tuberculosis.

Contraindications

Same as for a radical neck dissection.

Anesthesia

Same as for a radical neck dissection.

Surgical Technique

Dissection and elevation of the skin flap and the other steps are basically the same as in the radical neck dissection described above. But preserving at least one of the three nonlymphatic structures leads to special considerations that will be explored below in some detail.

Dissection of the sternocleidomastoid fascia. While the sternocleidomastoid muscle is generally preserved in this operation, its fascia is included in the surgical dissection (**Fig. 11.10**). Dissection of the fascia begins at the posterior border of the sternocleidomastoid muscle and proceeds anteriorly. Generally the dissection is done sharply with a scalpel or scissors. An experienced surgeon can also use electrocautery.

Preservation of the accessory nerve. The accessory nerve runs an anteroposterior, laterally downward course through the superior portion of the sternocleidomastoid muscle (**Fig. 11.11**). The nerve is exposed by spreading through the overlying fatty tissue with scissors. This is done on the medial aspect of the upper third of the sternocleidomastoid after careful medialization and elevation of that muscle with a blunt retractor. When large metastases are present, the nerve can be identified at its site of emergence caudal to the jugular foramen and lateral to the internal jugular vein. After the accessory nerve has been ex-

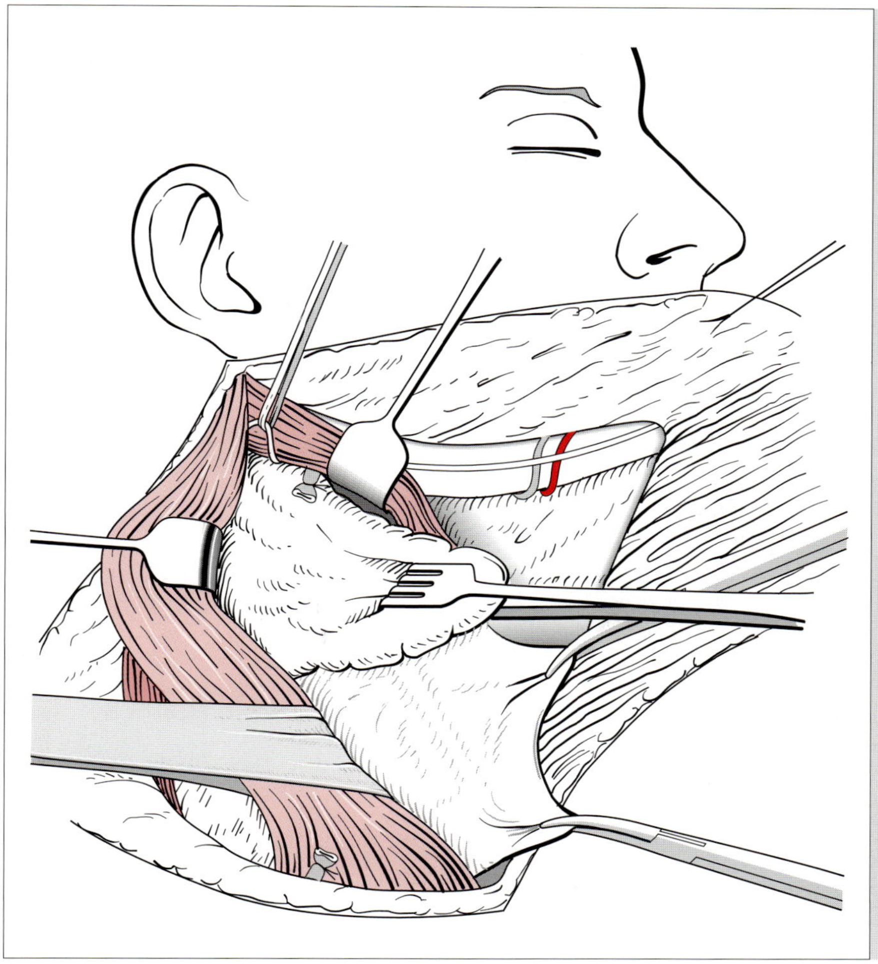

Fig. 11.11 Modified radical neck dissection. The superior portion of the accessory nerve is identified.

posed and identified, the nerve, which crosses the vein, is carefully snared with a soft tape between the skull base and sternocleidomastoid muscle and gently retracted from the operative field. A basic risk involved in using soft tapes is the sudden and inadvertent stretching of the snared nerve. The accessory nerve is also identified caudal to its site of emergence.

Dissection of the submuscular recess. Once the accessory nerve has been positively identified, removal of the lymph node-bearing fat at level IIB is begun. This is aided by maximum upward and lateral retraction on the sternocleidomastoid muscle. This maneuver also produces upward mobilization of the posterior belly of the digastric and the mandibular ramus. The fat between the sternocleidomastoid muscle and skull base is removed by pulling it forward and downward beneath the accessory nerve, aided by dividing the soft tissue at the boundary between levels IIA and B. As the dissection proceeds inferiorly, identifiable cutaneous branches of the cervical plexus are severed and nerve endings are coagulated to prevent neuroma formation. Dissection of level I and the submandibular gland is the same as in a radical neck dissection.

Dissection of the vascular sheath and levels II–IV. The sternocleidomastoid muscle is retracted laterally with a looped compress, and the lymph node-bearing fat is separated from the neurovascular sheath from above downward (**Fig. 11.12**). Avoid dissecting deep to the neurovascular sheath, as this could injure the sympathetic trunk. The inferior border of the cricoid cartilage marks the boundary line between levels III and IV. This is the approximate level at which the omohyoid muscle crosses the internal jugular vein. The muscle can be released from its clavicular attachment and included in the area to be dissected. It may also be preserved if its connection with the internal jugular vein is intact, as it can help maintain tension on the vessel wall and support its patency. The inferior margin of the block to tissue to be removed is clamped and ligated to prevent the development of a chyle fistula.

Dissection of level V. The accessory nerve, already exposed superomedially, is completely visualized in the posterior triangle by blunt dissection with a dissecting sponge (**Fig. 11.13**). The lymph node-bearing fat is mobilized toward the anterior border of the trapezius muscle. The posterior resection margin is clamped and ligated. Note that a level V dissection opens the posterior fascial layer of the posterior triangle, posing a risk of injury to branches of the brachial plexus, phrenic nerve, and transverse cervical artery. The wound is closed as previously described.

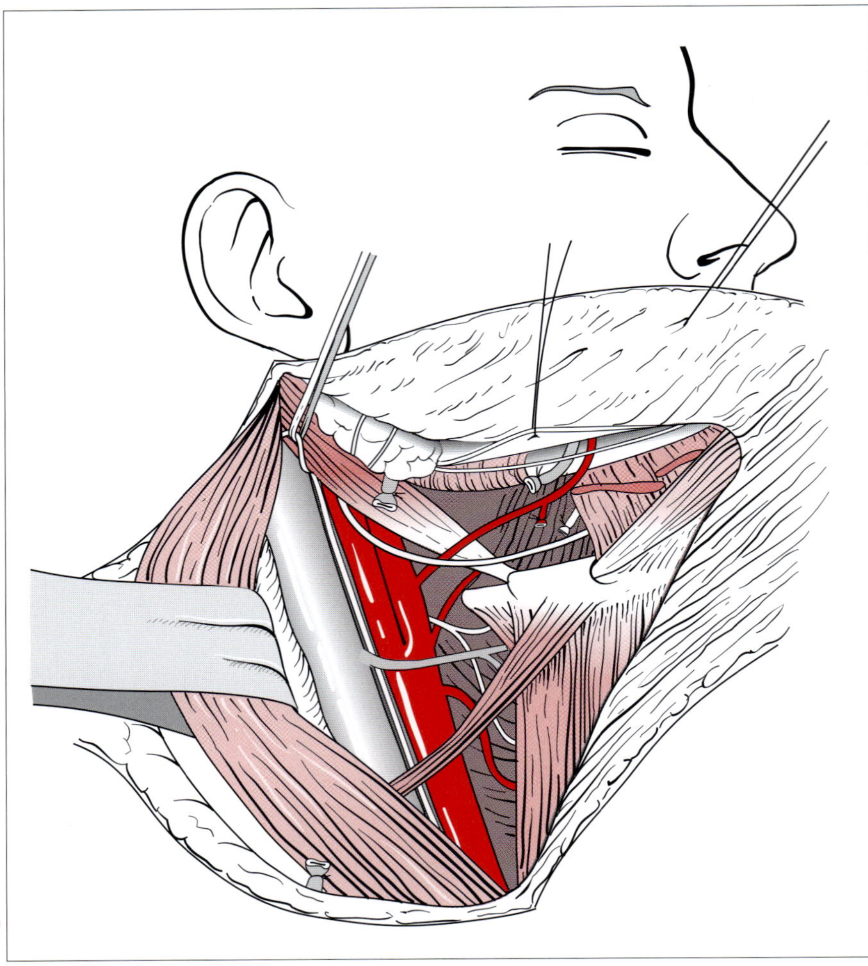

Fig. 11.12 Modified radical neck dissection. Appearance of the operative field after dissection of levels I–IV.

! Risks and Complications

Same as in a radical neck dissection.

Postoperative Care

Same as for a radical neck dissection.

Selective Neck Dissection

Surgical Principle

The resection is limited to selected cervical lymph node levels, depending on the primary tumor site. The sternocleidomastoid muscle, internal jugular vein, and accessory nerve are preserved. The incision is modified accordingly.

Indications

Clinical N0 neck, or even an N+ neck in selected cases.

Contraindications

None.

Surgical Technique

Selective neck dissection I–III (IV). The incision starts below the tip of the mastoid process, curves around the mandibular angle along skin creases, and ends parallel to the horizontal ramus of the mandible. Elevation of the skin flap, dissection of the submuscular recess, and exposure of the accessory nerve are the same as in a modified radical neck dissection. The lymph node-bearing fat is mobilized from above downward to the boundary of level IV (omohyoid muscle). The level I dissection is the same as previously described for a radical neck dissection while generally leaving the submandibular gland intact; wound closure is the same. Level IV can be included in the dissection without difficulty.

Selective neck dissection II–IV (V). The incision is like that described above but follows a skin crease in the lower neck or extends from the mastoid tip along the posterior border of the sternocleidomastoid muscle and ends ca. 2 cm above the jugular fossa. Dissection of the skin flap and submuscular recess and exposure of the accessory nerve are as previously described. The lymph node-bearing fat is dissected following mobilization

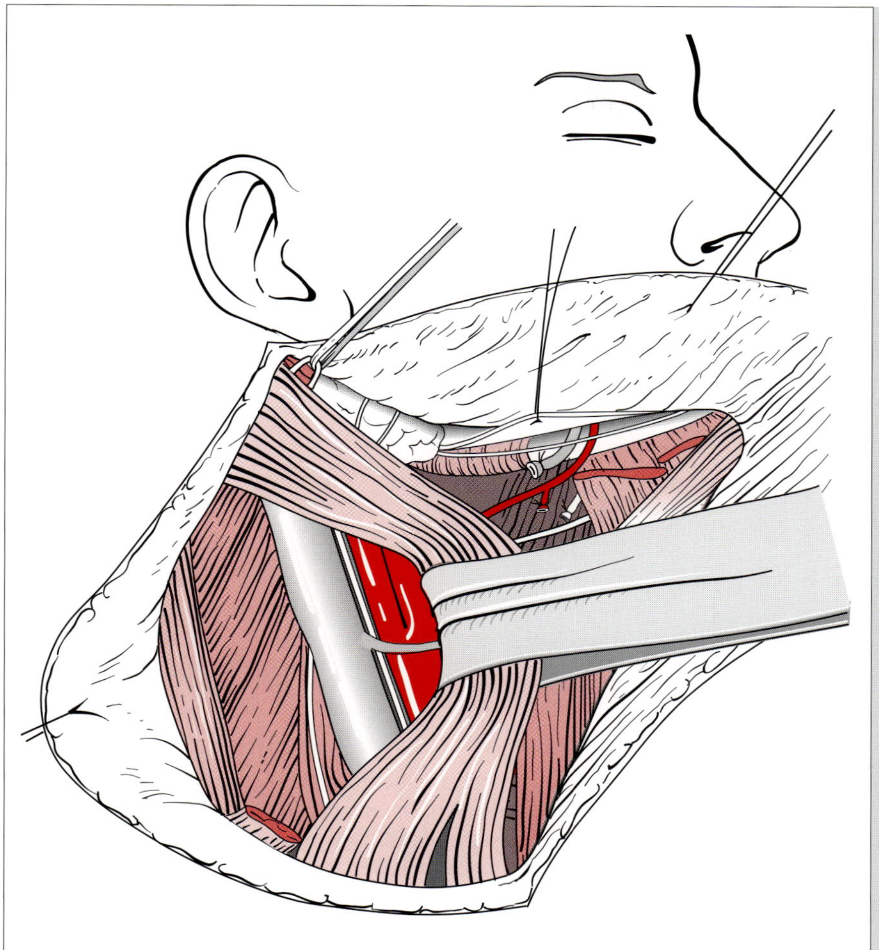

Fig. 11.13 Modified radical neck dissection. Appearance of the operative field after the dissection of level V.

of the sternocleidomastoid muscle, sparing the internal jugular vein and neural structures as described above. The omohyoid muscle can be preserved. Wound closure is the same as previously described. If the dissection includes level V, meticulous care should be taken to preserve the accessory nerve.

> **! Risks and Complications**
> Same as in a radical neck dissection.

Postoperative Care

Same as for a radical neck dissection.

Alternatives

Intensity-modulated radiotherapy (IMRT) can deliver high radiation doses to specific lymph node levels while sparing surrounding tissues based on the precise definition of predetermined target volumes. In the future, this technology may provide an effective alternative to classic radiotherapy.

Surgical Treatment of Thyroglossal Duct Cyst

Thyroglossal duct cysts are cysts in the cervical midline that arise from embryonic remnants of the thyroglossal duct. Conservative measures such as sclerosing injections and cauterization are of no value. The only definitive treatment is complete extirpation.

Surgical Principle

Complete surgical removal of the cyst and any associated tract or fistula including its attachment to the foramen cecum. A thyroglossal fistula may result from the surgical treatment of a thyroglossal duct cyst or from a spontaneously perforated cyst.

Indications

Any median neck cyst or cervical fistula.

Contraindication

Severe debilitation.

Specific Points Regarding Informed Consent

Neck Cyst or Lipoma, Thyroglossal Fistula

- Sensory disturbances involving the neck or ear.
- Paralysis of the accessory nerve, vagus nerve, phrenic nerve, hypoglossal nerve, facial nerve (marginal branch), and superior or inferior laryngeal nerve.
- Hoarseness or voice loss.
- Dyspnea, which may necessitate a tracheostomy.
- Poor cosmetic result, excessive scarring.
- Possible need to extend the skin incision.
- Mucosal injury, mediastinitis.
- Possible need to remove the body of the hyoid bone (thyroglossal duct cyst or fistula).
- Possible need to remove one tonsil.

Operative Planning

B-mode ultrasonography. Cysts may require fine-needle aspiration.

Special Instruments

Bulb-tipped probe.

Anesthesia

General endotracheal anesthesia.

Surgical Technique for a Thyroglossal Duct Fistula

Visualization of the fistula tract. A bulb-tipped probe is carefully introduced into the fistula tract, and a purse-string suture or circumferential ligature is placed around the external opening of the fistula. The suture is tightened over a blunt cannula, and methylene blue is injected into the tract.

Skin incision. When the fistula opening is located near the hyoid bone, a transverse skin incision is made that incorporates an ellipse of skin around the opening (**Fig. 11.14**). If the opening is at a lower level, a longitudinal midline incision starts above the hyoid bone and extends to a point just above the fistula opening, which is incorporated in an ellipse.

Dissection of the fistula tract to the hyoid bone. The platysma is divided. The fistula tract is identified by spreading through the surrounding soft tissues, exposing the strap muscles as far as the hyoid bone. The tract is snared and carefully elevated for further dissection.

Resecting the body of the hyoid bone. The central attachments of the strap muscles are released from the body of the hyoid bone with an electrocautery along with the muscles of the oral floor, and the hyoid bone is divided on both sides of the midline with cartilage scissors. The mid portion of the bone (**Fig. 11.15**) is adherent to the tract.

Dissection of the fistula tract behind the hyoid bone. The further course of the tract behind the hyoid bone is traced toward the foramen cecum. If the deeper continuation of the tract cannot be identified, the visible portion of the tract is removed along with directly adjacent tissue and the operation is concluded. If the tract can be traced to the foramen cecum, it is dissected to the level of the pharyngeal mucosa, and the foramen cecum is excised and removed in continuity with the tract. The pharynx is immediately repaired with heavy suture material. Tract dissection is facilitated by placing counter-pressure on the tongue base with a McIvor retractor introduced transorally and held at a slight angle by an assistant.

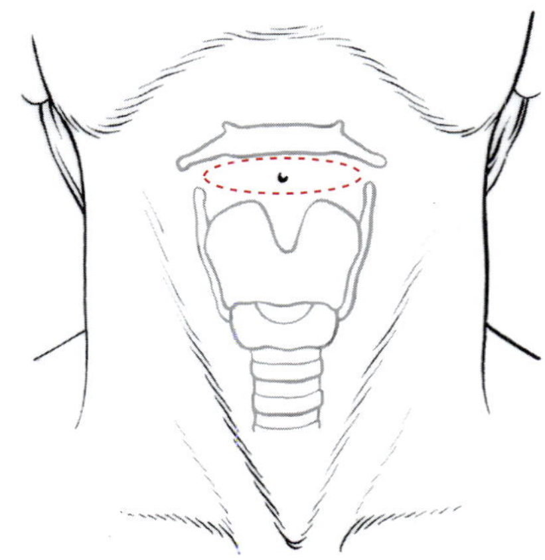

Fig. 11.14 Thyroglossal fistula, step 1.
An elliptical incision is made around the external opening of the fistula.

Wound closure. The wound is closed in layers over a suction drain, and a dressing is applied.

Surgical Technique for a Thyroglossal Duct Cyst

The technique is basically the same as for a thyroglossal fistula.

Skin incision and dissection of the cyst. A transverse skin incision is made above or below the cyst, dividing the skin and the platysma. The flaps are developed upward to a level above the body of the hyoid bone, and the cyst wall is dissected free. The body of the hyoid bone is resected.

Typically, a band of connective tissue extends from the cyst to the body of the hyoid bone, and so the body of the hyoid bone is resected as it is in the treatment of a thyroglossal fistula. Any tract remnants or branches are also identified and removed.

Rules, Tips, and Tricks
The removal of a thyroglossal duct cyst generally includes resection of the body of the hyoid bone. The dissection keeps to the midline to avoid damaging the hypoglossal nerve and superior laryngeal nerve. If cyst rupture occurs, the cyst wall should be packed with gauze during the rest of the dissection.

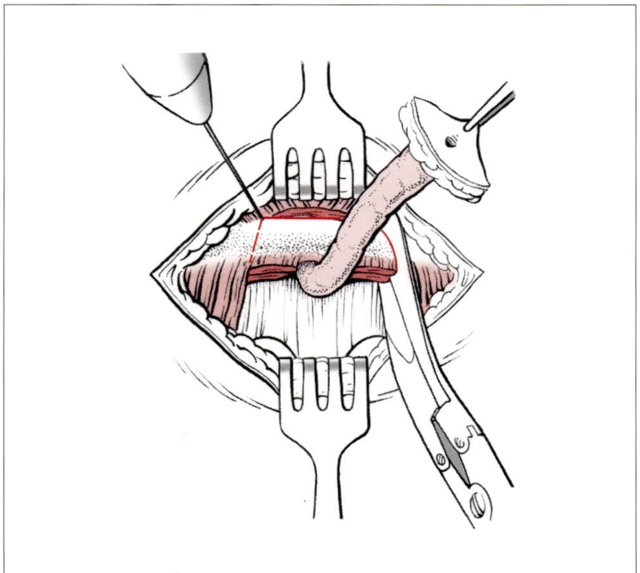

Fig. 11.15 Thyroglossal fistula, step 2.
The fistula tract is attached to the hyoid bone. The strap muscles and oral floor muscles are released, and the body of the hyoid bone is resected with cartilage shears.

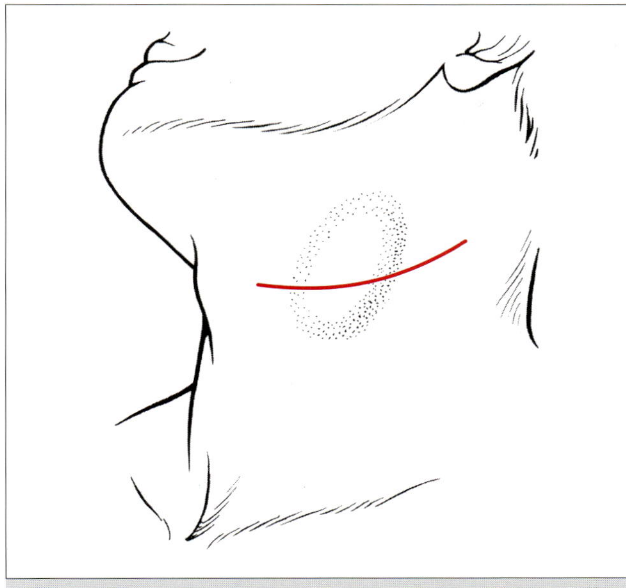

Fig. 11.16 Branchial cleft cyst, step 1.
The skin is incised at the anterior border of the sternocleidomastoid muscle or along an existing skin crease over the lower portion of the cyst.

! Risks and Complications

- An incomplete excision predisposes to recurrence. Resecting the body of the hyoid bone will generally have no adverse clinical effects.
- Keloid formation. Postoperative bleeding from the hyoid bone region (requires re-exploration). Dissecting the fistula close to the midline should avoid injury to the hypoglossal nerve and superior laryngeal nerve.

Postoperative Care

Antibiotic therapy beyond the perioperative period is necessary only if the fistula was opened or infected. The drain is removed according to output. If the excision extended to the tongue base, respiration should be monitored to detect any hematoma or edema formation about the laryngeal inlet. Recurrence of a thyroglossal duct cyst is managed by re-operation with wide excision of all abnormal tissue. There are cases that have required multiple surgical interventions, and an inadequate revision procedure predisposes to cyst or fistula recurrence.

Surgical Treatment of Branchial Cleft Cysts

Branchial Cleft Cyst

Branchial cleft cysts are usually manifested in young adults. Contrary to earlier theories of pathogenesis, it is now known that branchial cleft cysts arise from heterotopic epithelial inclusions in cervical lymph nodes ("tonsillogenic lymphadenopathy"), suggesting that the lesion results from the cystic transformation of a lymph node. The findings that support this hypothesis include patient age distribution, histologic findings, and especially the site of occurrence, as branchial cleft cysts are generally located at the level of the lateral hyoid cornu where the facial vein opens into the internal jugular vein. It is known that the posterior third of the tongue and the palatine tonsil drain into the jugulodigastric lymph node located at this site. According to this hypothesis, squamous epithelial cells travel with the lymph from the tonsillar crypts to the proximal lymph nodes in response to inflammatory processes. Recurrent infections over time may lead to the development of a cyst.

11

Surgical Principle

Complete removal of the cystic sac.

Indication

Any lateral neck cyst.

Contraindication

Severe systemic illness that would not justify the high anesthetic risk.

Surgical Technique

Skin incision. The skin is incised along an existing skin crease at the level of the cyst or one fingerwidth below the visible and palpable bulge (**Fig. 11.16**). The incision is deepened through the platysma, and the anterior border of the sternocleidomastoid muscle is identified while the wound margins are retracted.

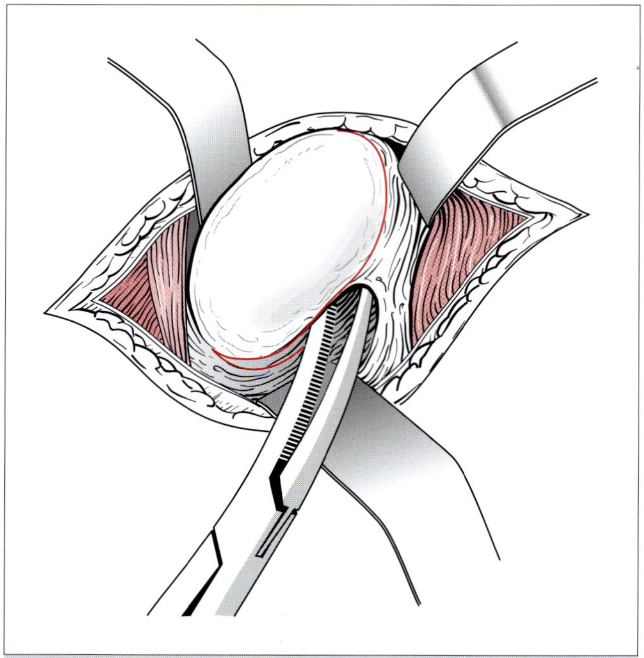

Fig. 11.17 Branchial cleft cyst, step 2.
The cyst sac is exposed by spreading open the surrounding soft tissues.

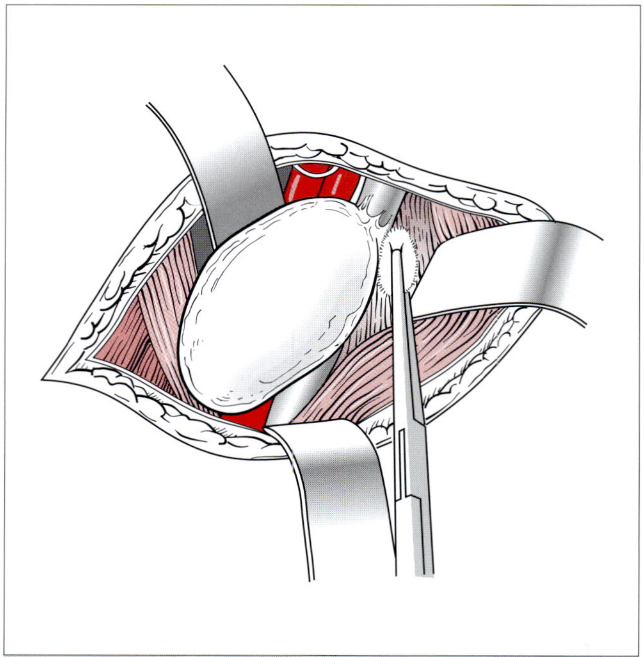

Fig. 11.18 Branchial cleft cyst, step 3.
When dense adhesions are present, the vascular sheath, hypoglossal nerve, and accessory nerve are isolated and preserved above and below the cyst.

11

Exposure of the cyst. The cyst sac is exposed by spreading and incising the adjacent connective tissue, aided by dissection with a mounted sponge (**Fig. 11.17**).

Mobilization of the cyst. The cyst sac is progressively mobilized and enucleated, aided by the insertion of packing strips, until it is completely freed from surrounding tissues (**Fig. 11.18**). *Dissecting directly on the cyst sac* will avoid inadvertent injury to neural structures (superior laryngeal nerve, recurrent laryngeal nerve, hypoglossal nerve, accessory nerve, mandibular branch of the facial nerve). If the cyst is tethered by significant adhesions due to previous inflammatory processes, we recommended first locating the vascular sheath below the cyst and mobilizing the cyst from below upward while carefully identifying the jugular vein, vagus nerve, and hypoglossal nerve. Isolation of these structures is also necessary in cases where cordlike processes extend from the cyst through the carotid bifurcation. If the cyst is ruptured, the tear site should be clamped off. With excessive drainage of cyst contents, the interior of the cyst should be tamponaded with packing material.

Wound closure. The wound is closed in layers over a suction drain.

Rules, Tips, and Tricks

If the cyst is large, its volume can be significantly reduced intraoperatively by aspirating its contents through a large-bore needle secured with a purse-string suture. This facilitates subsequent dissection and minimizes the risk of uncontrolled cyst rupture.

! Risks and Complications

The transection of cutaneous nerves may be followed by transient hypoesthesia about the cervical scar. Heavy scarring may occur in patients prone to keloid formation. Injury to the hypoglossal nerve, superior laryngeal nerve, recurrent laryngeal nerve, accessory nerve, or even the marginal mandibular branch of the facial nerve may occur in situations where anatomic landmarks are difficult to identify.

Postoperative Care

The suction drain is removed when the drainage volume falls to 30 mL or less. Antibiotic coverage should be continued beyond the perioperative period in patients with a secondary cyst infection. The sutures are removed on day 7.

Branchial Cleft Fistula

The pathogenesis of branchial cleft fistulas is quite different from that of branchial cleft cysts. A disturbance in the embryonic involution of the second through fourth branchial pouches may result in persistence of the cervical duct and its external opening. The opening of the pharyngeal fistula depends on the location of the second, third, and fourth branchial pouches. The second pouch gives rise to an opening located in the area of the supratonsillar recess. The third pouch is associated with an opening in the piriform recess anterior to the plica of the superior laryngeal nerve, and the fourth pouch with an opening in the piriform recess posterior to the plica. Thus, branchial cleft fistulas have a curved tract that ascends at varying angles to the external opening in the neck.

Excision of Branchial Cleft Fistula

Surgical Principle

Complete removal of the fistula tract from its external opening to the internal opening, which is generally located in the supratonsillar fossa or on the posterior pharyngeal wall.

Indication

Any lateral neck fistula, especially after previous infections. Surgery in these cases should be performed during an infection-free interval.

Contraindication

Severe debilitation.

Surgical Technique

Skin incision. A longitudinal incision is made along the anterior border of the sternocleidomastoid muscle to the external opening of the fistula, incorporating an ellipse of skin around the opening (**Fig. 11.19**).

Visualization and proximal dissection of the fistula tract. The platysma is divided. The tract is snared, having first been identified by the injection of methylene blue (or the insertion of a fine silver probe). The tract is followed while overlying soft tissues are divided. Meanwhile the dissection is deepened to the vascular compartment from the anterior border of the sternocleidomastoid muscle, and the jugular vein is identified. The tract passes more deeply in the area of the carotid bifurcation and usually emerges medially between the external and internal carotid arteries. With strong retraction on the sternocleidomastoid muscle, the vessels are isolated by blunt dissection and the hypoglossal nerve and vagus nerve are identified (**Fig. 11.20**).

Dissection of the distal fistula tract into the oral cavity. With the surrounding soft tissues retracted, the fistula tract is traced as deeply as possible through the cervical field. The external portion of the fistula is excised, and a bulb-tipped probe is introduced into the remaining tract until it enters the oral cavity. The tract is tied onto the probe proximal to its bulb end. The probe can now be advanced or pulled transorally to invert the fistulous tract into the oral cavity where it can be excised and ligated after insertion of a McIvor retractor (**Fig. 11.21**).

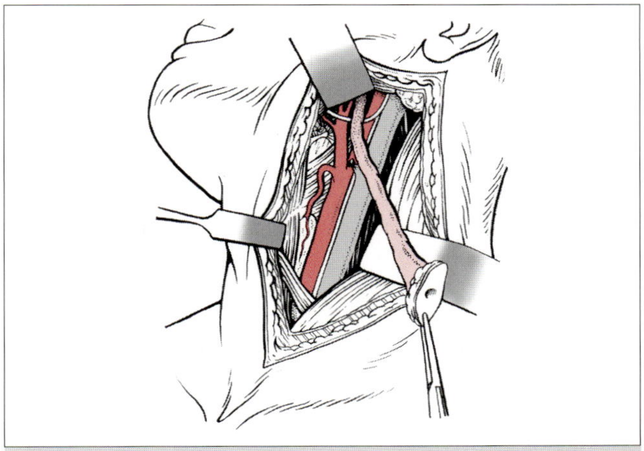

Fig. 11.20 Branchial cleft fistula, step 2.
Dissection of the fistula tract is continued, exposing the vascular sheath. In most cases the tract runs deeply through the carotid bifurcation.

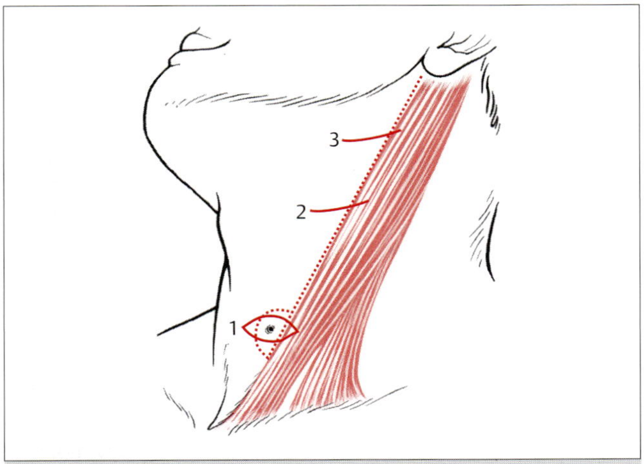

Fig. 11.19 Branchial cleft fistula, step 1.
The skin is incised along the sternocleidomastoid muscle, incorporating the fistula opening in an ellipse (dotted line). Another option is to access the fistula tract through two or three transverse incisions placed in existing skin creases (1–3).

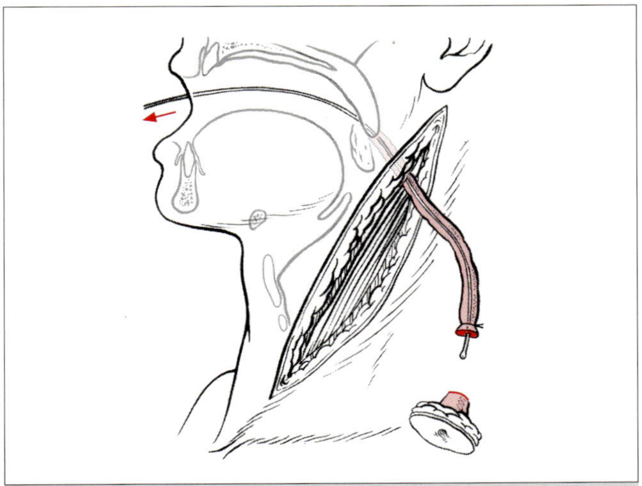

Fig. 11.21 Branchial cleft fistula, step 3.
The fistula tract is intussuscepted into the oral cavity with a bulb-tipped probe. The shortened duct is tied onto the probe and is inverted when pulled through.

Wound closure. The external wound is closed in layers over a small suction drain.

Modification

Instead of a longitudinal incision anterior to the sternocleidomastoid muscle, multiple transverse incisions can be placed in skin cleavage lines over the sternocleidomastoid. The intervening skin bridges are undermined, and the fistula is excised in typical fashion. This technique gives less exposure than the longitudinal incision but generally results in a more cosmetically favorable scar.

> **! Risks and Complications**
> The complications are basically the same as in the surgery of branchial cleft cysts. By practicing meticulous technique, the surgeon can avoid injuring the carotid artery when working through the carotid bifurcation.

Postoperative Care

The suction drain is removed when the drainage volume falls to 30 mL or less.

Excision of an External Laryngocele

- Extensive external and combined cysts are exposed through an external incision, traced to their attachment in the laryngeal ventricle, and excised.
- Large external laryngoceles that cannot be marsupialized transorally in adults should be excised if they are associated with significant complaints such as dyspnea or hoarseness or if they are cosmetically objectionable.

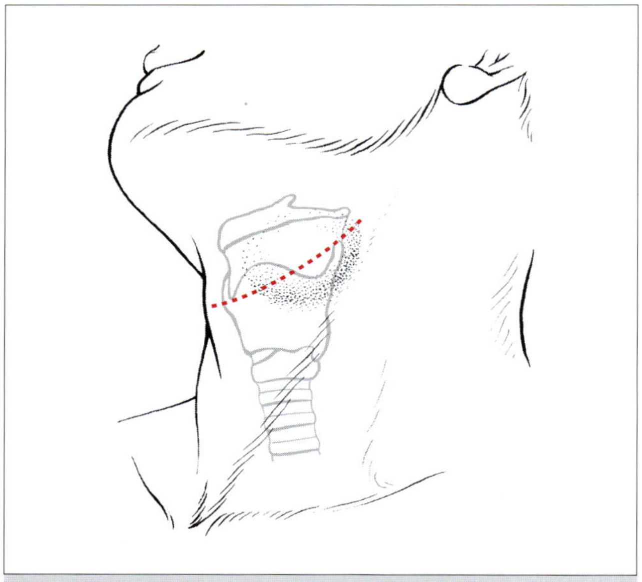

Fig. 11.22 Excision of an external laryngocele. Skin incision.

Surgical Technique

Skin incision. A slightly curved skin incision is made from the posterior border of the hyoid bone to the thyroid notch. The platysma and superficial cervical fascia are divided (**Fig. 11.22**).

Cyst identification. The strap muscles are divided along the hyoid bone (**Fig. 11.23a**). The laryngocele sac is bluntly dissected on the thyrohyoid membrane, proceeding carefully because of the friability of the sac. With an internal laryngocele, the thy-

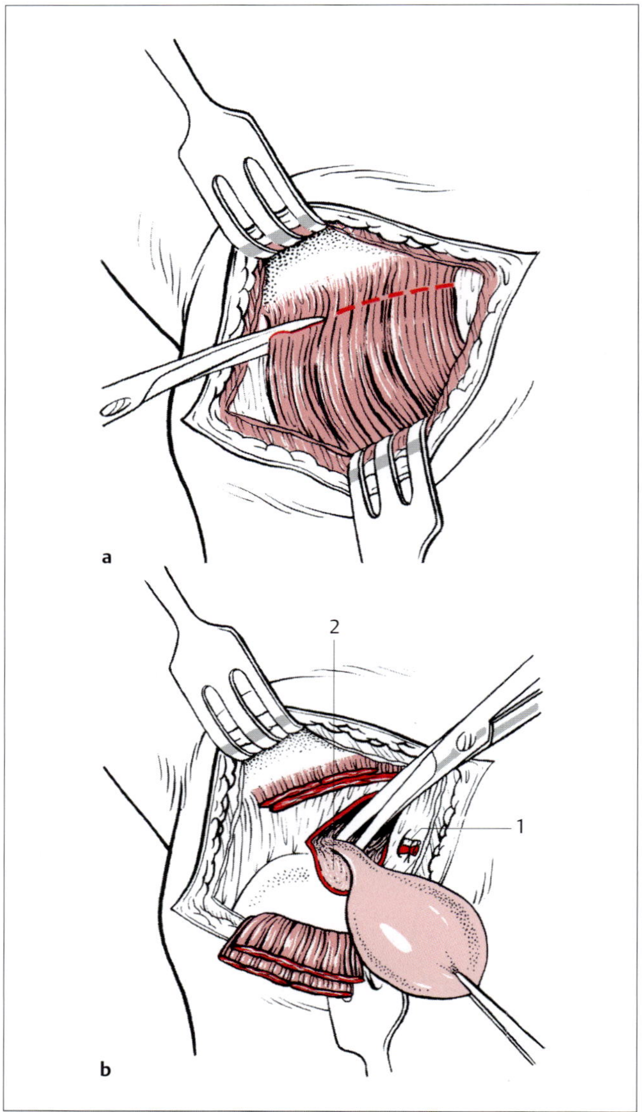

Fig. 11.23a, b Excision of a laryngocele.
a The strap muscles are detached from the hyoid bone.
b The cyst sac is bluntly mobilized. The superior laryngeal nerve (1) is identified, and the thyrohyoid membrane (2) is reflected downward.

11

rohyoid membrane is also detached from the hyoid bone and reflected inferiorly so that the surgeon can carefully dissect downward to the cyst sac. The base of the sac is traced to its opening into the ventricle, where it is resected and buried with a purse-string suture (**Fig. 11.23b**). If structures are difficult to identify, orientation is established by stripping the outer perichondrium and resecting a portion of the thyroid cartilage plate.

Wound closure. After excision of the laryngocele, the thyrohyoid membrane is returned and sutured into place. The wound is closed in layers over a suction drain.

Modification

Small external or combined laryngoceles and internal laryngoceles can be marsupialized through a transoral approach (see Chapter 10).

Rules, Tips, and Tricks

The superior laryngeal nerve must be preserved. Injury to the nerve can be consistently avoided by detaching the thyrohyoid membrane just below the hyoid bone and reflecting it downward.

! Risks and Complications

- Rare instances of deep neck infection.
- Cutaneous emphysema due to an incontinent purse-string suture.
- Dyspnea due to intralaryngeal hematoma formation (monitoring, tracheotomy if necessary).
- A carcinoma in the laryngeal ventricle may occasionally cause a laryngocele. This is confirmed by histologic examination of the pedicle.

Postoperative Care

The drain is removed on the second day. Postoperative care includes antitussive agents, antibiotics, and corticosteroid therapy as needed.

Cervical Lymphangioma

The great majority of lymphangiomas occur in the head and neck region. They may be isolated or associated with generalized abnormalities of the lymphatic system. Clinical evidence indicates that lymphatic malformations tend to grow slowly but show sudden enlargement in response to infections of the upper aerodigestive tract. Lymphangiomas typically grow by expansion but are also known to infiltrate surrounding structures such as the parotid gland or lingual muscles. This particularly applies to capillary lymphangiomas, which are considerably more difficult to treat.

Surgical Principle

The treatment of choice for lymphangiomas is conventional surgical excision. All portions of the lymphangioma must be removed to prevent recurrence. With lesions that infiltrate the lingual muscles, for example, an optimum trade-off must be found between functionality and an adequate resection based on individual functional and cosmetic considerations. Not infrequently, a lymphangioma in the parotid gland requires complete exposure of the facial nerve with intraoperative nerve monitoring. The number of surgical interventions should be kept to a minimum, as each procedure is followed by scarring that will hamper the next procedure. The best solution is a small number of operations, each achieving the best possible result. This particularly applies to the initial operation. In dealing with extensive cervical lymphangiomas that communicate with the floor of the mouth special care should be taken during the initial operation to reduce or even prevent subsequent traction from the lymphangioma on the mandible. The frequent development of mandibular hyperplasia is a major problem in children with giant lymphangiomas of the head and neck. It is usually associated with a backward-rotation growth pattern of the vertical rami, which is responsible for the open bite and malocclusion that develop in these patients.

Indications

Unlike hemangiomas, lymphangiomas do not undergo spontaneous resolution. Consequently, surgery is indicated for lymphangiomas that are causing functional and cosmetic complaints. Another treatment option is sclerotherapy with doxycycline or OK-432 (picibanil).

Contraindications

- None.
- If a lymphangioma is detected in utero and is causing a life-threatening obstruction, conventional surgical excision can be performed just a few days after cesarean delivery, making certain that facilities for intubation and tracheotomy are available if needed. In this context the ex utero intrapartum (EXIT) procedure, which is meanwhile performed in some specialized centers, should be mentioned.

Specific Points Regarding Informed Consent

The same points are emphasized as for a neck dissection and/or parotidectomy, depending on the findings.

Operative Planning

Palpation, ultrasonography, MRI. Incisional biopsy is contraindicated.

Special Instruments

Microscope, instruments for parotid surgery if needed, instruments for monitoring affected cranial nerves.

Anesthesia

General endotracheal anesthesia.

Surgical Technique

Skin incision. The skin is incised along the sternocleidomastoid muscle from the mastoid to the jugular fossa, depending on the extent of the lymphatic malformation. An auxiliary incision into the submandibular region may be added if needed. No further general guidelines may be given, as the incision will naturally depend on the individual extent of the angioma.

Exploration and excision. A cystic lymphangioma should be dissected along its outer wall. Often this type of lymphangioma can be completely extirpated without opening it. Capillary lymphangiomas can be much more difficult to remove. Some may broadly involve adjacent muscles or glands, and the extent of the resection should be based on the criteria outlined above.

Wound closure. The external wound is closed in layers over one or two suction drains.

Modification

The injection of doxycycline or OK-432 (picibanil) may be considered as a possible alternative to conventional surgical excision in some situations. Not yet approved for clinical use, OK-432 is a lyophilized incubation mixture of human α-hemolytic *Streptococcus pyogenes*. This agent incites a local inflammatory reaction resulting in adhesions that cause the lymphangioma to shrink. This therapy may be associated with significant complications (e.g., very high fever) in some patients.

> **! Risks and Complications**
> The complications are basically the same as those arising in major surgery of the neck and parotid gland. The principal risk is recurrence of the lymphangioma caused by a grossly complete but microscopically incomplete resection. Treatment of the recurrence carries a significantly higher surgical risk in terms of neurovascular injury.

Postoperative Care

The drains are removed when the drainage volume falls to 30 mL or less. Antibiotics should be continued past the perioperative period following extensive extirpations.

Surgery of Glomus Tumors (Paragangliomas)

Surgical Principle

The tumor is dissected in the carotid adventitia and removed while preserving the common and internal carotid arteries.

Indications

Glomus tumors (synonyms: paraganglioma, chemodectoma, carotid body tumor) are slow-growing tumors that should be managed surgically in patients aged 65 or younger. Surgery is also indicated after age 65 if malignant transformation is suspected or there is evidence or risk of complications due to continued tumor growth. The value of preoperative embolization for carotid body tumors is controversial, but a relatively new embolization material, Onyx, can apparently provide a marked improvement in embolization results. Of course, further experience is needed before the efficacy of this product can be definitively assessed.

Contraindications

- Debilitated patient.
- Patient over 65 years of age (relative contraindication).
- Very extensive tumor that no longer appears resectable or whose complete removal would require mutilating surgery.

Specific Points Regarding Informed Consent

- Sensory disturbances involving the neck or ears.
- Paralysis of the nerves supplying the trapezius, visceral muscles, diaphragm, lingual muscles, sublingual muscles, vocal cords, and facial muscles.
- Hoarseness or voice loss.
- Dyspnea, which may necessitate a tracheostomy tube.
- Poor cosmetic result, excessive scarring.
- Possible need to extend the skin incision.
- Mucosal injury, mediastinitis.
- Possible need to ligate blood flow to the brain, creating a risk of stroke symptoms (hemiplegia, aphasia, etc.)

Operative Planning

Palpation (pulsating mass that is movable only in the horizontal direction). Imaging workup may include ultrasonography, MRI,

MR angiography, and digital subtraction angiography. Incisional biopsy is contraindicated (profuse bleeding). The balloon inclusion test may be used to predict neurological status if the carotid artery must be ligated intraoperatively.

Special Instruments

Bulldog clamps, vascular prostheses, microcoagulation, microscope, otosurgical microinstruments.

Anesthesia

General endotracheal anesthesia.

Surgical Technique

Skin incision. The skin is incised along the sternocleidomastoid muscle, from the mastoid to the jugular fossa. An auxiliary incision into the submandibular region may be added if needed.

Vascular exposure. The vessels are exposed from below, and the tumor margins are isolated as far as the skull base. The hypoglossal nerve, vagus nerve, and accessory nerve may be isolated from the periphery and preserved.

Tumor mobilization. The tumor is very carefully freed from the carotid artery in the subadventitial plane aided by magnification, bipolar microcoagulation, and fine instruments. The branches of the external carotid artery may be ligated and divided to facilitate the dissection.

Control of tumor bleeding. Bleeding from the tumor can generally be controlled by packing the bleeding site, and a vasoconstrictor may be applied if desired. Dissection at a different site can be continued while the bleeding site is packed off. By proceeding carefully, the surgeon can usually remove the tumor intact without causing significant injury to the common or internal carotid artery.

Control of arterial bleeding. If significant injury occurs to the common or internal carotid artery, immediately compress or clamp off the initially exposed common carotid artery (note clamp time) and try to place a hemostatic clamp across the lesion. Then release the proximal clamp on the carotid artery and suture the arterial lesion over the clamp. This should be done by a vascular surgeon if the head and neck surgeon is inexperienced in vascular repairs.

Wound closure. The wound is closed in layers over a suction drain, and a dressing is applied.

! Risks and Complications

- Paralysis of the hypoglossal, accessory, or vagus nerve.
- Sympathetic nerve injury (Horner syndrome).
- Hemiparesis due to carotid artery ligation.
- Keloid formation, disturbance of cutaneous sensation in the neck, wound healing problems.

Postoperative Care

Remove the drain when residual output is 30 mL or less. Administer antibiotics.

Surgery of the Thyroid Gland

Anatomy and Relations

The thyroid gland consists of two symmetrical lobes joined by the isthmus ca. 2 cm below the laryngotracheal junction. The gland is wholly invested by a fibrous capsule, which is important in thyroid surgery as it permits the gland to be resected without significant risk of bleeding. The right and left lobes are attached to the anterior and lateral walls of the trachea by fibrous connective tissue. The superior pole of the thyroid gland is usually level with the center of the thyroid cartilage. The inferior border is typically located 1 cm below the site where the inferior thyroid artery enters the gland. The neurovascular sheath of the common carotid artery is posterolateral to the gland and the sternocleidomastoid muscle is anterolateral. The posterior border of the thyroid gland is approximately at the level of the tracheoesophageal groove (**Figs. 11.24, 11.25, 11.26, 11.27, 11.28, 11.29**).

Arterial supply. The superior thyroid artery enters the thyroid gland through its superior pole while the inferior thyroid artery enters at the inferior pole. The thyroid ima artery, present in 5% of the population, arises from the aortic arch and is generally unpaired.

Venous drainage. The inferior thyroid vein normally consists of two trunks. The right trunk runs anterior to the innominate artery to carry blood to the right brachiocephalic vein, or it may run anterior to the trachea to enter the left brachiocephalic vein. The left trunk opens into the left brachiocephalic vein. Both inferior thyroid veins occasionally form a common trunk called the thyroid ima, which opens into the left brachiocephalic vein. A plexus, known as the thyroid impar plexus, may also be present between the two inferior thyroid veins. It may be a source of bleeding in thyroid operations, occasionally necessitating a tracheotomy or other procedure in the suprasternal space.

Sympathetic innervation. Superior, medial and inferior thyroid nerves from the superior, middle and inferior cervical ganglia.

Parasympathetic innervation. Vagus nerve and laryngeal nerves (superior laryngeal nerve, recurrent laryngeal nerve).

Lymphatic drainage. Lymph from the thyroid gland drains beneath the fibrous capsule along the thyroid veins to the superior deep cervical lymph nodes, the submandibular lymph nodes and jugulodigastric nodes posterior to the digastric muscle, and the inferior deep cervical lymph nodes posterior to the internal jugular vein and anterior to the anterior scalenus

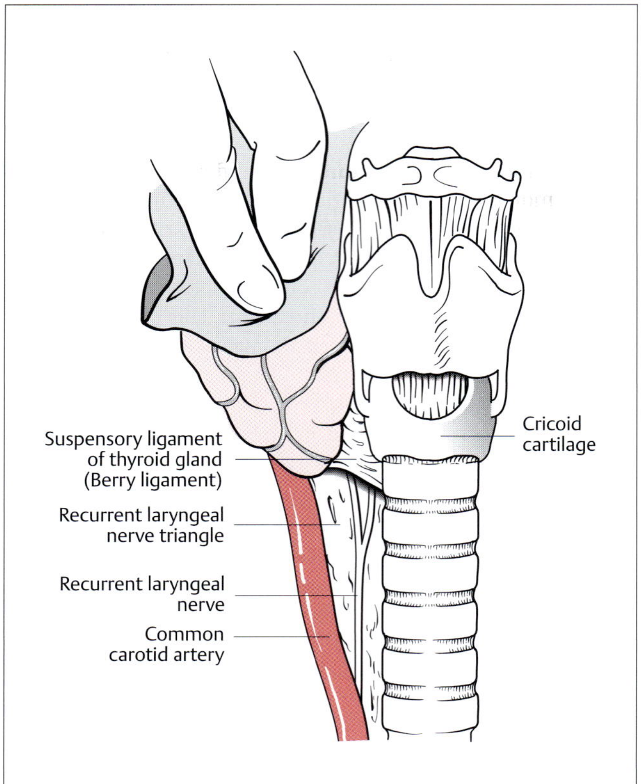

Fig. 11.24 Anatomy and relations of the thyroid gland. Anterior view of the recurrent laryngeal nerve.

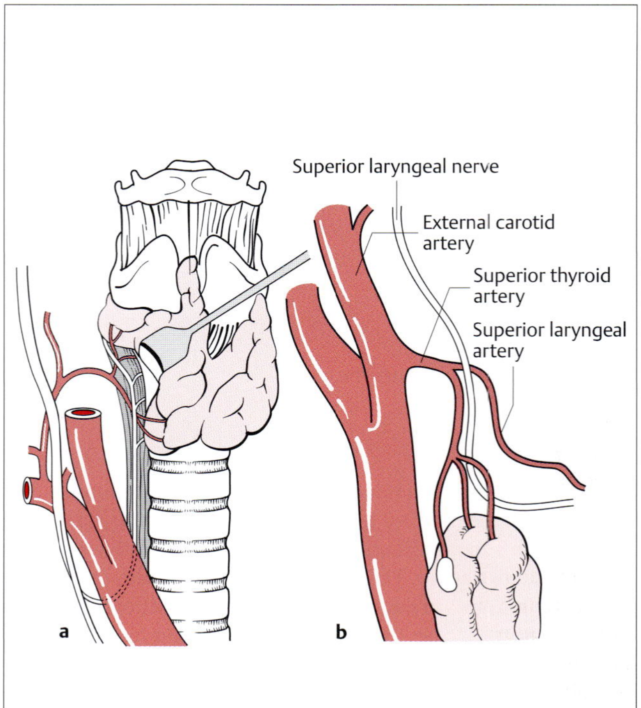

Fig. 11.25a, b Anatomy and relations of the thyroid gland.
a Relationship of the recurrent laryngeal nerve to the inferior thyroid artery.
b Relationship of the superior laryngeal nerve to the superior polar artery.

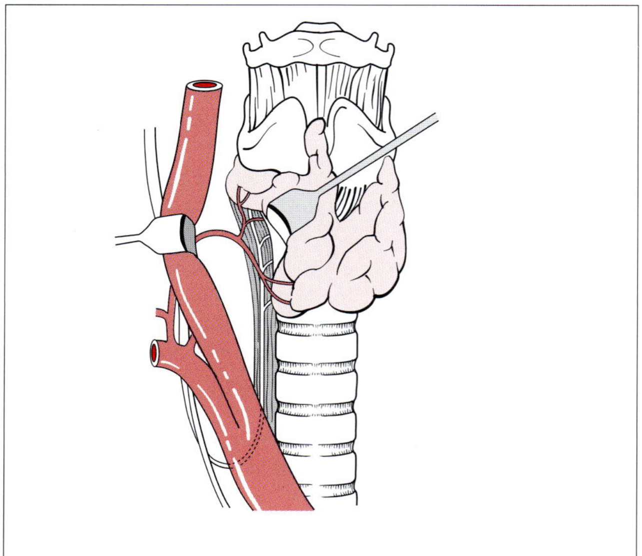

Fig. 11.26 Anatomy and relations of the thyroid gland. Variation in the course of the recurrent nerve near the gland.

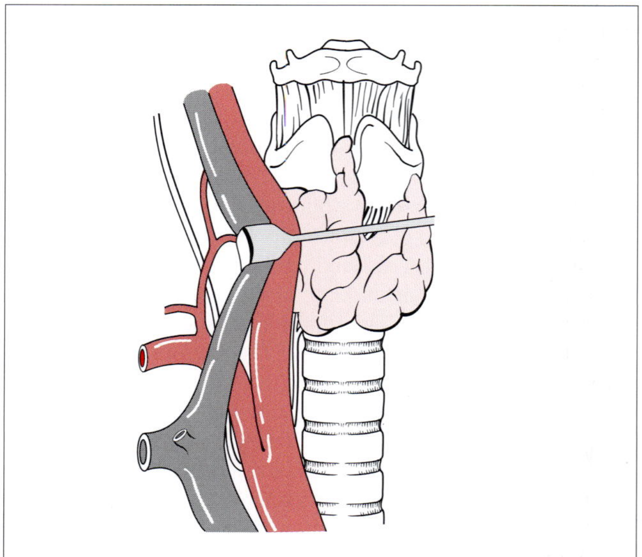

Fig. 11.27 Anatomy and relations of the thyroid gland. Variation in the course of the recurrent nerve near the gland.

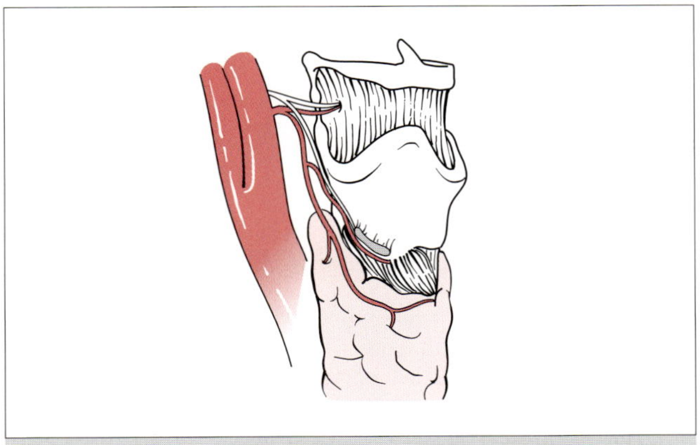

Fig. 11.28 Anatomy and relations of the thyroid gland. Common variation in the course of the external branch of the superior laryngeal nerve near the gland.

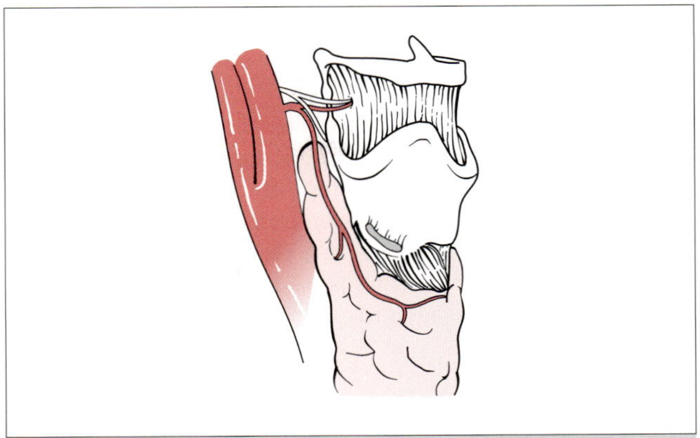

Fig. 11.29 Anatomy and relations of the thyroid gland. Common variation in the course of the external branch of the superior laryngeal nerve near the gland.

muscle and plexus fibers. The lymphogenous metastasis of thyroid carcinoma is influenced by the fact that the lymphatic regions draining the two thyroid lobes are not strictly separated between the sides. There is a branched network of lymphatic vessels that establishes anastomotic connections between the prelaryngeal and pretracheal lymph nodes. Connections also exist with retropharyngeal lymph nodes and with lymph nodes located in the superior mediastinum.

While head and neck surgeons in North America classify the cervical lymph nodes into six regions (p. 268), visceral surgeons use a classification based on the course of the head and neck vessels. This is a compartmental scheme in which the lymph nodes are arranged in a central compartment (C1), a right (C2) and left (C3) cervicolateral compartment, and a mediastinal compartment (C4) (**Fig. 11.30**). The central compartment (C1) encompasses the lymph node groups on both sides that are located medial to the neurovascular sheath and extend from the hyoid bone to the left brachiocephalic vein and right subclavian vein. This compartment is subdivided into a left central compartment (C1b) and a right central compartment (C1a). The trachea marks the boundary between the left and right central compartments. Two cervicolateral compartments are distinguished—a right cervicolateral compartment (C2) and a left cervicolateral compartment (C3). Each extends from the lateral aspect of the neurovascular sheath to the anterior border of the trapezius muscle. The mediastinal compartment encompasses the lymph node groups located caudal to the left brachiocephalic vein and right subclavian vein.

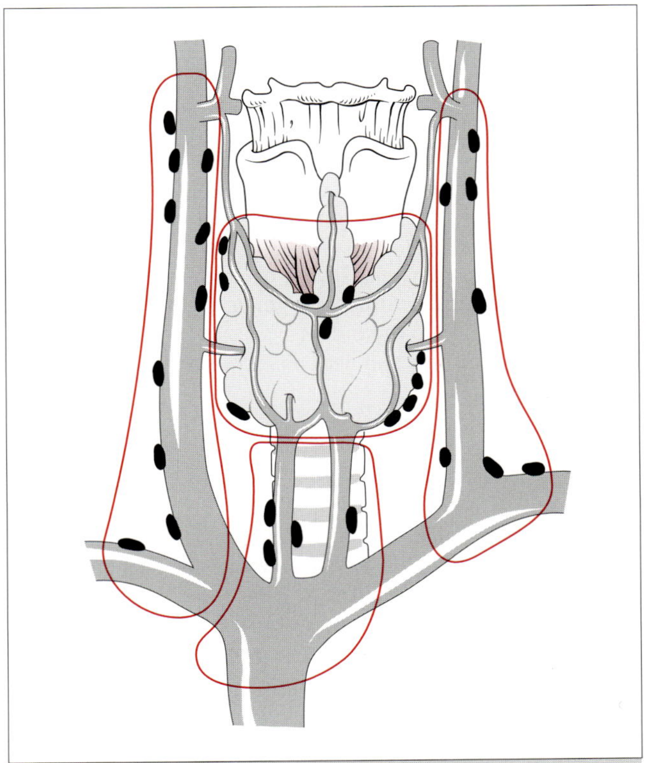

Fig. 11.30 Classification of cervical lymph node compartments with respect to metastatic involvement by thyroid cancer.

Thyroid Surgery

Approximately 5% of the population suffer from latent or overt thyroid dysfunction. As a result, thyroid disorders rank among the most common endocrine diseases. This section focuses on the surgical treatment of nodular goiters and thyroid malignancies. It is intended to give the trainee neck surgeon an appreciation of available surgical techniques and emphasize the importance of understanding the course of the recurrent laryngeal nerve, which is also essential in laryngectomies. It is equally important to understand the vascular relationships of the thyroid gland. Everyone who performs otolaryngologic surgery must deal with the thyroid gland in a variety of settings, including simple tracheotomies. Readers will find that a detailed study of thyroid neurovascular architecture will enhance their ability to complete many of the steps in surgical procedures.

11

Diagnosis

History

The surgeon should determine whether the patient has had prior contact with radioactive materials, especially in childhood, and must check for a family history of diseases such as medullary carcinoma and hypertension (e.g., in Sipple syndrome). Attention should also be given to a variety of symptoms such as globus sensation, pain (thyroiditis), swallowing difficulties, dyspnea, voice change, and growth changes.

Examination

- Size, shape, and consistency of the thyroid gland.
- Presence or absence of cervical lymphadenopathy.
- Laryngoscopy: vocal cord movement disorders that may suggest involvement of the recurrent laryngeal nerve.
- Tracheal deviation.
- Tumor fixation.
- Skin fixation.
- Thyroid scan.
- Aspiration cytology.

Surgical Principle

- Minimal operation consists of total thyroid lobectomy and isthmusectomy. This is recommended for unilateral or autonomous nodules.
- Total thyroidectomy with biopsy of central nodules is indicated for bilateral multinodular goiter, Graves disease, and bilateral Hashimoto thyroiditis.
- Total thyroidectomy and neck dissection are indicated for a thyroid malignancy.

Euthyroid Nodular Goiter

The multifocal, clonal, or polyclonal proliferation of thyroid cells with significant functional or morphologic heterogeneity of newly developed follicles or follicle-like structures is the pathomorphologic correlate of an enlarged thyroid gland, or nodular goiter. Recent publications emphasize the importance of removing all diseased thyroid tissue in goiter operations.

Surgical Principle

Resection of all nodular changes on both sides of the thyroid gland. A (total) thyroidectomy may be the best strategy for preventing a recurrence.

Indications

- Goiters with a thyroid volume greater than 60 mL (WHO grade II).
- Deficient iodine uptake on scintigraphy.
- Goiters causing mechanical problems (compression of the trachea and/or esophagus, WHO grade III).
- Pathohistologic confirmation of morphologically indeterminate findings.
- Suspicious nodules or definite suspicion of malignancy.
- Poor compliance with pharmacologic therapy.

Contraindication

Debilitated patient.

Specific Points Regarding Informed Consent

- Sensory disturbances involving the neck or ear.
- Growth lag of the skin flap.
- Paralysis of the accessory nerve, vagus nerve, phrenic nerve, hypoglossal nerve, facial nerve, or superior and inferior laryngeal nerves.
- Hoarseness or voice loss.
- Dyspnea, which may necessitate a tracheostomy.
- Poor cosmetic result, conspicuous scarring.
- Possible need to extend the skin incision.
- Mucosal injury, mediastinitis.
- Persistent drainage of lymphatic fluid.
- Possible conversion to a total thyroidectomy if carcinoma is found, or possible need for residual thyroidectomy based on specimen histology.
- Possible lifelong hormone replacement for postoperative hypothyroidism.
- Postoperative hypoparathyroidism.
- Need for prevention of recurrence.

Operative Planning

- Clinical examination and laboratory tests.
- Regional ultrasound examination (basic scans essential).
- Scintigraphy (not essential for euthyroid, endemic nodular goiter or suspected malignancy).
- Fine-needle aspiration cytology of clinically or sonographically suspicious nodules.
- Pre- and postoperative evaluation of vocal cord status (essential).
- Optional: tracheal spot film and esophagography, esophagoscopy, dynamic plethysmography.
- MRI in highly selected cases.

Special Instruments and Implants

- Roux retractor.
- Mixter clamp.
- Thyroid clamps.

Anesthesia

General endotracheal anesthesia.

Surgical Technique

Positioning. The patient is positioned supine with the upper body elevated 15–20° and the head and neck hyperextended. The head is supported on a ring or vacuum cushion.

Approach. Kocher incision of sufficient length dividing the skin, subcutaneous tissue, and platysma with a scalpel (**Figs. 11.31** and **11.32**).

Dissection of the cervical soft tissues. A skin–platysma flap is created by dissecting upward to the thyroid cartilage and downward into the subclavicular fossa. Dissection is aided by the use of a self-retaining retractor.

Development of the thyroid gland. The affected or predominantly affected side is turned toward the surgeon. The dissection initially proceeds from below upward (**Figs. 11.33** and **11.34**). The strap muscles are retracted laterally with a Roux retractor. The surgeon now identifies the second layer of the deep cervical fascia (parathyroid space or surgical space of de

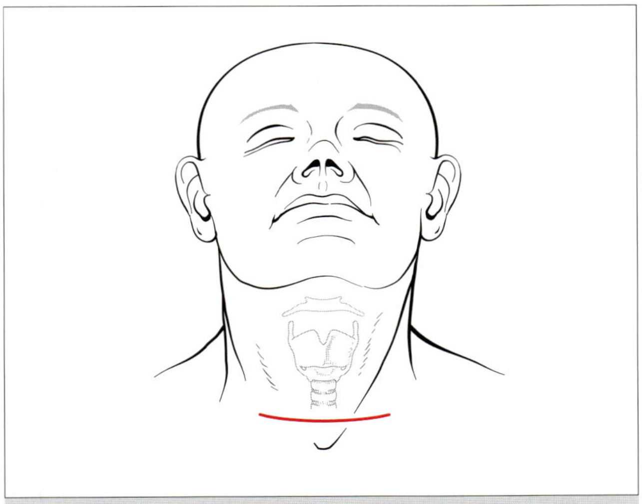

Fig. 11.31 Kocher incision for subtotal thyroidectomy.

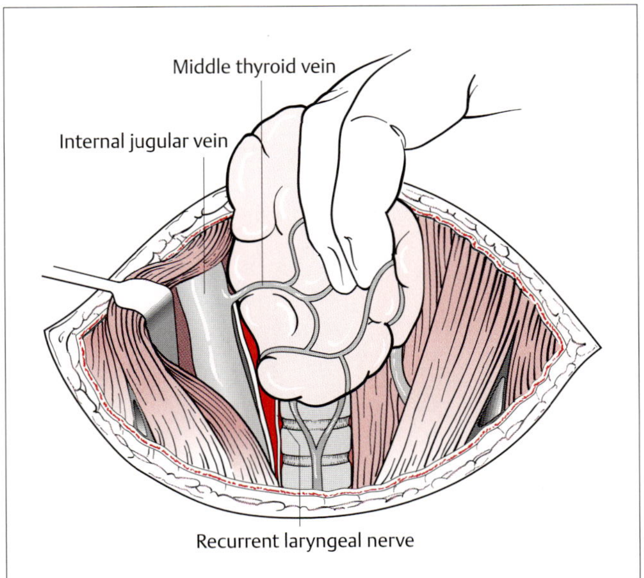

Fig. 11.32 Subtotal lobectomy.
The skin, subcutaneous tissue, and platysma are divided.

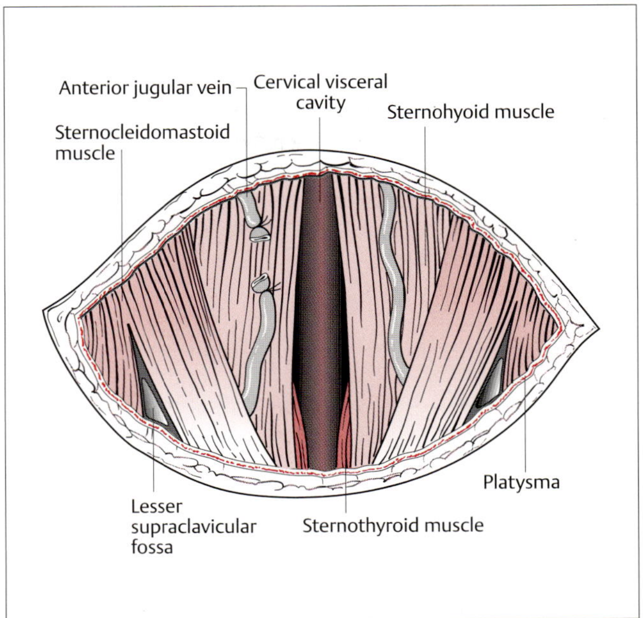

Fig. 11.33 Subtotal lobectomy.
The strap muscles are retracted laterally, and the de Quervain space is identified.

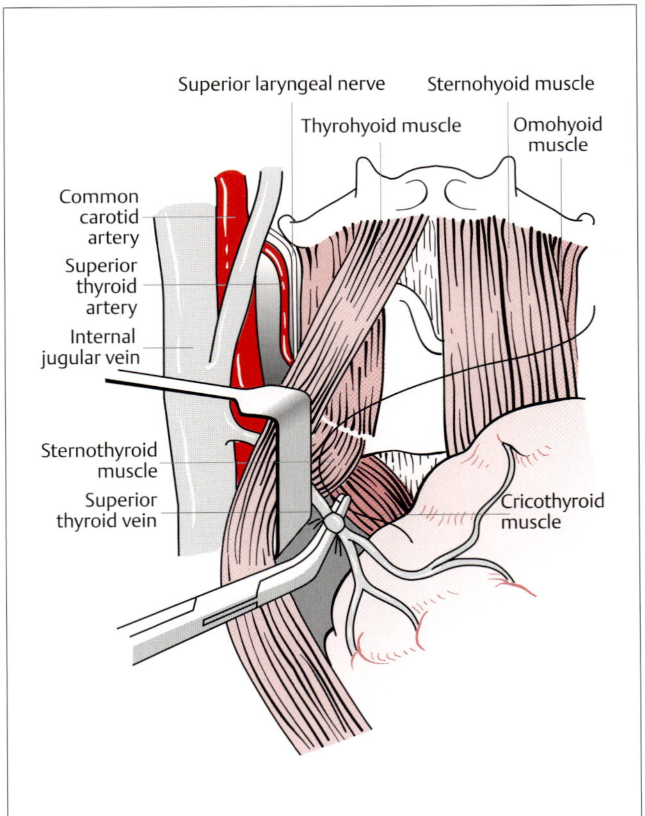

Fig. 11.34 Subtotal lobectomy.
The recurrent laryngeal nerve is identified. For clarity, the right sternohyoid muscle is not shown.

11

Quervain), which forms an avascular plane between the cervical fascia and thyroid capsule. The dissection is performed bluntly with a dissecting sponge, permitting almost the whole anterolateral aspect of the gland to be dissected bloodlessly while the lateral vein is ligated with fine, nonabsorbable sutures. Titanium clips may also be used (**Figs. 11.35, 11.36, 11.37**).

Now the recurrent laryngeal nerve is identified. This is most easily accomplished caudal to the site where the nerve crosses the inferior thyroid artery.

Next, the parathyroid glands are identified to establish orientation (**Fig. 11.38**). The inferior parathyroid gland appears as a brownish (caramel-colored), usually oval mass of flat tissue embedded in fat and usually located at the crossing of the artery and nerve. When all structures have been identified, the thyroid gland is bluntly dissected from below upward to the superior pole, using finger traction to progressively medialize the gland. The superior pole vessels are identified and successively ligated, placing the ligatures close to the thyroid capsule rather than ligating the vessels en bloc.

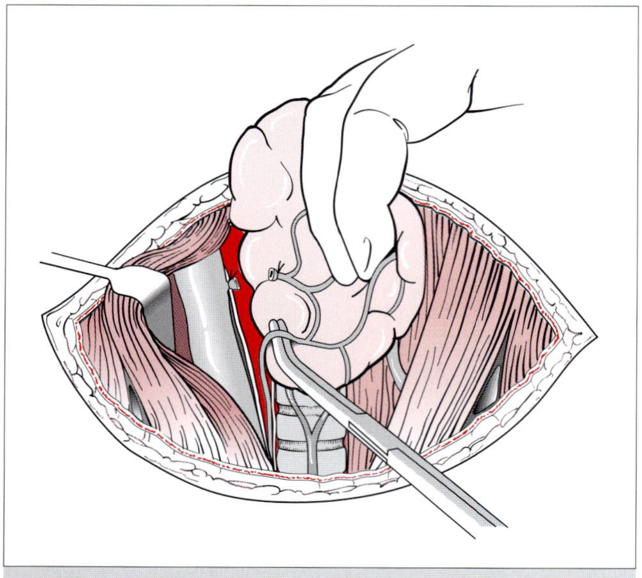

Fig. 11.35 Subtotal lobectomy.
The inferior thyroid artery is identified.

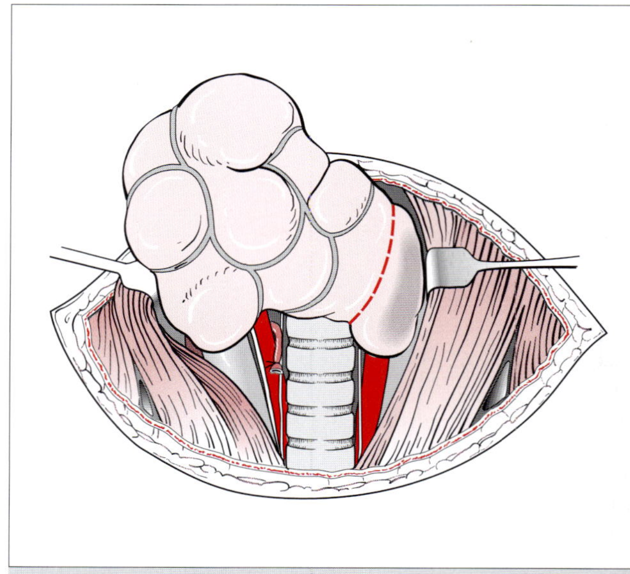

Fig. 11.37 Subtotal thyroidectomy.
Preparation for division of the isthmus.

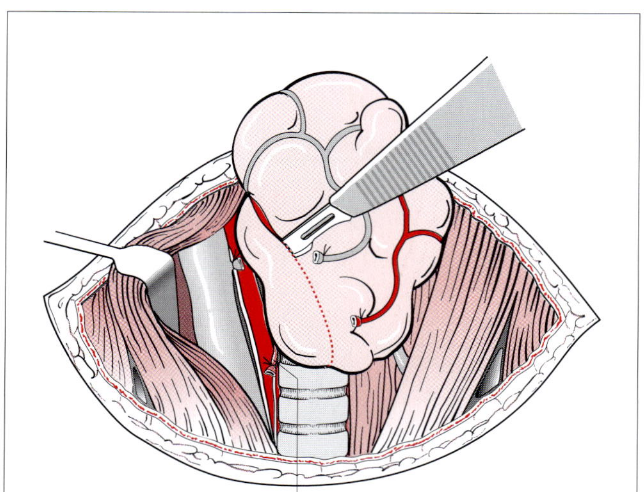

Fig. 11.36 Subtotal lobectomy.
The right side of the thyroid gland is incised after division of the inferior thyroid artery.

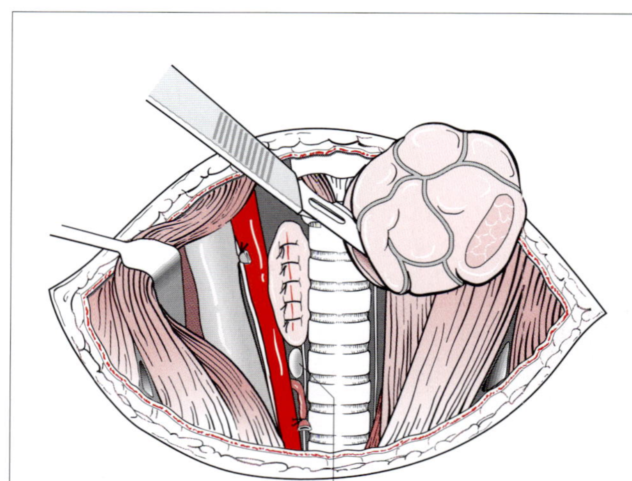

Fig. 11.38 Subtotal thyroidectomy.
The parathyroid glands are identified for orientation.

Caution
Ligating the vessels close to the thyroid capsule may damage the external branch of the superior laryngeal nerve if that branch runs close to the thyroid gland.

As the dissection proceeds and the gland is rotated medially, the recurrent laryngeal nerve can be traced to its entrance into the cricothyroid membrane, and the parathyroid glands are identified at their superior and inferior locations. The thyroid gland is further isolated from its blood supply and is separated from the anterior tracheal wall when the nerve and parathyroid gland have been positively identified (**Fig. 11.39**).

The isthmus and pyramidal lobe are under-run and divided following the careful placement of bilateral clamps. Both cut surfaces are secured with suture ligatures as in a tracheotomy (**Fig. 11.40**).

Wound closure. The wound is closed in layers, starting at the cervical midline and platysma, using simple interrupted sutures. The skin is closed with continuous intracutaneous sutures.

Rules, Tips, and Tricks
An absolutely bloodless field must be maintained throughout the operation. The recurrent laryngeal nerve should always be exposed, and tissue bordering the nerve should be dissected only after the nerve has been positively identified. Each parathyroid gland should be treated as if it were the last one. If its viability cannot be established beyond question, parathyroid autotransplantation should be performed. All relevant anatomic structures should be exposed and identified. Neuromonitoring of the recurrent laryngeal nerve is an option to be considered in selected cases.

Risks and Complications
- Postoperative bleeding that requires re-exploration. Generally this occurs within a few hours after surgery and warrants immediate exploration in patients with severe neck swelling and/or dyspnea.
- The incidence of recurrent laryngeal nerve paralysis depends on the type of operation. If there is postoperative suspicion of permanent unilateral damage, voice therapy should be instituted. Bilateral recurrent laryngeal nerve paralysis is generally manifested in the immediate postoperative period by progressive stridor and dyspnea. Instead of reintubation and/or tracheotomy, good results have been obtained with Lichtenberger reversible endo-extralaryngeal laterofixation (see Chapter 10) combined with corticosteroid therapy (e. g., 250 mg prednisolone IV).
- Hypoparathyroidism with tetany can be treated with oral or intravenous calcium (e. g., 2–8 g in divided oral doses of 1 g, or 1–10 g/day IV in 5 % glucose solution).

Postoperative Care

Respiration, circulation, and vigilance are monitored. Serum calcium is checked on the first postoperative day and if signs of hypocalcemia appear. The patient is positioned with the upper body elevated 30°.

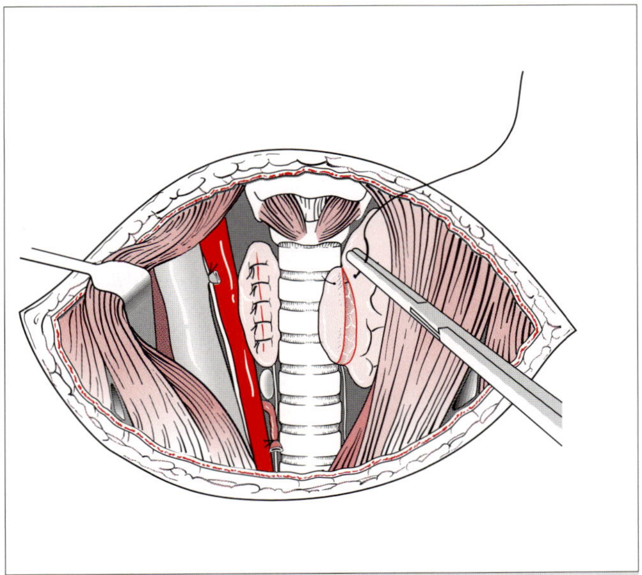

Fig. 11.39 Subtotal thyroidectomy.
The thyroid gland is freed from the anterior tracheal wall after the nerve and parathyroid gland have been positively identified.

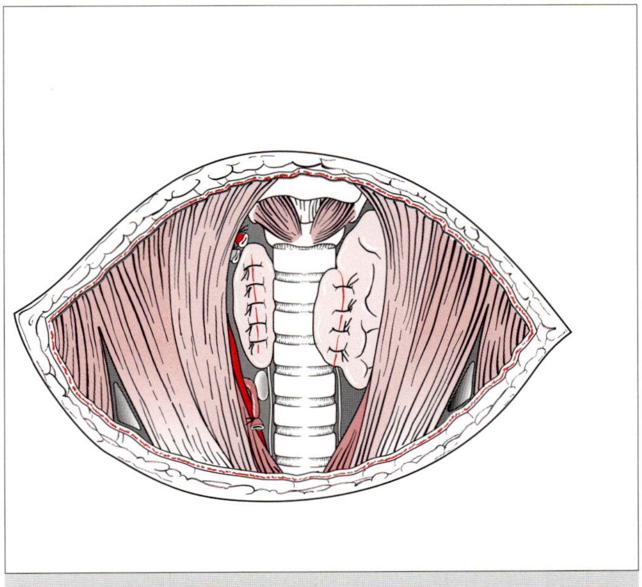

Fig. 11.40 Subtotal thyroidectomy.
The wound is closed in layers.

11

Surgery of Thyroid Malignancies

General

The most common entity is papillary thyroid carcinoma, which accounts for 50–80% of all thyroid malignancies. It is significant that papillary thyroid cancers are multicentric in ca. 20% of all cases. Unlike follicular thyroid cancers, papillary cancers tend to undergo lymphogenous metastasis, initially involving the cervical lymph nodes and later metastasizing to mediastinal nodes. Hematogenous metastasis, especially to the lung, occurs only in later stages of the disease. Despite its propensity for lymphogenous spread, papillary thyroid carcinoma generally has a very favorable prognosis that differs little from survival curves in the normal population, especially in its early stages.

Follicular thyroid carcinoma is much less common, accounting for 5–15% of all thyroid malignancies. Its pathomorphologic features are highly variable and have a significant impact on diagnosis. It metastasizes by the hematogenous route, spreading chiefly to lung, liver, skeleton, and brain. Cervical lymph node metastasis is rare.

Undifferentiated thyroid carcinoma is a very aggressive neoplasm. Given its rapid, destructive local growth and fulminant lymphogenous and hematogenous metastasis, the prognosis is very grave and patients rarely survive for more than a few months.

C-cell carcinoma, which is derived from the calcitonin-producing C cells of the thyroid gland, accounts for ca. 10% of all thyroid malignancies. In ca. 30% of patients this tumor is one manifestation of a condition known as type II multiple endocrine neoplasia (MEN2). Survival depends chiefly on the tumor stage. Primary thyroid carcinomas are rare and include squamous cell carcinoma, adenocarcinoma, signet ring carcinoma, mucoepidermoid carcinoma, and clear-cell carcinoma.

11

Surgical Principle

The surgical treatment principle for well-differentiated thyroid carcinomas consists of the surgical resection of all neoplasms with adequate margins, low morbidity, and little, if any, mortality. This principle applies to papillary, follicular and papillary–follicular carcinomas as well as medullary carcinomas and Hürthle cell carcinomas of the thyroid gland. It also applies to resectable anaplastic tumors and squamous cell thyroid cancers.

Indications

Well-differentiated papillary and follicular carcinomas, anaplastic carcinomas, and squamous cell carcinomas of the thyroid gland.

Contraindications

Advanced systemic diseases.

Specific Points Regarding Informed Consent

- See under goiter surgery; also risk of vagus nerve paralysis.
- Hoarseness or voice loss.
- Dyspnea, which may necessitate a tracheostomy.
- Possible need for radioiodine therapy.
- Postoperative hypoparathyroidism.

Operative Planning

Clinical examination, ultrasound, aspiration cytology, preoperative chest radiographs, pre- and postoperative vocal cord function tests.

Anesthesia

General endotracheal anesthesia.

Surgical Technique

Thyroidectomy

Positioning. Same as for a goiter resection.

Incision and dissection of the cervical soft tissues. A Kocher incision is extended upward along the anterior border of the sternocleidomastoid muscle. If a lateral neck dissection is planned, the platysma is divided and the skin–platysma flap is developed superiorly.

Exposure of the thyroid gland. The strap muscles are dissected from the outer capsule of the thyroid gland through a longitudinal midline incision and are retracted laterally. If a lateral neck dissection is planned for the same sitting, the sternocleidomastoid muscle is snared and retracted laterally upward.

Thyroidectomy. First the neck is carefully palpated for enlarged lymph nodes. They are most commonly located in the area of the cricothyroid ligament, parathyroid glands, tracheoesophageal region, or along the internal jugular vein and superior mediastinum. If the lymph nodes cannot be adequately assessed preoperatively, they should be examined at operation.

With a Langenbeck retractor on the inferolateral part of the skin incision, the inferior pole of the thyroid gland is carefully mobilized by blunt dissection and is pulled upward with the aid of moist cotton between the surgeon's finger and the gland.

The lobe is separated from the trachea, and the branches of the inferior thyroid artery are doubly ligated. The main trunk of the inferior thyroid artery should not be ligated to maintain adequate blood flow to the parathyroid glands. The various attachments between the artery and nerve can be directly identified as the gland is mobilized further.

The lobe is tethered by its superior vessels and by the posterior suspensory ligament, which passes from the inner or medial aspect of the gland to the trachea. This dense, thick portion of the suspensory ligament is called the "pedicle" or adherent zone of the thyroid gland. It connects the thyroid gland to the trachea. The branches of the recurrent laryngeal nerve run beneath the ligament. A prolongation of the thyroid gland that attaches to the esophagus is generally present below and posterolateral to these recurrent nerve fibers. This extension, which may be up to 4 cm long or longer, is removed in continuity with the bulk of the gland. A small arterial vessel, a branch of the inferior thyroid artery, runs along the inferior border of the adherent zone and is accompanied by a frequently complex network of veins and arteries. This region requires meticulous dissection, giving particular attention to preserving the nerve fibers while the total lobectomy is performed.

The adherent zone is mobilized by undermining it with a small Mixter clamp. If bleeding occurs from the artery or vascular plexus along the posterior ligament, it is too risky to clamp the vessels due to the proximity to the nerve fibers. Careful pressure will usually stop the bleeding and allow the vessels to be ligated in a bloodless field. It is common to find several vessels attached to the posterior suspensory ligament. Extreme care should be taken to avoid injuring the nerves. The vessels should not be cauterized, as this could damage the laryngeal nerve or its branches.

The thyroid lobe is now pulled downward to continue exposure of the vessels and superior pole. The external branch of the superior laryngeal nerve may be interwoven with or adherent to these vessels. The vessels of the superior pole are occluded with one proximal and one distal suture. Clamps are not placed on the proximal stump of the vessels. The artery and vein should be ligated separately whenever possible to prevent the formation of an arteriovenous fistula. This also helps prevent injury to the external branch of the superior laryngeal nerve.

The wound is closed as described above.

Lateral Neck Dissection

A lateral neck dissection is indicated in patients with clinical suspicion of lymph node metastases and/or positive lymph node involvement (**Figs. 11.41** and **11.42**). Generally it is recommended that the medial compartment also be cleared in patients with large primary tumors.

Postoperative Care

The surgical excision of malignant thyroid tumors with resection of the medial and lateral compartments constitutes the basic treatment for thyroid malignancies. The subsequent need for radioiodine therapy, radiotherapy and/or replacement therapy and the scheduling of oncologic follow-up are determined on an interdisciplinary basis.

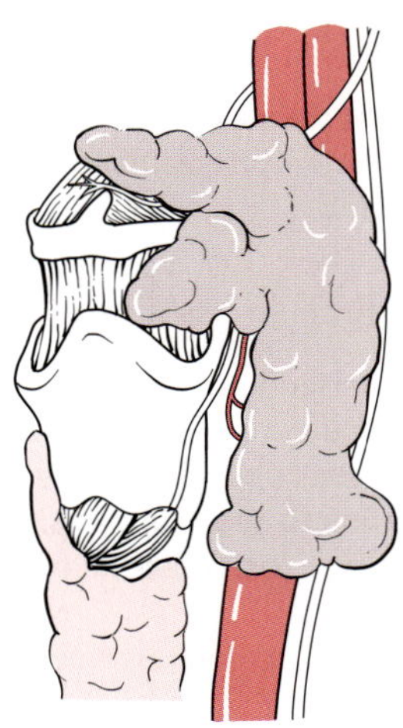

Fig. 11.41 Level of the neck dissection.
Appearance prior to dissection for a thyroid malignancy.

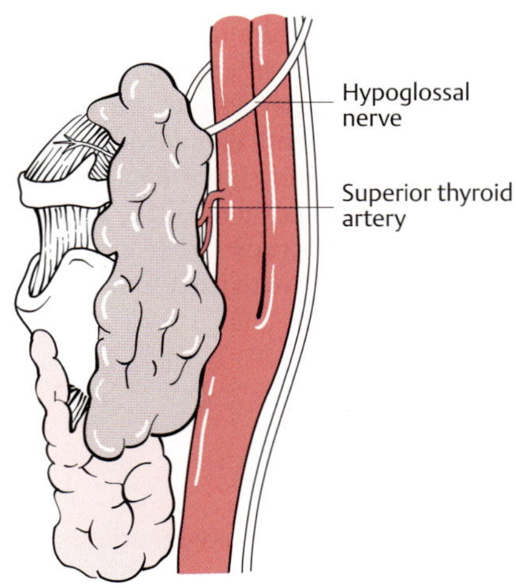

Fig. 11.42 The dissected neck tissue is mobilized, exposing the hypoglossal nerve and superior thyroid artery.

12 Surgery of the Esophagus and Mediastinum

Endoscopic Surgery

Anatomical Data

The length of the esophagus ranges from 20 to 34 cm in adults. The esophagus has three physiologic constrictions that are relevant to endoscopy. The first constriction, caused by the tone of the constrictor muscles, is located at the esophageal inlet approximately 14 cm (12–16 cm) from the upper incisor teeth. The middle constriction, formed by the aortic arch and left main bronchus, is located ca. 27 cm (22–29 cm) from the upper incisor teeth, and the lower constriction (cardia) is located at ca. 41 cm (32–50 cm).

Esophagoscopy can be performed with a rigid tube or flexible esophagoscope. The indications for both methods overlap somewhat, but the choice of an endoscope will depend partly on the preference and experience of the surgeon. The rigid esophagoscope can be used both diagnostically and therapeutically and is the instrument of choice for foreign body extractions. Fiber-optic instruments, on the other hand, are better for performing diagnostic endoscopy under local anesthesia. This technique is often combined with gastroduodenoscopy.

Rigid Esophagoscopy

Surgical Principle

A rigid tube is introduced transorally into the esophagus for dilation, inspection, incisional biopsy, or foreign body extraction.

Indications

- Suspected foreign body in the esophagus.
- Esophageal polyps.
- Dilation of strictures or webs.
- Suspected esophageal neoplasm.
- Investigation of wall changes due to caustic ingestion.
- Cardiospasm.
- Suspected esophageal varices or for sclerotherapy (flexible esophagoscopy is generally preferred).

Contraindications

- Severe changes in the cervical or thoracic spine.
- Severe systemic diseases that would contraindicate general anesthesia.

Specific Points Regarding Informed Consent

- Dental injury or tooth loss.
- Dysphagia, gastric intubation.
- Hoarseness or voice loss.
- Dyspnea, which may necessitate a tracheostomy.
- Mucosal injury, perforation of the esophageal wall.
- Pneumonitis with associated lung changes.
- Mediastinitis.
- Paralysis of the lingual nerve and hypoglossal nerve.
- Subcutaneous emphysema in the neck.

Operative Planning

Contrast radiography of the esophagus. Barium should be withheld if there is possible esophageal wall injury from a foreign body or risk of aspiration.

Special Instruments

Esophagoscopes of assorted lengths and diameters. Endoscopic forceps, cup forceps, suction tips, dilators, optical esophagoscope with telescopes (if needed), optical forceps, and apparatus for air insufflation. The tube length and diameter should conform to patient anatomy (height, age, sex, condition of cervical spine).

Anesthesia

General endotracheal anesthesia (relatively large endotracheal tube with minimal cuff inflation, complete muscular relaxation).

Surgical Technique

Positioning. Supine with the head initially elevated for introducing the endoscope. As the endoscope is advanced, the head is lowered. Protection of the upper teeth is mandatory.

Exposure of the larynx and piriform sinus. The head is slightly elevated and tipped back (as for intubation or bronchoscopy). The laryngoscope handle is drawn straight back so that the blade presses downward on the tongue, exposing the epiglottis and arytenoid processes (**Fig. 12.1a, b**). Saliva is removed by suction.

Insertion of the esophagoscope. The esophagoscope is introduced at the right oral commissure and inserted behind the arytenoid processes, which are easily lifted forward with the instrument tip in this position. Meanwhile an assistant draws back the upper lip to protect it from pressure injury. The rigid esophagoscope is gently advanced to a site just proximal to the esophageal inlet, which appears as an oblong slit. As the tube passes behind the arytenoid cartilage, further observation is done through the endoscope and the laryngoscope blade is removed.

Entering the esophagus. To advance the scope across the esophageal inlet, the patient's head is slightly lowered until the transverse opening of the inlet is centered in the field of view. With the patient fully relaxed, the surgeon can easily advance the tube into the esophagus with just two fingers and without having to apply force.

Stabilizing the tube. The left hand stabilizes the tube against the dental arch while simultaneously protecting the teeth and retracting the lips.

Further insertion and inspection of the esophagus. The tube is advanced further under constant vision, and secretions are aspirated as needed. The lumen of the esophagus should always be kept at the center of the field; this is accomplished by lowering the head further and slightly elevating the tip of the tube as it advances (**Fig. 12.1a–f**). The tip of the scope will also tend to follow the natural curve of the esophagus toward the left side. Gastric acid reflux often occurs when the endoscope passes through the cardia.

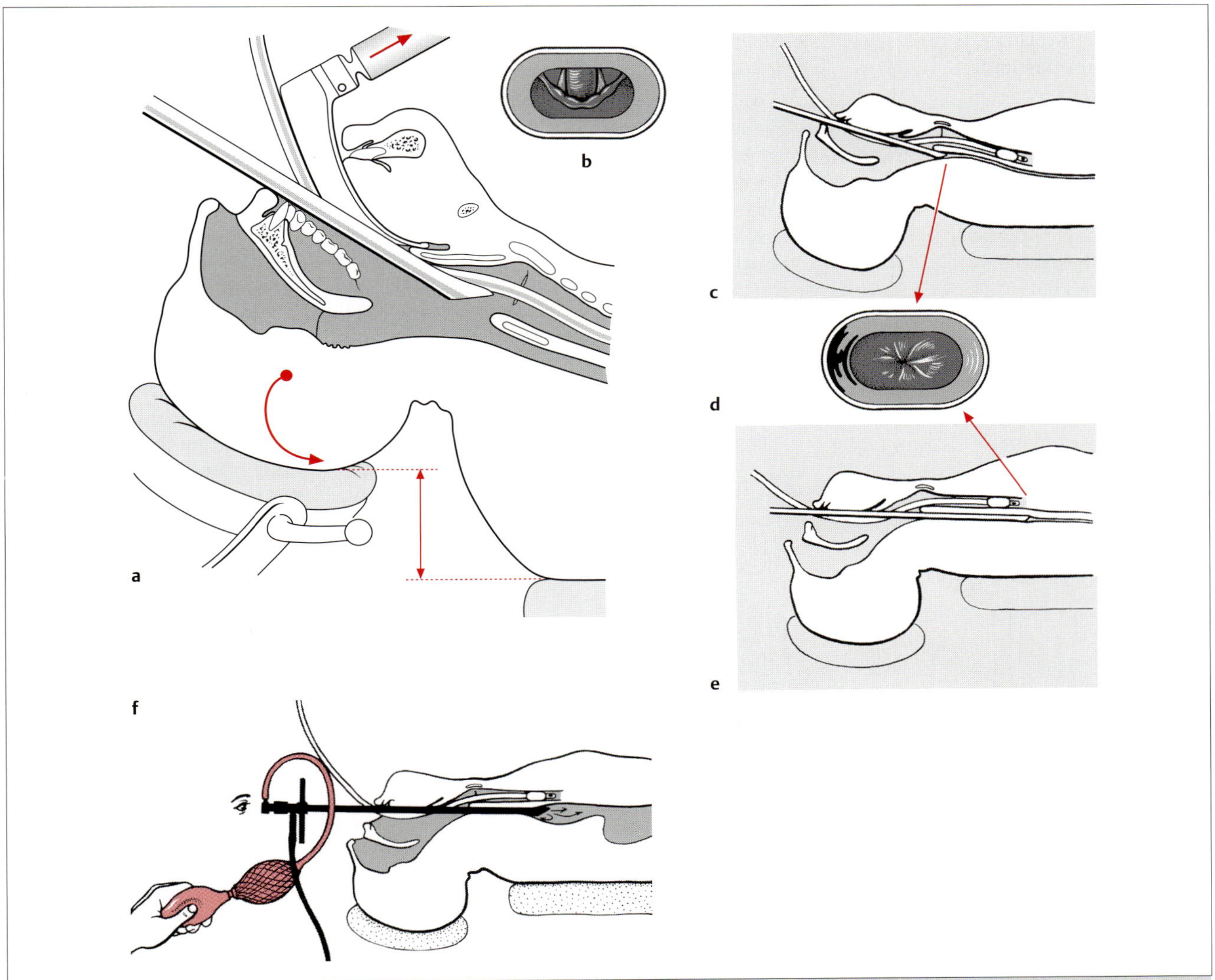

Fig. 12.1a–f Rigid esophagoscopy.
a The head is elevated and tilted back for insertion of the esophagoscope. The pharynx is expanded with a laryngoscope blade.
b The tip of the tube is carefully advanced behind the visible arytenoid cartilages.
c When the tip of the scope has passed through the esophageal inlet, the head is lowered.
d This permits the tube to remain centered on the esophageal lumen.
e At deeper levels the head is lowered further and the tip of the tube is elevated slightly in the anterior direction.
f With a pneumatic esophagoscope, visualization is improved by insufflating air into the esophagus.

! Risks and Complications

- Perforation of the hypopharynx or esophagus leading to mediastinitis, pleural or pericardial injuries, or peritoneal injury. Previously undetected hypopharyngeal diverticula increase the risk of perforation.
- Dental injury or tooth loss, especially in patients with pre-existing tooth damage.
- Dislocation of the arytenoid cartilage.

Postoperative Care

No special measures are necessary after esophagoscopy. Oral intake may have to be withheld in patients with mucosal lesions. Antibiotic coverage is generally withheld as it could mask an incipient mediastinitis.

A suspected perforation should be investigated immediately by oral contrast examination with a water-soluble contrast medium (detection of extravasation) and soft lateral neck radiographs (air detection, increased prevertebral density). A suspected deeper perforation should be investigated by chest radiographs (pleural effusion) and standing abdominal radiographs (air crescent). Thoracic CT scans may be ordered in consultation with a radiologist. Palpation of the neck will disclose cutaneous emphysema. Watch for signs of sepsis. The detection of an esophageal perforation generally requires immediate intervention, usually aided by a thoracic surgeon.

Foreign Body Extraction from the Esophagus

Foreign bodies most frequently become lodged at the first esophageal constriction and less commonly at the second or third constriction. Predisposing factors are esophageal strictures due to caustic ingestion or neoplasia.

Surgical Technique

Exposure of the foreign body. The esophagoscope is introduced as described above, and the foreign body is visualized. The tip of the scope is brought to bear on the foreign body, which should be centered in the tube. Occasionally the foreign body is lost to view when the tube is advanced but is reacquired by withdrawing the tube slightly.

Extraction of smooth-surfaced foreign bodies. Smooth-surfaced foreign bodies such as coins and buttons are grasped with an alligator forceps or other suitable instrument, pulled against the end of the tube, and carefully extracted along with the tube. The scope is then reintroduced to inspect the esophagus for injuries or additional foreign bodies.

Extraction of impaled foreign bodies. Impaled foreign bodies such as needles and bone fragments must first be oriented transversely. The esophagoscope tip is initially trained on the less impaled end, which is grasped with an alligator forceps and will become the leading edge during removal. The impaled end is then visualized and carefully extracted with the tube. The interior of the esophagus is then reinspected (**Fig. 12.2a–c**).

Foreign body extraction using special instruments. Special instruments are available for the extraction of certain foreign bodies. Straight pins can be bent to aid removal (**Fig. 12.2d**), and safety pins can be closed within the esophagus using a dedicated instrument. Denture plates and other large foreign bodies can be removed piecemeal with forceps, punches, or serrated scissors.

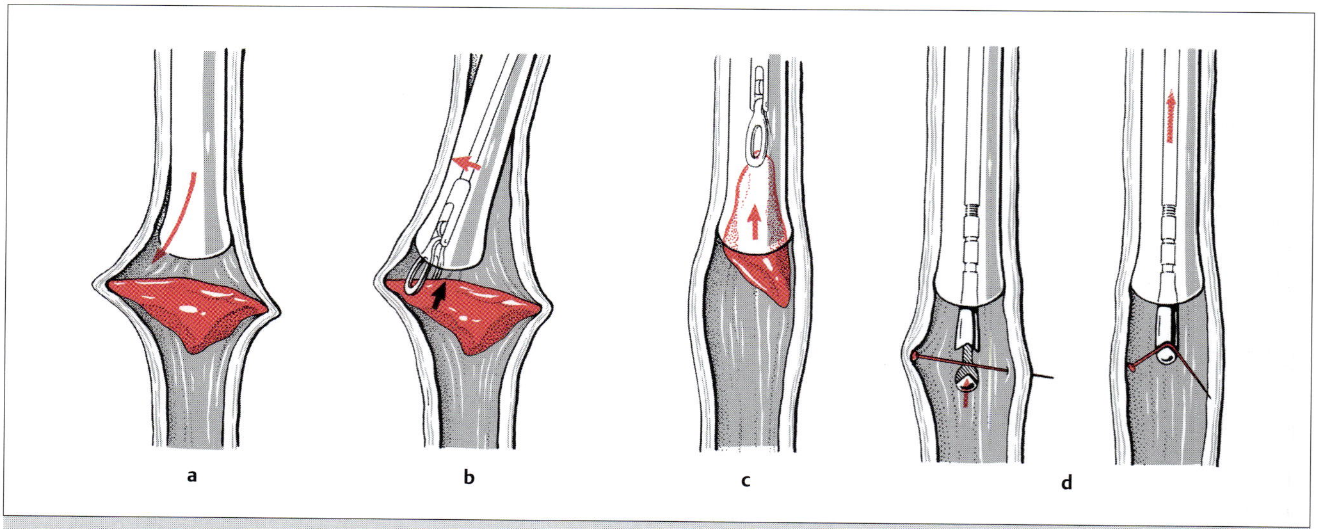

Fig. 12.2a–d Foreign body extraction from the esophagus.
a The tip of the tube is trained on the ingested foreign body.
b The tip of the tube is angled laterally, and one end of the foreign body is grasped with a suitable instrument.
c The leading end of the foreign body is pulled into the esophagoscope and extracted under the protection of the tube.
d An impaled straight pin is bent in situ with a special instrument to facilitate extraction.

Modification

If an esophageal foreign body cannot be extracted by the transluminal route, or if a relatively large perforating injury is present, the neck can be opened externally through a cervical or thoracic esophagotomy, depending on the level of entrapment. Even with a successful foreign body extraction, there may still be a large perforating injury that requires primary repair through a cervical mediastinotomy to prevent mediastinitis.

> **! Risks and Complications**
> Same as in esophagoscopy. The risks depend on the nature of the foreign body, its location, the presence or absence of impalement, and especially on previous extraction attempts and the time delay until extraction is performed.

> **Rules, Tips, and Tricks**
> Swallowed partial dentures often contain hooks that become impaled in the esophageal wall. The hooks must be clipped off with a forceps and removed separately before the rest of the denture is extracted.

Postoperative Care

Patients with esophageal wall injuries from impaled foreign bodies should be closely monitored to exclude periesophagitis or mediastinitis. It may be necessary to withhold oral intake of food and liquids.

Esophageal Biopsy

Esophageal biopsies are taken with a fine cup forceps or punch. An endoscopic forceps or an optical esophagoscope with air insufflation permits highly accurate tissue sampling. Any bleeding is controlled by dabbing the bleeding site with a vasoconstrictor.

Esophageal perforation may occur in incisional biopsies. But because the underlying changes are generally associated with significant wall thickening, there is relatively little risk of perforation when careful technique is used.

Flexible Esophagoscopy

Surgical Principle

A fiber-optic endoscope can be passed transorally into the esophagus under topical anesthesia with very little patient discomfort. It can also be advanced into the stomach and duodenum (esophagogastroduodenoscopy).

Indications

- Panendoscopy of the esophagus, stomach, and duodenum.
- Diagnostic endoscopy, incisional biopsy, or the removal of smooth foreign bodies (coins, etc.) in cases where general anesthesia or rigid endoscopy (rigid spinal column or kyphosis) is contraindicated.
- Bleeding esophageal varices.

Contraindications

Changes located high in the postcricoid region or at the esophageal inlet are relative contraindications. Flexible esophagoscopy should be performed cautiously in patients with hypopharyngeal diverticula (risk of perforation).

Operative Planning

Preoperative planning may require oral contrast radiographs of the esophagus.

Special Instruments

Fiber-optic endoscope with viewing, suction and instrument channels, light source, and suction–irrigation system.

Anesthesia

The patient is premedicated with atropine, and triflupromazine may be added if necessary. The pharynx is anesthetized with lidocaine. Intravenous sedation may also be appropriate in some patients.

Surgical Technique

Preparations and positioning. Dentures are removed. The patient is positioned in *left lateral decubitus* with the head flexed slightly forward.

Introduction of the esophagoscope. The head is tilted slightly forward, and a bite guard is inserted. The examiner stabilizes the instrument tip with the index and middle fingers of the left hand and pulls the tongue forward. The instrument is introduced from the side with the right hand while the patient is told to take a deep breath and swallow. If a springy resistance is encountered at ca. 15 cm, the instrument has deviated into a piriform sinus; it should be slightly withdrawn and re-advanced as the patient is again instructed to swallow.

Passage through the esophageal inset and further insertion. After the instrument tip has passed through the esophageal inlet, it is carefully advanced further under vision. The visual field should be kept clear at this stage by *suction and air insufflation*. As the instrument continues to advance, the distal end of the esophagoscope should always be directed toward the esophageal midline with the control handle. As in rigid esophagoscopy, the interior of the esophagus should be carefully inspected, especially during withdrawal, and air should be insufflated as needed to maintain luminal expansion (**Fig. 12.3**).

Tissue sampling or foreign body removal. Biopsies are taken under vision with special forceps passed through the instrument channel of the endoscope. Special loops and attachments for foreign body retrieval, for use through the instrument channel, have also been developed.

> **! Risks and Complications**
> Flexible esophagoscopy has basically the same risks as rigid endoscopy. There is definitely less risk of esophageal perforation, although a flexible endoscope may still perforate the esophageal wall.

Treatment of Acute Caustic and Scalding Esophageal Injuries and Strictures

Caustic and scalding injuries of the esophagus are characterized in the acute stage by necrosis and edema of the oropharynx, larynx, and esophagus with stridor, very severe pain, shock, and subsequent signs of systemic intoxication. Patients surviving the acute stage will develop esophageal strictures in approximately the third week.

Treatment of an Acute Caustic Injury

Milk or water (200–300 mL in adults, ca. 100 mL in children) should be given orally within 10–30 minutes after caustic ingestion. The following measures are *contraindicated*: emesis, gastric lavage (exacerbates the injury by re-exposing the esophagus to the caustic agent), neutralization therapy (may cause heat generation or foaming), and the administration of activated charcoal (ineffective).

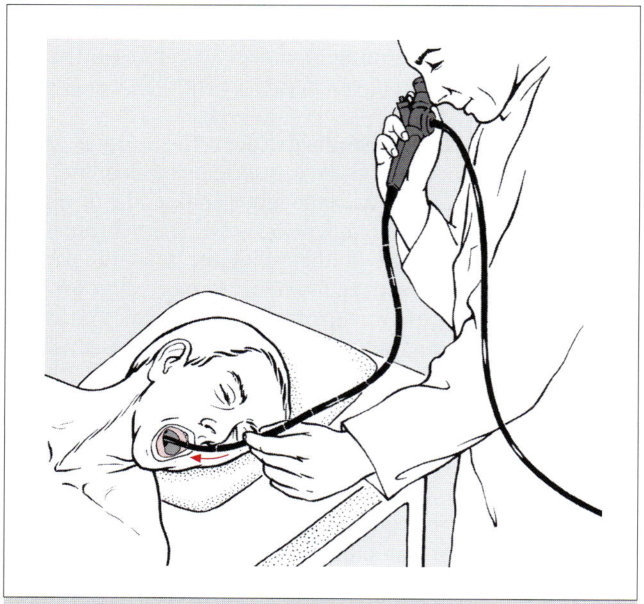

Fig. 12.3 Flexible esophagoscopy.
The patient is in left lateral decubitus with the head supported and flexed slightly forward. The examiner stands next to the patient and introduces the endoscope into the mouth from the side.

The patient should be treated for shock by instituting a continuous intravenous drip. High-dose antibiotics are administered. High corticosteroid doses are generally recommended (250–500 mg). They should not be given for very severe caustic injuries with high risk of gastric perforation or for minor caustic injuries (unnecessary), where steroids should be withheld until the fifth day.

Esophagoscopy is only occasionally necessary in the initial stage in cases where the extent of esophageal wall involvement is uncertain. Initial esophagoscopy is generally performed at ca. 4–6 days. Corticosteroids should be discontinued if only minor wall changes are found. It should be continued if esophagoscopy reveals hyperemia or edema of the esophageal mucosa or more extensive changes. Corticosteroid therapy is generally maintained for a total of 4 weeks.

Esophageal dilation is performed at ca. 7–12 days in patients who have significant crusting and ulceration. Dilations are scheduled daily (up to 20 Fr in children, up to approximatly 30 Fr in adolescents or approximately 40 Fr in adults), and the size of the dilator may be increased over time as needed. Regular esophagoscopic and radiographic follow-ups should be performed during the course of the treatments.

Treatment of Esophageal Strictures

Late esophageal dilation is indicated in cases where an esophageal stricture has formed despite steroid therapy and early dilation. It can be performed through an esophagoscope under visual guidance by introducing the dilator tip into the stricture and carefully advancing it or by advancing the dilator blindly over a preplaced string.

Technique of Esophageal Dilation over a Guide String

Making the guide string. A small, perforated lead shot is tied to the end of a silk string ca. 6–7 m long. Multiple small beads may be used for a tight stricture.

Introducing the guide string. A silk string is preplaced in the gastrointestinal tract to guide the dilator. The lead shot tied to the string is introduced transnasally in children and transorally in adults. As segments of the rolled-up string are paid out, the patient drinks liquid to advance the swallowed string down the esophagus. The lead shot can then be advanced further with the esophagoscope.

Initial dilation. Esophageal dilation is begun after the string has advanced ca. 5 m into the gastrointestinal tract. This process may take several days. If there is doubt, the location of the lead shot can be checked radiographically before the dilator is introduced. Occasionally the string may become tangled in the upper aerodigestive tract, only to be expelled when dilation is attempted.

Dilation technique (with a hollow dilator). The string protruding from the patient's mouth is threaded through the hollow dilator with a thin looped wire. The dilator should have a tapered tip conforming to the size of the stricture.

The string is now manually pulled taut and the dilator is carefully advanced down the esophagus with the other hand. The distance from the upper incisor teeth to the cardia is premarked on the dilator so that the insertion depth can be deter-

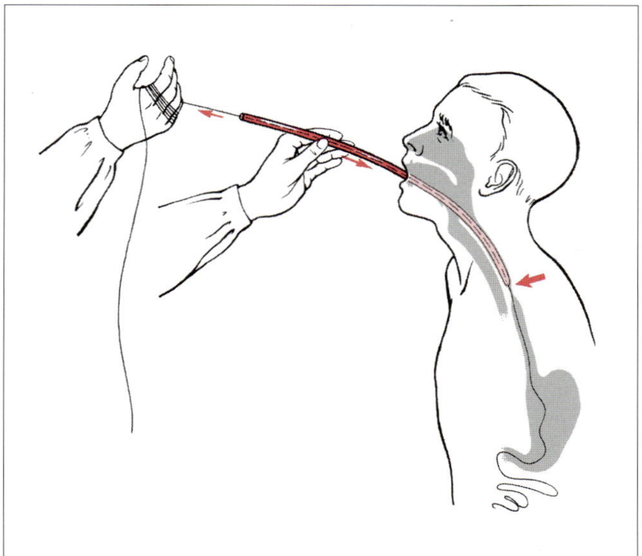

Fig. 12.4 Dilation of the esophagus over a guide thread. The thread is pulled taut with one hand while the other hand carefully advances the dilator.

mined. No more than two or three dilator sizes should be used in any one sitting (**Fig. 12.4**).

Change to a solid dilator and self-dilation. When the esophagus has been dilated to 40 Fr in adults (less in children and adolescents), the hollow dilator is replaced by a solid dilator. Exceptions may occur. Start with a solid dilator that is slightly smaller than the last string-guided dilator. Both the hollow and solid dilators should be smeared with lubricant. If solid dilation goes smoothly, further dilations can be performed by the patient or (for a child) by a parent or caregiver.

Modifications

In cases where a gastrostomy has been created, retrograde dilation can be performed.

Esophagus reconstruction (e.g., by jejunal transplantation or gastric pull-up) should be performed in cases where strictures and stenoses cannot be managed conservatively.

Rules, Tips, and Tricks

Esophageal dilation must be continued for some time—perhaps for an indefinite period in patients with very tight strictures. Dilatation at intervals is sometimes an option and will depend on the degree of the stenosis.

! Risks and Complications

- Esophageal perforation with mediastinitis or pleuritis following the use of a solid dilator may require immediate surgical intervention.
- Small mucosal tears may occur during string-guided dilation and usually are not a cause for concern. As a rule, there is no significant risk of perforation in string-guided dilations if the string is held taut. Rupture of the esophageal wall may occur in exceptional cases, however, and will require immediate surgical intervention.
- When dilations are performed over a long period of time in children, the size of the dilator should be increased every 2–3 years to allow for growth.
- A neoplasm should be excluded when dealing with strictures or stenoses from an unknown cause. Neoplasia should also be considered in recurrent strictures following an early childhood caustic injury, and if necessary should be excluded by biopsy.

Cervical Esophagotomy

Surgical Principle

Exposure of the cervical esophagus or hypopharynx through an external incision in the neck. Foreign bodies that cannot be extracted endoscopically can be removed by esophagotomy.

Indications

- Failed endoscopic attempt at extraction of esophageal foreign body.
- Removal of sharp foreign bodies that have migrated through the esophageal wall and are no longer accessible to esophagoscopy.

Contraindication

Debilitation is only a relative contraindication to cervical esophagotomy.

Anesthesia

General endotracheal anesthesia.

Surgical Technique

Positioning. The head is turned to the side as for a neck dissection. A roll is placed beneath the shoulders to hyperextend the neck.

External approach. The esophagus and hypopharynx are generally exposed through the left side of the neck unless an impaled foreign body has been identified on the right side.

Incision. The incision is made along the anterior border of the sternocleidomastoid muscle from the mandibular angle to the jugular fossa, or a lower transverse incision may be made in an existing skin crease.

Dissection and exposure of the vascular sheath. The fat, platysma, and superficial cervical fascia are divided. The vascular sheath is exposed from the site where it is crossed by the omohyoid muscle.

Exposure of the prevertebral fascia. The prevertebral fascia is exposed by blunt dissection medial to the vascular sheath, initially by spreading through the soft tissues and then by dissection with a mounted sponge. The veins passing to the thyroid gland are ligated. The location of the foreign body may also require ligation of the superior thyroid artery and, if necessary, the inferior thyroid artery. *Caution: protect the recurrent laryngeal nerve*, which runs close to the thyroid capsule. Ligate and divide the inferior thyroid artery at a far lateral site (**Fig. 12.5**).

Opening the esophagus and extracting the foreign body. The thyroid gland and larynx are rotated to the opposite side with a Langenbeck retractor, allowing the esophagus to be easily separated from the prevertebral fascia with mounted sponges. The foreign body is located by palpation. The esophagus is incised longitudinally at the level of the foreign body, and the object is removed.

Wound closure. The incision is immediately closed with absorbable sutures, inverting the mucosal edges as in a pharyngeal closure after laryngectomy. The suture is covered with a second row after the placement of a feeding tube. Finally the wound is closed in layers over a suction drain (**Fig. 12.6**).

> **! Risks and Complications**
> Wound infection, mediastinitis, esophagocutaneous fistula, recurrent laryngeal nerve palsy, erosive hemorrhage from the carotid artery caused by the drain, postoperative bleeding from the inferior or superior thyroid artery.

Postoperative care

The feeding tube is maintained for 8 days, at which time water-soluble contrast radiographs are obtained. The suction drain is removed according to drainage volume. Antibiotics are administered.

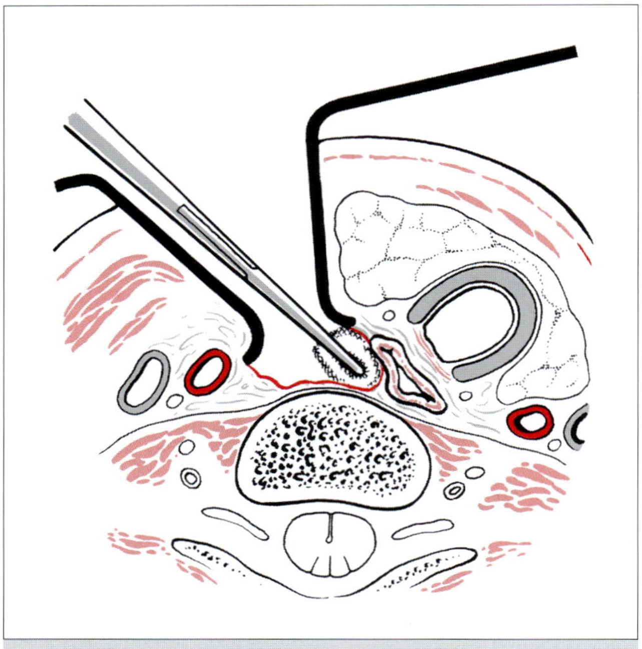

Fig. 12.5 Cervical esophagotomy.
The larynx, thyroid gland, and strap muscles are retracted medially toward the opposite side. The vascular sheath and sternocleidomastoid muscle are retracted laterally. The deep cervical fascia between the retracted structures is approached by blunt dissection.

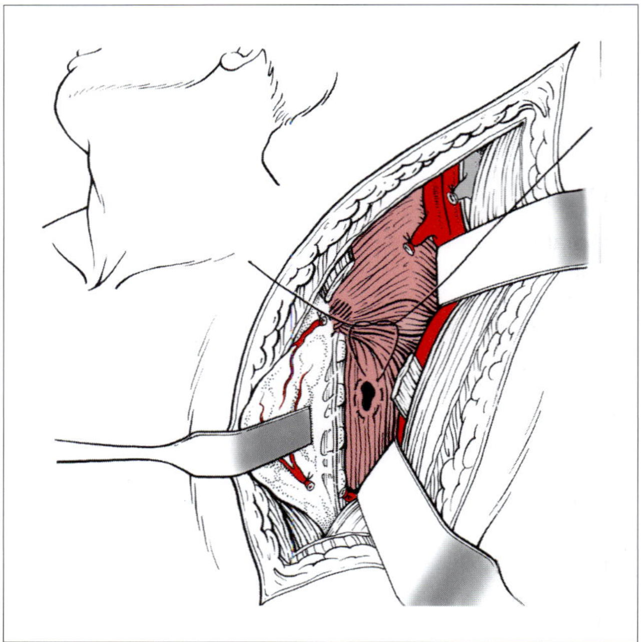

Fig. 12.6 Cervical esophagotomy.
The thyroid vessels are ligated, and the esophagus is exposed. The esophagus is incised after placement of a purse-string suture.

Cervical Mediastinotomy

Surgical Principle

The mediastinum is opened through the neck for the drainage of mediastinal abscesses arising from the neck, pharynx, or esophagus. The operation may include repairing a causative perforation in the esophagus.

Indications

- Mediastinitis arising from the neck (buried tonsillar, parapharyngeal or tongue-base abscess).
- Perforating injuries of the hypopharynx or upper esophagus.
- Abscess formation after transoral diverticulotomy for a hypopharyngeal (Zenker) diverticulum.

Contraindications

None, because surgery is life-saving.

Operative Planning

Radiographs of the superior mediastinum, soft lateral radiograph of the neck. Some cases may require oral water-soluble contrast examination or CT scans.

Anesthesia

General endotracheal anesthesia.

Surgical Technique

External approach. Usually on the left side, but the neck may be opened on the right side for a right-sided lesion.

Incision. The skin is incised along the anterior border of the sternocleidomastoid muscle from the clavicle to the mandibular angle or along a lower, pre-existing transverse skin crease.

Exposure of the vascular sheath. The fat, platysma, and superficial cervical fascia are divided. The vascular sheath is exposed at the site where the jugular vein crosses the omohyoid muscle.

Exposure of the prevertebral fascia. The prevertebral fascia is exposed by blunt dissection medial to the vascular sheath, which is retracted laterally with a Langenbeck retractor. Usually it is necessary first to ligate transverse veins that drain the thyroid gland. The superior and inferior thyroid arteries may be ligated if necessary. The larynx and thyroid gland are held aside with a blunt retractor.

Drainage of the mediastinal abscess. The esophagus is separated from the prevertebral fascia by blunt dissection with the finger or mounted sponge. The mediastinum is entered, and the mediastinal abscess is drained. This may be aided by passing a long-bladed Killian speculum or short esophagoscope down to the prevertebral fascia.

Closure of an esophageal perforation. Any esophageal perforation must be identified. This is done by mobilizing the adventitia and pushing aside the heavy fibrinous deposits that are usually present to expose the perforation site. A probe may be advanced to the site endoscopically to aid localization in the presence of severe inflammatory changes. The perforation is closed as described under esophagotomy, bearing in mind that the inflammatory friability of the tissue often causes significant problems. It may be necessary in some cases to cover the site with a pedicled muscle flap after placing a feeding tube. Denecke (1962) also recommends adding a myotomy of the fundiform part of the cricopharyngeus and the cervical esophageal muscle to reduce pressure on the oversewn perforation site during swallowing.

Drainage and wound reduction. A heavy rubber suction drain is placed in the abscess cavity, and the upper and lower ends of the wound are reduced with sutures. Iodoform gauze packing is placed in the central portion of the wound, which is left open.

> **! Risks and Complications**
>
> - Surgical injury to the recurrent laryngeal nerve (which often cannot be positively identified due to extensive inflammatory changes).
> - Risk of bleeding from small and large vessels, which are often difficult to ligate securely due to their general friability.
> - Risk of pneumothorax, pyopneumothorax, and systemic sepsis. Esophageal fistulas may develop. Heavy external scarring may occur as a result of secondary healing.

Postoperative Care

High-dose broad-spectrum antibiotic therapy is indicated. The drain is left indwelling as long as drainage is returned. Packing should be changed until the wound is fully granulated. Follow-up thoracic and mediastinal radiographs should be obtained, and esophageal integrity should be assessed later by oral contrast examination.

13 Surgery of the Salivary Glands

Surgery of the Submandibular Salivary Gland

Incision of the Submandibular Duct

Surgical Principle

Incision of the duct from the caruncle or over the stone, followed by extraction of the stone.

Indication

Stones in the distal excretory duct.

Contraindications

- Intraglandular stones.
- Recurrent multiple lithiasis.
- Reactive chronic inflammatory glandular changes following prolonged stone obstruction or sialadenitis.

Specific Points Regarding Informed Consent

- High incidence of recurrence.
- Salivary stasis due to duct stricture.
- Wound infection.
- Numbness due to lingual nerve injury.

Operative Planning

The stone is identified and localized by palpation and ultrasonography. Plain radiographs or sialography may be necessary in some cases. CT scans are rarely required.

Special Instruments

Blunt-tipped scissors for incising the duct. Salivary duct probes or dilators may be required. Microscope or binocular loupe.

Anesthesia

Topical anesthesia followed by infiltration with a local anesthetic containing epinephrine.

Surgical Technique

Incision. A probe or dilator is introduced into the caruncle under microscopic vision. The lower blade of a blunt-tipped scissors is inserted, and the overlying tissue is incised to the stone. Another techniquae is to incise the mucosa directly over the stone and spread the tissue apart to expose the duct, which is incised on the stone (**Fig. 13.1**).

Extraction. The stone is easily shelled out with a small hook advanced to a point behind the stone. It may also be helpful to

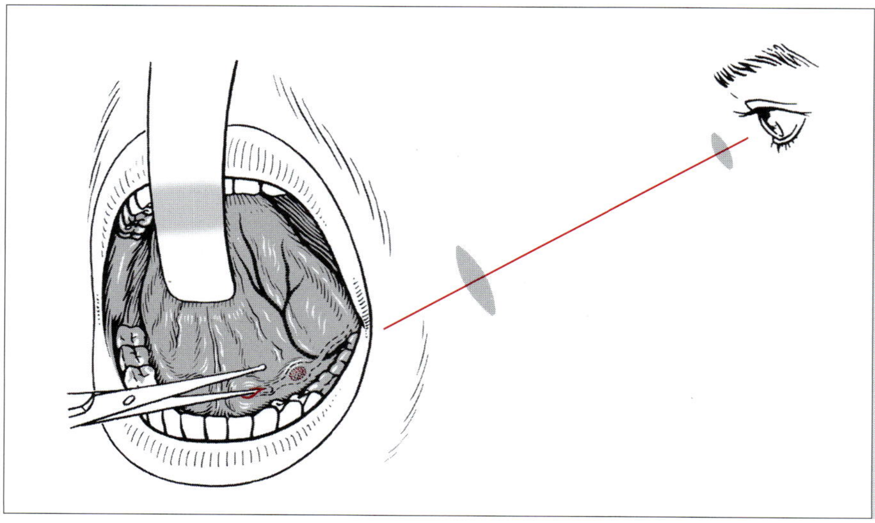

Fig. 13.1 Incision of the submandibular duct.
One blade of a blunt-ended scissors is introduced into the duct from the caruncle, and the intervening tissue is divided.

use a slender suction tip to retrieve a stone near the hilum without extensive tissue division. External pressure on the gland will keep the stone from receding. None of the incisions are sutured. Sialendoscopy has meanwhile achieved a high clinical relevance. Hereby a thin sialendoscope is inserted into the duct system (submandibular gland and parotid gland), the lesion is diagnosed, and even interventions can be performed such as transsections of synechia, stone extraction, etc.

Rules, Tips, and Tricks

- The lingual nerve crosses beneath the submandibular duct near the gland and runs anteromedial to the excretory duct. To protect the nerve, incise only the tissue perpendicular or just lateral to the duct rather than near the hilum.
- Distal stones require splitting the duct, while more proximal stones can be removed through an incision directly over the stone.

! Risks and Complications

- Sensory disturbances due to lingual nerve injury.
- Duct obstruction due to stricture or stenosis.
- Occasional cellulitic inflammation of the oral floor.

Postoperative Care

Antibiotic therapy.

Alternatives

- Excision of the submandibular gland.
- Lithotripsy.
- Basket extraction.
- Sialendoscopy.

Excision of the Submandibular Gland

Surgical Principle

Complete removal of the submandibular gland from the neck while preserving the marginal mandibular branch of the facial nerve.

Indications

- Chronic recurrent submandibular sialadenitis.
- Recurrent sialolithiasis or intraglandular stone formation.
- Benign and malignant tumors of the submandibular gland.
- Part of a regional neck dissection.

Contraindications

- Severe systemic disease.
- Massive, acute sialadenitis with cellulitis. Surgery is indicated only after unsuccessful antibiotic therapy or previous incision.

Specific Points Regarding Informed Consent

- Wound infection.
- Injury to the marginal mandibular branch of the facial nerve with associated sensory disturbances.
- Rare instances of lingual or hypoglossal nerve palsy with associated sensory or motor deficits.
- Postoperative bleeding, possibly associated with laryngeal edema or hematoma.

Operative Planning

- Palpation, especially bimanual.
- Ultrasonography.
- If necessary: sialography, CT, or MRI.

Anesthesia

General anesthesia is preferred.

Special Instruments

Standard neck tray.

Surgical Technique

Incision. A curved incision ca. 4–5 cm long is made two fingerwidths below the mandible, extending to the anterior border of the sternocleidomastoid muscle. The fat and platysma are divided in a strictly perpendicular plane (**Fig. 13.2**).

Exposure of the gland. The superficial cervical fascia deep to the platysma is spread apart at a relatively low level. The facial vein in the posterior part of the field is isolated, ligated, and reflected upward. The fascia and vessel are bluntly dissected upward to the mandibular border, proceeding directly on the gland surface. The facial artery is usually encountered at this point; it is bluntly isolated on the gland, doubly ligated, and reflected upward. This maneuver also retracts the marginal mandibular branch of the facial nerve, which crosses over both vessels, out of the operative field (**Fig. 13.3**).

Mobilization. The gland is mobilized from its compartment from the posterior side. The tissue at the posterior border is spread open and the cavity bluntly deepened with two mounted sponges, exposing the proximal portion of the facial artery in front of the posterior belly of the digastric. If the vessel enters the gland, it is doubly ligated and divided (**Fig. 13.4**). At this point the body of the gland can be freed from its compartment from the posterior aspect. The hypoglossal nerve is visible above the digastric loop in the deeper portion of the field. Smaller veins can now be accurately identified and ligated.

Anterior mobilization. The anterolateral pole of the gland that overlies the mylohyoid muscle is bluntly mobilized. The part of the gland that extends medially forward around the edge of the mylohyoid muscle is freed with a dissecting forceps while several veins are coagulated.

Division of the duct. At this point the gland is still attached by its excretory duct, and it is attached by the submandibular ganglion to the lingual nerve, which runs deeply parallel to the duct. With traction on the gland, the submandibular ganglion is

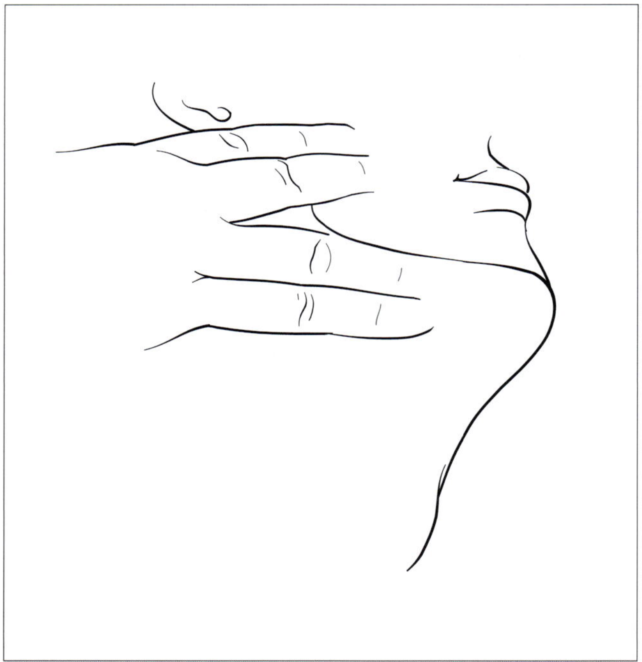

Fig. 13.2 Excision of the submandibular gland.
The skin is incised two finger-widths below the mandible.

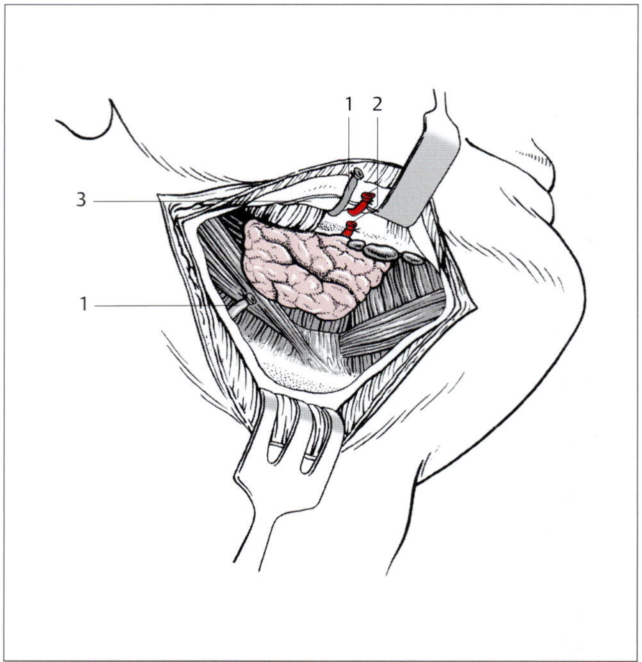

Fig. 13.3 Excision of the submandibular gland.
The facial vein (1) is ligated and reflected upward. The facial artery (2) is also ligated at the superior border of the gland, below the mandible, and reflected upward. Both superior vascular stumps hold the marginal mandibular branch of the facial nerve out of the operative field (3).

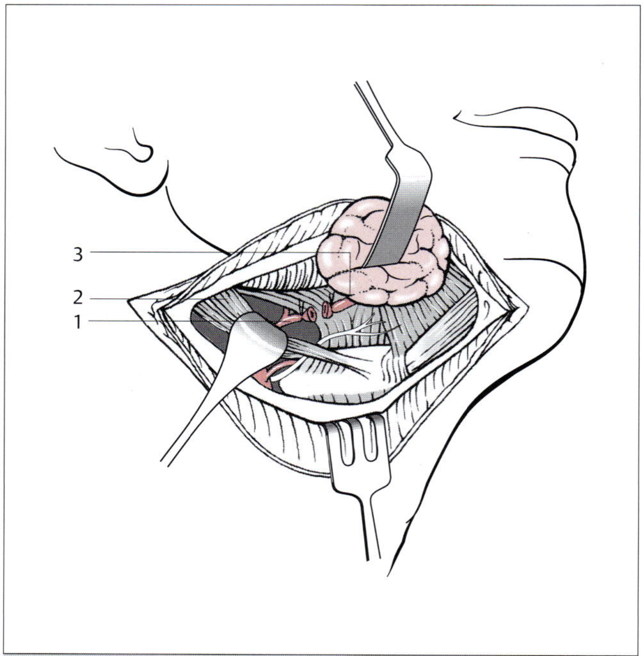

Fig. 13.4 Excision of the submandibular gland.
The proximal facial artery (1) is ligated above the posterior belly of the digastric muscle (2) before it enters the gland (3).

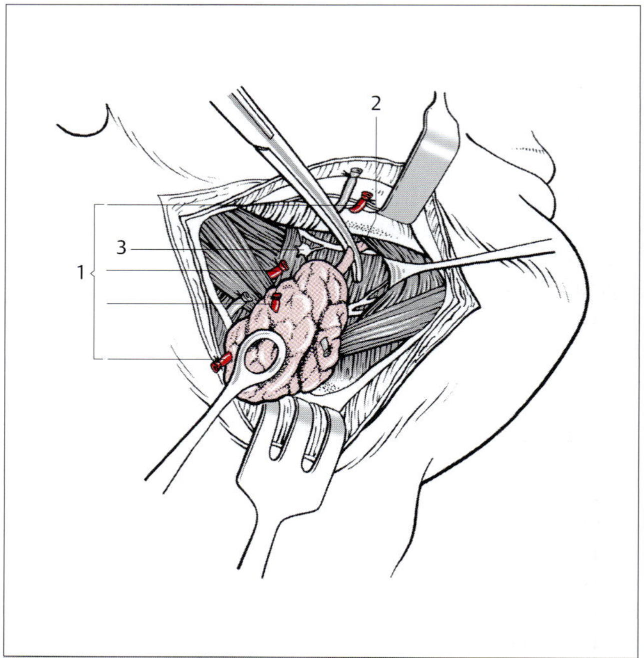

Fig. 13.5 Excision of the submandibular gland.
1 Vascular stumps of the facial artery
2 Division of the duct
3 Submandibular ganglion

transected and the lingual nerve is bluntly retracted. The duct is doubly ligated and divided, and the gland is removed (**Fig. 13.5**).

Wound closure. The wound is closed in layers over a suction drain.

Rules, Tips, and Tricks

- The marginal mandibular branch of the facial nerve can be directly identified and protected by facial nerve monitoring. This is safer than reflecting the nerve branch upward with the vascular stumps. The tissue above the ligated facial vein is explored with a stimulating electrode, and the nerve is identified and protected by spreading through the tissue in the direction that the nerve is expected to run.
- Indirect thermal injury is avoided by using only bipolar coagulation in proximity to neural structures.
- The hypoglossal nerve is located below the gland and excretory duct. It is visible above the tendon of the digastric muscle.
- Stones from the hilar area may become displaced anteriorly into the duct during the dissection. In some cases they can be "milked" back into place, but otherwise the duct should be dissected further and, if necessary, resected through the oral cavity.
- Arterial vessels should be at least doubly ligated to prevent the slippage of ligatures. Suture ligation is preferred to prevent significant postoperative bleeding with risk of hematoma formation and laryngeal edema.

! Risks and Complications

- Injury to the marginal mandibular branch of the facial nerve; sensorimotor disturbances due to hypoglossal or lingual nerve injury.
- Scarring, keloid formation, possible hollowing of the submandibular contour.
- Postoperative wound infection, postoperative bleeding from arterial and venous vessels necessitating reintervention; risk of edema at the laryngeal inlet.

Postoperative Care

The suction drain is removed according to drainage volume. Antibiotic coverage is indicated perioperatively or if signs of inflammation appear.

Alternatives

Lithiasis can be treated by duct incision, basket extraction, or lithotripsy. Increasing application of interventionl sialendoscopy.

Surgery of the Sublingual Gland

The most frequent surgical intervention refers to the treatment of the ranula that allows several therapeutic options, such as complete extirpation, sometimes also broad marsupialization. In each case, special attention must be paid to the lingual nerve, which must always be identified and preserved in surgery of the lateral floor of the mouth.

Surgery of the Parotid Gland

Treatment of Parotid Gland Injuries

Injuries of the parotid gland may be superficial with a parenchymal fistula, may involve ductal injury, or may be deep with associated profuse arterial bleeding and facial nerve disruption.

Parotid Parenchymal Fistula

Superficial injuries are treated by accurate suture re-approximation of the parenchymal lesion. The repair should include the parotid capsule, which is accurately closed with a purse-string suture or continuous plicating suture depending on the location and pattern of the injury. If salivation returns and atropine administration does not relieve salivary pressure on the suture line, the repair will have to be repeated.

The extensive destruction of parotid tissue is managed by parotidectomy with preservation or reconstruction of the facial nerve.

Injury to the Parotid Duct

Surgical Principle

Reconstruction of the parotid (Stenson) duct over a catheter stent.

Indication

Fresh injury of the excretory duct outside the parotid gland.

Contraindications

Intraglandular duct injury or extensive glandular injury (an indication for parotidectomy).

Specific Points Regarding Informed Consent

- Risk of facial nerve injury.
- Fistula formation.
- Stricture formation in the excretory duct with stasis and recurrent parotiditis.

Special Instruments

Microscope, salivary duct catheter made of vinyl or silicone.

Anesthesia

Local or general anesthesia.

Surgical Technique

After the wound has been cleaned and the wound edges debrided, a catheter is inserted into the excretory duct from the buccal side. The appearance of the catheter in the wound serves to identify the distal limb of the parotid duct.

The operating microscope is brought to bear, and the proximal duct stump is identified by salivary discharge during milking of the duct. The proximal stump is also threaded onto the catheter and re-approximated to the distal stump with microsutures. The wound is closed.

Rules, Tips, and Tricks

Obtain meticulous hemostasis after identifying the duct. Firmly retract and expose the cut surface to help identify the duct.

! Risks and Complications

Facial nerve injury, infection, stricture, cutaneous salivary fistula in the cheek.

Postoperative Care

- Antibiotic therapy.
- Leave the catheter indwelling for 2–3 weeks. Administer atropine as required.

Alternatives

Extensive injuries or inability to locate the proximal duct stump will necessitate a parotidectomy with facial nerve dissection.

If a buccal fistula develops as a late sequela, the fistula should be outlined with an elliptical incision. The attached fistula tract is mobilized, drawn into a mucosal incision and sutured there. Another option is parotidectomy.

Facial Nerve Injury

Surgical Principle

Reconstruct the nerve by performing an end-to-end anastomosis or interposing a nerve graft.

Indication

Any facial nerve injury, preferably within a short time after the trauma.

Contraindications

Severe underlying systemic disease, coma, severe head trauma, shock.

Specific Points Regarding Informed Consent

See under Parotidectomy.

Operative Planning

Documentation of preoperative findings.

Special Instruments

Same as for a parotidectomy, plus microsurgical scissors, a needle holder and forceps. Bipolar cautery. Operating microscope. Nerve stimulation device.

Anesthesia

General anesthesia is preferred.

Surgical Technique

Exposure. If the peripheral and central facial nerve stumps cannot be clearly identified in the open wound to allow for a tension-free repair, the injury is generally managed by performing a superficial parotidectomy (q. v.) and then dissecting the nerve trunk and peripheral branches. If necessary, the main trunk of the facial nerve can be identified by retrograde dissection from the anterior border of the gland.

Facial nerve reconstruction. The proximal and distal facial nerve stumps are identified and mobilized. If the stumps cannot be re-approximated without tension, an interposition graft should be used. The graft can be harvested from the great auricular nerve, which is visible at the posteroinferior edge of the parotid gland in a superficial parotidectomy. The great auricular nerve is easily dissected and harvested at that site and can provide multiple branches if needed. The interposition graft is fitted into place, approximated to the stumps, and fixed with epineural sutures.

Facial nerve repair. The peripheral and central stumps are lightly freshened, and the epineural sheaths are accurately re-approximated on all sides with 9–0 or 10–0 nonabsorbable monofilament suture material until nerve fascicles are no longer seen. Before dissecting the stumps and performing the actual repair, we recommend tacking each nerve end to the underlying wound bed with a 7–0 epineural stay suture. This will facilitate the dissection and relieve tension on the anastomosis (**Fig. 13.6**).

Wound closure. Generally the wound is closed in layers over a simple Penrose drain.

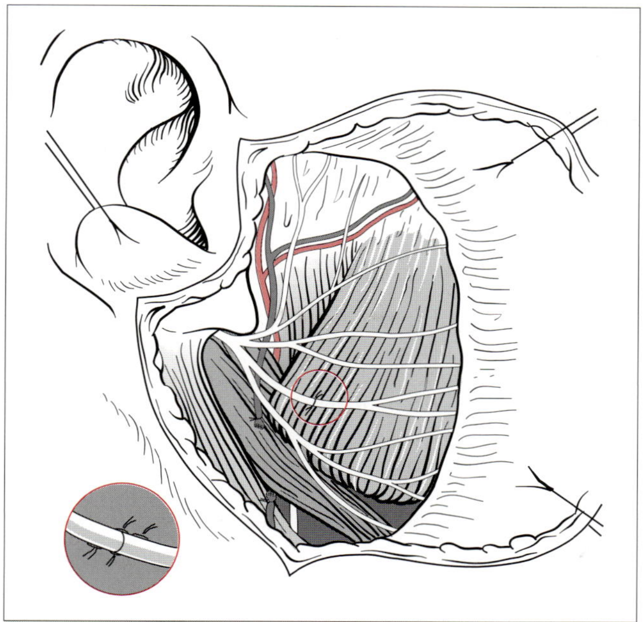

Fig. 13.6 Facial nerve repair.
Epineural stay sutures fix the stumps to the underlying tissue before the epineural repair sutures are placed.

Rules, Tips, and Tricks

- A primary repair or reconstruction should be performed whenever possible.
- If a primary repair cannot be performed because of overriding considerations, nerve stumps that are visible in the wound should be tagged with colored sutures.
- Repairs done more than 1 week after the injury are more difficult because of scarring and yield a less favorable result.
- Interposition grafts should be no longer than necessary to bridge the defect without tension. Longer grafts tend to have poorer functional results.

Postoperative Care

Same as after a parotidectomy.

Alternatives

The paralyzed face can be rehabilitated by secondary reconstructive plastic surgery.

Treatment of Parotid Abscess

Surgical Principle

Drainage of the abscess.

Specific Points Regarding Informed Consent

Risk of facial nerve injury.

Operative Planning

- Superficial parotid abscess is palpable as a fluctuating mass.
- Deeper abscesses can be detected sonographically or by CT.

Special Instruments

Dissecting forceps or dressing forceps for spreading tissues.

Anesthesia

Local anesthesia is an option for superficial parotid abscesses. General anesthesia is preferred for deep abscesses.

Surgical Technique

Incision. The incision conforms to the location of the abscess. A direct, superficial incision is appropriate only for an abscess that is about to break through the skin. Otherwise a preauricular incision is made anterior to the tragus, or an abscess at a lower site can be exposed by incising downward from the tip of the mastoid process. This incision can be curved around the mandibular angle if needed (**Fig. 13.7**).

Blunt dissection. The abscess is bluntly exposed by carefully spreading through the overlying tissues with a dressing forceps or dissecting forceps, working parallel to the presumed course of the facial nerve. The abscess capsule is identified and widely opened. A smear is taken, the contents are aspirated, and a Penrose drain is inserted.

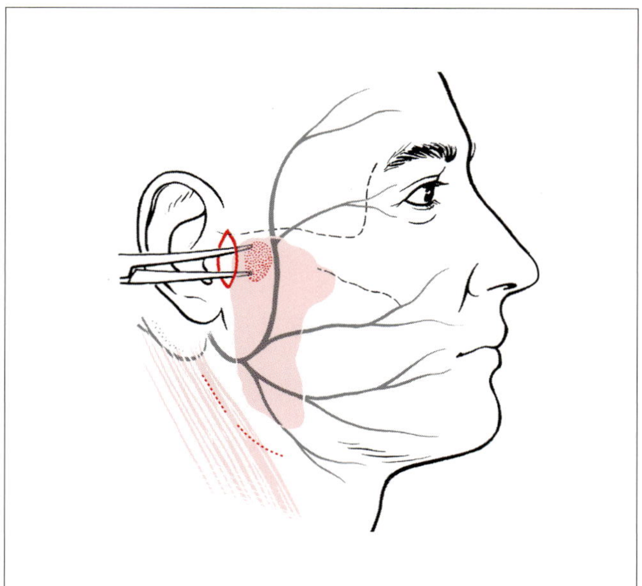

Fig. 13.7 Parotid abscess.
The placement of the skin incision and the plane of the blunt dissection depend on the location of the abscess.

13

Rules, Tips, and Tricks

- The abscess is widely opened by introducing the tip of the dissecting forceps and spreading open the blades.
- If it proves difficult to locate the deep portion of the abscess, pus can be aspirated with a needle and the abscess can then be spread open along the aspirating needle to define the course of the abscess.

! Risks and Complications

- Facial nerve injury.
- Persistent salivary fistula, bleeding.
- Spread of inflammatory changes into the parapharyngeal space or vascular compartment with septic complications, especially in debilitated patients.

Treatment of Parotid Stones

If the parotid stone does not pass spontaneously with conservative therapy (sialagogues, glandular massage) and if attempted extraction with a stone-retrieval basket is unsuccessful, a papillotomy can be performed from within the oral cavity. Following topical anesthesia plus infiltration of a local anesthetic with epinephrine, the ostium is dilated with a salivary duct probe and the duct is incised at the papilla over the indwelling probe or opened with a fine blunt-tipped scissors. Stones lodged near the papilla can be enucleated with a small hook. This technique is associated with a definite risk of stricture formation. Sialendoscopy is currently undergoing rapid developments and is on its way to becoming a standard procedure. By means of this procedure ductal stenosis and even concrement extractions may be performed with a complete view on the site.

Another option, which is currently preferred, is extracorporeal lithotripsy performed under sonographic guidance.

Parotidectomy is an option in patients with multiple stones that have not resolved with extracorporeal lithotripsy.

Parotidectomy

Superficial Parotidectomy

Surgical Principle

En bloc resection of the superficial (lateral) lobe of the parotid gland with preservation of the facial nerve.

Indications

- Benign tumors (monomorphic adenoma, pleomorphic adenoma, cystadenolymphoma, lymphangioma).
- Sialolithiasis of the gland that has not responded to conservative therapy.
- Extensive, irreparable injuries of the parotid gland.

Contraindications

- Debilitated patients who are a poor surgical risk.
- Pre-existing facial paralysis with a suspected malignant tumor (radical resection).
- Lesions arising in or involving the deep parotid lobe (indication for total parotidectomy).

Specific Points Regarding Informed Consent

- Sensory disturbance at the surgical site, rare instances of significant scar pain.
- Risk of facial nerve injury, rarely permanent, occasionally transient, with persistent deficits.
- Salivary fistula.
- Keloid formation, contour change due to tissue loss.
- Frey syndrome.
- Postoperative bleeding, wound infection.
- Recurrence.
- Reoperation, or need to extend the operation if unexpected lesions are found.
- Chewing difficulties, usually transitory.

Operative Planning

- B-mode ultrasonography. CT or MRI may be appropriate in selected cases.
- Fine-needle biopsy.
- Electrophysiologic facial nerve testing in selected cases.

Anesthesia

General anesthesia is preferred. Infiltration of the incision site with a vasoconstrictor will reduce bleeding and improve visualization of the operative field.

Special Instruments

Binocular loupe or operating microscope, bipolar cautery, fine dissecting forceps and scissors. Facial nerve monitoring device may be required.

Surgical Technique

Positioning and preparation. Supine with the head turned to the opposite side, hyperextended and tilted slightly back. In many hospitals the intraoperative electrophysiological monitoring of the facial nerve has become a routine procedure. This turns out to be very helpful, e.g. in the context of second or third interventions in the area of the then scarred parotid region.

Skin incision. An S-shaped incision is made in the skin crease anterior to the tragus, extending from the zygomatic arch around the earlobe and over the mastoid, then downward following a skin crease behind the mandibular angle (**Fig. 13.8**). If necessary, curved extensions can be added superiorly and anteriorly. The lower part of the incision is deepened to the anterior border of the sternocleidomastoid muscle, and the glistening white capsule of the parotid gland is exposed by spreading through the tissues with a dissecting forceps. The resulting skin flap is retracted laterally from the gland with small retractors, rather than toward the anterior border of the gland. The plane between the gland capsule and deep buccal fascia is progressively developed very close to the parotid capsule with a dissecting scissors, a tangentially directed scalpel, or mounted sponge. Strands of tissue from the tragal perichondrium are sharply divided, and then the superior portion of the soft-tissue flap is elevated by a combination of blunt and sharp dissection. The facial nerve branches emerging from the anterior border of the gland are protected by relying mainly on blunt dissection with a mounted sponge or by blunt tissue spreading in the direction of the nerve branches. The skin flap is reflected forward and secured with stay sutures.

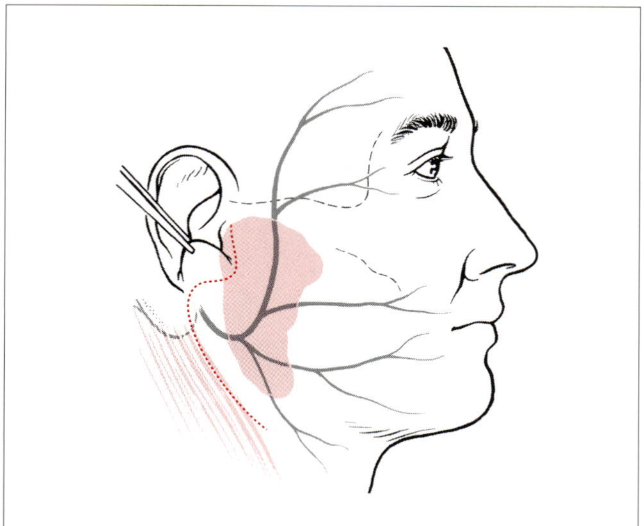

Fig. 13.8 Superficial parotidectomy.
Skin incision.

Mobilization. The gland is separated from the sternocleidomastoid muscle by a combination of blunt and sharp dissection, opening up a gap in which the posterior belly of the digastric muscle can be seen. The retromandibular vein is ligated and divided, and the great auricular nerve is at least partially divided (**Fig. 13.9**). Meanwhile the superior portions of the gland are separated from the cartilaginous ear canal with a dissecting forceps and mounted sponge. Next, the earlobe is retracted posterosuperiorly with a stay suture. While the gland body is pulled forward with a blunt retractor, the tough fibers stretching from the anterior border of the mastoid and ear canal to the gland are transected. Tissue separation from the mastoid is completed from below, aided by the operating microscope.

Facial nerve exposure. The tip of the tragal cartilage, called the pointer, marks the location of the facial nerve trunk, which is ca. 8 mm below the cartilage tip. The second key landmark is the posterior belly of the digastric muscle, as the facial nerve emerges and becomes more superficial at its superior border (**Fig. 13.10**). The stylomastoid foramen is reached from the medial end of the tympanomastoid fissure. The dissection is aided by broadly separating and retracting the tissue laterally with

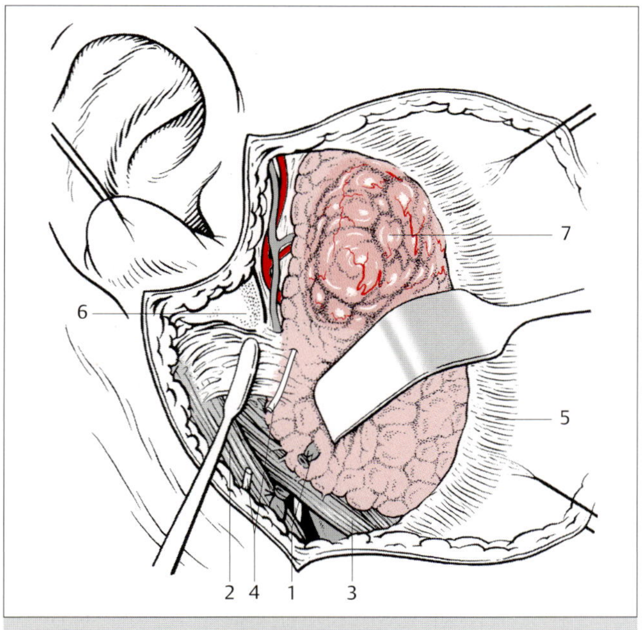

Fig. 13.9 Superficial parotidectomy.
Mobilization of the gland. Tough strands of connective tissue between the mastoid and gland are divided.

1 Retromandibular vein
2 Sternocleidomastoid muscle
3 Digastric muscle
4 Great auricular nerve
5 Platysma
6 Tragal cartilage
7 Tumor

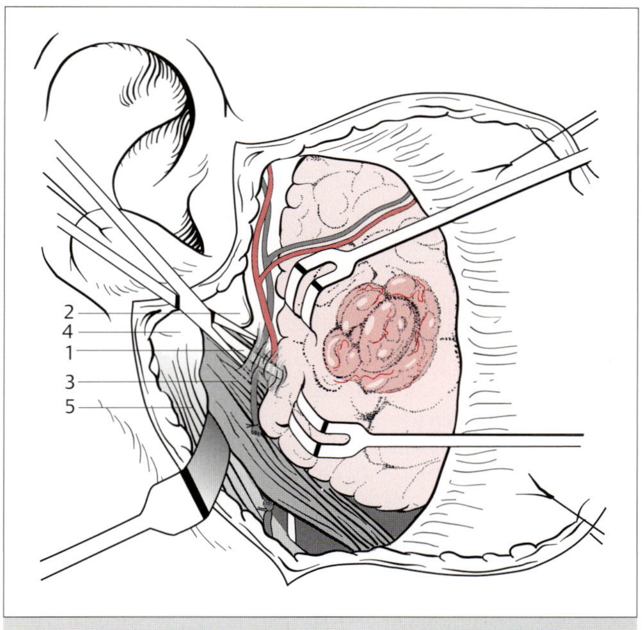

Fig. 13.10 Superficial parotidectomy.
The facial nerve trunk is identified.

1 Facial nerve trunk after division of connective-tissue bands in the parotidomastoid fascia
2 Tip of tragal cartilage ("pointer")
3 Posterior belly of digastric muscle
4 Mastoid
5 Sternocleidomastoid muscle

small retractors while working under the microscope or magnifying loupe. Strands of connective tissue around the facial nerve are progressively isolated and divided parallel to the course of the nerve. This is done with small mounted sponges, a Freer elevator, and baby mosquito forceps until finally the nerve is visible as a distinct white cord passing laterally forward and downward from above (**Fig. 13.11**). Generally at this point the nerve is crossed by the stylomastoid artery, which is ligated. Any identification problems can be resolved by facial nerve monitoring with a nerve stimulator.

Isolation of the superficial lobe. The tissue overlying the nerve is spread apart and opened laterally with a dissecting forceps, working directly on the facial nerve trunk. This creates a larger, funnel-shape opening whose edges are firmly retracted while the tissue is bluntly dissected to the bifurcation of the facial nerve. Further dissection may proceed upward along the frontal branch or downward along the marginal mandibular or cervical branch, depending on the tumor site. The nerve branches are progressively exposed by spreading through and pushing aside the glandular tissue and separating the intervening parenchyma between the deep and superficial lobes. Exposure of the facial nerve branches is constantly hindered by small vessels crossing over the nerve, and these vessels are coagulated and divided as they are encountered. The gland is then mobilized from above downward or from below upward as far as its anterior margin, culminating in the ligation and division of the parotid duct emerging from the front of the gland. At this point the superficial lobectomy specimen is removed en bloc (**Fig. 13.12**).

Wound closure. The wound is closed in layers over a suction drain. If necessary, a superiorly based flap from the sternocleidomastoid muscle can be reflected into the deep portion of the surgical cavity.

Rules, Tips, and Tricks

- Avoid violating the tumor capsule to prevent seeding of the wound. This is why an en bloc dissection of the superficial lobe is preferred to a "sectoral" dissection in which the tissue over the nerve is incised.
- Frozen section histology should be obtained if malignancy is suspected.
- To prevent Frey syndrome, keep very close to the capsule when dissecting the skin flap to preserve the deep buccal fascia, which creates a natural barrier to autonomic dysfunction. Swinging a sternocleidomastoid muscle flap into the wound bed at the end of the operation is another effective countermeasure against Frey syndrome.
- Use only bipolar coagulation in the gland region.

! Risks and Complications

- Intraoperative tumor cell dissemination.
- Risk of facial nerve injury.
- Frey syndrome.
- Salivary fistula.
- Postoperative bleeding.

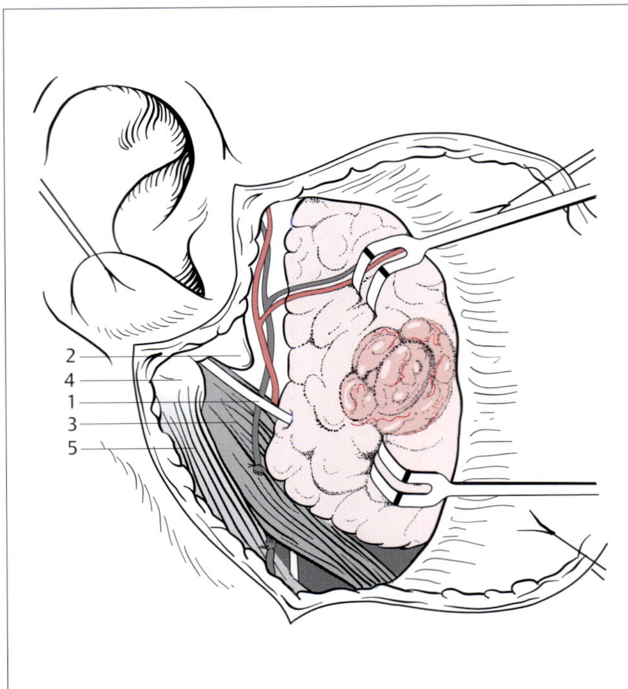

Fig. 13.11 Superficial parotidectomy.
1 Facial nerve trunk
2 Pointer
3 Posterior belly of digastric muscle
4 Mastoid
5 Sternocleidomastoid muscle

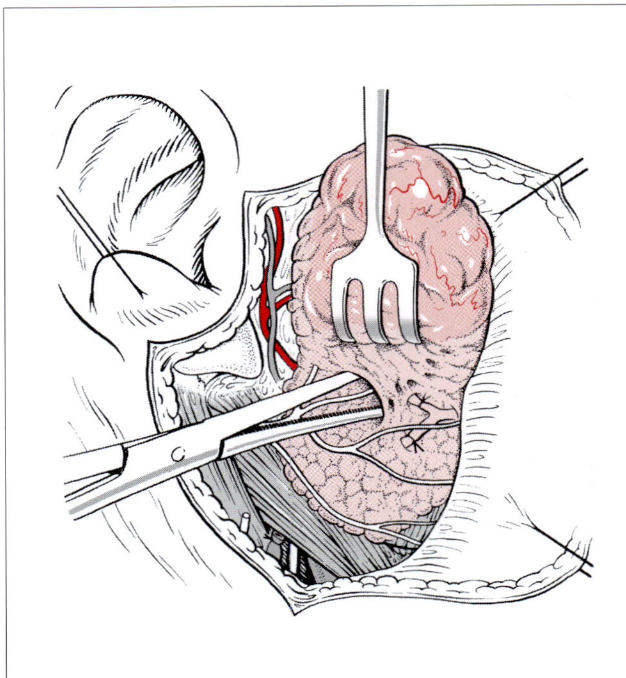

Fig. 13.12 Superficial parotidectomy.
Dissection of the nerve branches in preparation for en bloc removal of the superficial lobe.

13

Postoperative Care

The drain is removed as the drainage volume decreases. Perioperative antibiotics are administered.

Alternatives

Retrograde Facial Nerve Dissection

In cases where the tumor directly overlies the facial nerve trunk, the pointer method often cannot be used to identify the main trunk. Instead, the nerve divisions are dissected back toward the trunk in retrograde fashion from the sites where the branches emerge from the parotid capsule (**Fig. 13.13**). When the gland has been isolated to its anterior border, the soft tissues are bluntly dissected with a Freer elevator or mounted sponge toward the expected course of the facial nerve, aided by facial nerve monitoring, until the branch is identified and traced back along its course by blunt tissue spreading and retraction. The facial nerve divisions must be treated with meticulous care using blunt dissection wherever possible. This permits the gland to be developed en bloc, as in the antegrade dissection technique.

Subtotal or Total Parotidectomy with Preservation of the Facial Nerve

Surgical Principle

The initial part of the operation is the same as in a superficial lobectomy, then the parotid tissue medial to the facial nerve is additionally removed. A subtotal parotidectomy is appropriate for benign lesions. Malignant tumors that have not invaded the facial nerve are managed by a total parotidectomy that removes all of the deep parotid tissue while preserving the facial nerve divisions.

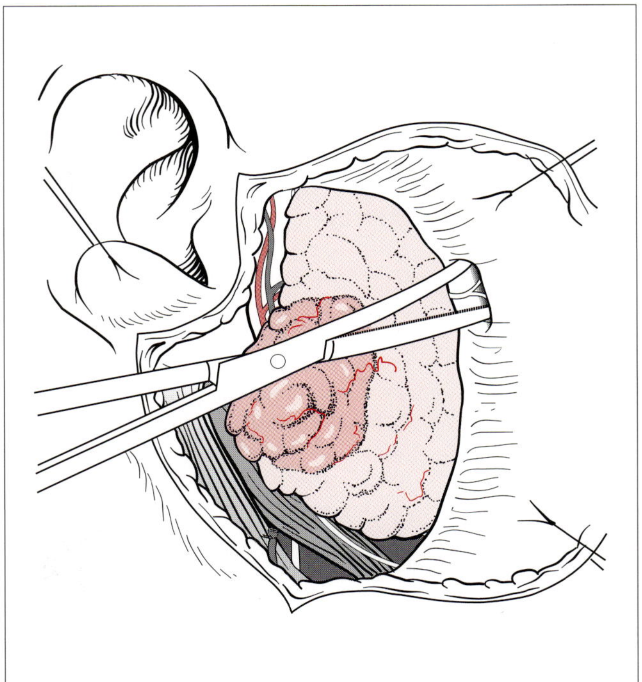

Fig. 13.13 Superficial parotidectomy.
Retrograde dissection. The nerve branches are identified at their site of emergence from the gland.

Indications

- Basically the same as for a superficial lobectomy. A subtotal parotidectomy is indicated for changes arising in the deep lobe of the gland.
- Chronic recurring parotiditis that cannot be managed conservatively (subtotal parotidectomy).
- Sjögren syndrome, suspected non-Hodgkin lymphoma (subtotal parotidectomy).
- T1 and T2 low-grade acinar cell carcinomas, also T1 and T2 low-grade mucoepidermoid carcinomas, even when confined to the superficial lobe (total parotidectomy).
- Malignant mixed tumors located entirely within a pleomorphic adenoma and not invading the parotid tissue outside the adenoma (total parotidectomy). Some tumors may require a neck dissection and radical parotidectomy.
- T1 and T2 adenocarcinomas, T1 and T2 squamous cell carcinomas without facial nerve involvement (total parotidectomy and neck dissection).

Specific Points Regarding Informed Consent

- Sensory disturbance at the operative site, rare instances of significant scar pain.
- Risk of facial nerve injury, palsy, persistent deficits.
- Salivary fistula.
- Keloid formation, contour change due to tissue loss.
- Frey syndrome.
- Postoperative bleeding, wound infection.
- Recurrence, metastasis.
- Reoperation, or need to extend the operation if unexpected lesions are found.
- Chewing difficulties, usually transitory; temporomandibular joint dysfunction.
- Risk to cranial nerves IX, X, XI, and XII.

Operative Planning

- B-mode ultrasonography. CT or MRI may be performed in selected cases.
- Assessment of regional lymph node status.
- Fine-needle biopsy.
- Electrophysiologic facial nerve testing in selected cases.
- Exclusion of distant metastasis.

Anesthesia

General anesthesia. Infiltration of the incision site with a vasoconstrictor will reduce bleeding and improve visualization of the operative field.

Special Instruments

Binocular loupe or operating microscope, bipolar cautery, fine dissecting forceps and scissors. Facial nerve monitoring may be required.

Surgical Technique

Standard Superficial Parotidectomy

Isolation. The facial nerve branches are isolated from underlying tissue as necessary with dissecting forceps and scissors and elevated with a rubber tape.

Separation. Glandular components are separated from the mandible and masseter muscle with dissecting scissors and also by blunt dissection along the cleavage plane. Branches of the external carotid artery will be encountered, most notably the maxillary artery and superficial temporal artery. To prevent heavy bleeding, the external carotid artery is exposed and ligated above the facial artery but still caudal to the posterior belly of the digastric, behind which the vessel continues its medial course. The medial boundary of the dissection is formed by the digastric muscle, stylohyoid muscle, and styloid process, behind which the internal carotid artery and hypoglossal, glossopharyngeal and vagus nerves are located (**Fig. 13.14**).

Extirpation. After the deep portion of the parotid gland has been freed from all surrounding structures including the cartilaginous and bony lateral skull base and the upper portion of the sternocleidomastoid muscle, it is mobilized from beneath the facial nerve branches and extirpated.

Subtotal and total parotidectomy differ only in the degree of residual tissue removal, subtotal parotidectomy being the less radical operation.

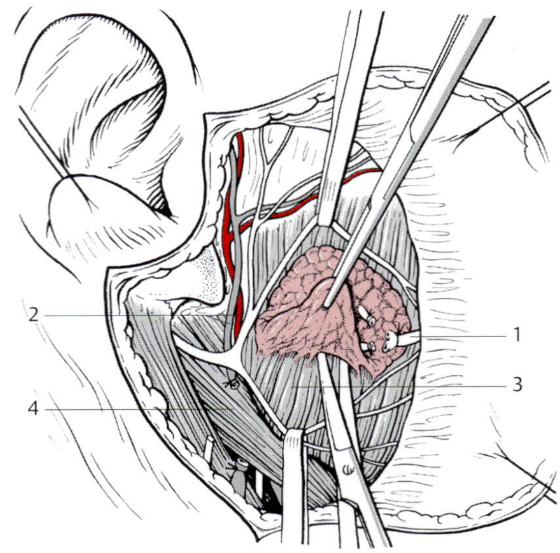

Fig. 13.14 Total parotidectomy.
The deep portions of the parotid gland are mobilized after isolation of the facial nerve branches.
1 Parotid duct
2 Superficial temporal vessels
3 Masseter muscle
4 Digastric muscle

! Risks and Complications

- Risk of facial nerve injury, risk of at least transient paralysis; significantly higher than in superficial parotidectomy.
- Risks to cranial nerves IX, X, XI, and XII.
- Frey syndrome.
- Salivary fistula.
- Postoperative bleeding, injury to internal carotid artery.
- Temporomandibular joint dysfunction.

13

Postoperative Care

The drain is removed as the drainage volume decreases. Perioperative antibiotics are administered. Some patients may require postoperative radiotherapy.

Alternatives

Iceberg tumors with predominant pharyngeal extension cannot be removed through a transparotid approach without violating the tumor capsule. In these cases the parapharyngeal space can be accessed by extending the external neck incision and exposing the vascular compartment and relevant neural structures, then mobilizing the medial portion of the tumor from below by blunt dissection with the index finger or mounted sponge. If access is still insufficient, it can be increased by temporary resection of the posterior portion of the mandible behind the trigeminal alveolar nerve.

In future, endoscopic techniques may be an available option.

Radical Parotidectomy

Surgical Principle

Complete removal of the parotid gland with the resection of facial nerve branches involved by a malignant parotid tumor. Generally the procedure is combined with a neck dissection and may be followed by facial nerve reconstruction where indicated or feasible.

Indications

- Large T3 or T4 parotid malignancies and tumors with facial nerve involvement.
- Adenoid cystic carcinoma in cases not treatable by total parotidectomy due to tumor size, patient age, tumor distance from facial nerve, etc.
- Infiltrating adenocarcinoma.
- Malignant tumors that have already caused preoperative facial nerve paralysis.

Contraindications

- Debilitated patient.
- Distant metastasis (relative contraindication).
- Invasion of structures that would no longer permit a local resection.

Specific Points Regarding Informed Consent

- As in parotidectomy, but with emphasis on facial nerve palsy if reconstruction is not possible or successful; permanent sequelae.
- Neck dissection (see Chapter 11).
- A graft may have to be harvested from the sural nerve or hypoglossal nerve, with associated motor or sensory deficits.
- Extension of the procedure to the mandible or mastoid with associated risks and sequelae.
- Tumor-dependent risks to the lower cranial nerves and internal carotid artery.

Operative Planning

- Detailed imaging evaluation by B-mode ultrasonography, CT, and MRI.
- Search for distant metastases.
- Fine-needle biopsy.
- Electrophysiologic facial nerve testing in selected cases.

Special Instruments

Instruments for parotid surgery, facial nerve monitoring, operating microscope, nerve repair set.

Anesthesia

General anesthesia.

Surgical Technique

Exposure. Initially the same as for a superficial parotidectomy, but the incision is extended upward and especially downward (for neck dissection) as needed. Further modifications are situation-dependent in cases where the resection must include areas of skin invasion.

Facial nerve reconstruction. If a facial nerve reconstruction is planned, the nerve is exposed by antegrade or retrograde dissection to within a short distance of the tumor and is isolated as described above. It is partially separated from the deep and superficial lobes only at peripheral sites uninvolved by tumor. Further dissection requires ligation of the external carotid artery, and it may also be necessary to resect portions of the mandibular ramus or mastoid, depending on the extent of tumor involvement. Finally the tumor is removed in continuity with the parotid gland and neck dissection specimen.

Nerve reconstruction follows the neck dissection. Cutaneous defects may require a regional skin flap for coverage.

Rules, Tips, and Tricks

- Detailed preoperative imaging is necessary to confirm the indication for radical parotidectomy. Frozen section histology is obtained intraoperatively to determine the limits of the resection (including the facial nerve).
- Facial nerve reconstruction is tumor- and stage-dependent.

! Risks and Complications

- Same as in a total parotidectomy.
- Potential for permanent facial paralysis.
- Possible sensory disturbances in the second and third trigeminal nerve divisions with invasion of the retromaxillary space.
- Sequelae of neck dissection.
- Temporomandibular joint dysfunction.

Postoperative Care

Chemoradiotherapy may be indicated, depending on the tumor entity and its extent.

Alternative

Palliative chemoradiotherapy.

Parotid Revision Surgery

Given the extreme difficulty and risks of nerve exposure following a superficial or total parotidectomy, generally it is best to look for *indication-dependent alternatives* to a revision parotidectomy with nerve exposure:

- *Recurrence of pleomorphic adenoma* is enucleated by blunt and sharp dissection through an incision over the tumor(s), combined with skin excision as needed. Surgery is aided by the operating microscope, facial nerve monitoring, and dissecting parallel to the facial nerve branches to reduce the risk of paralysis.
- *Circumscribed malignant tumor remnants* with a more favorable prognosis are resected in the same way but with a generous margin of surrounding tissue.
- With an *extensive but still resectable malignant tumor recurrence*, exposure of the nerve may be attempted using retrograde and antegrade techniques. Radical resection is preferred from an oncologic standpoint, however.

14 Surgery of the Ear

Preoperative Measures and Preparations

Preoperative Measures

Indications

Indications and preoperative planning are based on the following:

- History.
- Otomicroscopy, cleansing, smears for bacteriological analysis (if required).
- Testing of eustachian tube patency, facial nerve function.
- Test for fistula sign, spontaneous nystagmus, vestibular function.
- Pure-tone threshold (hearing loss), speech audiometry, impedance audiometry.
- Radiographic views (Schüller, Stenvers, high-resolution CT).
- Local findings in the nose, nasopharyngeal, and paranasal sinuses.

Informed Consent

Otologic surgery requires an informed consent procedure, which should include the disclosure of rare risks and allow time for an informed decision:

- Facial paralysis.
- Meningitis.
- Hearing loss or deafness.
- Tinnitus.
- Dizziness.
- Disturbance of taste sensation.
- Recurrent perforation.
- Otorrhea.
- Sensory disturbances and neuralgia about the ear.
- Change in auricular shape, keloid formation.
- Reoperation.
- Other possible treatment options.
- Success rates, postoperative care, and special instructions.

Preoperative Preparations

Preoperative Treatment

Patients with drainage from chronic otitis media or an old radical surgical cavity should receive preoperative treatment to resolve inflammatory changes, as this will promote wound and graft healing and facilitate intraoperative dissection. Two weeks before the planned operation, the spectrum of infecting organisms is determined by taking a smear and testing antibiotic sensitivity. Local cleaning of the ear should be followed by the placement of an ear wick to which antibiotic drops (e.g., ciprofloxacin or ofloxacin) are applied. Selective polyp removal with preservation of structures at risk can help to relieve drainage and inflammation. An effective oral antibiotic is also administered. Extensive cholesteatomas are occasionally resistant even to intensive preoperative treatment and respond only to surgical evacuation.

Preoperative Preparations

The operative site should be adequately shaved according to the selected approach (endaural or retroauricular). Before the area is aseptically prepared, the external ear canal is occluded with a strip to keep out potentially ototoxic antiseptic solution.

Positioning

The patient lies flat on the operating table with the head turned to the side and secured in a headrest or ring.

Postoperative Care

- Perioperative antibiotic therapy. Systemic antibiotics instituted during preoperative preparations are continued until the sixth postoperative day.
- Hearing and balance are monitored daily by tuning fork testing and nystagmus goggles. A bone conduction audiogram is obtained if necessary.
- Sutures are removed on the sixth postoperative day.
- Packing is removed on the sixth day after stapes surgery, tympanoscopy, or myringoplasty; otherwise at 3 weeks. Ointment strips should be replaced if a fetid odor is present.
- Gelatin sponge and silicone film are removed under the microscope using a suction tip and microforceps.
- Any granulations are removed with a curette or fine cup forceps. Patchy granulations or swellings of the ear canal are treated with triamcinolone tincture, and an ear wick may be placed if desired.
- Early Valsalva maneuvers are encouraged in patients with eustachian tube dysfunction.
- Bed rest is enforced on the first day after procedures that open the vestibule.
- Tinnitus, hearing loss, or vestibular signs are managed with infusion therapy, corticosteroid therapy, and by loosening aural packing.

Anesthesia

General anesthesia is recommended in *children*. Short procedures such as paracentesis are usually performed under propofol, ketamine, or a similar agent with mask ventilation.

Minor procedures in *adults* are often performed with topical anesthesia of the tympanic membrane. Infiltration anesthesia is suitable for several other procedures in adults. General anesthesia is recommended for sensitive patients and in cases where extensive drilling is proposed. Local infiltration of a vasoconstrictor is always recommended, even in general anesthesia, for the reduction of bleeding.

Topical Anesthesia

A small cotton pledget drenched in 4% lidocaine solution is applied directly to the tympanic membrane. To ensure direct contact with the eardrum, the pledget should be small enough to pass all the way to the membrane without wedging in the ear canal. It is gently molded to the tympanic membrane with a curette.

Local Anesthesia (Infiltration Anesthesia)

Premedication

- Benzodiazepine (e.g., Tranxilium 10–20 mg in an adult dose) is given orally on the eve of the operation.
- Pethidine (e.g., Dolantin, 0.5–1 mg/kg body weight) is given by intramuscular injection 30–45 minutes before the start of the operation.
- Midazolam can be administered intravenously during the operation (always place an IV line) at an individualized dose.

Anesthetic Agents

Ready-to-use solutions such as lidocaine with 1:200 000 epinephrine (eliminates dilution errors).

A relatively high epinephrine concentration is sometimes needed to reduce bleeding in otologic surgery. The total dose of epinephrine should not exceed 4 drops per 5–10 mL of local anesthetic, resulting in a final concentration between 1:100 000 and 1:50 000 (stock solution is 1:1 000).

- Vascular injection.
- Overdose due to dilution errors.
- Do not use epinephrine in conjunction with cyclopropane or halothane anesthesia. Take hypertension into account when dosing. Drug interactions may occur.

Technique

- The concha is pulled forward, and the retroauricular fold is infiltrated with local anesthetic. The needle is advanced beneath the elevated concha to the inlet of the posterior ear canal, which visibly bulges when the depot is injected. The needle is withdrawn slightly and advanced to the floor of the ear canal and then to the roof, placing additional depots at each site (**Fig. 14.1**).
- The ear canal is spread open with a nasal speculum, and anesthetic is injected at posterosuperior, inferior, and anterior sites while the needle is in contact with the bone.
- The intercartilaginous fissure and tragus are infiltrated, and the root of the helix is infiltrated from the anterior side.
- The mastoid surface is also infiltrated when a retroauricular approach is used.
- Optimum onset of action occurs at 8–10 minutes.

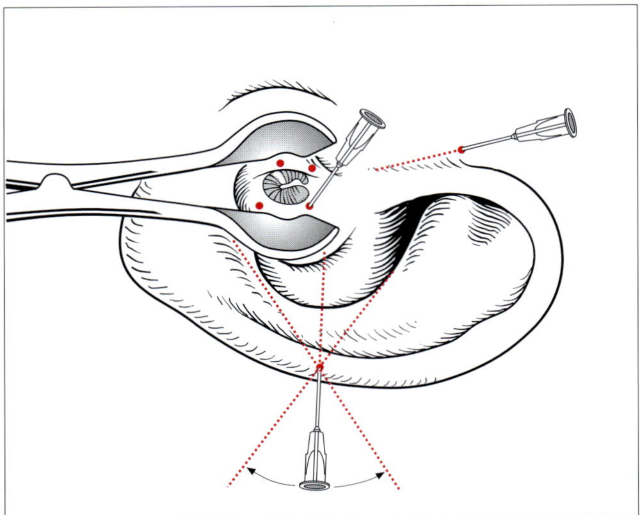

Fig. 14.1 Local anesthesia.
The aural crease and meatal opening are infiltrated with a needle inserted from the retroauricular fold. Anesthetic is also infiltrated along the crus of the helix to the intercartilaginous fissure and in the tragus. With the needle in contact with bone, depots are placed at posterior, superior, anterior, and inferior sites in the ear canal.

! Risks and Complications
See Chapter 2, pages 4 and 5.

General Anesthesia

A vasoconstrictor should be infiltrated to reduce bleeding, as in local anesthesia.

When the graft is introduced, nitrous oxide inhalation should be suspended as a precaution against graft displacement.

15 Surgery of the Auricle and Ear Canal

Basic Principles and General Measures

Surgical Anatomy—Muscles, Nerves, and Vessels

The auricle, or pinna, develops from the fusion of six auricular hillocks of the first and second branchial arches (mandibular and hyoid arches). The ear canal derives from the first branchial cleft located between the arches. The range of variation of auricular shapes and deformities can be attributed to growth abnormalities or a failure of fusion of the auricular hillocks. A well-known example of an anatomic variant is the auricular tubercle, known also as Darwin's tubercle, which corresponds to the point of the ear in mammals.

External Ear

The external ear consists of the auricle, the external ear canal (external auditory canal, external acoustic meatus), and the lateral surface of the tympanic membrane. The lateral contours of the ear are defined by prominences (eminences) and depressions (fossae) in the elastic auricular cartilage, which is directly apposed to the outer skin with no intervening fat. Only the earlobe and the free auricular border posterosuperior to the earlobe are formed by a noncartilaginous skin duplication that contains connective tissue and fat. Because there is no subcutaneous tissue layer, the anterior skin of the auricle is almost immovable relative to the perichondrium, which makes the auricle highly vulnerable to tangential trauma. This contrasts with the posterior side of the auricle, especially near the auricular root, which has a thick layer of subcutaneous fat.

The lateral aspect of a normally shaped auricle presents typical surface features (**Fig. 15.1a–d**). The rim of the auricle, called the helix, forms a laterally curled ridge that terminates inferiorly in the tail of the helix, which is continuous with the earlobe (lobule). The helical skin widens anteriorly and blends with the skin over the zygomatic arch, while the tip of the helix curves downward and backward to terminate as the helical crus. Anterior and parallel to the helix is the antihelix, which divides superiorly into two crura (anterior and posterior). The depression between the crura is the triangular fossa. The variable depression between the helix and antihelix is called the scapha (scaphoid fossa). The external ear canal is covered anteriorly by the tragus. Opposite to the tragus, and separated from it by the intertragic notch, is the antitragus, which forms a tubercle at the inferior root of the antihelix. The deep central cavity of the auricle is the concha. The helical crus, which features a sharp anterior protrusion (the helical spine), divides the concha into the cymba conchae (between the anterior crus of the antihelix and the helical crus) and the conchal cavity, which is the actual vestibule leading to the external ear canal. The acoustic meatus, then, is framed by the cartilage of the conchal cavity, by the tragus anteriorly, and by the helical crus superiorly. Between the tragus and helical crus is a cartilage-free space (anterior notch) covered only by connective tissue and muscle (superficial: auricularis anterior muscle; deep: temporalis muscle). This makes it a useful site for an "endaural auxiliary incision" to enlarge the meatal opening.

The auricular cartilage basically defines the surface anatomy of the auricle (**Fig. 15.1b, d**) except for the earlobe, the cartilage-free gap between the antitragus and helical tail, and the anterior notch. The medial (posterior) surface of the auricular cartilage (**Fig. 15.1c**) forms a less prominently developed "negative" of the lateral surface contours (**Fig. 15.1b**).

> **Rules, Tips, and Tricks**
> The variable anterior and posterior surface anatomy of the auricle can hamper anatomical orientation in surgical procedures, which are most commonly performed on the medial ("posterior") cartilage surface to modify the shape of the lateral ("anterior") surface.

Thus, characteristic depressions in the lateral surface of the auricle (triangular fossa, auricular concha, scapha) correspond to prominences (eminences) on the medial surface. Conversely, prominences in the lateral surface (helical crus, antihelix) correspond to depressions (fossae) in the medial cartilage surface. These prominences and depressions can be difficult to identify during posterior dissection of the auricle because they are compensated by the variable thickness of the auricular cartilage and because depressions are bridged by connective tissue or even muscle (between the concha and scapha).

> **Rules, Tips, and Tricks**
> The anterior auricular surface presents conspicuous surface features while the posterior surface is mostly featureless. As a result, corresponding points on the anterior and posterior surfaces can be positively identified only by piercing the auricle with marking needles.

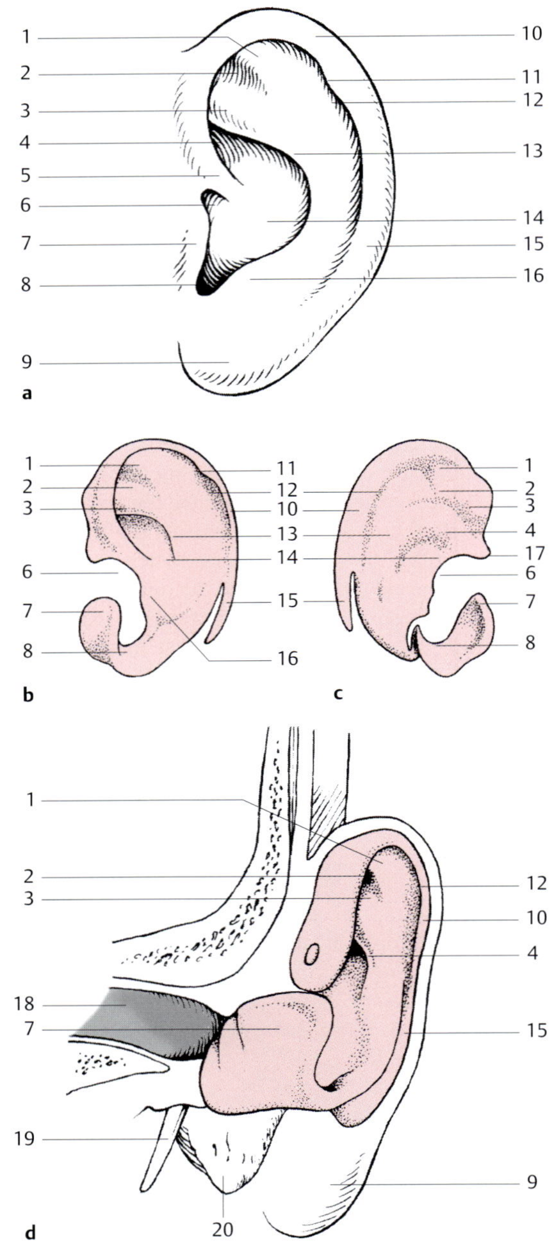

Fig. 15.1a–d Infrastructure of the auricle and ear canal (left side).
a Auricular surface anatomy, lateral view.
b Cartilaginous framework, anterior view.
c Cartilaginous framework, posterior view.
d Coronal section through the auricle and ear canal.

1 Posterior crus of antihelix
2 Triangular fossa
3 Anterior crus of antihelix
4 Cymba conchae
5 Crus of helix
6 Anterior notch
7 Tragus
8 Intertragic notch
9 Earlobe (lobule)
10 Helix
11 Darwin tubercle
12 Scapha
13 Antihelix
14 Conchal cavity
15 Tail of helix
16 Antitragus
17 Spine of helix
18 Ear canal
19 Styloid process
20 Mastoid tip

The posterior auricular skin is relatively smooth and forms an angle only between the scapha and concha (scaphoconchal angle). The fold located at the junction with the mastoid skin is called the postauricular sulcus. The normal surface area of the posterior auricular skin is considerably smaller than on the anterior side because the anterior surface presents conspicuous surface features and because fibrofatty tissue and the auricularis posterior muscle occupy the angle between the concha and mastoid (**Fig. 15.2a, b**). Nevertheless, redundant skin is usually present on the posterior side of the auricle in patients with prominent ears.

Ear Canal

The ear canal (**Fig. 15.1d**) consists of a medial bony part, which occupies approximately one-third of its total length, and a lateral cartilaginous framework. The floor and sidewalls of the bony ear canal are formed by the tympanic part of the temporal bone, the roof by the squamous part. The meatal cartilage is not a closed tube but forms a trough that is open posteriorly and superiorly and has additional gaps in its floor. These cartilage-free gaps are covered by connective tissue, which completes the tubular shape of the cartilaginous canal.

15

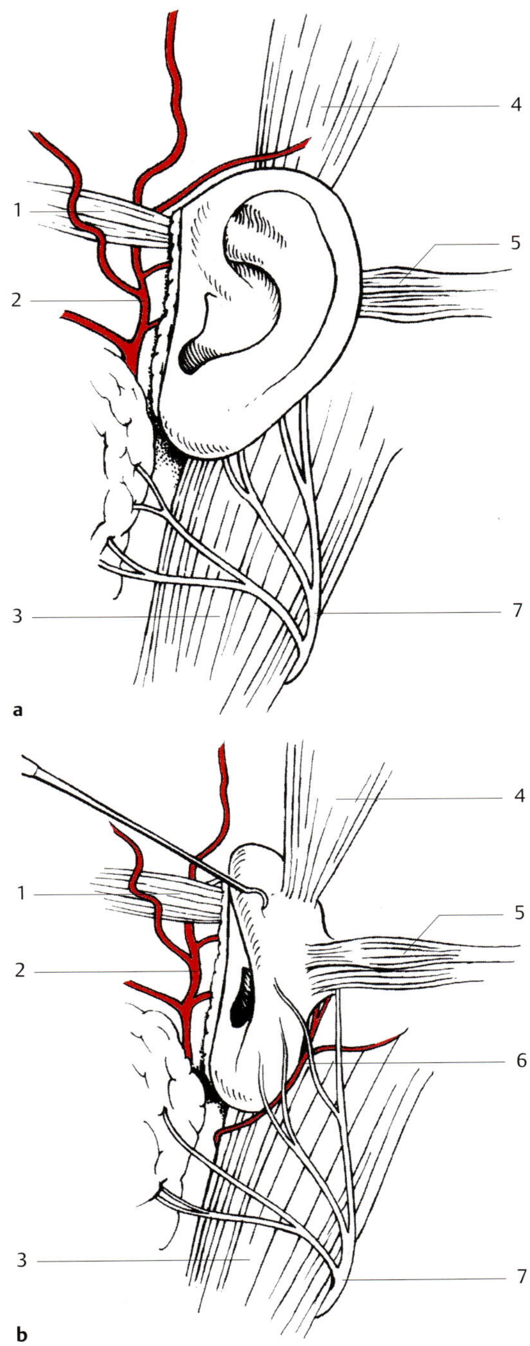

Fig. 15.2a, b Muscles, nerves, and blood vessels of the auricle (left side).
a Lateral view.
b Posterior view.
1 Auricularis anterior muscle
2 Superficial temporalis muscle
3 Sternocleidomastoid muscle
4 Auricularis superior muscle
5 Auricularis posterior muscle
6 Posterior auricular artery
7 Greater auricular nerve

Rules, Tips, and Tricks

The tragus is the direct lateral continuation of the meatal cartilage, which is connected to the auricle itself only at its inferior end (intertragic notch).

Because the tympanic membrane is at an oblique angle relative to the long axis of the ear canal, the anterior wall of the ear canal is longer (approx. 26 mm) than the posterior wall (approx. 21 mm). The auricular skin is continuous with the skin lining the ear canal. It is very thin in the bony ear canal, adherent to the periosteum, and covers the lateral surface of the tympanic membrane. The skin at the meatal opening contains hairs with sebaceous glands and cerumen glands (specialized sweat glands) whose pigments are responsible for the brown coloration of the cerumen.

Muscles

The auricle, like all openings in the face, is surrounded by muscles that are classified as mimetic muscles and are supplied by the facial nerve (**Fig. 15.2a, b**). They have no functional significance but may have to be exposed and, if necessary, divided or resected in some surgical procedures. They are interconnected by the galea aponeurotica to form a muscular system. The galea is a tendinous expansion beneath the scalp that stretches between the occipitalis and frontalis muscles. A mobile tissue plane, the subaponeurotic layer, separates the galea from the periosteum of the cranial vault (pericranium). The muscles converge toward the auricular cartilage in a stellate pattern from the posterior, superior and anterior sides. The auricularis anterior muscle inserts on the helical spine.

Nerves

The auricular skin derives most of its sensory innervation from the great auricular nerve. This main branch of the cervical plexus becomes superficial at the posterior border of the sternocleidomastoid muscle (punctum nervosum), descends on the muscle, and divides into an anterior and posterior branch. Smaller branches from the vagus nerve and auriculotemporal nerve (branch of the mandibular nerve) supply portions of the anterior auricular surface, the ear canal, and the temporal skin.

Vessels

The auricle receives its blood supply from the posterior auricular artery (branch of the occipital artery) and from the superficial temporal artery (superficial terminal branch of the external carotid artery). The vascular network is so rich that even small tissue bridges left by trauma to the ear are sufficient to maintain adequate blood flow to the auricle. The arterial blood supply is compromised less by superior tears than by inferior tears.

Preoperative Diagnosis, Documentation, and Counseling

The auricle is generally evaluated with respect to its size, position, and shape. The *size* of a normal auricle from the superior helical rim to the earlobe (**Fig. 15.3**) is approximately equal to the distance from the glabella (at the level of the eyebrows) to the subnasale (junction of the columella and upper lip). *Macrotia* refers to an auricle that significantly exceeds that size. Often this condition affects only the superior third (scapha) or inferior third (lobule) of the auricle. An abnormally small auricle (*microtia*) can have a variety of presentations ranging from excessive overhang of the upper helix ("cup ear") to a rudimentary auricle. Pronounced forms are associated with meatal atresia.

The *position* of the auricle relative to the head is evaluated from the anterior, lateral, and superior aspects (see **Fig. 15.6**). When the head is viewed in profile (**Fig. 15.3**), the longitudinal axis of the auricle forms a ca. 30° angle to a perpendicular line through the Frankfurt horizontal (imaginary line connecting the infraorbital rim to the roof of the ear canal). Thus it is roughly parallel to the vertical ramus of the mandible. When *viewed from the front* (**Fig. 15.4b**), the antihelix and helix should be at approximately the same level or the helix should be just outside the antihelix. The auricle is described as "prominent" if the helix is conspicuously visible from the front and projects more than 1.5 cm from the mastoid plane. These relationships are described by two angles that are measured in the *superior view* (**Fig. 15.4c**). The angle between the concha and scapha behind the ear should be ca. 90°. If the angle is greater than 90°, the antihelical fold is absent and the helix is protuberant. If the angle is less than 90°, the helix is curled medially and is hidden by the antihelix when viewed from the front. The relationship of the auricle to the skull is described by the concha–mastoid angle (cephaloauricular angle). The cross-sectional axes of the auricle and mastoid normally form a ca. 30° angle.

Analysis of the *auricular shape in the lateral view* should include at least four structures (**Fig. 15.4a**):

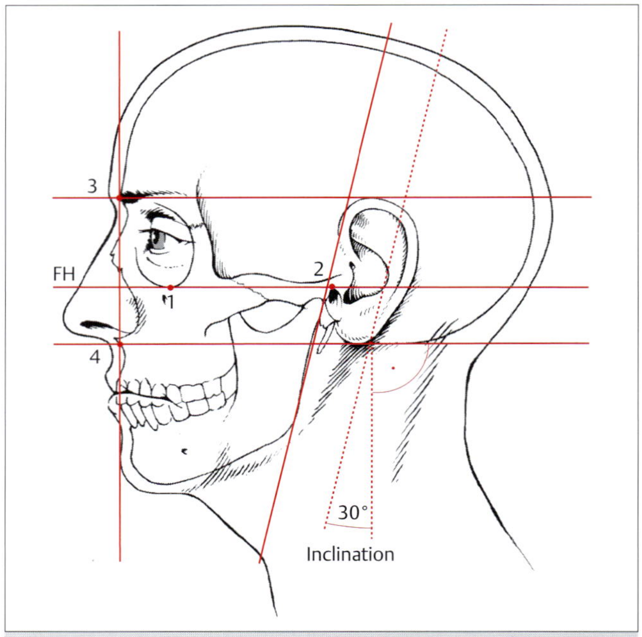

Fig. 15.3 Anatomical relations of the auricle.
FH = Frankfurt horizontal through the infraorbital rim (1) and roof of the ear canal (2). The longitudinal axis of the auricle runs at an angle of ca. 30° (inclination) to the frontal plane (perpendicular to FH), making it roughly parallel to the vertical ramus of the mandible. The height and position of the auricle are defined by lines parallel to the FH through the supraorbitale (the most prominent part of the forehead between the eyebrows = 3) and the subnasale (junction of the columella and upper lip = 4).

Rules, Tips, and Tricks

- Helix: helical rim is flattened or unfolded (scapha too large). Helical circumference is too short, causing lateral overhang of the upper helix (cup ear, lop ear).
- Antihelix: prominent helix due to absence of the antihelical fold, especially its posterior crus.
- Concha: deepening of the conchal bowl causing middle-third protrusion of the auricle (viewed from the front).
- Earlobe: large and pendulous, absent, or "attached."

Otoplasty to correct an auricular deformity should create normal anatomical relationships whenever possible. It is important to avoid overcorrection in the form of flat ("pinned back") ears or a helical rim that is not visible from the front.

When findings have been described according to this scheme, preoperative *photographic documentation* is strongly recommended. The forehead and chin should be visible in photographs taken from the front and side. The workup should include an occipital view to document auricular position and full-frame lateral photographs of the auricles to document surface anatomy. Clips should be used to hold back the hair, if necessary.

Because elective surgical procedures on the auricle are generally done for aesthetic improvement, preoperative counseling is essential. In case of total or subtotal auricular reconstruction the patient should not have *unrealistic expectations* about the outcome of an auricular reconstruction. It should always be emphasized that reconstructions can approximate a natural auricle but can rarely, if ever, achieve it. The alternative of a bone-anchored auricular prosthesis should be discussed. If autologous grafts are needed, the patient should understand the potential for donor site morbidity when the grafts are harvested (e.g., costal cartilage).

Anesthesia and Preoperative Preparations

Anesthesia

Principle

Auricular surgery is easily performed under *local anesthesia*. If the operation lasts less than 1 hour, local anesthesia is even appropriate for cooperative children 12 years of age or older. Auricular surgery requires an intravenous line, premedication

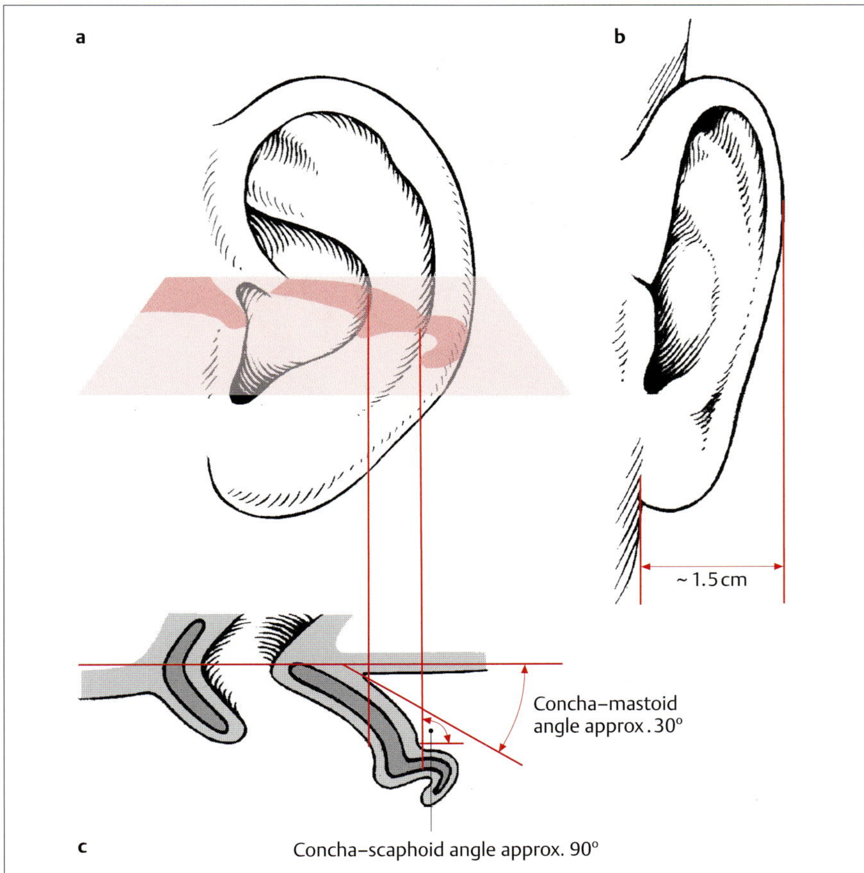

Fig. 15.4a–c Position of the auricle and angular measurements in cross-section (left auricle).
a Lateral view showing the transverse plane (**c**) at the level of the ear canal. Corresponding vertical lines indicate the position of the antihelix and scapha.
b Normally the helix projects no more than 1.5 cm from the head when viewed from the front.
c Cross-section at the level of the ear canal. The retroauricular angle between the concha and scapha (scaphoconchal angle) is ca. 90°. The angle between the auricle and mastoid plane (concha–mastoid angle) is ca. 30°.

(e.g., midazolam), and appropriate monitoring (ECG, pulse oximetry, blood pressure in older patients).

General anesthesia is recommended in patients with heavy scarring of the operative site, in long operations involving extensive reconstruction, and in small children.

Contraindications

- Severe cardiovascular disease with arrhythmia and hypertension.
- Allergy to local anesthetics.
- Anticoagulant therapy.
- Platelet aggregation inhibitors should be discontinued at least 2 weeks before surgery.

Timing of Surgery

Rules, Tips, and Tricks
Preschool age (4–5 years) is an excellent time for the surgical correction of prominent ears.

This is recommended because very little auricular growth occurs after 5 years of age and because the auricular cartilage is still soft and pliable in this age group. The possibility of combining the otoplasty with other necessary procedures (adenoidectomy, paracentesis, inguinal hernia, phimosis) should be discussed with the parents.

Technique of Local Anesthesia (Fig. 15.5)

Local anesthesia is induced by injecting up to 10 mL of 1 % lidocaine solution with epinephrine (1:200 000). The needle is inserted in the retroauricular skin, and the anesthetic is injected in a fan-shaped pattern. The sensory branches of the vagus nerve and auriculotemporal nerve are blocked by an additional injection anterior to the tragus, directing the needle tip toward the floor of the ear canal. This may induce temporary, reversible *facial paralysis*, and this possibility should be disclosed during informed consent.

15

Preoperative Preparations

Whenever possible, avoid shaving the scalp hairs for a standard otoplasty. It is sufficient to apply adhesive surgical drapes, and if necessary the (freshly washed) hair should be pulled back from the operative field and secured with clips or tied in a ponytail. Despite the potential for contamination, perioperative antibiotic prophylaxis is necessary only for complex reconstructions and graft procedures. It is also advisable in these cases to trim the hairs short in the operative area. Close shaving would obscure the hairline, which is an essential landmark in many reconstructive procedures.

Instruments and Suture Materials

Instruments

Instruments should permit the atraumatic handling of skin and cartilage. Subcutaneous fat and skin should be grasped with a fine surgical forceps, and cartilage with an Adson–Brown forceps. Dissection should be done with a pointed scissors. A single-pronged or small three-pronged hook should be used for the fixation of soft tissues and cartilage.

Suture Materials

Proper suture materials are essential for achieving a permanent result and avoiding complications. Cartilage incisions are sutured with absorbable material (e.g., 4–0 Vicryl). Nonabsorbable material should be used for cartilage-shaping sutures. Braided sutures predispose to infection and fistula formation due to their wicking action, so monofilament is preferred (e.g., 4–0 Ethibond). Clear sutures will be invisible through the thin skin.

The removal of retroauricular skin sutures is often painful and difficult because the postoperative auricle cannot be retracted far from the head. Absorbable sutures that dissolve within approximately 8 days are advantageous, especially in children, but some subcutaneous sutures (e.g., 4–0 Vicryl) should also be used to stabilize the skin sutures.

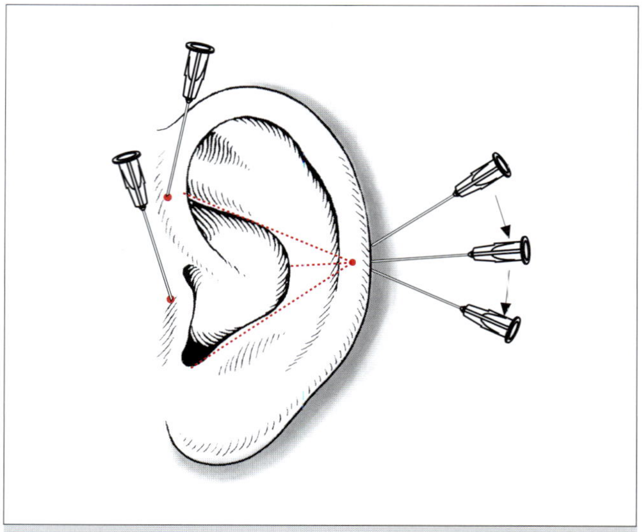

Fig. 15.5 Local anesthesia of the auricle and ear canal. The needle is inserted behind the postauricular sulcus, and local anesthetic is injected in a fan-shaped pattern to infiltrate the posterior auricular surface and especially the posterior circumference of the meatal opening. Local anesthetic is also injected anterior to the helical crus if an endaural auxiliary incision will be placed in the anterior notch. Surgery in the ear canal or skin mobilization anterior to the tragus also requires injection anterior to the tragus toward the temporomandibular joint.

Correction of Prominent Ears

Surgical Principle

15

A prominent ear is generally corrected by *reduction* of the concha, the *creation* of an antihelical fold or roll, and *setback* of the corrected auricle. Conchal reduction is achieved by cartilage resection. An antihelix roll is created by approximating corresponding points on the auricular cartilage, with or without previous cartilage scoring, and general auricular setback is accomplished by suture fixation toward the mastoid plane.

Rules, Tips, and Tricks
An antihelical fold is created by approximating pairs of anterior "cartilage points" with posteriorly placed sutures (with or without previous cartilage scoring).

Historically, the methods for creating an antihelical fold are based on three major principles, all of which were published in 1963:

- Scoring only (Stenström).
- Sutures only (Mustarde).
- Combination of scoring and sutures (Converse).

Stenström (1963) found that simple manual reshaping of a prominent auricle could produce a normal-appearing ear. He believed it was unnecessary to remove cartilage and relied instead on creating an imbalance of stresses within the cartilage. In their pioneering study of hyaline rib cartilage, Gibson and Davis (1958) found that expansile forces generated by the matrix at the center of a cartilage cross-section counteracted the contractile forces exerted by the layer of close-packed chondrocytes on the cartilage surface. They called this the "balanced cross-section." The perichondrium does not contribute to this balance of forces. When a layer of superficial cartilage is removed on one side, the balance is disrupted and the contractile force from the undamaged surface becomes dominant, causing the cartilage to curl in that direction. When Stenström did similar studies on auricular cartilage, he found that hyaline rib cartilage and elastic auricular cartilage behaved in the same way. He questioned the explanation of Gibson and Davis regarding contractile and expansile forces, however. The Stenström principle involves superficial scoring of the anterior surface of the antihelical cartilage. He separated the tail of the helix from the concha through a retroauricular skin incision and split the conchal cartilage in the direction of the helical crus. Access for cartilage scoring was gained by subcutaneous tunneling over the body of the antihelix, the posterior crus, and if necessary the anterior crus. He scored the cartilage using the blade of an Adson–Brown forceps with a curved and elongated tip. An elliptical retroauricular skin excision at the level of the antihelix was an essential part of the Stenström procedure. Another method is to expose and score the anterior surface of the antihelical cartilage "under vision" through a cartilage incision in the scapha (Chongchet 1963).

The Scottish plastic surgeon *Mustarde* created an antihelix roll with posterior cartilage sutures made of soft silk (1963). This technique avoids the creation of sharp cartilage edges, and the cartilage is shaped by adjusting the tension under which the sutures are tied. He felt it was unnecessary to resect and reduce the conchal cartilage since the antihelix can be "rolled back" with sutures. Luckett in New York had noted the possibility of shaping the antihelix with sutures in a much earlier publication (1910). He also claimed that the correction of auricular prominence by reducing the cephaloauricular angle did not address the underlying pathology, which required the creation of an antihelical fold. Potential problems of suture technique include suture fistula formation, recurrence due to "migration" of the cartilage sutures, and visibly tight sutures (like a violin bow) below the skin surface.

Converse (1963) fashioned an antihelix and posterior crus by making parallel cartilage incisions in the scapha, triangular fossa, and concha and then joining the incisions with shaping sutures (chromic catgut or nylon). For very heavy cartilage, the correction was supported by thinning the retroauricular cartilage with a rotating wire brush. A posterior elliptical skin excision at the level of the antihelix completed the procedure.

Our concept involves a graded approach. We use a suture-only technique when dealing with soft, malleable cartilage that does not show significant elastic recoil. Rigid cartilage is also weakened at selected sites by making incisions in the anterior cartilage surface (as practiced by Stenström and Chongchet). Once the auricle has been reshaped and the concha has been reduced if needed, the auricle is set back with concha–mastoid sutures (Furnas 1968).

Indications

- The indications depend on the degree of deformity. The criteria cited earlier, such as the concha–mastoid angle, scaphoconchal angle, lateral projection of the helix, and size of the conchal bowl, should be well outside the normal range.
- Generally the more pronounced the abnormality, the more rewarding the surgical procedure. The correction of very mild deformities is difficult, but rarely gratifying for either patient or surgeon.
- It is common to find differences in the degree and location of deformities between the two ears. It is still advisable in these cases to perform a *bilateral* correction, as experience has shown that the uncorrected ear will usually appear prominent relative to the operated side.

Contraindications

- A very mild degree of cosmetic deformity would contraindicate otoplasty, especially in adults. Patients seeking corrective surgery in this situation will generally have a *significant psychological component*, and in most cases the auricle is not the real problem. Even with a technically excellent otoplasty, the patient is likely to be dissatisfied with the result.
- Otoplasty may be contraindicated for medical reasons including a high *susceptibility to infections* due to immune deficiency (diabetes, HIV infection, corticosteroid therapy) and proneness to hypertrophic *scarring* or keloids. The auricular skin is a site of predilection for keloid formation, which may occur in response to surgery or injury. Keloids appear as raised, lobulated, bluish-gray scars that transgress the boundaries of the original injury to involve healthy skin. Hypertrophic scars are also raised above the skin surface but are always confined to the injured area. Patients with pre-existing keloids are assumed to be prone to keloid formation and should not undergo auricular surgery—though it is not always helpful to make an individual risk assessment based on scars in other body regions, because a retroauricular skin incision may form a keloid even in patients with a normal-appearing appendectomy scar, for example.

Specific Points Regarding Informed Consent

Besides general surgical risks such as infection (perichondritis) and bleeding (hematoma), the patient should understand the risks of excessive scarring (hypertrophic scars, keloids), auricular deformity, recurrence, and suture fistulas.

Operative Planning

A "prominent ear" does not present simply as a protruding auricle with an otherwise normal morphology. The affected auricle generally shows anatomical abnormalities, which is why this condition is considered a deformity rather than a normal variant (see **Table 15.2**). There are *three typical deformities of auricular structure* that require specific surgical correction to achieve a "normal" ear (**Fig. 15.6a–c**).

When viewed from the front, the helix projects more than 1.5 cm from the lateral facial region. Protrusion of the upper two-thirds of the helix is caused mainly by absence or deficiency of the antihelical fold, especially the posterior crus. Middle-third prominence is accentuated by a deep concha, and lower-third prominence by frequent lateral protrusion of the earlobe. If the antihelix roll is absent and the concha is continuous with the scapha, a bowl-shaped auricle results. This deformity is characterized by prominence of the middle third of the auricle, which usually stands well away from the mastoid plane (concha–mastoid angle = 90°).

The auricle should also be analyzed for additional deformities correctible with surgical techniques that go beyond a "standard otoplasty." This would include the correction of a *large scapha*, which is usually associated with an absent or diminished helical fold (see **Fig. 15.27**).

A lop ear may present initially as a simple auricular deformity. In reality, though, it is based on an abnormally short helical rim, which requires an entirely different surgical approach (see **Fig. 15.28**).

Another problem is disproportion of the lower third of the auricle caused by excessive length of the earlobe. This problem can also be corrected with special techniques (see **Fig. 15.24**).

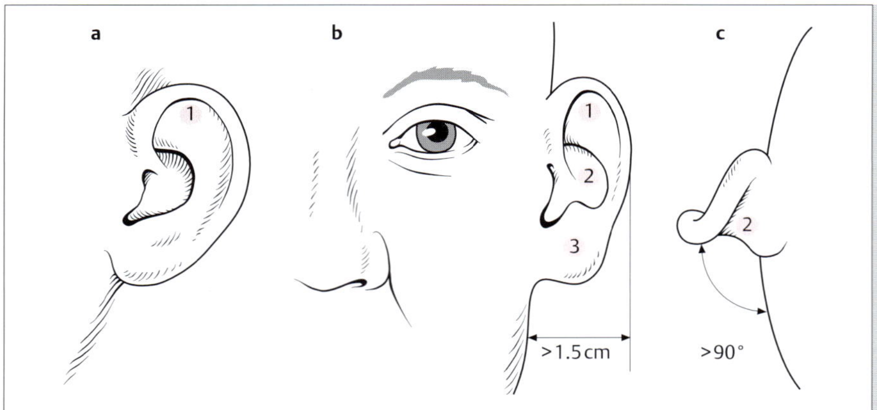

Fig. 15.6a–c Analysis of the prominent auricle.
a Lateral view.
b Anterior view.
c Superior view.
1 Absence of the antihelical fold
2 Prominent conchal bowl
3 Protruding earlobe
The helix projects more than 1.5 cm from the mastoid plane. The concha–mastoid angle is approximately 90°.

Lateral protrusion of the antitragus is a technically difficult problem to correct. Surgical correction should not be attempted without a compelling indication, which is rarely present. Patients should be advised of this special circumstance so that they will not attribute pre-existing prominence of the antitragus to the surgery itself.

Timing: Prominent ears are usually corrected at 4–5 years of age, before the child begins school. The auricle should not undergo significant additional growth after age 5.

Surgical Technique

In typical cases that require correction of the size, shape, and position of the auricle, the surgical procedure can be divided into several steps. These "building blocks" are largely independent of one another and can be assembled in a modular fashion to meet individual requirements. The operative steps are listed below and illustrated in **Fig. 15.7**.

Rules, Tips, and Tricks

- Retroauricular incision.
- Excision of conchal cartilage.
- Creation of an antihelical fold.
- Correction of the earlobe.
- Setback of the reduced and reshaped auricle.
- Retroauricular sutures.

15

Additionally, the planning and conduct of the surgery should follow this principle:

The correction is planned on the anterior auricular surface and performed on the posterior auricular surface.

Retroauricular incision, exposure of the posterior cartilage surface and mastoid plane (**Fig. 15.8a–c**). The skin incision is made ca. 1 cm lateral and parallel to the postauricular sulcus. This will make the scars less conspicuous than an incision closer to the helix and will provide broad skin coverage for the antihelix shaping sutures (to prevent suture fistulas). The incision should extend far enough superiorly to furnish easy access to the posterior crus of the antihelix. The lower part of the incision should terminate on the posterior surface of the earlobe. The skin incision should not violate the cartilage or perichondrium. The skin is mobilized in the epiperichondrial plane as far as the helical rim, leaving the skin attached to the rim itself. It is important to undermine the skin completely so that the auricular cartilage can be everted through the incision, exposing all of its posterior surface (**Fig. 15.8b**). Small bleeding sites can be accurately controlled with bipolar coagulating forceps. The dissection is extended medially and posteriorly to expose the periosteum of the mastoid plane. The auricularis posterior muscle is resected to make room for the conchal setback (**Fig. 15.8c**). The posterior auricular artery is coagulated at this time. Care is taken to obtain adequate posterior mobilization of the mastoid skin. The mobilized area should approximately equal the area covered by the posterior auricular surface.

Reduction of the concha by cartilage excision (**Figs. 15.9, 15.10, 15.11**). The concha is reduced by excising a crescent-shaped strip of cartilage. Generally the concha is most prominent in the middle third, and so the cartilage resection should be widest at that level (**Fig. 15.9a**). In a few cases the concha is most prominent in its upper third (**Fig. 15.9b**) or lower third, and the widest part of the excised crescent is shifted accordingly.

The retroauricular cartilage incision is planned on the anterior auricular surface. The proposed cut edge of the cartilage should be "in the shadow" of the antihelix (**Fig. 15.10a**). Viewed in cross-section, an S-shaped transition will be created from the antihelix to the conchal bowl, with the cartilage incision placed at the transitional curve (**Fig. 15.10b**). The cartilage along this transition zone is pierced with three No. 16 hypodermic needles inserted from the anterior side of the auricle (**Fig. 15.10a**). The superior needle is inserted below the anterior crus, the middle needle at the site of maximum lateral protrusion, and the inferior needle below the antitragus. Next, the perichondrium and cartilage surface are incised from the retroauricular side with a No. 15 scalpel blade along an imaginary semicircular line connecting the needles. This initial incision should be superficial for marking purposes (**Fig. 15.10c**). Then the needles are removed. Actual division of the cartilage is now performed in one step while the middle finger of the free hand provides counter-pressure and helps to keep the scalpel from penetrating the anterior perichondrium and skin (**Fig. 15.10d**). The full

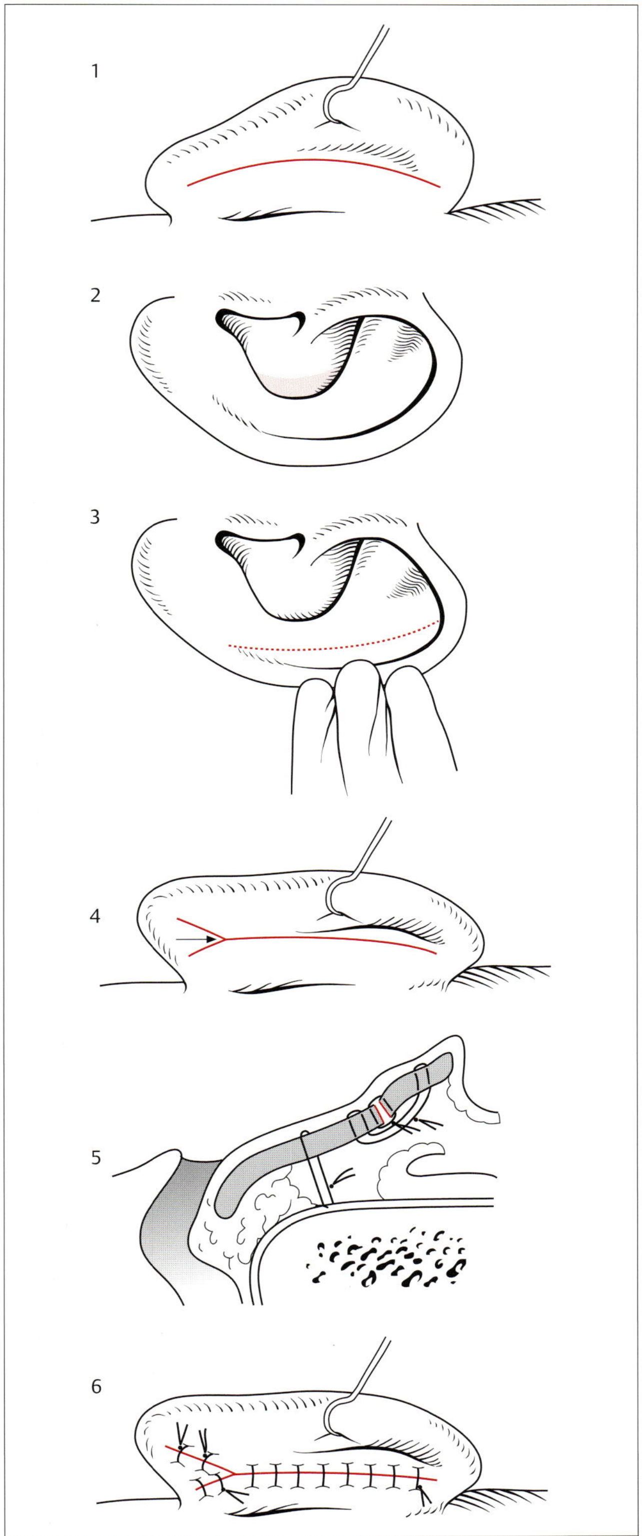

Fig. 15.7 Individual steps in the surgical correction of prominent ears:
1 Retroauricular incision
2 Excision of conchal cartilage
3 Creation of an antihelical fold
4 Correction of the earlobe
5 Setback of the corrected auricle
6 Retroauricular sutures

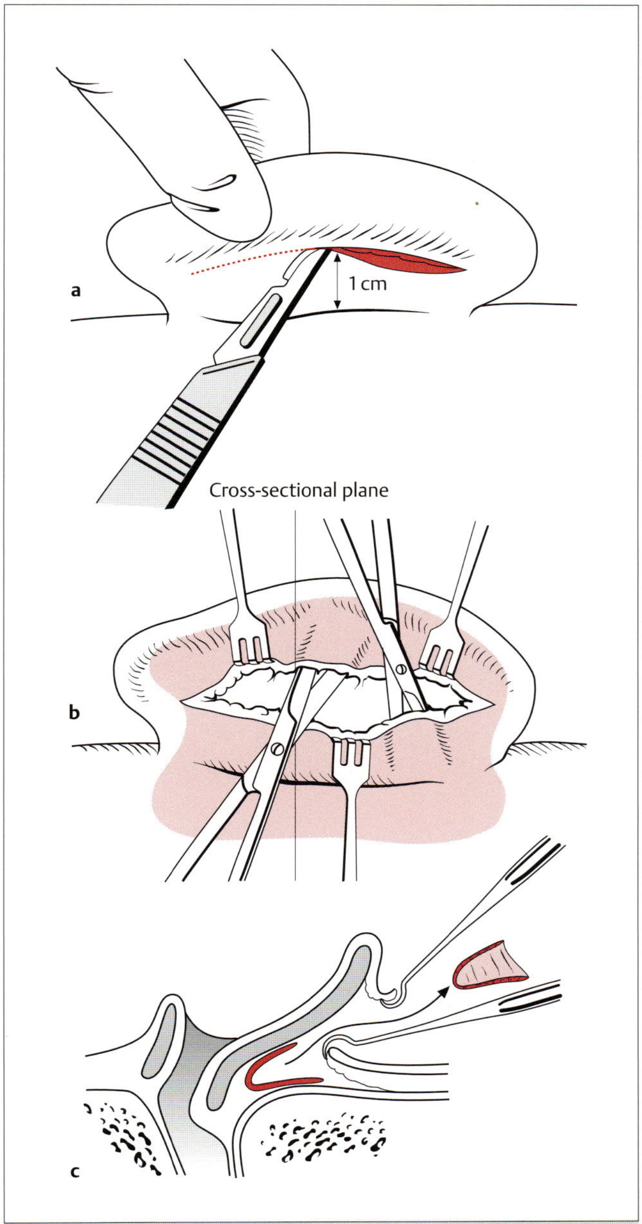

Fig. 15.8a–c Incision and exposure of the posterior auricular surface.
a The skin is incised ca. 1 cm lateral to the postauricular sulcus.
b The skin is undermined on the posterior cartilage surface while preserving the perichondrium.
c Cross-section at the level of the ear canal (corresponding to **Fig. 15.4**). The skin is elevated from the mastoid, leaving the periosteum intact. The auricularis posterior muscle may be resected to facilitate later setback of the auricle.

cartilage thickness should be divided in one action; a jagged line may result if the initial cut is superficial and then deepened by additional cuts. When the cartilage is properly incised to the anterior perichondrium, the cut edges of the cartilage can be cleanly separated. If the incision does penetrate the anterior skin despite precautions, the wound is oversewn with 6–0 monofilament suture material.

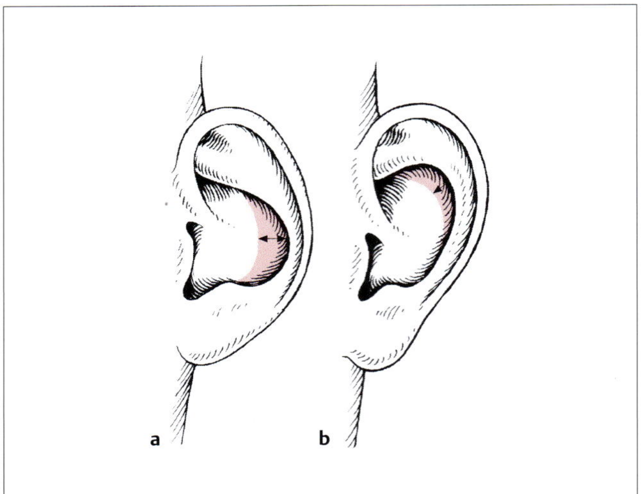

Fig. 15.9a, b Types of conchal prominence.
a Middle-third prominence.
b Upper-third prominence.
The strip resection is widest at the level where the concha is most prominent.

The cartilage resection may proceed only after the skin has been elevated from the anterior cartilage surface. This begins by stripping the perichondrium from the anterior cartilage surface at a circumscribed site until the cartilage can be broadly grasped with an Adson–Brown forceps. This broad purchase is necessary to hold the cartilage securely for further dissection. If only a very circumscribed tissue area is grasped, it may easily tear or slip out of the forceps. Further dissection of the skin proceeds in the subperichondrial plane with a pointed scissors or elevator, mobilizing the skin as far as the meatal opening and the crus of the helix (**Fig. 15.11a, b**).

Rules, Tips, and Tricks

This extensive mobilization is necessary due to the relative skin excess that will form after the cartilage resection. Broad undermining can distribute the redundant skin over a larger area with less (transient) folding of the skin.

Next, a crescent-shaped cartilage strip of the desired size is resected from the concha with a curved, pointed scissors (**Fig. 15.11c, d**). Over-resection should be avoided. It is better to reduce the concha to the desired size progressively by a series of smaller strip resections. All bleeding sites on the perichondrial surface are carefully coagulated with bipolar forceps before the cartilage sutures are placed.

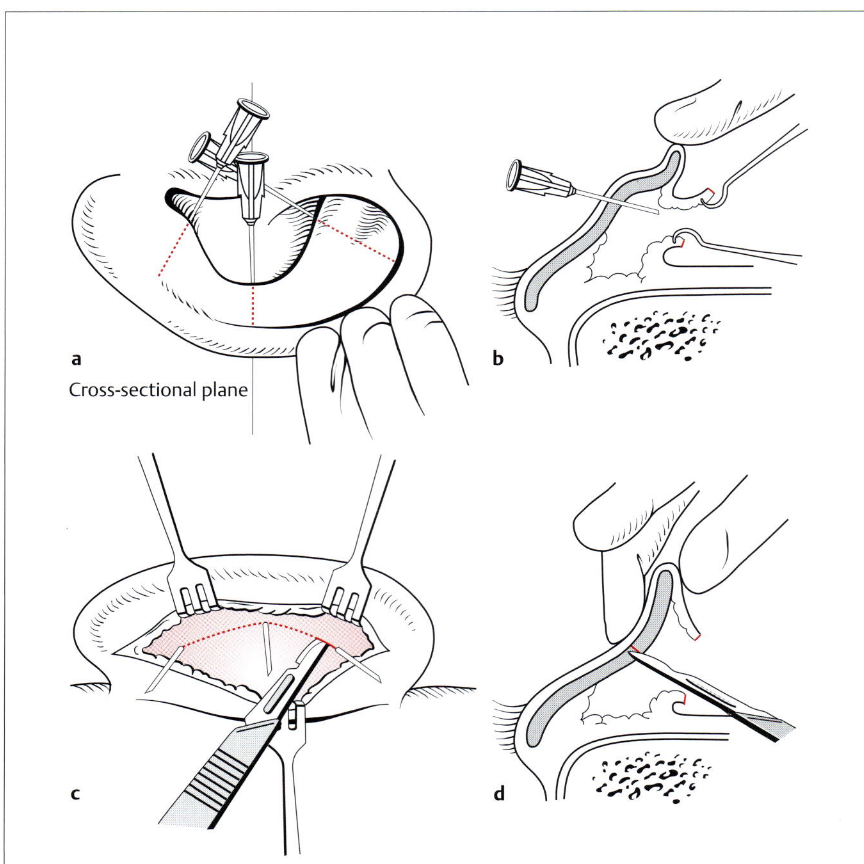

Fig. 15.10a–d Reduction of the concha: planning, cartilage exposure, and incision.
a Needles mark the line of the retroauricular cartilage incision. One each is passed through the cartilage at the center of the concha, below the antitragus, and below the anterior crus.
b Corresponding cross-section at the level of the ear canal. The needle is placed in the shadow of the antihelix that will be formed.
c The cartilage is marked by superficial retroauricular incision of the perichondrium along an imaginary line connecting the three needles.
d Corresponding cross-section. The cartilage is divided with a No.15 scalpel blade while the finger of the free hand protects the anterior skin.

15

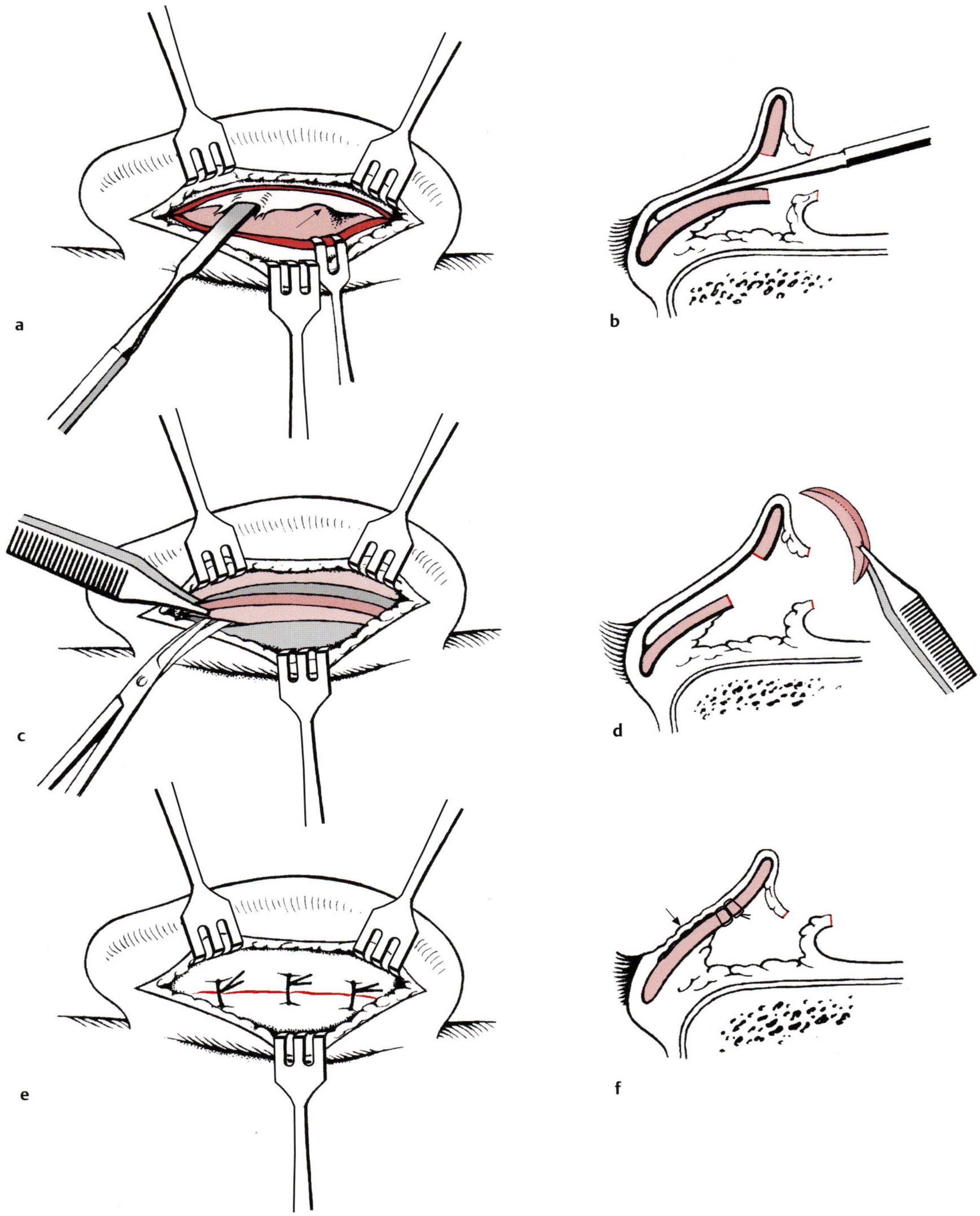

Fig. 15.11a–f Dissection of the anterior conchal surface, cartilage resection, and cartilage sutures.
a The anterior auricular skin is mobilized in the subperichondrial plane to the meatal opening while exposing the helical crus (arrow).
b Corresponding cross-section.
c A crescent-shaped strip of cartilage is resected with scissors. The width of the cartilage strip should be greatest at the level of maximum conchal prominence.
d Corresponding cross-section.
e The cartilage edges are approximated with absorbable figure-of-eight sutures.
f Corresponding cross-section. The relative skin excess forms small, temporary folds along the anterior surface (arrow).

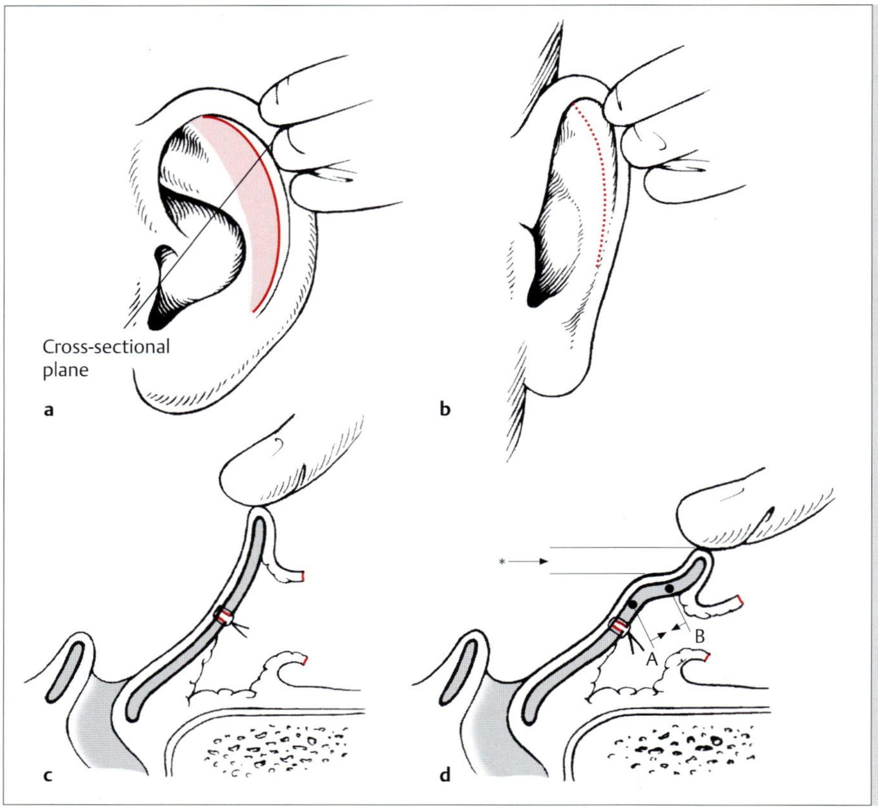

Fig. 15.12a–d Creation of an antihelical fold.

a Creation of antihelical fold by manual setback of the helix in the lateral view. The straight line marks the location of the cross-sectional planes in **c** and **d**.

b Anterior view.

c, d Auricular cross-section before and after setback of the helix. The goal of corrective surgery is to set back the helix so that it just visible outside the antihelix (*). This is accomplished by approximating the two cartilage points A and B.

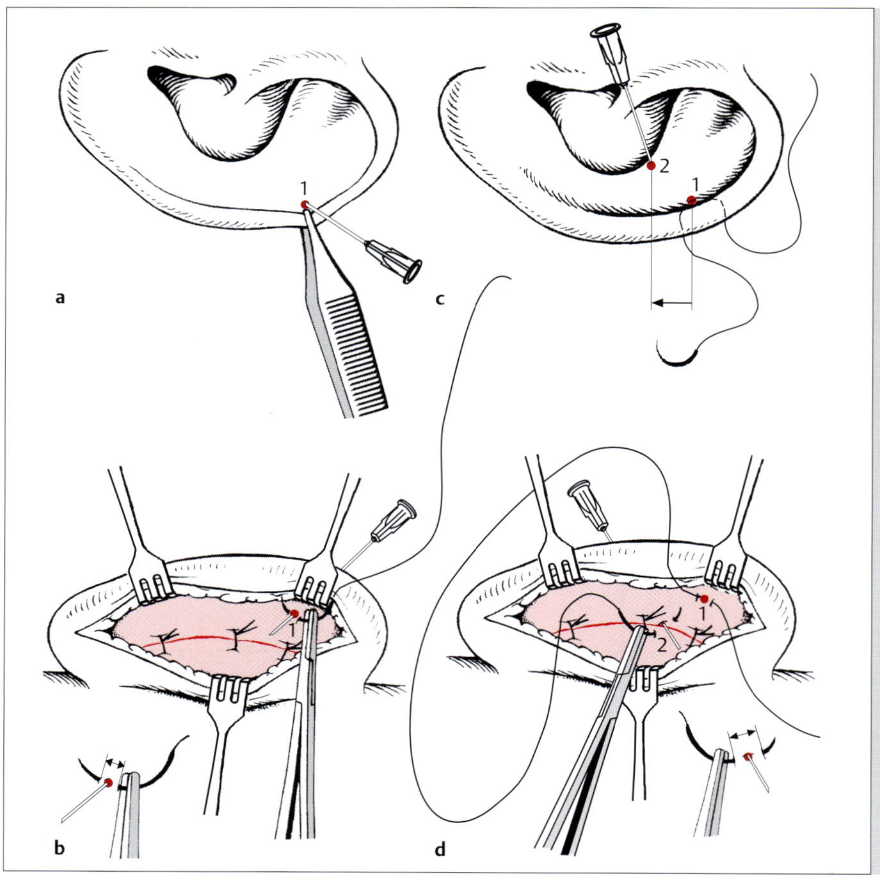

Fig. 15.13a–d Defining a pair of points on the anterior auricular surface. The shaping sutures are placed on the posterior surface.

a Point 1 on the anterior surface of the scapha is located by forceps pressure and marked with a needle.

b A suture is passed through point 1, piercing the cartilage at a single point (see arrows at lower left).

c Opposing point 2 is located in the shadow of the antihelix. It is then shifted slightly toward the earlobe (see arrow).

d A wide suture bite is taken through the cartilage, generally in the area of the previous conchal incision (see arrows at lower right).

The cut edges are re-approximated with cartilage sutures (**Fig. 15.11e, f**) using an absorbable braided material such as 4–0 Vicryl. The cartilage edges should be precisely approximated to avoid any superior or inferior shifting or overriding of the edges. Figure-of-eight sutures are best for achieving an accurate coaptation. At least three sutures should be used that take wide bites through the cartilage.

Creation of an antihelical fold (**Figs. 15.12, 15.13, 15.14, 15.15**). The desired antihelix roll can be raised by manual setback of the helix (**Fig. 15.12a, b**). Viewed in cross-section , it is clear that this roll is created by the approximation of two corresponding cartilage points (**Fig. 15.12c, d**). The location of these points is most accurately determined on the anterior auricular surface and marked with needles. The first cartilage point is defined in the scapha in the upper third of the auricle by applying pressure with forceps tips, and a needle is passed through the anterior and posterior surface at that point (**Fig. 15.13a**). A nonabsorbable monofilament suture (e.g., 4–0 Ethibond) is then passed through the full cartilage thickness *at that single point* from the posterior side (**Fig. 15.13b**).

Rules, Tips, and Tricks

The anterior auricular surface is checked to make sure that the suture does not catch the anterior skin.

The point corresponding to this initial suture is located in the shadow of the antihelix and is then shifted slightly oblique toward the earlobe (**Fig. 15.13c**). Generally this point corresponds to the site of the previous conchal incision. This point, too, is marked with a needle and monofilament suture, which takes a *wide bite* through the cartilage without piercing the anterior skin. It may encompass the existing incision in the conchal cartilage (**Fig. 15.13d**). The offset of these two suture points will produce the desired slight curvature of the longitudinal antihelix axis. The surgeon now ties the suture ends with double slip-proof knots while evaluating the antihelix roll (**Fig. 15.14a, b**). When viewed from the front, the helix should be just outside the antihelix, or at least at the same level (**Fig. 15.14d**). Marked posterior deviation of the helix is unnatural and should be avoided. This central suture is supplemented by at least two additional sutures placed superior and inferior to it (**Fig. 15.14c**). It is possible to place all sutures before tightening, but immediate tightening after placing each suture allows the new shape to develop so that the position of the following suture can be adjusted accordingly.

Rules, Tips, and Tricks

The antihelix-shaping suture passes through a single point in the scapha but should widely engage the conchal cartilage.

If a perpendicular fold appears in the scaphal cartilage when the suture is tied, this means that the suture at that location engaged a wider area, not just a single point, or that adjacent sutures have caused “bunching” of the intervening cartilage (see **Fig. 15.12**). The sutures should be replaced (see **Fig. 15.22**). When the sutures are tied, the retroauricular skin should be

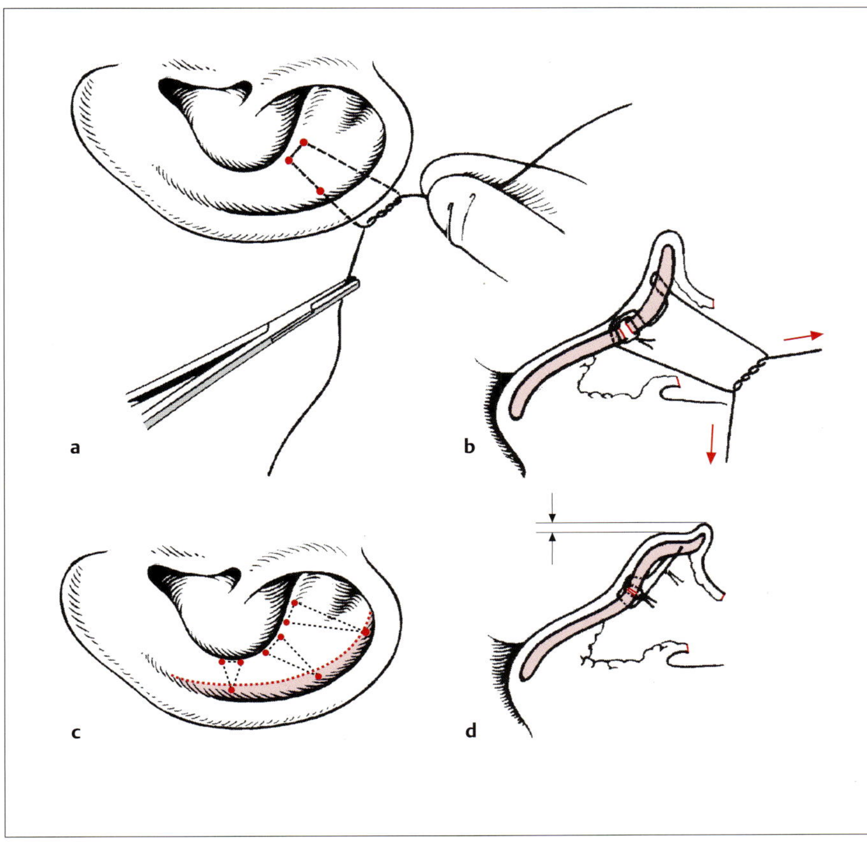

Fig. 15.14a–d Creation of an antihelical fold.

a Placement of a double knot. The surgeon evaluates the antihelix roll that forms in the anterior auricular surface when the knots are tightened.
b Corresponding cross-section.
c The central retention suture is supplemented by two additional sutures. The cartilage suture in the concha should be shifted toward the earlobe. The suture should pierce the scaphal cartilage at a single point while taking a wider bite in the conchal bowl.
d Corresponding cross-section. Setback of the helix should leave the helical rim slightly outside the antihelix (arrows) or should place both features at the same level.

slightly elevated with a single-pronged hook to keep it clear of the knot.

The lower third of the antihelix merits special attention. At that site the helical cartilage separates from the antihelix and may cause protrusion of the earlobe (see **Fig. 15.16**). An approximating cartilage suture between the helix and antitragus may be sufficient to move the earlobe to the desired position. This suture should not deform the antitragus or rotate it laterally, however. It is better in such cases to use a Y–V plasty for earlobe setback, as described below (see **Fig. 15.17**). Additionally, the shaping sutures should not exert undue tension on the antihelix. This may produce a very sharp-edged antihelix susceptible to skin necrosis, and a transverse cartilage fold may occasionally form (see **Fig. 15.22**). At the same time, accurately placed shaping sutures may compensate for an antihelix that still seems too high in this area by incorporating the vertical part of the concha into the new antihelix. This requires considerable adjustment in the level of the corresponding pair of points: While the scaphal point is defined as usual, the second point is placed more on the floor of the concha. Tying the suture will cause the vertical part of the concha to roll outward until both cartilage points are at approximately the same level. This maneuver is technically difficult, and often requires several attempts. It is easier to reduce the concha by using the resection technique described above.

Modification for stiff cartilage (**Fig. 15.15**). Stiff, heavy auricular cartilage (mainly in adults) has a great deal of "spring" or recoil, and shaping the antihelix with sutures alone may cause the sutures to erode through the cartilage. In these cases the shaping sutures should be supplemented by *weakening and di-*

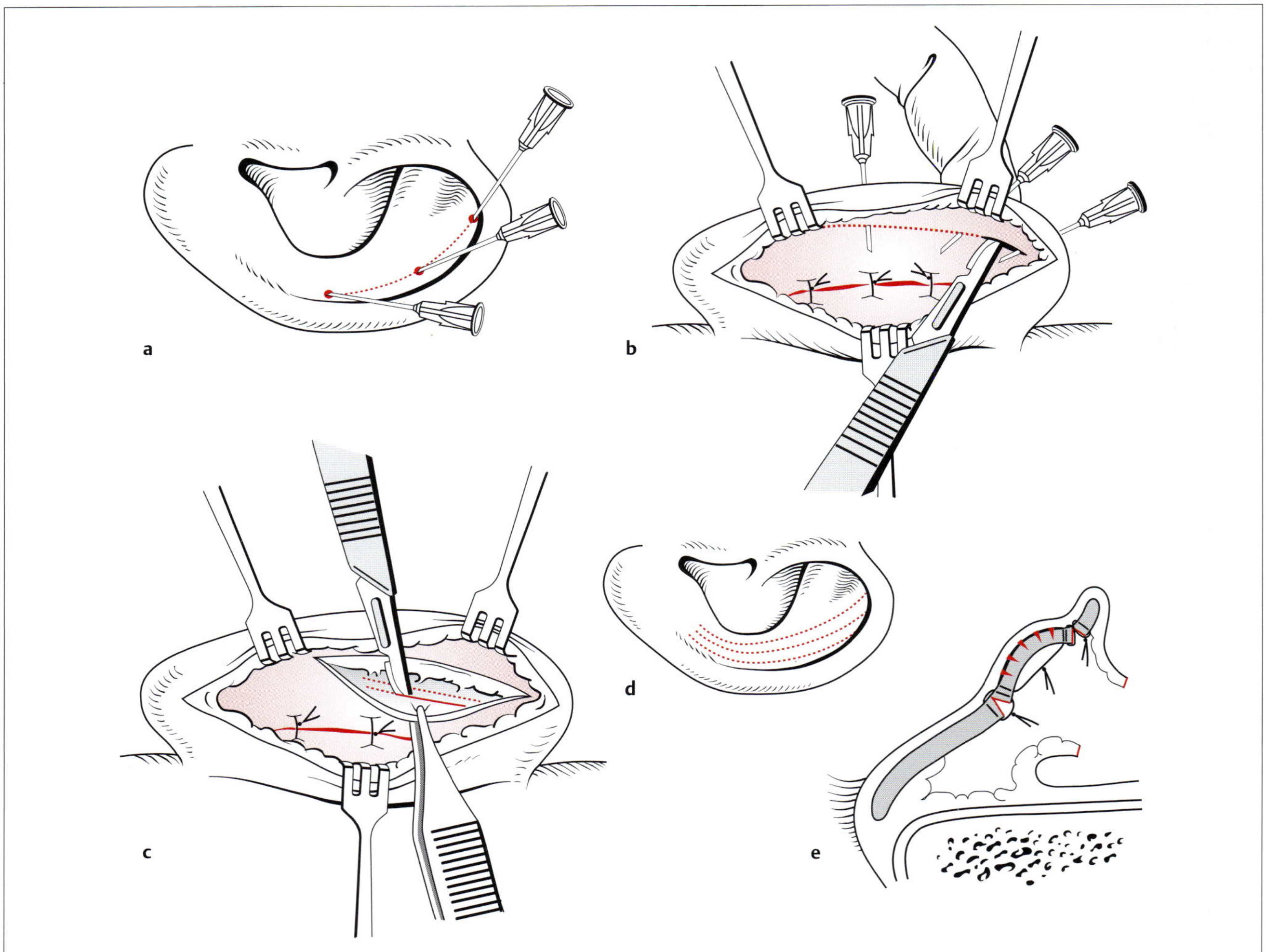

Fig. 15.15a–e Creation of an antihelical fold in stiff, heavy cartilage.
a The planned cartilage incision in the scapha is marked with needles inserted from the anterior side.
b The posterior perichondrium is incised superficially in continuity with the marking needles from the posterior crus of the antihelix to the helical tail.
c The exposed cartilage edge is grasped with Adson–Brown forceps, and the perichondrium is stripped from the anterior surface to the triangular fossa and conchal bowl. Shallow scoring incisions are then made parallel to the antihelical axis with a No. 15 scalpel blade.
d Transparent view of the scoring incisions through the anterior auricular skin.
e Shape of the antihelix after the placement of a retention suture, cross-sectional view. Caution: If the scoring incisions are too deep, sharp cartilage edges will result.

rect modeling of the cartilage. This can be done by scoring the anterior cartilage or thinning the posterior cartilage with a round diamond bur. Cartilage thinning should encompasses the entire surface of the antihelix on the posterior side. The advantage of this technique is that is does not require cartilage incisions. On the other hand, the Stenström technique of cartilage scoring utilizes the biomechanical properties of the cartilage. Making superficial incisions in one side of the cartilage creates a preponderance of cartilage tension on the opposite side, causing the cartilage to warp toward the scored surface (i.e., the scored surface becomes convex).

The anterior surface of the antihelix is exposed through a posterior cartilage incision. The correct position of the incision in the posterior cartilage surface is again defined with marking needles introduced from the anterior side. They are placed through the scapha at three points along the transitional curve between the concave scapha and convex antihelix (**Fig. 15.15a**). The needle sites are interconnected on the posterior surface by scoring the perichondrium with a No. 15 blade to mark the location of the incision (**Fig. 15.15b**). The full-thickness cartilage incision is made in one continuous action, again using the finger of the free hand to apply counter-pressure and protect the anterior auricular skin.

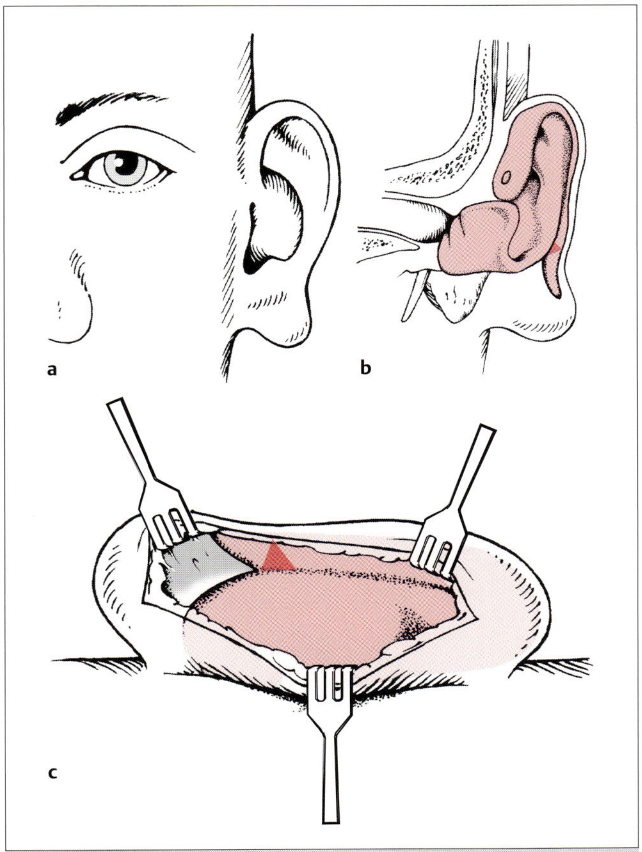

Fig. 15.16a–c Earlobe correction by repositioning the helical tail.
a The earlobe protrudes laterally when viewed from the front.
b Although the earlobe itself does not contain cartilage, the helical tail may cause it to deviate laterally (proposed cartilage resection is marked).
c A medially based cartilage wedge is excised from the helical tail to alter its alignment.

The perichondrium is elevated from a circumscribed area on the anterior surface, the cartilage is firmly grasped with an Adson–Brown forceps, and the perichondrium is stripped from the entire area of the proposed antihelical fold. The anterior cartilage is then scored parallel to the antihelical axis (**Fig. 15.15c, d**).

Rules, Tips, and Tricks

The scoring incisions should be very superficial. If they are too deep, visible cartilage edges will result. Another option is to crosshatch the cartilage surface.
This weakening technique will produce the desired antihelix roll without any additional measures, but definitive, controlled shaping of the antihelix with nonabsorbable retention sutures should still be performed (**Fig. 15.15e**). The cartilage incision for exposing the anterior surface of the antihelix should be closed with absorbable sutures as described above for the conchal incision.

Setback of the earlobe (**Figs. 15.16** and **15.17**). At this stage of the operation the surgeon should always check to see whether the earlobe is still prominent after the auricular setback and requires correction. A prominent earlobe is especially conspicuous following correction of the auricle (**Fig. 15.16a**). This protrusion may be caused by a fleshy, bulky earlobe or by lateral rotation of the helical tail (**Fig. 15.16b**). This is assessed by placing gentle manual pressure on the base of the earlobe. If marked

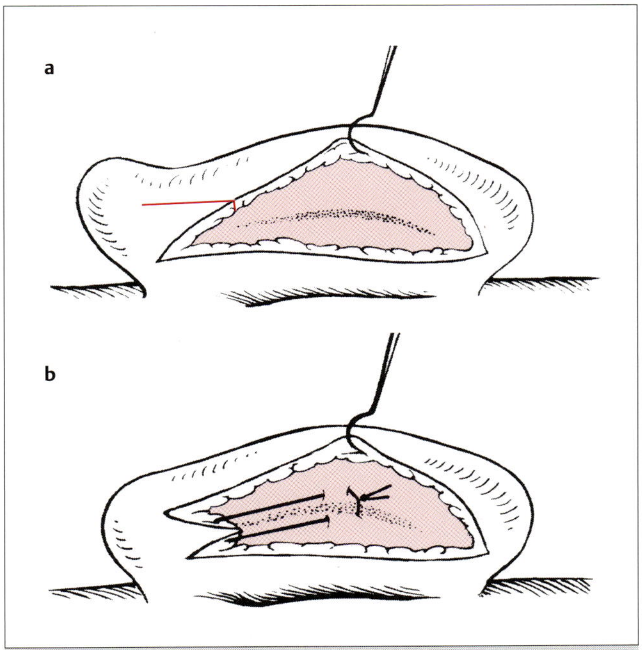

Fig. 15.17a, b Earlobe correction by a Y–V plasty.
a A soft-tissue protrusion of the earlobe can be corrected by skin advancement. This is done by placing an auxiliary incision at an angle to the existing retroauricular incision, transforming the linear incision into a Y-shaped incision. The earlobe is undermined, and a mattress suture is placed between the triangular skin flap and posterior cartilage surface.
b Tightening the knot shifts the triangle superiorly, allowing for controlled medial displacement of the earlobe.

15

cartilage recoil is present, the helical tail can be transversely divided. First the cartilage-free area between the antitragus and helical tail is dissected free from the posterior side and the tail is exposed. Completely dividing the tail at the end of this cartilage-free segment, combined if necessary with a small cartilage wedge excision, may be sufficient to bring the tail of the helix into line with the longitudinal helical axis (**Fig. 15.16c**). As with an isolated soft-tissue protrusion of the auricle, a Y–V plasty can then be added to achieve a *controlled* setback.

In contrast to a V–Y plasty, which employs a V-shaped skin incision, skin advancement, and a Y-shaped suture line to lengthen the skin, a *Y–V plasty* produces the opposite effect of *tissue shortening* (**Fig. 15.17**). In this technique the skin on the back of the earlobe is incised by an auxiliary incision placed at an acute angle to the existing retroauricular incision, and an inferiorly based triangular skin flap is raised. If the apex of this triangle is now grasped with a forceps and pulled slightly in the cephalad direction, it will produce a visible setback of the earlobe when viewed from the anterior side. A 4–0 subcutaneous mattress suture is now passed through the apex of the skin flap and then through the perichondrium on the posterior surface of the conchal cartilage (**Fig. 15.17b**). The correct tension vector is determined by pulling upward on the suture ends in various directions before passing the suture through the perichondrium. When the suture has been tied, the surgeon can view the ear from the front while slowly tightening the knot to determine the optimum degree of earlobe correction.

Setback of the auricle (**Fig. 15.18**). Following reduction of the concha, the creation of an antihelical fold, and correction of the earlobe, the auricle should be set back to achieve a normal concha–mastoid angle of ca. 30°. Forceps are again placed on the anterior auricular surface to determine which point in the concha is best for moving the auricle closer to the mastoid plane. This cartilage point is usually located just superior to the center of the concha, and the best setback effect is obtained by exerting slight posterosuperior traction. That point is marked with a needle, and a nonabsorbable monofilament suture (e.g., 4–0 Ethibond) is passed through the cartilage and perichondrium from the retroauricular side (**Fig. 15.18a, b**). Again, traction on the suture ends will determine the direction of pull that produces the optimum desired effect. The mastoid periosteum is now pierced in that direction to create a U-shaped suture path

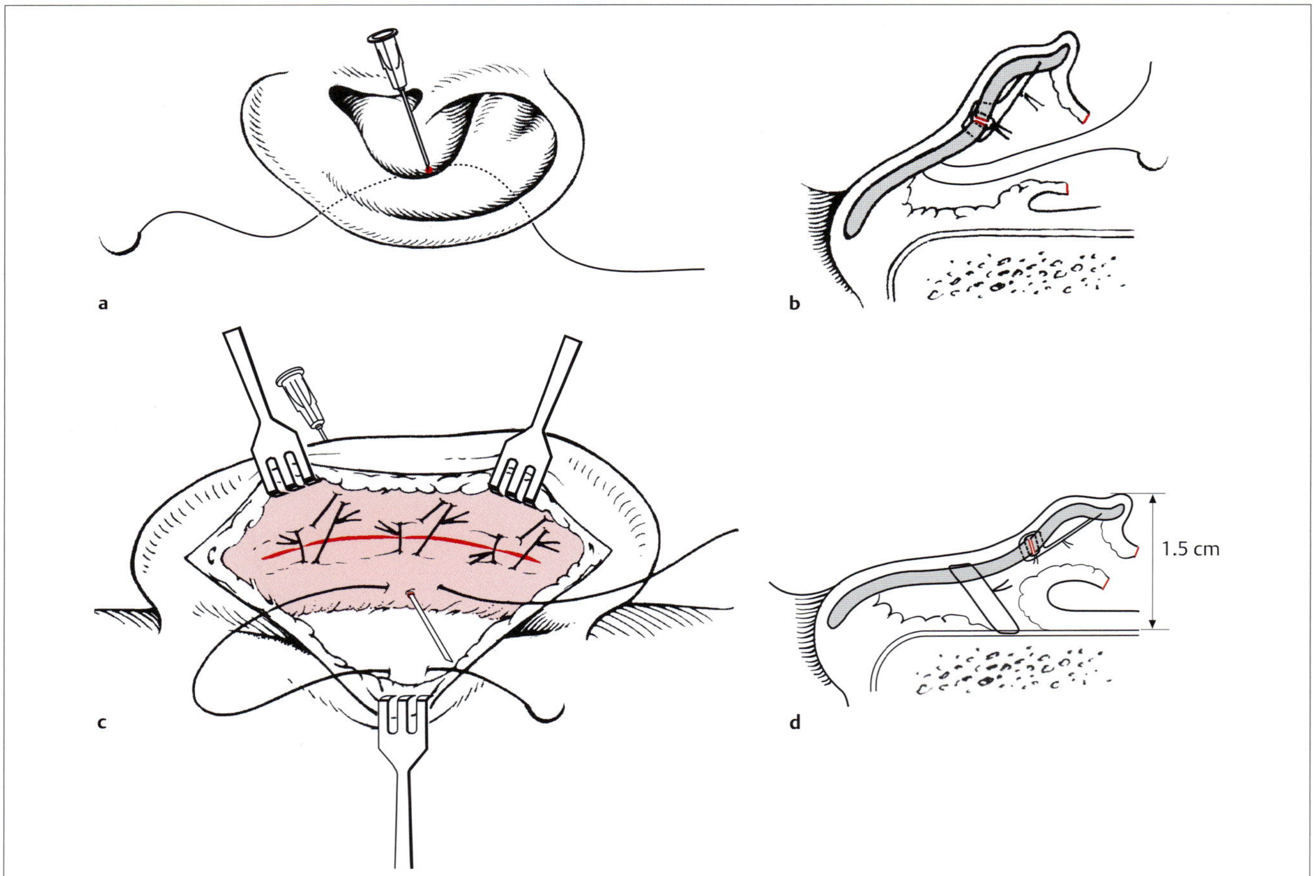

Fig. 15.18a–d Auricular setback with a concha–mastoid suture.
a The appropriate cartilage point in the concha is marked with a needle, and a suture is placed from the posterior side.
b Corresponding cross-section. The suture takes a wide cartilage bite.
c The suture is passed through the periosteum over the mastoid in a mattress configuration.
d Corresponding cross-section. The suture should shorten the helix-mastoid distance to ca. 1.5 cm while reducing the concha–mastoid angle to 30°. The concha–mastoid suture should be shifted posteriorly to ensure that the displaced conchal cartilage does not narrow the meatal opening.

15

(**Fig. 15.18c**). This anchoring suture should be placed as far posteriorly as possible during retraction of the mastoid skin. This is necessary to ensure that the force vectors will produce the desired setback effect on the auricle.

Rules, Tips, and Tricks

If the mastoid suture is placed too close to the ear canal, it will tend to pull the conchal cartilage toward the canal opening and may cause meatal stenosis.

Thus, fixation of the conchal cartilage to the mastoid periosteum not only produces a general setback of the auricle but also straightens the conchal cartilage and maintains patency of the ear canal. A potentially adverse effect of this suture is to shift the postauricular sulcus posteriorly, placing it at the approximate level of the periosteal suture (**Fig. 15.18d**). The symmetrical correction of both auricles is facilitated by checking the setback with a ruler placed against the mastoid (1.5 cm from midhelix to the mastoid scalp).

Skin resection and closure (**Fig. 15.19**). The setback of the auricle, combined with the posterior shift of the postauricular sulcus, leads to an excess of postauricular skin (**Fig. 15.19a**). Redundant skin is carefully resected with scissors, bearing in mind that the tightened postauricular skin cannot permanently protect the auricular setback against any cartilage recoil force that may still be present. The greater the preoperative concha–mastoid angle, the greater the skin excess following the correction. When the skin has been resected, the subcutaneous wound edges are first re-approximated with several absorbable sutures. The skin surface should also be closed with absorbable sutures (**Fig. 15.19c**). This is advantageous in both children and adults because of the difficulty of accessing the suture line.

Dressing and aftercare (**Fig. 15.20**). It is important to prevent the accumulation of subperichondrial blood (hematoma), especially when the anterior auricular skin has been mobilized. This is aided by packing the auricular contours with gauze strips that are precisely molded to the newly formed concavities. This can be done for instance with pledgets that have been impregnated with ointment (e.g., petroleum jelly containing an antibiotic) so that they can be more easily molded into the lateral contours of the ear. Particular care is taken to pack the scapha and concha (**Fig. 15.20a**). Next, a sterile compress is folded into

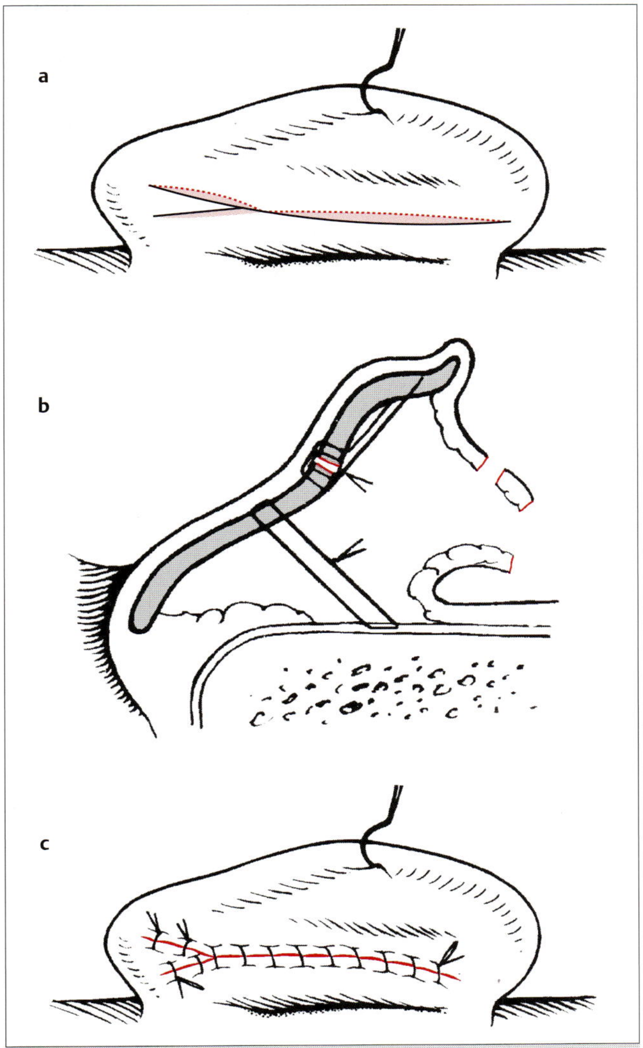

Fig. 15.19a–c Retroauricular wound closure.
- **a** The setback of the auricle and earlobe creates redundant postauricular skin that should be resected before skin closure.
- **b** Cross section: The concha–mastoid suture causes a posterior shift of the postauricular sulcus.
- **c** The skin is closed with a running suture, the auxiliary earlobe incision with interrupted sutures.

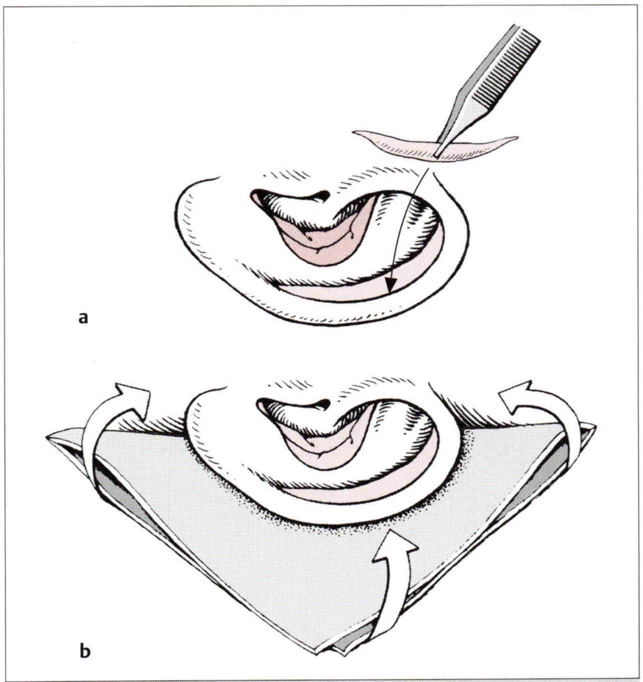

Fig. 15.20a, b Dressing after otoplasty.
- **a** Ointment-impregnated gauze strips are molded into the scapha, concha, and if necessary the triangular fossa.
- **b** A compress is folded into a triangle and placed over the postauricular skin. The ends are folded over the auricle (arrows).

a triangle and its longest side, also impregnated with ointment, is placed behind the ear (**Fig. 15.20b**). The purpose of this compress is to exert a gentle anterior pressure on the mobilized retroauricular and mastoid skin to create a postauricular sulcus. The corners of the triangle dressing are then folded over the auricle and covered with an additional sterile pad. Finally the head is wrapped with a circumferential elastic bandage, taking care that the bandage is *not wrapped too tightly*.

Generally this dressing remains in place for 5 days. When it is removed, the auricle is checked for hematoma, pressure points, infection, or retroauricular dehiscence. After the gauze strips have been removed, the auricle may remain uncovered for a time. The hair may be shampooed after 8 days, by which time the retroauricular sutures will have dissolved and the skin incision should be impervious to bacterial contamination. The patient is advised to wear a circumferential head dressing or elastic headband to keep the ears from accidentally bending forward during sleep, and should avoid participation in sports for a total of 6 weeks. Follow-up visits are generally scheduled for 2 weeks after the operation and ca. 3–6 months later for a final examination that includes photographic documentation.

Rules, Tips, and Tricks: Correction of Postoperative Problems

Residual deformities after otoplasty may be noted at typical sites. Ideally they should be recognized and corrected intraoperatively. Prompt surgical intervention within 1–2 weeks also has a high success rate, as the cartilage deformity has not yet become fixed due to scarring. Shaping sutures can still be removed, replaced, or added during this period.

If the central third of the auricle has been well corrected (or even overcorrected) but the earlobe or upper third of the helix still shows relative prominence, a *"telephone deformity"* is present. In this case a shaping suture should be added to set back the upper helix (**Fig. 15.21**). Like all retention sutures, it should consist of nonabsorbable monofilament material that is placed in mattress fashion beneath the anterior crus of the antihelix at the optimum correction point previously marked in the anterior scapha. This suture is tightened only until the helix appears normally positioned when viewed from the front.

Other helical rim deformities near the posterior crus may occur in cases where the last shaping suture was placed too close to the helical rim, causing the crest of the antihelix to become continuous with the helix. This is prevented by placing the last suture far enough from the helix to flatten the termination of the antihelix roll. Otherwise the antihelix can be "uncoupled" from the helix by making a short incision in the scaphal cartilage perpendicular to the long axis of the antihelix (**Fig. 15.21b**). This keeps the convexity of the posterior crus from being transmitted to the helical rim. The following rule should be noted, however:

> **Rules, Tips, and Tricks**
> Always avoid excessive setback of the helix "behind the antihelix."

Two other residual deformities involve the antihelix and scapha. Tightening the antihelix shaping sutures may raise a *transverse fold* in the scaphal cartilage (**Fig. 15.22**). This may result from the fact that the suture bite in the scaphal cartilage was too wide during creation of the antihelix. The needle should pierce the anterior cartilage and perichondrium *at a single point*. If this transverse cartilage fold is present and does not disappear when light pressure is placed on the anterior surface, the cartilage suture should be removed and replaced.

It is desirable to have a slight curve in the longitudinal axis of the antihelix. Despite the use of an offset mattress suture to

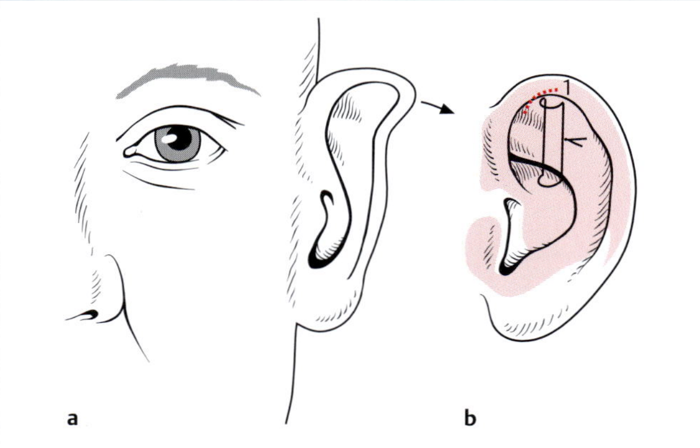

Fig. 15.21a, b Residual deformity after otoplasty.
a "Telephone ear." The posterior crus of the antihelix has not been adequately formed, causing protrusion of the upper helix.
b This problem is corrected by placing an additional posterior cartilage suture that extends from the upper pole of the helix to the anterior crus of the antihelix. A transverse cartilage incision may have to be added to separate the helix and posterior crus (1).

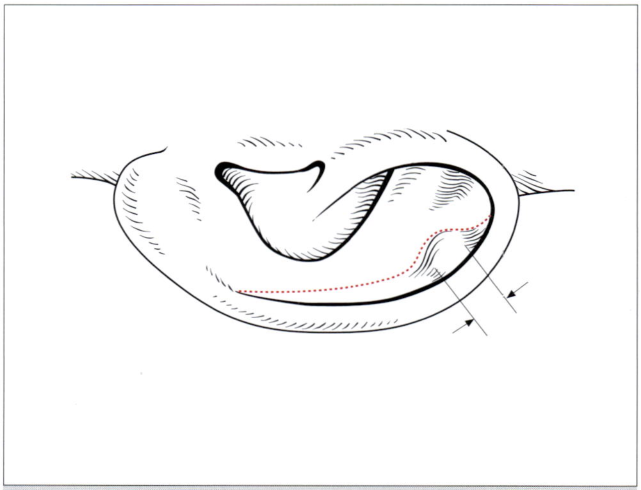

Fig. 15.22 Cartilage fold in the scapha.
The suture bite in the scaphal cartilage was too wide (arrows) during creation of the antihelix, causing a ridge to form when the suture was tied. This problem is corrected by removing and placing the antihelix retention sutures.

15

produce this curve (**Fig. 15.14c**), the antihelix often includes a relatively straight segment that looks unnatural (**Fig. 15.23a**).

Rules, Tips, and Tricks

An accurately placed concha–mastoid suture can produce auricular setback as well as a curved antihelical axis.

Again, the apex of the desired curve is located by probing the anterior surface with a forceps (**Fig. 15.23b**). The point should lie within the shadow of the antihelix. Pressure from the forceps can easily determine whether the desired antihelical curve will be obtained. This cartilage point is then engaged from the posterior side with a nonabsorbable suture. Traction on the suture ends defines the most favorable direction of pull. The needle is passed in that direction through the mastoid periosteum and tied (**Fig. 15.23c**).

Besides deformities noted in the immediate postoperative period, there are other deformities that may develop during the subsequent healing period and are thus classified as *late complications* in the broadest sense of the term (**Table 15.1**).

Contour irregularities usually occur in the form of sharp edges over the antihelix. They result from too-deep scoring of the cartilage surface, which was initially masked by postoperative edema. Revision is difficult and should be done no earlier than 6–12 months after the operation. Tangential removal of the cartilage edges is generally insufficient, and it is best to cover the entire antihelix with an autologous temporal fascial graft. The graft can be placed through an incision in the scaphoid fossa.

A continuum exists from minor *asymmetries* that do not require treatment to a unilateral *recurrence* of auricular prominence. The upper third of the auricle is most commonly affected in cases where a permanent antihelical fold was not produced. If the shaping suture was placed against a high resistance, the constant traction may cause the cartilage suture to migrate, causing a recurrence of helical protrusion. Again, revision should not be attempted before 6–12 months postoperatively. It is essential to weaken the cartilage by adequate anterior scoring before a new shaping suture is placed. With *recurrence or persistence of a prominent earlobe*, the helical tail should be divided and a triangular skin flap developed on the posterior surface of the earlobe, carrying the dissection close to the lobular border.

Table 15.1 Complications of otoplasty (after Weerda 1994)

Early complications	Late complications
Pain	Deformity
Bleeding	Asymmetry
Hematoma	Recurrence
Pressure ulcer	Keloid
Perichondritis	Defect
Meatal stenosis	
Suture fistula	
Residual deformity	

The postauricular skin is also susceptible to skin bulges, hypertrophic scars, and even keloids. *Skin bulges* result from a surplus of redundant skin that is too great to resolve spontaneously. Secondary resection of the redundant skin can usually be accomplished without difficulty.

Hypertrophic scars are rare and usually do not require surgical treatment because their proximity to the postauricular sulcus does not cause cosmetic deformity and because they may regress over a period of years.

Keloids, on the other hand, differ from hypertrophic scars by forming a tumorlike growth that expands beyond the original wound area to involve normal skin. Besides individual disposition (more common in dark-skinned individuals), it has been suggested that keloids may result from wound tension following an excessive skin resection.

Rules, Tips, and Tricks

An excessive retroauricular skin resection to shape the auricular contour leads to skin tension that increases the risk of keloid formation.

15

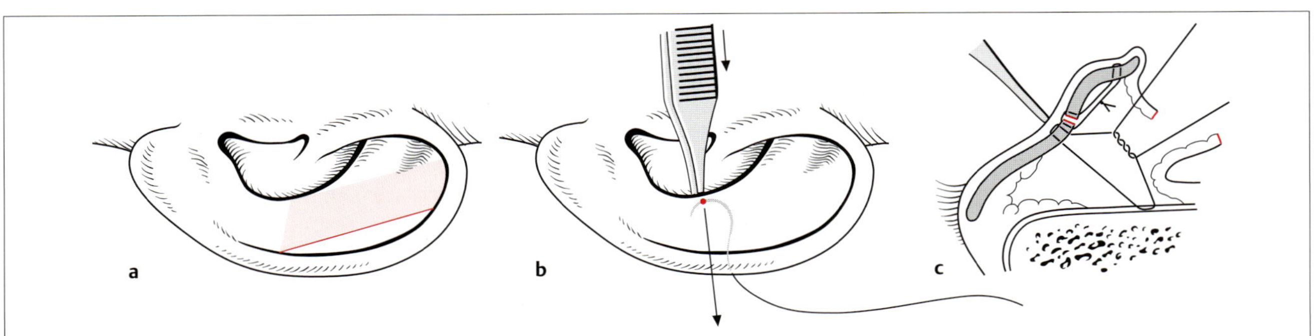

Fig. 15.23a–c Straight segment in the antihelical fold.
a If the antihelix shaping sutures were not properly spaced, the normally curved longitudinal axis of the antihelix may include a relatively straight segment.
b The antihelix can be curved by proper placement of the concha–mastoid suture. Forceps pressure defines the point in the concha that is best for imparting a curve (arrow).
c Corresponding cross-section. The suture has two effects: it sets back the auricle and produces curvature of the antihelical fold.

The treatment of this nodular hyperplasia is problematic and should be withheld in mild, cosmetically acceptable cases because of the high incidence of recurrence. On the other hand, retroauricular keloids may expand from their original site and become visible. One option that may be tried is to resect the affected skin and resurface the area with a full-thickness skin graft from the groin. Another option is the intradermal injection of a corticosteroid crystal suspension. A pressure dressing is worn for several months after treatment.

Auricular defects caused by resection or perichondritis range from mild to catastrophic. They can be treated with reconstructive techniques developed for microtia, but it is likely that significant residual deformities will remain. Prevention is crucial, therefore, and the surgeon should understand the risks of irreversible auricular deformity, especially in association with cartilage resections.

Risks and Complications (Table 15.1)

The complications of otoplasty, which include residual deformities in the broadest sense, can be divided into early and late complications. Early complications occur during the first 4 weeks postoperatively. Late complications may occur for up to one year after surgery.

Minor postoperative *wound pain*, especially after local anesthesia has subsided, is generally of no concern and can be treated with analgesics. Aspirin products should be avoided because they inhibit platelet aggregation; it is better to use nonsteroidal anti-inflammatory agents such as phenylbutazone or ibuprofen. More severe pain is usually caused by a bandage that has been wrapped too tightly. This may also cause a *pressure ulcer* in the skin on the anterior auricular surface. Pain is relieved by loosening the bandage. Prevention consists of applying the initial dressing without undue pressure.

Postoperative bleeding on the day of the surgery may be adequately controlled with a pressure dressing, but this pressure should not be maintained for more than 2 hours. Most cases will require revision of the retroauricular wound, especially with bleeding from branches of the posterior auricular artery in the lower part of the wound. The risk of postoperative bleeding is particularly high following the use of a local anesthetic with epinephrine. The vasoconstriction suppresses intraoperative bleeding, which is then manifested after the effect of the medication has worn off. Prevention consists of meticulous hemostasis with bipolar coagulation forceps, especially in the area of the postauricular sulcus.

Subperichondrial hematoma develops only at sites where the skin has been separated from the cartilage surface. Subperichondrial hematomas on the anterior auricular surface have the greatest clinical importance. They are most commonly located in the conchal area. Generally it is sufficient to remove the blood by percutaneous aspiration and apply a pressure dressing for 5 days. Antibiotic therapy is also recommended. If the hematoma persists for more than 5 days, there is a danger of cartilage necrosis with disruption of auricular contours. In this case the conchal skin on the anterior auricular surface should be incised and the hematoma aspirated with a needle. Any cartilage that has already become necrotic should be removed. To prevent recurrence, a gauze bolster is placed over the wound and fixed to the posterior auricular surface with all-layer mattress sutures. It remains in place for 3–4 days (see **Fig. 15.30**).

Severe inflammation of the auricle, especially of the perichondrium, is rare following otoplasty. Often the cause is simply an infected retroauricular hematoma, which is opened and irrigated. Care is taken to maintain adequate drainage after the placement of a Penrose drain. Inadequate treatment of the inflammation may lead to a "smoldering" perichondritis manifested by patchy skin redness and often accompanied by blistering and tenderness to pressure. Early cases may respond well to parenteral antibiotics (cephalosporins) and local alcohol compresses. If cartilage necrosis has already occurred, operative treatment is required (see **Figs. 15.30** and **15.31**).

Meatal stenosis (narrowing of the ear canal) may be caused by an inadequate concha–mastoid suture for auricular setback. If the periosteal suture is placed too far anteriorly, the conchal cartilage will be shifted toward the meatal opening and will narrow it from behind. It is advisable, then, to check the width of the meatal opening intraoperatively after auricular setback and adjust the suture placement if necessary. If the stenosis goes unnoticed until later, the meatal opening can be enlarged by a circumscribed cartilage excision from its posterior wall, performed through a small skin incision in the anterior surface of the concha.

Suture fistulas are manifested by nonhealing, punctate granulations and occur almost exclusively on the posterior auricular surface. A suture end is often visible within the granulation tissue. In these cases the nonabsorbable suture must be removed. Suture fistulas can be prevented by cutting the suture ends very short after tying and not placing the cutaneous suture directly over a retention suture. The suture material also plays a role, and plastic monofilament has proven particularly successful despite its rigidity. Another (more costly) option is to use a Gore-Tex suture. If at least 6 weeks have passed since the surgery, removal of the suture will rarely cause significant deformity, especially if cartilage scoring or abrasion has also been performed. Retention sutures are no longer needed if scar tissue has already formed between the approximated cartilage edges on the posterior auricular surface.

Alternatives

The procedures described above are subject to numerous modifications. Before any modifications are used, it should be determined whether the result is controllable (without having to rely on predicted scar traction), permanent (even after absorbable sutures have dissolved), and natural (with no sharp cartilage edges). If these criteria are met, there should be no objection to using simpler, less invasive techniques. For example, cartilage retention sutures can be placed through a skin incision without broad retroauricular exposure if they enter and exit the skin at a single point. This would be an option only in patients with pure antihelical deformities and soft cartilage, however, and this is not a common situation.

Surgery of the Earlobe

Reduction of the Earlobe (Fig. 15.24)

A "fleshy earlobe" may be markedly out of proportion to the auricle and may be particularly conspicuous when viewed from the front below a nonprotruding auricle. Volume reduction can be achieved by resecting a full-thickness (skin–fat–skin) wedge of tissue. Placing the resection in the free border of the earlobe would create a surface discontinuity with a conspicuous scar. A wedge resection at the base of the earlobe yields a better aesthetic result (**Fig. 15.24a**) and will place the scar in a skin fold below the tragus (**Fig. 15.24b**).

Correction of an "Attached Earlobe" (Fig. 15.25)

In most cases an "attached earlobe" is broadly adherent to the buccal skin and is often hypoplastic as well (**Fig. 15.25a**). It is then necessary to augment the anterior part of the earlobe with a mobilized flap of buccal skin. For this purpose a curved incision is made through the buccal skin below the base of the earlobe (**Fig. 15.25b**), creating a skin flap that is advanced anteriorly to epithelialize the anterior surface of the new earlobe (**Fig. 15.25c, d**). This gives the border of the earlobe a rounded shape while leaving a skin defect below the lobule (**Fig. 15.25e**). Direct re-approximation of the defect usually leaves a conspicuous scar but is possible in principle. A better solution is to lengthen the pre- and retroauricular wound margins. Following skin mobilization and the excision of the Burrow triangles (**Fig. 15.25e**), the skin can be advanced superiorly to make the infra-auricular defect invisible (**Fig. 15.25f, g**).

A sufficient amount of subcutaneous fat should be included in the infra-auricular skin flap to produce adequate fullness of the earlobe.

Reconstruction of the Earlobe (Fig. 15.26)

If the earlobe is absent due to a congenital malformation, trauma, or tumor excision, the anterior and posterior surface can be reconstructed from infra-auricular skin (as described by Gavello). The auricular base of the earlobe is freshened, and a transposition flap is outlined that has two small lobes at its inferior end (**Fig. 15.26a**). These lobes will form the free border of the reconstructed earlobe. The posterior lobe of the flap (the posterior surface of the earlobe) should be slightly smaller than the anterior lobe so that the suture line will be slightly behind the visible earlobe margin. Generally the axis of the transposition flap is directed obliquely and posteroinferiorly so that the distal end of the flap is outside the hairline. The mobilized skin flap (which includes subcutaneous fat for "fullness") is folded over on a vertical axis and sutured to the auricle. When the free border of the earlobe is sutured, small dog ears can be resected to eliminate redundant skin. The resulting donor defect can be closed primarily after skin mobilization or may be closed using the technique shown in **Fig. 15.25e, f**.

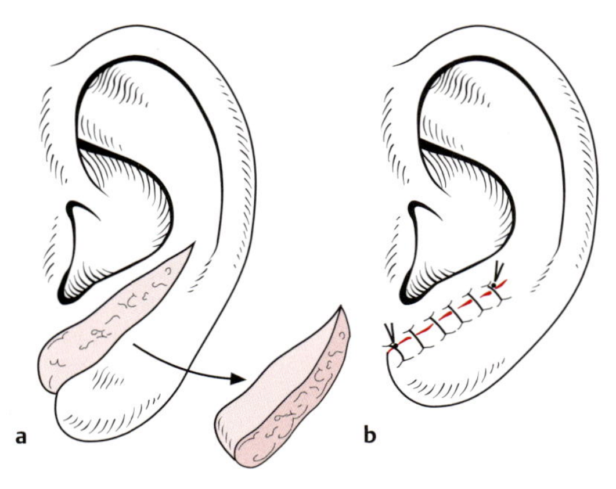

Fig. 15.24a, b Reduction of the earlobe.
a A full-thickness, anteriorly based soft-tissue wedge is resected.
b The resulting scar lies below the antitragus, avoiding suture placement in the free edge of the earlobe.

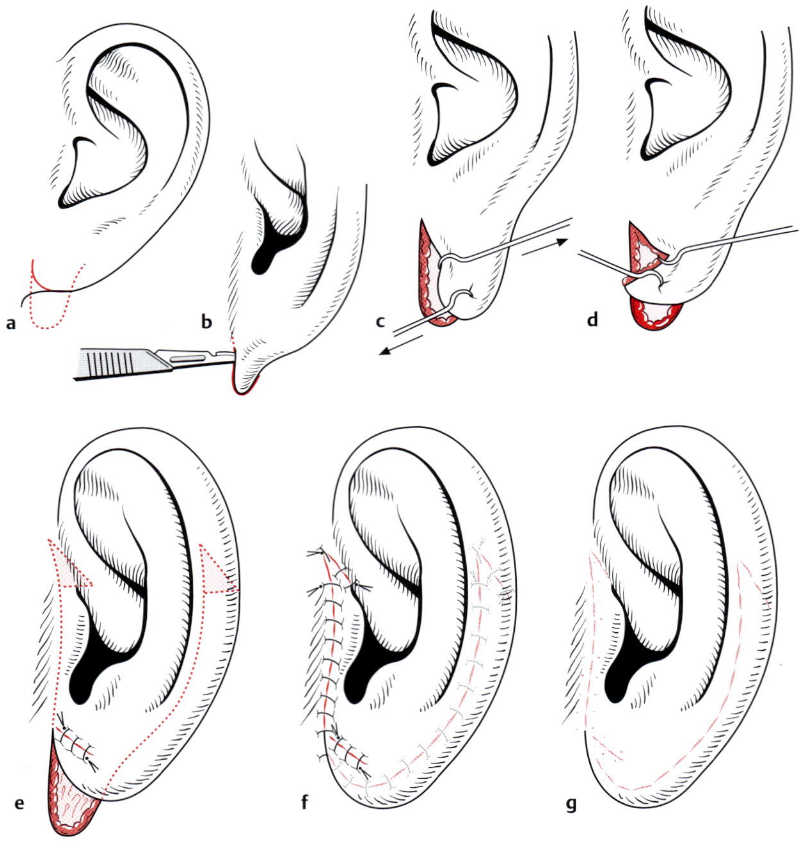

Fig. 15.25a–g Correction of an "attached earlobe."

- **a** In most cases the earlobe is also hypoplastic. The desired correction and planned incision are indicated.
- **b** U-shaped incision of the buccal skin and base of the earlobe.
- **c, d** The U-shaped flap of buccal skin is advanced to cover the wound surface at the anterior border of the earlobe.
- **e** Posterior oblique view. The flap has been sutured to the lobule. The donor defect can be closed primarily after skin mobilization. Another option is skin advancement (auxiliary incision with necessary skin resections is shown).
- **f** Appearance after superior advancement of the pre-, sub-, and retroauricular skin.
- **g** The resulting scars are placed in RSTLs.

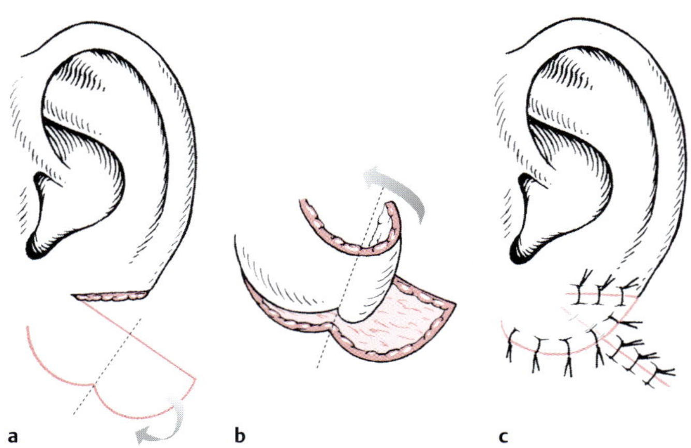

Fig. 15.26a–c Reconstruction of the earlobe.

- **a** The location and shape of the anteriorly based transposition flap are shown. The longitudinal axis is slightly oblique to keep the distal end of the flap outside the hairline. The posterior part of the flap may be slightly smaller than the anterior part. The proposed fold-over axis and direction are shown. The proposed area of attachment to the auricle has been freshened.
- **b** The flap is elevated and folded over.
- **c** Appearance after flap transfer and suture fixation. The primary wound area can be closed primarily (as shown) or closed by skin advancement (**Fig. 15.25e–g**).

Auricular Malformations

Classification

Congenital malformations of the auricle may be extremely diverse. This particularly applies to minor changes that fall under the heading of grade 1 dysplasia. The classification in **Table 15.2** distinguishes three grades of severity based on basic structural changes and surgical implications (after Marx 1926, Tanzer 1977, Weerda 1988). Characteristic forms are often designated by special names.

Prominent ears are also classified as a malformation. They were discussed earlier in this chapter. The correction of grade 2 dysplasia and especially grade 3 dysplasia is extremely challenging, and details may be found in specialized surgical textbooks.

Some malformations, on the other hand, are more common and should not be confused with prominent ears because their correction requires a completely different approach.

Macrotia

In principle all of the auricular structures may be abnormally enlarged, but macrotia commonly affects only the upper third. The antihelical fold (especially the posterior crus) and helical fold are absent, and the helix is flattened, resulting in an enlarged scapha (**Fig. 15.27a, b**). The helix may appear to be pointed at its upper pole (*satyr ear*). An oversized conchal bowl combined with soft auricular cartilage is called a *Machiavellian ear*.

Surgical Principle

The main problem in macrotia is the excessive length of the helical rim, which must be shortened. A simple antihelix plasty would not alter the dimensions of the helix and scapha and would only improve the position of the helix relative to the head. A different approach is needed to reshape the helix and reduce the scapha.

Surgical Technique (after Davis, Fig. 15.27)

An incision is made through the anterior auricular skin and cartilage parallel to the helical rim, extending from the crus to the tail of the helix (**Fig. 15.27a**). Another incision is made along the notch between the helix and tragus, skirting the helical crus in a V shape and extending to the posterior auricular surface. This incision divides the skin only (**Fig. 15.27b**). These incisions separate the helix from the scapha while leaving the lower por-

Table 15.2 Classification of congenital auricular deformities (after Weerda 1988, Tanzer 1977, Marx 1926)

Grade 1 dysplasia	
Principle	Almost all structures of a normal auricle are present. Ear canal is generally normal
Correction	Does not require augmentation by skin or cartilage
Forms	Macrotia
	Prominent auricle
	Cryptotia (cup ear)
	Absence of the upper helix
	No deformities: absent tragus, "satyr ear" ("Machiavellian ear"), "Darwin tubercle," "Stahl ear" (third antihelical crus)
	Coloboma
	Earlobe deformities: attached, large, absent, bifid
	Cup ear deformity: Type I: mild overhang of the antihelix + hypertrophic concha + constricted helix ("lop ear") Type II: marked overhang of the upper helix
Grade 2 dysplasia	
Principle	Some normal auricular structures are present. Meatal stenosis may be present
Correction	May require some augmentation by skin or cartilage
Forms	Type III cup ear: auricular deformity in all three dimensions (constricted ear)
	Mini-ear
Grade 3 dysplasia	
Principle	Complete absence of normal auricular structures. Meatal stenosis or atresia is usually present
Correction	Total reconstruction of the skin and cartilaginous framework
Forms	Unilateral
	Bilateral
	Anotia

tion of the helix still attached to the posterior auricular surface. The scapha is now reduced as needed by resecting a strip of skin and cartilage over the antihelix (**Fig. 15.27c, d**). If necessary, the posterior cartilage surface can also be exposed through this approach and an antihelical fold can be created with sutures or by scoring the anterior cartilage surface. The posterior surface of the mobilized helical cartilage is now exposed and scored with small incisions to create an anterior concavity that reproduces the natural roll of the helical rim (**Fig. 15.27d**). The helix is then returned and the helical crus is shortened to reduce the helical circumference (**Fig. 15.27e**). The skin incisions are closed with running monofilament sutures (**Fig. 15.27f, g**).

Microtia (Fig. 15.28)

A common form of microtia is the *lop ear* or *cup ear*, which is classified as a grade 1 or grade 2 dysplasia depending on its severity. Here we shall describe only the principle for correcting a type I or type II deformity (**Table 15.2**). In contrast to macrotia described above, the cup ear is characterized by an abnormally short helical rim.

Rules, Tips, and Tricks

In a cup ear the helical circumference is too short, causing the auricle to become bunched together or constricted.

The shortened length of the helix creates a lateral overhang in which the superior helical rim is hooded over the scapha or antihelix (**Fig. 15.28a**). An antihelix plasty is not sufficient to correct this type of deformity. Any attempt to move the helix manually to a corrected position will evoke a significant recoil force due to the high tissue tension. Surgical lengthening of the helix by tissue augmentation is the only way to definitively correct the underlying problem.

Surgical Principle

The principle of corrective surgery is to lengthen the helical circumference with a pretragal transposition flap.

Surgical Technique (Davis Modification, Fig. 15.28)

The incision is like that described above for macrotia correction, except for two details. In the overhanging part of the helix, the incision does not follow the scapha but cuts across the skin of the overhang to match the thickness of the newly formed helix. The anterior part of the incision does not skirt the helical crus, but outlines a superiorly based transposition flap anterior to the tragus (**Fig. 15.28a**).

After cartilage division and mobilization, the newly defined helical rim and deformed cartilage framework are exposed at the level of the scapha and antihelix (**Fig. 15.28b**). The overhanging cartilage is resected, preserving the skin, and is stored for subsequent use (**Fig. 15.28c**). The superior helical rim is

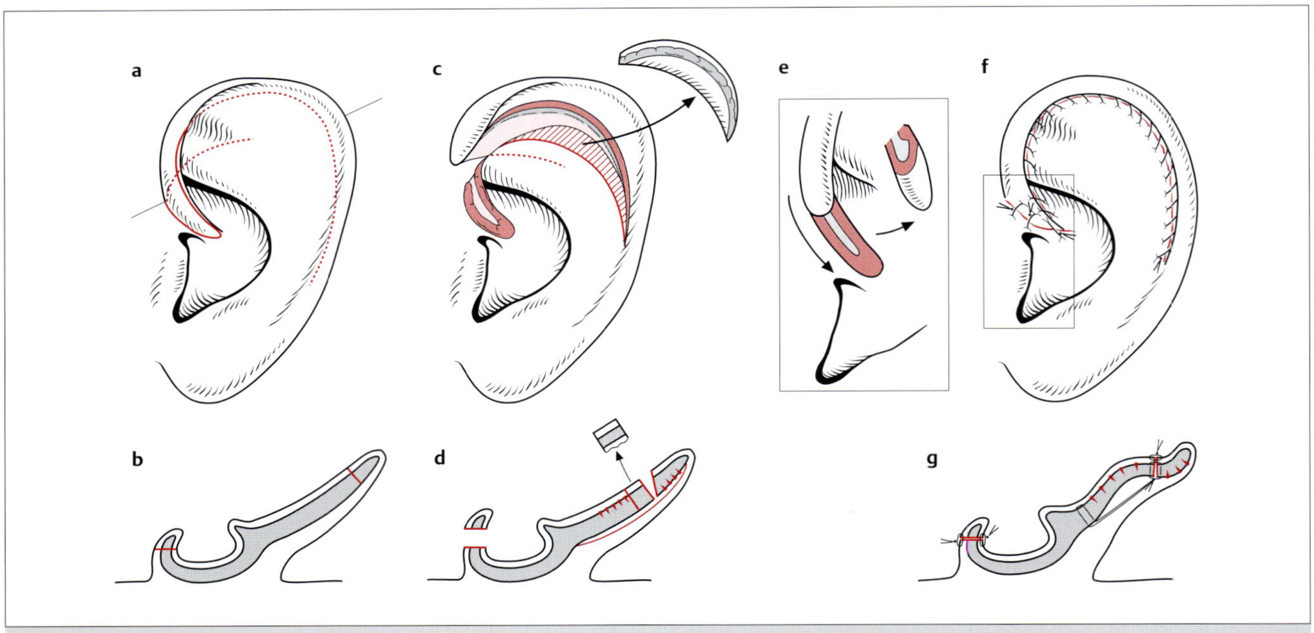

Fig. 15.27a–g Correction of macrotia (Davis technique).
- **a** The upper third of the auricle is too large due to absence of the posterior crus and a broad scapha with effacement of the helical fold. The proposed incision line in the anterior and posterior auricular surfaces is shown. The cross-sectional plane in **b**, **d**, and **g** is also shown.
- **b** Corresponding cross-section.
- **c** Detachment of the helix. The scapha is reduced by a chondrocutaneous resection.
- **d** Corresponding cross-section. Cartilage scoring incisions are placed posteriorly and anteriorly, respectively, to create helical and antihelical folds.
- **e** Close-up view of how helical length is decreased by partial resection of the crus.
- **f** Appearance after suturing. A helical fold has been created by posterior cartilage scoring and shortening of the helix.
- **g** Corresponding cross-section with the antihelix shaping suture.

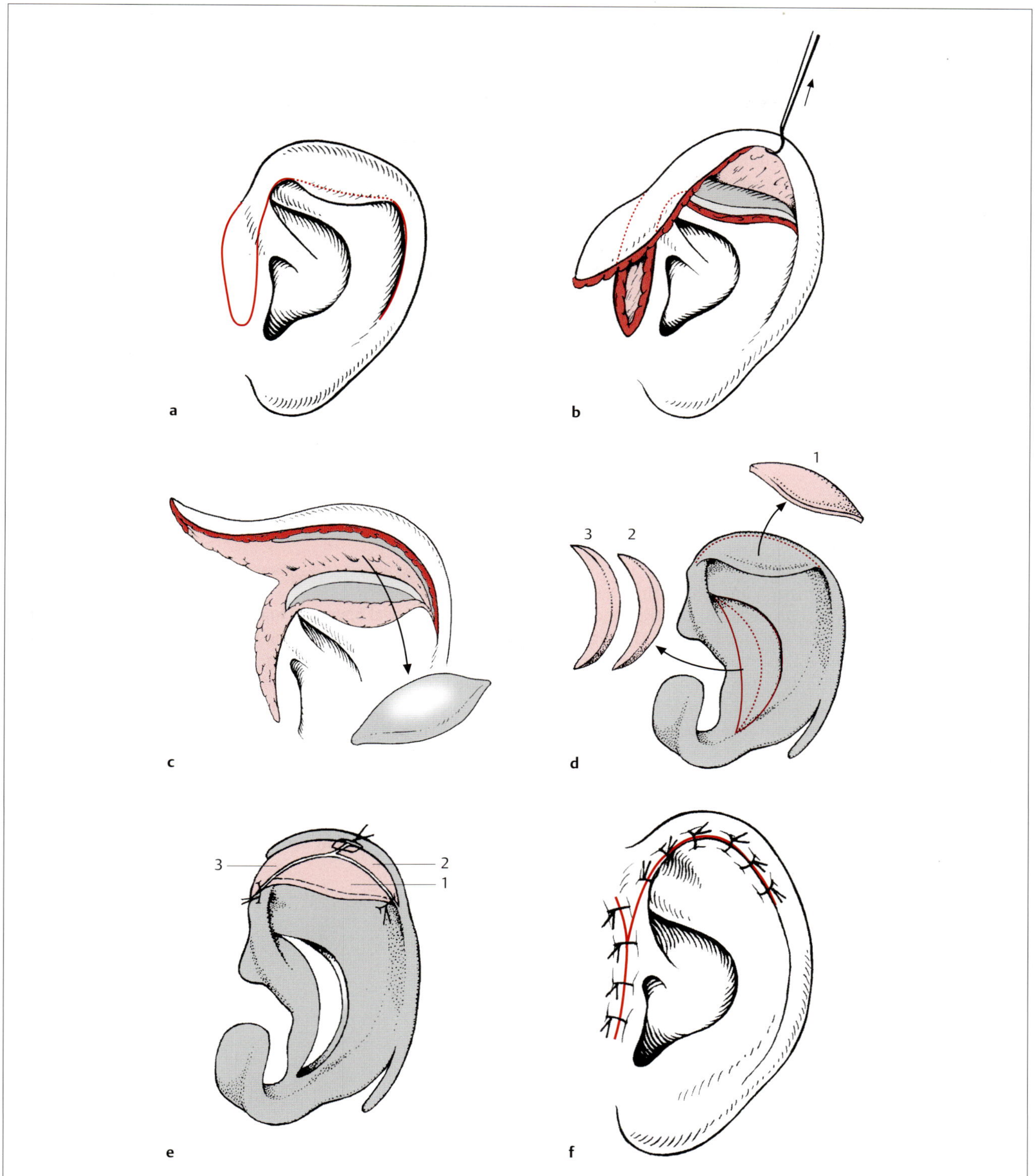

Fig. 15.28a–f Correction of microtia.

a The helical circumference is too short, causing the upper third of the helix to fold laterally over the antihelix. The helix is divided along the scapha and lengthened by pretragal flap advancement (V–Y plasty).

b Elevating the helix (arrow) moves the end of the flap superiorly.

c The hooded cartilage segment is separated from the skin and removed.

d This segment (1) is used along with two cartilage strips (2, 3) from the conchal bowl to reconstruct the helix.

e The helix and scapha are reconstructed with three cartilage grafts.

f Appearance after wound closure. The donor defect anterior to the tragus is closed in Y-shaped fashion.

then reconstructed using two additional cartilage strips taken from the conchal bowl and is supported by inset of the resected cartilage overhang (**Fig. 15.28d, e**).

In a type II or type III cup ear, the skin on the anterior auricular surface is generally not sufficient to cover the new cartilage framework. In this case a composite graft can be taken from the anterior surface of the concha and used to reconstruct the skin and cartilage framework in the scaphal region (see Reconstruction of Nasal Defects in Chapter 5).

Next, the helix is placed onto the new cartilage framework, and the transposition flap is advanced superiorly and inset (**Fig. 15.28f**). The donor defect anterior to the tragus is closed by mobilizing the surrounding skin.

Alternatives

Milder forms of cup ear may be corrected by simple resection of the overhanging helical cartilage combined with an antihelix plasty.

Auricular Appendages and Auricular Fistulas

Auricular Appendages

Auricular appendages ("ear tags") are redundant tissue structures that form at the junction between the first and second branchial arches (mandibular and hyoid arches). Generally they are located in front of the tragus but occasionally occur in the buccal region. They are removed purely for aesthetic reasons. The skin duplications are usually pedunculated and are treated by elliptical excision and removal. The axis of the elliptical incisions should be oriented along vertical, preauricular RSTLs. The defect is closed primarily by undermining the surrounding skin.

Auricular Fistulas and Cysts

Auricular fistulas and cysts have similar sites of occurrence. Fistula openings and cysts are frequently found in the area of the helical crus (**Fig. 15.29a**). Cysts are considerably less common and often result from the development of inflammatory adhesions in a fistula tract. Fistulas generally extend toward the ear canal and terminate blindly, but in rare cases they may open into the ear canal itself (**Fig. 15.29b**). The precise course of the fistula can be determined by probing or by the injection of methylene blue. It should be noted that probing of the fistula may be hampered by inflammatory adhesions.

Surgical Principle

Broad exposure and complete removal of the epithelium of the fistulous tract.

Indication

Recurrent inflammations. Surgical treatment should be performed when the fistula is not infected.

Surgical Technique (Fig. 15.29)

Surgical removal begins by making an elliptical incision around the fistula opening, following the above general guidelines for placement of the incision (**Fig. 15.29a**). The incision may be extended superiorly and inferiorly in RSTLs to gain additional exposure. This corresponds to the endaural auxiliary incision used for tympanoplasty and exposes the bony roof of the ear canal. A probe is introduced to define the fistula tract, and the fistula is dissected free with the probe in place. All fistulous epithelium must be removed to prevent a recurrence. The lateral part of the resection is closed primarily, and any opening in the external meatus is left to heal by spontaneous epithelialization.

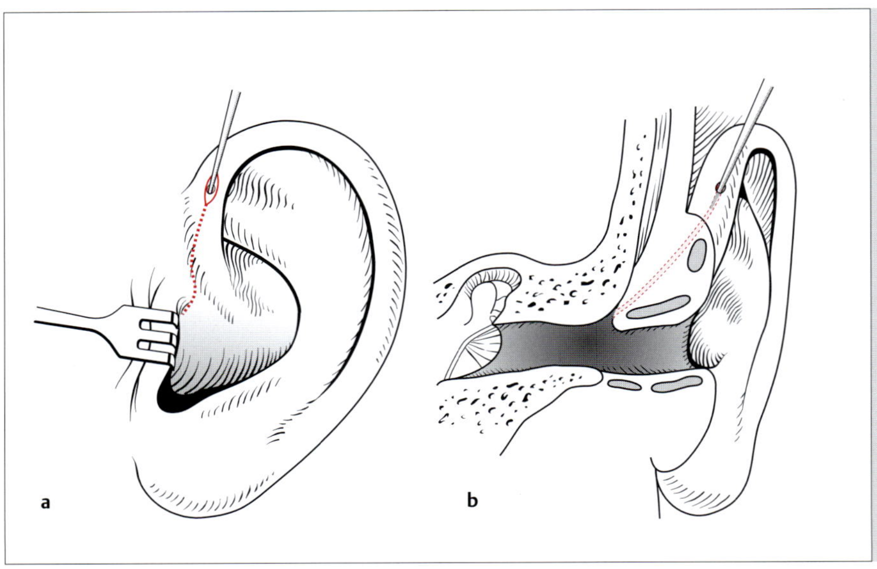

Fig. 15.29a, b Auricular fistula.
a The opening of the fistula at the root of the helix is probed with a blunt-tipped probe. An elliptical incision is made around the fistula opening and extended to the roof of the ear canal in the form of an endaural auxiliary incision.
b Frontal view: the fistula extends to the roof of the ear canal.

15

> **Rules, Tips, and Tricks**
> It is crucial to expose and identify all portions of the fistulous tract. Dissecting along a blunt-tipped probe inside the tract is more accurate than methylene blue instillation—for if the dye leaks into surrounding tissue, the tract can no longer be positively identified.

Ear–Neck Fistulas

Preauricular fistulas should be strictly distinguished from fistulas that create a communication between the ear and neck. In this case the fistula openings are located in the ear canal and anterior to the sternocleidomastoid muscle. The communicating tract may pass above or below the facial nerve, and the nerve must be protected by exposing it prior to dissection and resection of the fistula. Thus, ear–neck fistulas require more extensive surgery than preauricular fistulas, and the additional technical details must be considered during preoperative planning.

Auricular Injuries and Tumors

Lacerations

Lacerations at the root or border of the auricle are repaired with cutaneous sutures using an everting technique to prevent discontinuities. Larger cartilage tears are re-approximated with absorbable sutures to prevent sharp cartilage edges. Even a subtotal tear should heal as long as the auricular flap is still connected to the rest of the auricle by a small bridge of skin. Hence the skin bridge should be carefully preserved and the flap sutured back in its original position. Thereafter the wound should be closely watched to confirm proper healing.

> **Rules, Tips, and Tricks**
> If the repaired auricle does not appear viable (white in color), the surgeon should promptly intervene and save as much auricular cartilage as possible for performing a secondary reconstruction (see **Fig. 15.32**).

Skin Defects

Skin defects with exposed cartilage must be covered to maintain cartilage nutrition and prevent chondritis. The defect may be covered with a free full-thickness skin graft or an island flap (see **Fig. 15.34**). Superficial skin erosions, on the other hand, may heal spontaneously when treated with antibiotic ointment and covered with a sterile dressing.

Hematoma of the Pinna

A *hematoma* of the pinna is characterized by a collection of blood, a *seroma* of the pinna by a fluid collection between the perichondrium and cartilage. They are usually caused by trauma in which the auricle is subjected to a violent tangential force (e.g., in boxing or wrestling). The anterior auricular surface does not have a subcutaneous fat layer to create mobility between the skin and cartilage. Thus, hematomas generally occur on the anterior surface when a shearing force between skin and cartilage causes the perichondrium, which is firmly attached to the skin, to tear away from the cartilage. A hematoma or seroma is dangerous because it may disrupt the nutrition of the underlying cartilage. When the cartilage in the affected area is deprived of nutrition by diffusion, it becomes soft and loses its shape (parallels with septal hematoma).

> **Rules, Tips, and Tricks**
> A hematoma should always be treated because of the potential for cartilage destruction.

Conservative therapy may be tried in acute cases by evacuating the hematoma with a percutaneous needle and applying a pressure dressing for 3 days. These measures should be done under antibiotic coverage (most superinfections are caused by Gram-negative bacteria). When dealing with a recurrence or an older hematoma or seroma, surgical treatment is indicated (**Figs. 15.30** and **15.31**).

Surgical Principle

Drainage of the hematoma through an anterior skin incision. Nonviable cartilage should be resected. Bolstered mattress sutures are placed to prevent a recurrence.

Surgical Technique (Figs. 15.30 and 15.31)

If the hematoma is located in the conchal area (**Fig. 15.30**), the skin is incised in the shadow of the antihelix. The skin flap is dissected toward the ear canal. The hematoma is evacuated and any granulations are removed with a curette. If the cartilage has already been affected (become soft), it should be resected into healthy (firm) surrounding cartilage. The skin flap is returned and sutured, and several full-thickness sutures are placed through the anterior and posterior auricular surfaces and tied over bolsters to prevent a recurrence. With the affected cartilage removed, the anterior perichondrium is directly apposed to the posterior perichondrium and will become adherent to it.

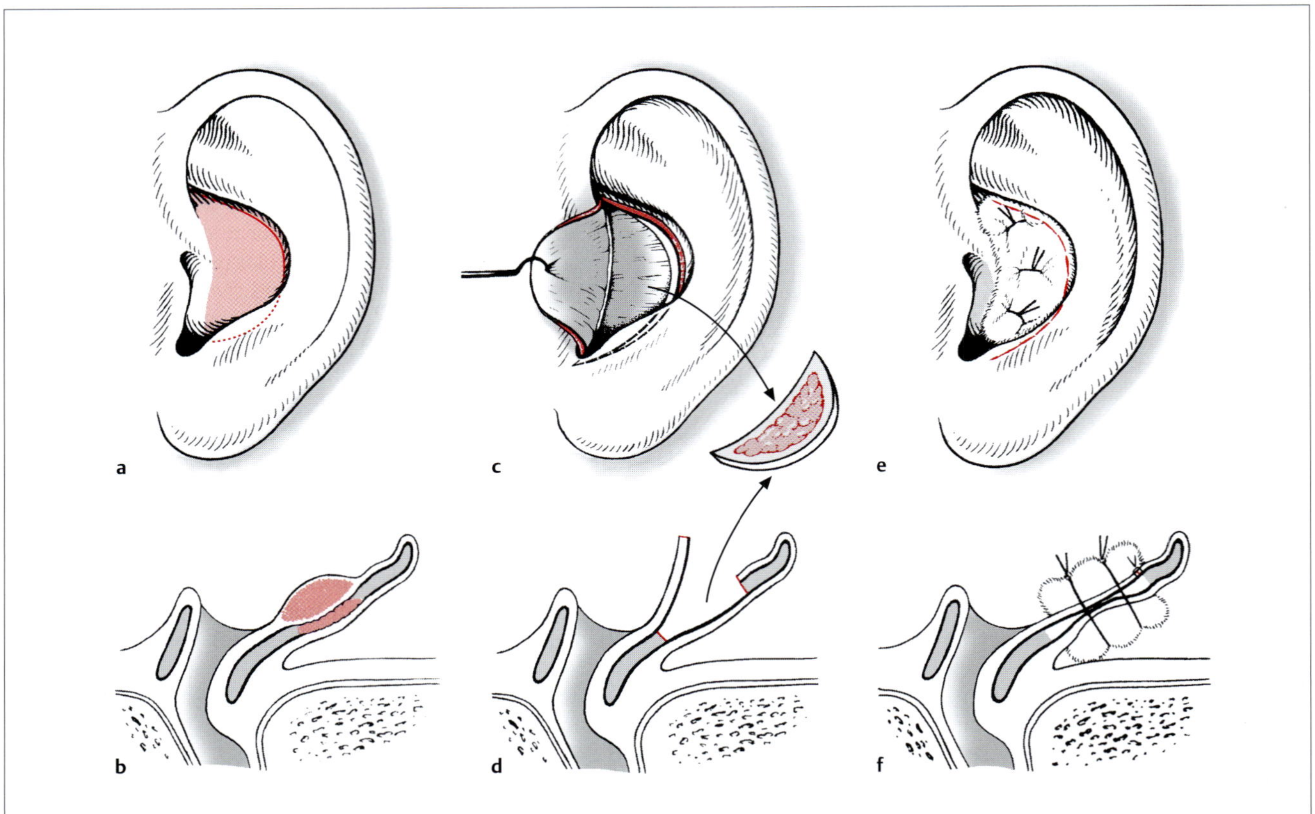

Fig. 15.30a–f Treatment of conchal hematoma.
a A subperichondrial hematoma has produced a rounded bulge in the conchal skin.
b Corresponding cross-section at the level of the ear canal. The hematoma has already caused circumscribed necrosis of the conchal cartilage.
c The conchal skin is incised, and an anteriorly based skin flap is raised. The hematoma is evacuated, and softened cartilage is removed.
d Corresponding cross-section.
e The flap is replaced, and mattress sutures are placed over gauze bolsters to prevent a recurrence.
f Corresponding cross-section.

Rules, Tips, and Tricks
The cartilage resection will not significantly affect auricular shape when a stable cartilage framework is left behind (i. e., do not remove cartilage from the auricular border).

The *antihelix* and *scapha* are also common sites of occurrence for hematomas (**Fig. 15.31**). In this case the anterior skin incision runs below and parallel to the helix. The rest of the procedure is like that for a conchal hematoma. If cartilage excision is necessary, care should be taken to leave a sufficiently wide strip of cartilage along the helical rim. If this is not possible, the helix should be reconstructed at once by implanting autologous cartilage from the concha of the same or opposite ear. This will prevent scar contraction of the skin over a deficient cartilage framework, which would no longer be reversible in a later reconstruction.

Rules, Tips, and Tricks
Chronic hematomas have a firm consistency due to calcium deposits ("wrestler's ear," "cauliflower ear"). If the framework has not contracted too much and the cartilage is merely thickened, it can be treated by thinning. In this case the cartilage is exposed through anterior skin incisions as in an acute injury.

Auricular Perichondritis

Auricular perichondritis may develop after trauma or surgery (tympanoplasty, otoplasty for prominent ears). It may also result from ear scratching or even insect stings. The main causative organisms are *Pseudomonas aeruginosa*, staphylococci, and streptococci. Perichondritis is manifested by inflammatory auricular redness and pain, with occasional skin blistering and regional lymphadenopathy. Swelling of the auricular skin effaces the normal lateral contours of the ear.

Treatment in the acute inflammatory stage is conservative and consists of alcohol compresses and systemic, preferably

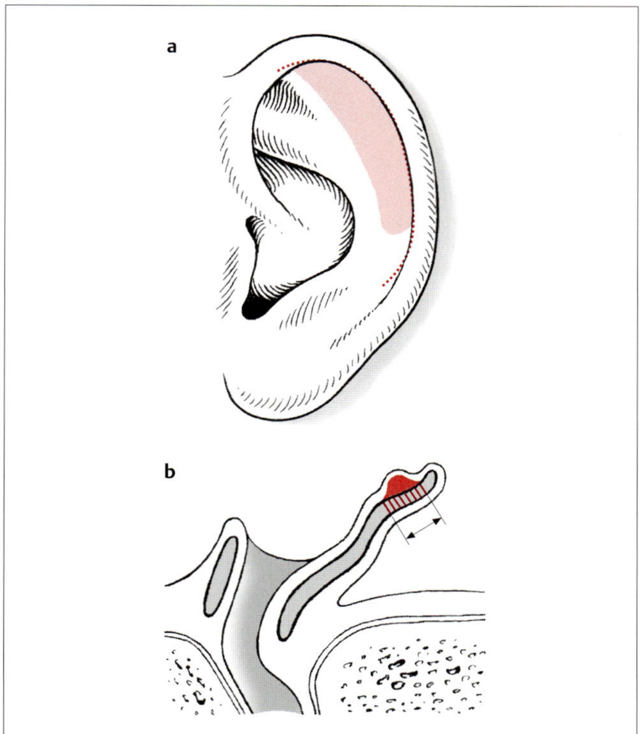

Fig. 15.31a, b Hematoma in the region of the scapha and antihelix.
a A hematoma caused by tangential trauma is often located in the scapha, whose normal contours are effaced. The anterior skin incision runs below and parallel to the helical fold.
b Corresponding cross-section. Necessary cartilage resection from the antihelix (arrow) creates a contour defect that is immediately reconstructed with autologous auricular cartilage from the same or opposite ear.

parenteral antibiotics that are active against Gram-negative organisms.

If cartilage necrosis has occurred, the infected cartilage must be removed through a retroauricular incision.

Surgical Principle

Rules, Tips, and Tricks
In perichondritis with cartilage destruction, all the softened cartilage must be cut right back, leaving only the healthy cartilage.

Surgical Technique

Although the surgeon should be reluctant to resect too much, all affected cartilage should definitely be removed. Unless all infected cartilage is resected, the inflammation will progress and may culminate in complete loss of the cartilaginous framework.

Unlike a noninfectious hematoma or seroma, bacterial perichondritis does not call for immediate reconstruction with autologous cartilage. If significant portions of the cartilage framework are absent, especially along the helix, reconstruction with autologous costal or auricular cartilage should be undertaken at ca. 8 weeks, before there has been time for significant skin contraction to occur.

Auricular Avulsion

When part or all of the auricle has been avulsed as a result of trauma, a simple reattachment with sutures will rarely succeed. The same applies to an attempted microvascular anastomosis. Generally we are dealing with a detached auricular segment of variable size, and planning the reconstruction will establish the parameters for the end result.

Surgical Principle

The detached auricle is refashioned by cartilage resection into a viable "composite graft" while leaving the skin on the anterior cartilage surface intact.

Surgical Technique (after Weerda, Fig. 15.32)

A chondrocutaneous composite graft should heal if the diameter of the cartilage does not exceed 1.5–2 cm. Accordingly, the posterior cartilage surface of the avulsed auricle is exposed by dissecting away the skin and is windowed at the scapha, concha, and triangular fossa (**Fig. 15.32e**). The recipient bed is prepared by raising a posteriorly based flap of mastoid skin, and the avulsed auricle is sutured into place. It is crucial for the posterior cartilage surface to have broad contact with the mastoid wound surface and reflected mastoid skin. The mastoid skin and posterior auricular skin are then sutured together (**Fig. 15.32f, g**).

When the auricular framework has healed at ca. 3–6 weeks, the retroauricular skin duplication is divided and the auricle is elevated from the mastoid. The skin is thinned and used to cover the posterior auricular surface and mastoid. A residual skin defect is usually present in the postauricular sulcus and is closed either with full-thickness retroauricular skin from the opposite side or with full-thickness skin harvested from the groin (**Fig. 15.32h, i**).

Better aesthetic results can often be achieved with an orthotopic cartilage framework than with autologous rib cartilage. Thus, it is always worth a try to preserve the cartilage framework using the technique described above. Reconstruction of the auricle with autologous rib cartilage is a complex procedure that requires multiple operative steps and exceeds the scope of this concise surgical textbook. A bone-anchored auricular prosthesis might also be considered as an alternative to surgical reconstruction.

Auricular Tumors

It is rare to encounter benign auricular tumors that require surgical treatment. This would most likely be considered for a keratocanthoma, a hard nodule with a central keratin plug.

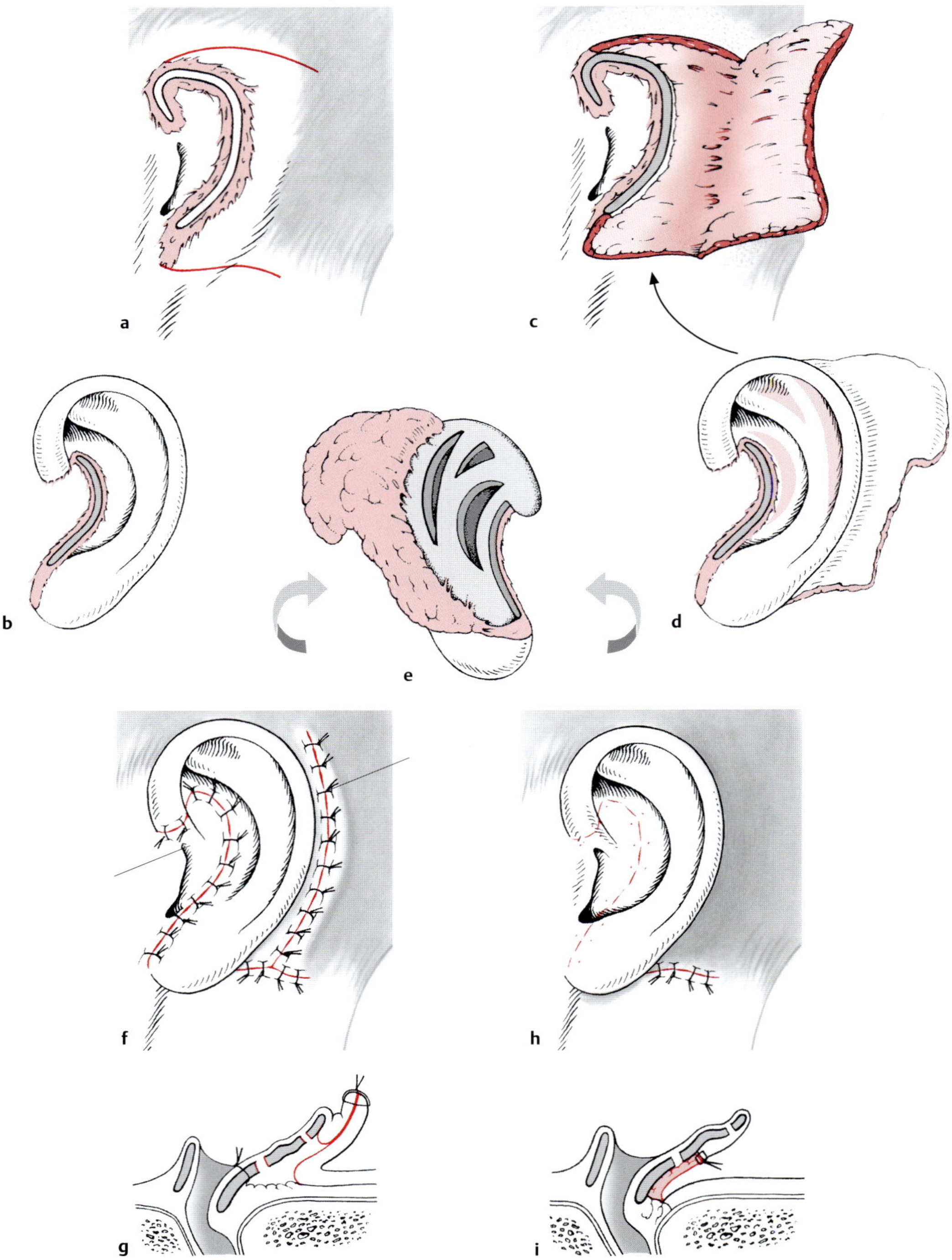

Fig. 15.32a–i Reattachment of a complete auricular avulsion (Weerda technique).

a, b The auricle has been completely avulsed at the concha and intertragic notch (**b**). The tragus is preserved. The mastoid surface is exposed through two auxiliary incisions (**a**).

c The skin over the mastoid is reflected posteriorly, preserving the periosteum.

d, e The skin is dissected from the posterior surface of the avulsed auricle, and windows are cut in the cartilage of the scapha, concha, and triangular fossa from the posterior side (**e**). Prepared in this way, the auricle is approximated to the avulsion site and to the posterior surface of the recipient bed created over the mastoid (**d**).

f, g All the wound lines have been sutured. The cross-sectional view in **g** (plane indicated by the line in **f**) shows how the skin on the posterior auricular surface and the mastoid skin have been approximated and sutured together.

h, i Appearance after inset of the retroauricular skin and reconstruction of the postauricular sulcus with a full-thickness skin graft.

Surgery is usually reserved for malignant tumors, most notably basal cell carcinoma, squamous cell carcinoma, and melanoma. There is always the potential for metastasis with squamous cell carcinoma and melanoma, and lymph node dissection and radiotherapy should be considered in addition to local excision.

Hemangiomas of the auricle are best treated by embolization or laser coagulation, depending on their extent and the equipment available. If a subtotal auricular resection is necessary, an effort should be made in older patients to preserve the upper portion of the helix to support the earpiece of reading glasses. Partial resection and immediate reconstruction are an option in cases where intraoperative frozen-section histology has confirmed negative margins.

Tumors of the Concha

Surgical Principle

Skin tumors in the conchal bowl are excised with adequate margins that include an island of underlying cartilage (**Fig. 15.33**). The resection exposes the posterior layer of perichondrium. The defect can be covered with a full-thickness retroauricular skin graft, but a more elegant solution is to reconstruct the defect with a retroauricular island flap (**Fig. 15.34**).

Surgical Technique (Figs. 15.33 and 15.34)

First, the retroauricular skin at the base of the wound is divided vertically at the approximate center of the defect ((**Fig. 15.34a, b**). This incision defines half the circumference of the skin island. Further dissection now proceeds on the posterior auricular surface. The existing incision is extended to an ellipse toward the postauricular sulcus (**Fig. 15.34c**). The skin island should be wider inferiorly than superiorly to match the size of the defect. A beginner should use a template to ensure that the skin island is cut to an adequate size.

Further dissection is crucial for maintaining an adequate blood supply to the flap:

> **Rules, Tips, and Tricks**
> The mastoid skin should not be undermined toward the ear canal, but parallel to the mastoid surface.

This technique preserves a vascular pedicle near the posterior circumference of the ear canal (**Fig. 15.34d**). Bridging connective tissue must be divided superiorly and inferiorly so that the skin island can be swung forward into the defect and sutured into place. The retroauricular donor defect is closed primarily in two layers (**Fig. 15.34e–g**).

Tumors of the Helix (Figs. 15.35 and 15.36)

Besides malignancies, helical tumors consist mainly of "painful ear nodules" (chondrodermatitis nodularis helicis). The defect created by excision of a small tumor can be covered by helical advancement. This is done by dividing the lower helix in two layers (anterior skin and cartilage) at its junction with the scapha and also resecting a chondrocutaneous wedge below the antitragus (**Fig. 15.35**). The mobilized helix, still attached to the posterior skin, is now approximated and sutured to the superior edge of the defect, preferably using an everting technique (intracutaneous mattress suture) to avoid a conspicuous notch. While this method does make the auricle slightly smaller by shortening the helical circumference, it yields a good aesthetic result for defects up to 1 cm long.

Larger tumors require an auricular wedge resection (**Fig. 15.36**). Since the edges of a wedge resection cannot be re-approximated without tension, chondrocutaneous "dog ears" must additionally be resected from the scapha. Again, the free border of the helix should be closed with intracutaneous mattress sutures. Because the defect is closed without tissue replacement, the upper half of the auricle is significantly reduced in size.

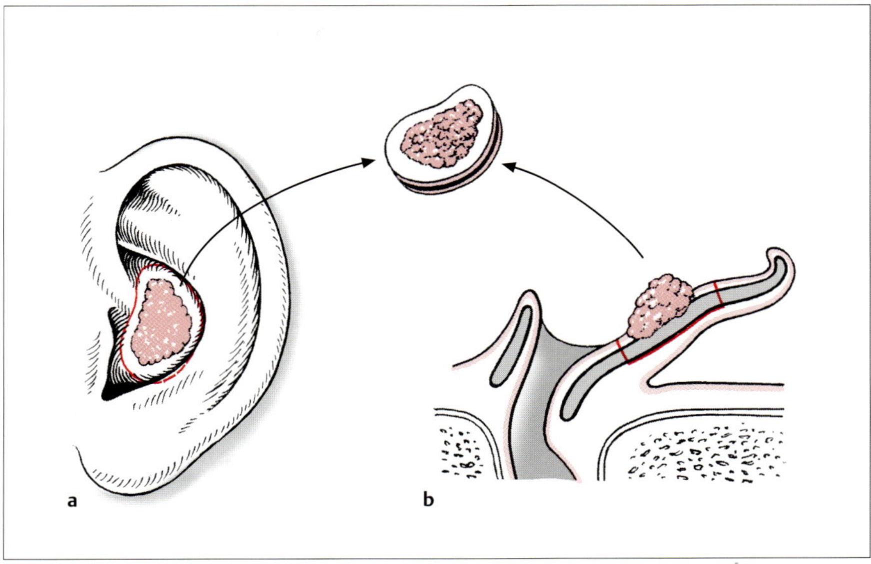

Fig. 15.33a, b Resection of a conchal tumor.
a The skin tumor and underlying cartilage are excised with adequate margins, preserving the posterior perichondrium.
b Cross-section at the level of the ear canal. The posterior skin and perichondrium remain intact.

15

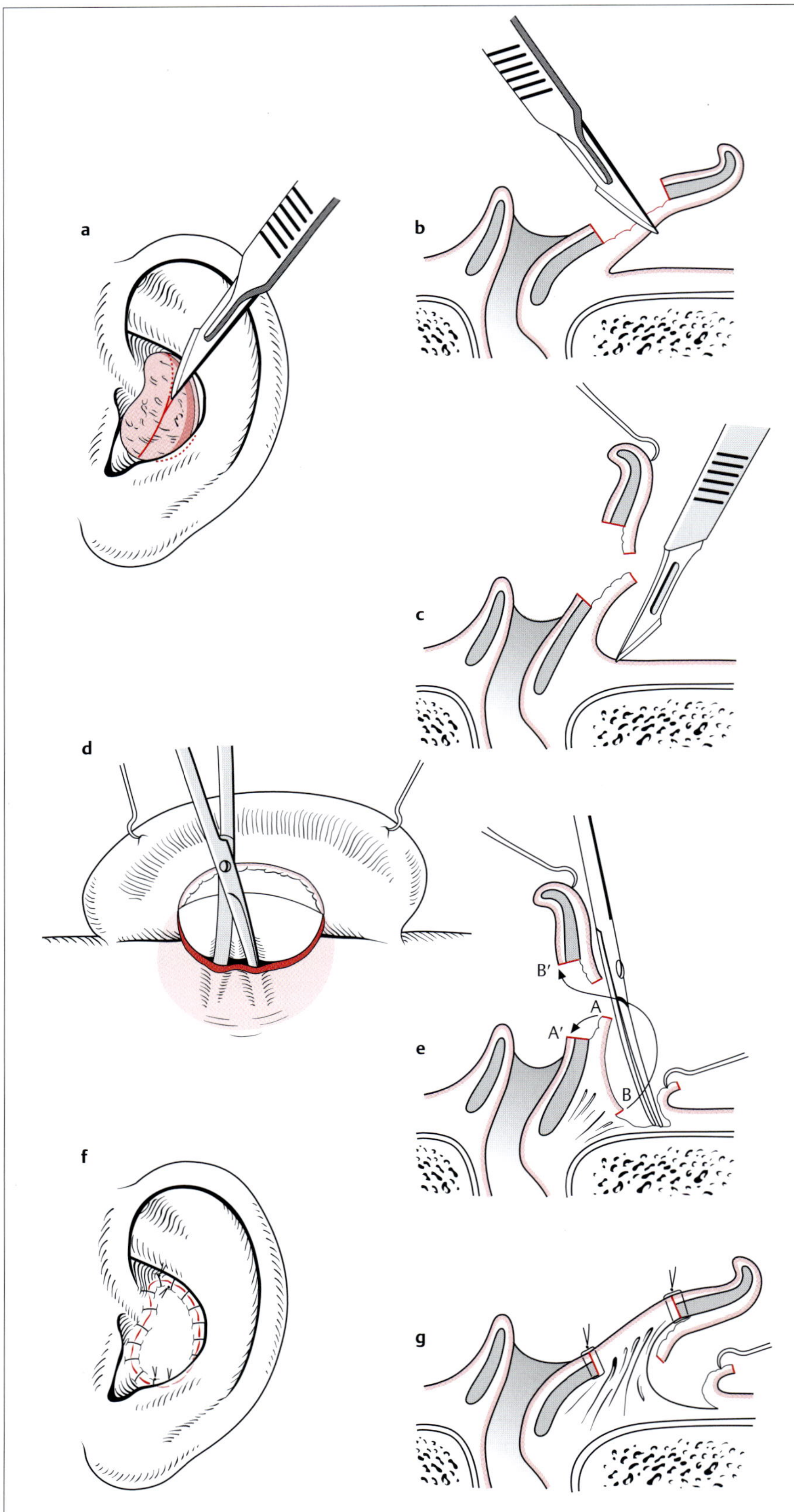

Fig. 15.34a–g Reconstruction of the conchal skin defect with a retroauricular island flap.

- **a** The posterior auricular skin is incised at the center of the defect with a No. 11 scalpel blade.
- **b** Corresponding cross-section. This incision creates a full-thickness defect while also defining the lateral circumference of the cutaneous island flap.
- **c** The flap is completed by incising the skin over the mastoid lateral to the postauricular sulcus.
- **d** Posterior view. The skin island has been outlined. The full-thickness defect is visible over the superior edge of the island. The flap pedicle should be dissected toward the mastoid.
- **e** Cross-section. The scissors dissection is directed parallel to the mastoid surface, preserving a connective tissue pedicle toward the ear canal. The objective is to approximate point A to A′ and point B to B′.
- **f, g** Having been mobilized in all directions, the skin island is rotated 180° into the anterior defect and sutured into place. Cross-sectional view (**g**) shows the position of the island flap. The donor defect can be closed primarily owing to the broad mobilization of the mastoid skin.

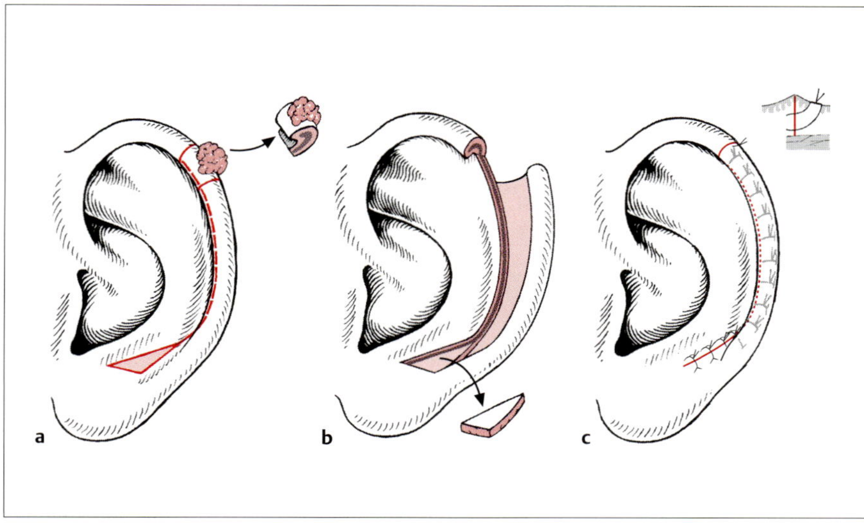

Fig. 15.35a–c Reconstruction of a small helical defect after tumor resection.
- **a** A helical skin tumor is removed by chondrocutaneous resection. The defect will be closed by helical advancement. An incision is marked along the scapha at its junction with the helical rim. A wedge of skin and cartilage will be resected below the antitragus.
- **b** After the anterior skin and cartilage have been incised (leaving the posterior skin intact), the helix is mobilized down to the helical tail, and a tissue wedge is removed at the lower end of the incision.
- **c** The helix has been advanced superiorly and sutured into place. An everting intracutaneous mattress suture (detail) prevents notching of the helical rim.

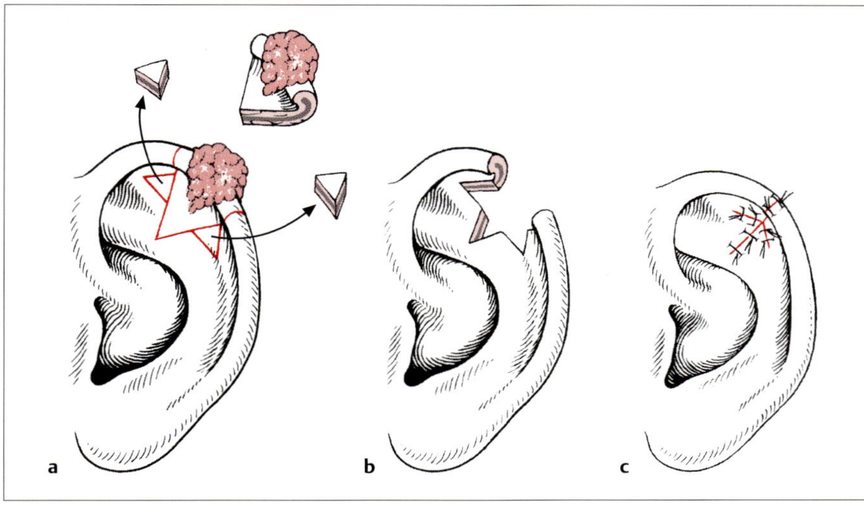

Fig. 15.36a–c Wedge resection for a large skin tumor of the helix.
- **a** The tumor is removed by a full-thickness resection, creating a wedge-shaped defect. Full-thickness dog ears are also removed from the scapha to allow for primary closure.
- **b** Appearance after the cartilage resections.
- **c** Appearance after closure. The resections have reduced the height and width of the upper auricle.

Ear Canal

Earlier sections dealt with the surgical anatomy of the ear canal and with preauricular and ear–neck fistulas (see **Fig. 15.29**). Because the operative treatment of meatal exostosis and other tumors basically follows the techniques used in middle ear surgery, it is described under that heading.

Foreign Bodies

Foreign bodies that are not lodged within the ear canal can be removed with a small hook inserted behind the foreign body. This requires general anesthesia in children because of the risk of tympanic membrane injury. Local anesthesia may be adequate in adults (see **Fig. 15.5**). If the foreign body has been lodged in the ear for some time, a stricture may have formed lateral to the object due to inflammation and scarring. In this case the foreign body cannot be removed without enlarging the ear canal. This can be done through an endaural auxiliary incision (**Fig. 15.37a**), which allows the soft tissues on the roof of the ear canal to be spread open.

Stenoses (Figs. 15.37 and 15.38)

Most stenosing lesions of the cartilaginous ear canal are strictures due to post-traumatic or postoperative scarring, and most are located near the meatal opening (**Fig. 15.37a**). Bony narrowing is often present in malformations. If the ear canal is completely occluded, cerumen and cellular debris may accumulate between the stricture and tympanic membrane, causing a gradual pressure rise similar to a cholesteatoma.

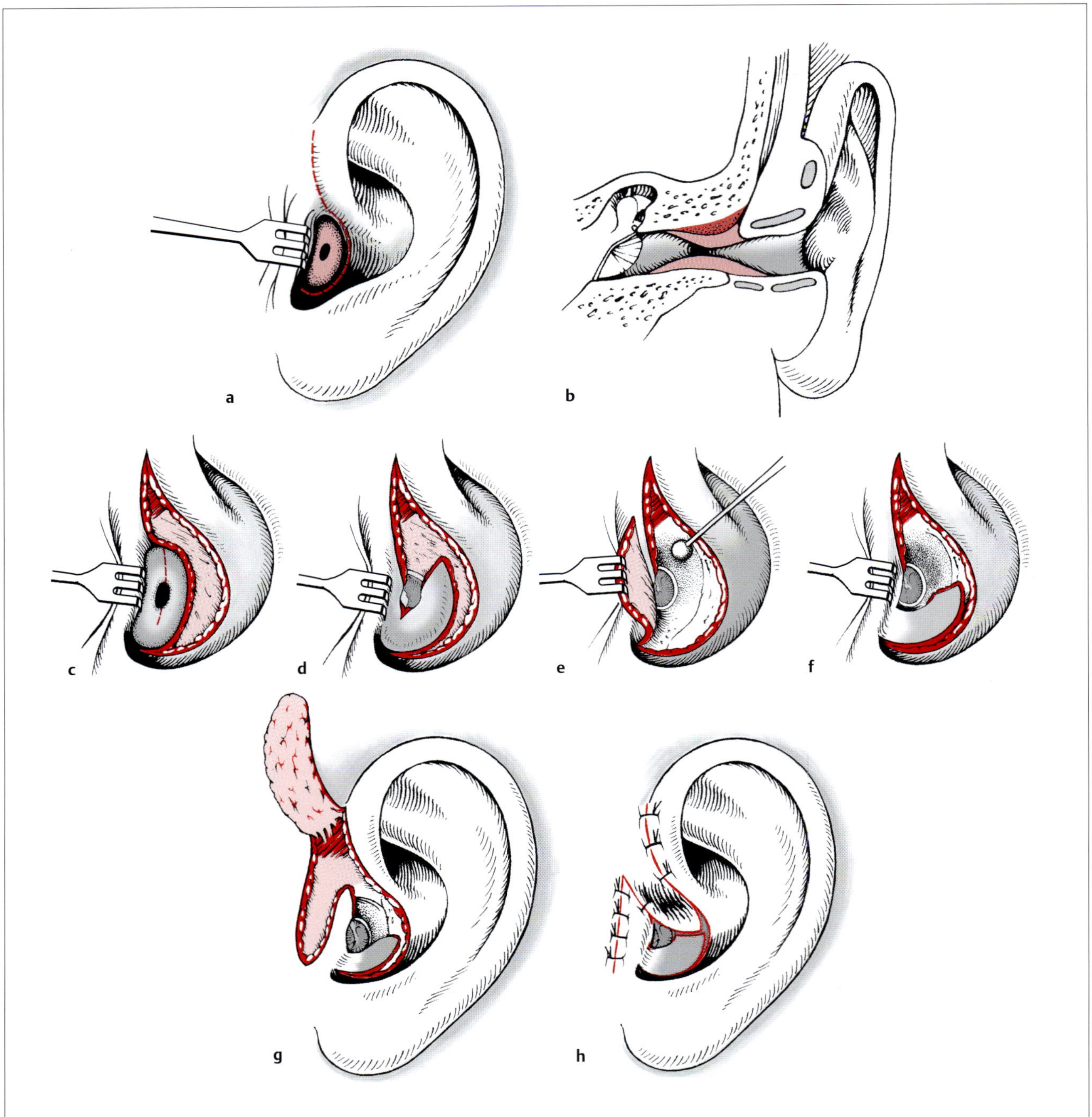

Fig. 15.37a–h Stricture at the junction of the cartilage and bony ear canal.

a Buttonhole stricture located deep in the auditory canal. Lines indicate the endaural auxiliary incision in the anterior notch and an extension down the posterior meatal wall.

b Coronal section: A thick pad of scar tissue has formed beneath the annular cutaneous stricture. The ear canal must be enlarged by removing part of the bony roof (shaded).

c The meatal bone is exposed superiorly and posteriorly. The strictured meatal skin is incised at the roof and floor of the ear canal.

d A counter-incision is added near the tympanic membrane, and the skin is separated from the bone, leaving it attached to the anterior wall.

e The bony ear canal is enlarged posteriorly and superiorly with a burr.

f When the available meatal skin is spread out, bare bone is still visible on the roof and posterior wall of the canal.

g A superiorly based flap is outlined and raised anterior to the tragus. It is swung into the ear canal through the endaural auxiliary incision.

h The tip of the flap is within the canal, and its base has been sutured at the meatal opening. The donor defect can be closed primarily by skin mobilization. The flap pedicle increases the distance between the helical crus and tragus. This can be corrected secondarily by skin resection after the flap has healed.

Surgical Principle

A stricture caused by subcutaneous circumferential scarring of the ear canal is always associated with a deficiency of skin. It is therefore necessary to increase the endaural skin area.

If treatment is limited to scar excision leaving large epithelial defects in the cartilaginous ear canal, a recurrence is inevitable. Moreover, several months of treatment with a meatal dilator often yields a poor result and is distressing for the patient.

Various techniques are available for augmenting the meatal skin:

- Skin replacement with thin full-thickness or split-thickness skin grafts.
- Replacing the skin on the meatal roof with a pretragal transposition flap (**Fig. 15.37**).
- Replacing the skin on the posterior meatal wall with a retroauricular, partially de-epithelialized transposition flap (**Fig. 15.38**).

Surgical Technique

Pretragal Transposition Flap (Fig. 15.37).

An endaural auxiliary incision is made through the cartilage-free gap between the helix and tragus and extended along the posterior bony circumference of the meatal opening to the floor of the ear canal. The skin in the meatal roof is then incised to create a communication with the semicircular skin incision (**Fig. 15.37a**). Another incision splits the inferior edge of the stricture to the floor of the ear canal, leaving the meatal skin attached only to the anterior wall and tympanic membrane. Next, the skin is additionally incised several millimeters lateral and parallel to the edge of the tympanic membrane on the posterior wall and floor so that it can be advanced toward the canal floor (**Fig. 15.37d**). This exposes the bone on the roof and posterior wall of the ear canal, and these portions of the bony canal are widely enlarged with a burr. This is necessary to accommodate the skin flaps that will be swung into the ear canal, as they are considerably thicker than the normal meatal skin. After the bony canal has been enlarged, the orthotopic meatal skin is thinned and spread out over the canal floor, leaving a portion of the posterior bony meatal wall uncovered. This area on the roof and posterior wall will be covered with a superiorly based, thinned transposition flap raised anterior to the tragus and swung into the ear canal through the endaural auxiliary incision. This flap will also increase the distance between the tragus and helix, which may require a minor secondary correction after the flap has healed. The donor defect is closed primarily by mobilizing the skin. While the flap transposed to the cartilaginous ear canal can be inset with sutures, the flap covering the meatal bone must be secured with packing. This is best accomplished with gelatin sponge after first lining the circumference of the ear canal with silicone film. The gelatin sponge and silicone film should remain in place for 3 weeks. The meatal opening is additionally packed with strips impregnated with antibiotic ointment.

Retroauricular, Partially De-epithelialized Transposition Flap (Fig. 15.38)

A retroauricular flap can be used in the treatment of extensive stenosis and especially meatal atresia. A retroauricular incision is made just lateral to the postauricular sulcus, and the meatal opening is reached by dissection on the periosteum. The subsequent periosteal incision is based on the meatal opening (**Fig. 15.38a**). The posterior auricular skin is incised parallel to the posterior circumference of the meatal opening, and a perpendicular incision is made in front of the tympanic membrane. After a counter-incision is made near the edge of the tympanic membrane, superiorly and inferiorly based flaps of meatal skin are dissected from the underlying bone and elevated (**Fig. 15.38c**). The bony posterior meatal wall and suprameatal spine are burred down to expose the cellular system. The skin defect created by the bone resection and unfolding of the meatal skin is covered with a retroauricular transposition flap. This flap is obtained by incising the mastoid skin parallel to the incision in the postauricular sulcus and joining both incisions at the level of the earlobe. When the flap is elevated from the periosteum, it forms a superiorly based transposition flap whose apex is thinned by the removal of subcutaneous fat, as the flap will be placed close to the tympanic membrane. Now the flap is swung into the ear canal over the newly created bony rim, and the area requiring de-epithelialization is marked. This area is de-epithelialized, leaving a layer of dermis intact. Two sutures are placed between the proximal border of the epithelial island and the posterior border of the lateral meatal skin, and the sutures are tied after the auricle has been returned to its normal position. The dissected periosteal flap is fixed as far posteriorly as possible to obtain posterior enlargement of the meatal opening. The donor defect created by the transposition flap is closed in two layers by mobilizing the mastoid skin. Finally the skin of the transposition flap is packed against the bone of the posterior meatal wall with gelatin sponge over a layer of silicone film. As with the pretragal flap, the packing is left in place for 3 weeks.

Rules, Tips, and Tricks

A great many options exist for surgical procedures to improve the shape or position of the auricle, or to reconstruct auricular defects. Some are appropriate for very specific situations but not for a broad range of indications. The procedures presented in this chapter are effective basic techniques that can be adapted as needed to meet individual requirements.

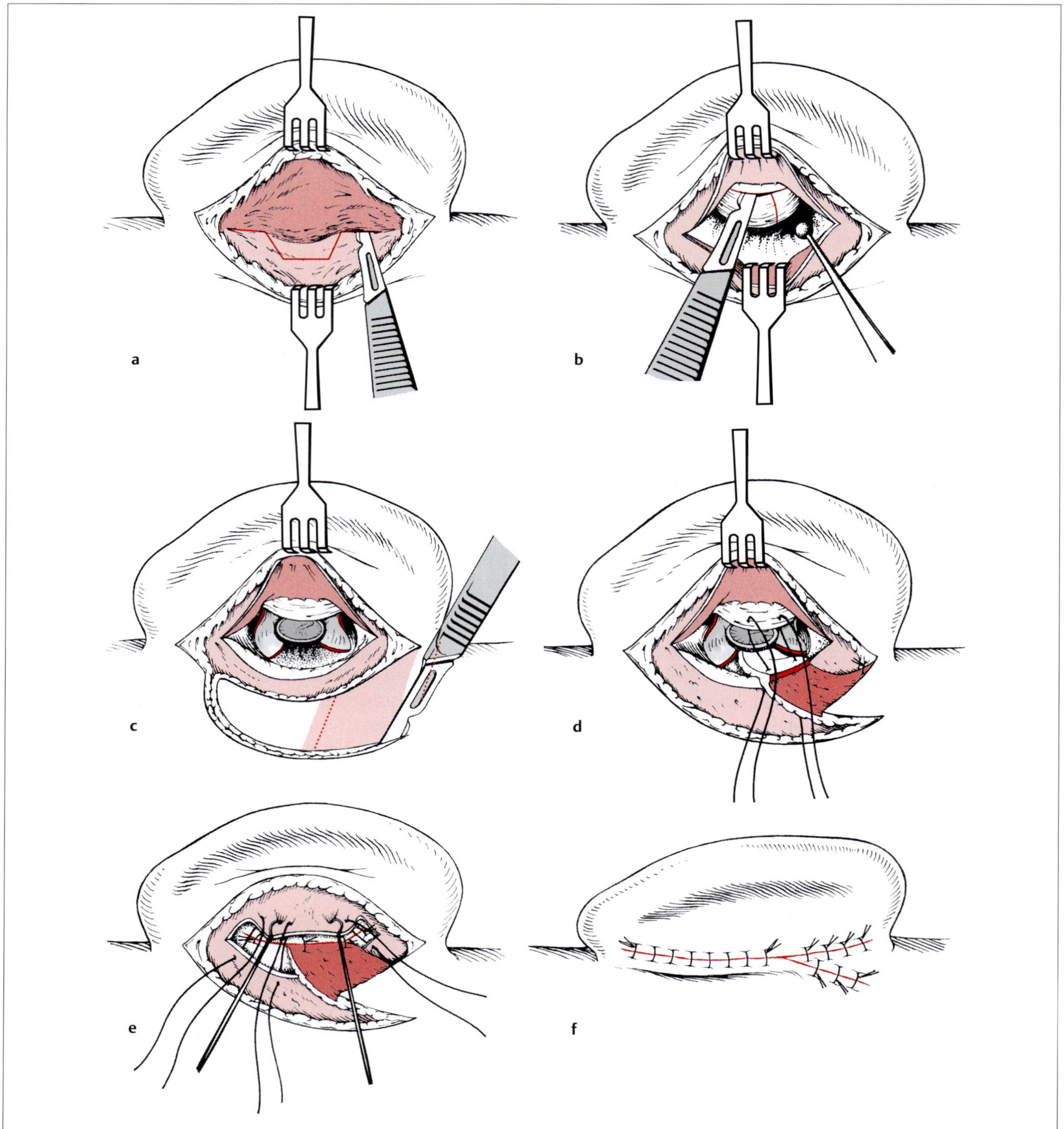

Fig. 15.38a–f Epithelialization of a defect in the posterior meatal wall with a partially de-epithelialized retroauricular transposition flap.

a A retroauricular incision is made in the postauricular sulcus, and the soft tissues are dissected from the meatal opening while sparing the periosteum. A periosteal flap based medially on the posterior meatal wall is outlined.

b A semicircular skin incision is made in the posterior wall with a scalpel. After subperiosteal dissection of the meatal skin, a second, perpendicular skin incision is made toward the tympanic membrane. The bony ear canal is then enlarged by burring down the bone. If atresia is present, an artificial meatus is created with the burr.

c Aided by a counter-incision near the tympanic membrane, the superiorly and inferiorly based skin flaps are spread open. This leaves a large area of bare bone on the posterior meatal wall, which would lead to recurrence of the stenosis without epithelial coverage. A superiorly based retroauricular transposition flap is outlined, and the desired area that will be de-epithelialized is marked.

d After the proximal portion of the flap pedicle has been de-epithelialized and the tip of the flap thinned, the tip is swung into the ear canal. The lateral posterior wall of the ear canal is fixed to the transposition flap with two sutures.

e Appearance after the epithelial island of the transposition flap has been joined to the skin of the posterior meatal wall. The sutures have been placed for reattaching the periosteal flap.

f Appearance after retroauricular wound closure.

15

16 Surgery of the Bony Ear Canal and Tympanic Membrane

Exostosis

Surgical Principle

The bony overgrowth is removed until the circumference of the tympanic membrane is fully visible.

Indication

- Stenosing exostosis with recurrent otitis media.
- Direct bone contact with tympanic membrane causing impaired sound conduction.
- Interference with hearing aid fitting.
- Restricted access for middle ear surgery or myringoplasty.

Contraindication

Auricular malformation (relative).

Specific Points Regarding Informed Consent

- Tympanic membrane perforation.
- Hearing loss, tinnitus.
- Facial nerve injury.
- Stricture due to scarring.
- Salivary fistula.
- Temporomandibular joint injury.

Anesthesia

Local or general anesthesia.

Surgical Technique

- The patient is positioned supine with the head turned to the side and immobilized on a headrest or ring.
- An endaural incision is made and retractors are placed.
- An H-shaped skin flap is created over the exostosis. It may be in continuity with the endaural incision if desired.
- The meatal skin is separated superiorly and inferiorly from the exostosis with an angled round incision knife (**Fig. 16.1**). With a very large, broad-based exostosis that almost completely obstructs the ear canal, the skin is mobilized in stages while exposed portions of the exostosis are progressively removed. The superior flap is reflected outward while the inferior flap is retracted away from the drilling site with the suction tip.
- The bone is removed with a diamond burr using progressively smaller burr diameters. Alternatively, an exostosis with a narrow base can be removed with a gouge.
- Any remaining bony edges can be removed with a House curette (**Fig. 16.2**).
- The meatal skin is reapproximated.
- Silicone film and packing are placed into the ear canal.
- The wound is closed.

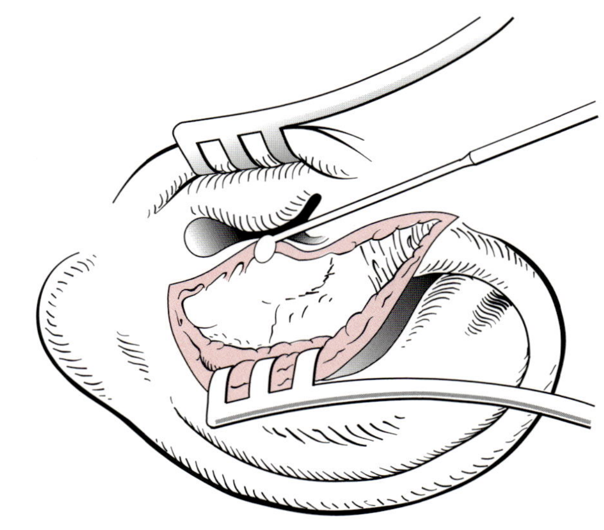

Fig. 16.1 Removal of exostosis.
An endaural incision is made, and the skin over the dome of the exostosis is incised. The incision is extended to form H-shaped flaps. The meatal skin is elevated superiorly and inferiorly with a round incision knife.

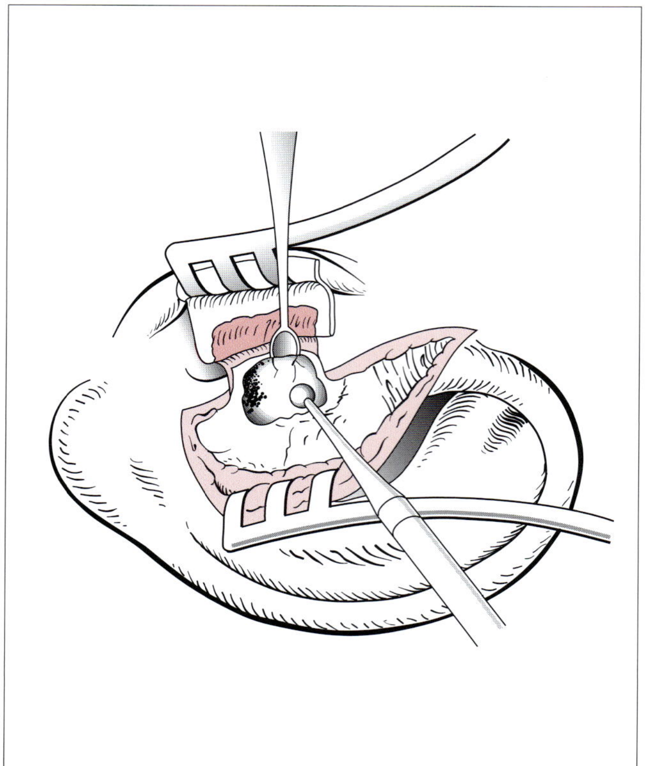

Fig. 16.2 Removal of exostosis.
A large exostosis can be hollowed out with a burr, and the remaining shell can then be fractured with a House curette. The meatal skin is approximated to the anterior wall with a Silastic strip.

Rules, Tips, and Tricks

- The entire circumference of the tympanic membrane must be visible.
- Do not drill below the level of the tympanic membrane (mainly an issue when excising a posterior wall exostosis).
- Do not drill through the anterior canal wall. The mastoid air cells may be opened but should be covered with meatal epidermis or fascia before closing.
- With a very large exostosis, it is better to remove and reimplant meatal skin than damage the skin with a burr.
- Elevated meatal skin can be kept away from the burr with adhesive strips (e. g., Silastic).
- A very large exostosis can be hollowed out and the remaining shell fractured with a House curette (**Fig. 16.2**).
- Bony edges projecting over the tympanic annulus can be removed with a House curette, working parallel to the annulus.

! Risks and Complications

- Wrapping of meatal skin around the spinning burr.
- Facial nerve injury (keep above the level of the tympanic membrane).
- Inner ear damage caused by drilling, accidental contact with the short process of the malleus, ossicular dislocation, tympanic membrane perforation, salivary fistula in the ear canal caused by drilling through the bony anterior canal wall (may also damage the temporomandibular junction), meatal stricture due to extensive skin loss.

Postoperative Care

Perioperative antibiotics. Packing should remain in place for 2–3 weeks. Any granulations that form should be removed.

Removal of Small Tumors in the Ear Canal

Surgical Principle

Circumscribed tumors are excised with healthy margins, followed if necessary by coverage of the surgical defect.

Indications

Superficial benign and malignant tumors of the external ear canal.

Contraindications

Local excision is contraindicated for tumors that have infiltrated deeper tissues, invaded surrounding tissues, or cannot be clearly visualized.

Specific Points Regarding Informed Consent

See Exostosis.

Anesthesia

Local or general anesthesia.

Surgical Technique

- The patient is positioned supine with the head turned to the side and immobilized on a headrest or ring.
- An endaural incision is made, and retractors are placed.
- The tumor is circumscribed with adequate margins.
- The specimen is freed from underlying bone with an angled round incision knife (**Fig. 16.3**).
- The underlying bone is smoothed with a diamond burr.

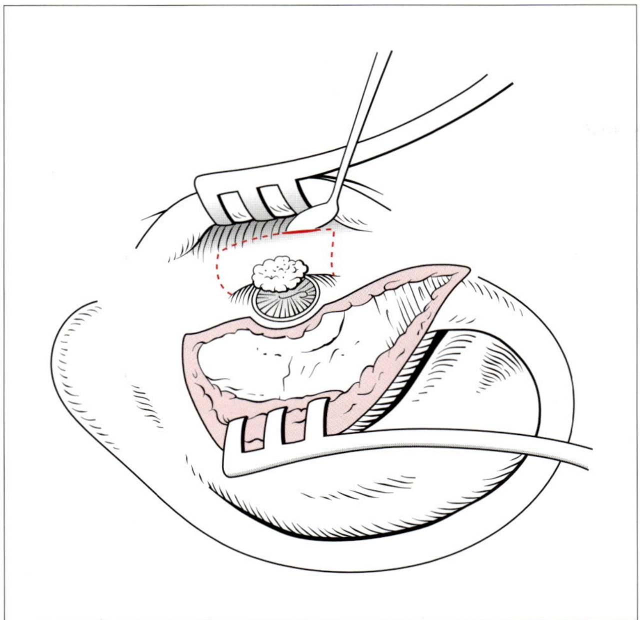

Fig. 16.3 Excision and removal of a meatal tumor.

- If necessary, the defect is covered with split-thickness postauricular skin.
- Silicone film and packing are placed into the ear canal.

Rules, Tips, and Tricks

- The tumor must be completely excised.
- The specimen is mounted and sent for pathologic examination.
- With a narrow ear canal that offers poor access and vision, the bony inlet of the ear canal can be enlarged posteriorly with a burr. For bone exposure, see Endaural Approach.

! Risks and Complications

Residual tumor. Meatal stricture due to scarring.

Postoperative care

Perioperative antibiotics. Packing should remain in place for 2–3 weeks.

Minor Surgery of the Tympanic Membrane

Myringotomy and Tube Insertion

Surgical Principle

The tympanic membrane is incised in the anteroinferior quadrant for decompression and drainage of effusion, followed if necessary by the insertion of a drainage tube.

Indications

- Refractory acute otitis media, especially in patients with early facial nerve palsy or vertigo.
- Persistent otitis media with effusion, impaired eustachian tube ventilation, significant autophony due to a patulous eustachian tube or cleft lip and palate (tube insertion).

Contraindications

High position of the jugular bulb, carotid artery anomaly, glomus tumor (pulsating mass visible behind the tympanic membrane), coagulation disorder (relative).

Specific Points Regarding Informed Consent

- Postoperative development of acute otitis media.
- Recurrence of otitis media with effusion.
- Persistent tympanic membrane perforation, possibly with recurrent bouts of otitis; cholesteatoma formation.
- Loss or slippage of the drainage tube into the middle ear cavity.
- Permanent conductive or sensorineural hearing loss or tinnitus. Facial nerve paralysis and vertigo are usually transient effects caused by local anesthesia.

Anesthesia

Local or general anesthesia. Topical anesthesia may be adequate in selected cases.

Surgical Technique

- **Positioning.** Local anesthesia: sitting position with the upper body tilted back and the head immobilized (assistant). General anesthesia: supine on the operating table with the head turned to the side and immobilized on a headrest or ring.
- **Approach.** Transcanal (an endaural auxiliary incision is occasionally necessary).
- The largest aural speculum that can be accommodated is used.
- Viewing through the operating microscope, the surgeon makes an incision in the anteroinferior quadrant of the tympanic membrane with a sickle knife (or in the posteroinferior quadrant if the anteroinferior quadrant is difficult to see). The incision is directed radially from the center of the membrane toward the periphery (**Fig. 16.4**). In patients with acute otitis media, the incision may also be placed at

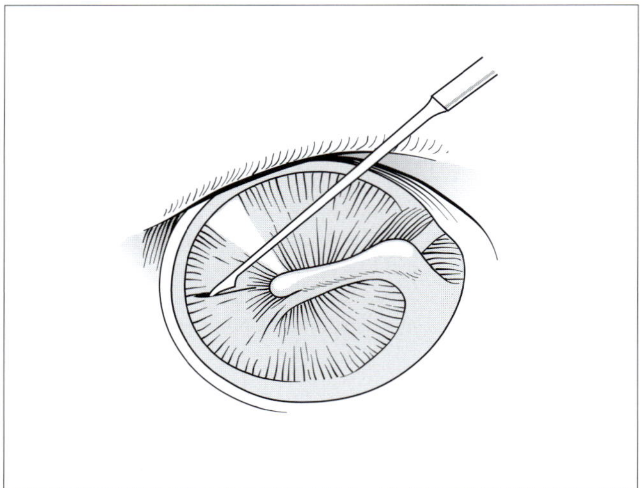

Fig. 16.4 Myringotomy.
A radial incision is made in the anteroinferior quadrant of the tympanic membrane with a sickle knife.

the most prominent site in the bulging membrane, provided it is not too close to the ossicular chain.

- Fluid is suctioned from the middle ear.
- A drainage tube is inserted if necessary (e.g., gold or titanium grommet). The tube is grasped with a microforceps or applicator, tipped slightly forward, and passed to the myringotomy site. The leading edge of the inner flange is slipped beneath the anterior edge of the incision. The forceps or applicator is withdrawn, and a sickle knife or slightly curved needle is used to push the rest of flange beneath the posterior edge of the incision (**Fig. 16.5a–c**).
- Bleeding can be controlled by local application of naphazoline if necessary.
- A T-tube is inserted with a special applicator. The T-shaped tabs are advanced past the tympanic membrane and then expand to hold the tube in place (**Fig. 16.6a–c**). The tube can also be introduced with a microforceps that holds the tabs straight until they are ready to deploy.

Rules, Tips, and Tricks

- Confirm correct placement of the tympanostomy tube.
- If the device has a pull string, it should be adequately shortened before insertion.
- Suctioning very thick mucus from the middle ear can be a slow and tedious process. Sometimes it is helpful to make a second myringotomy incision to equalize the negative pressure that develops when aspirated mucus completely fills the myringotomy.
- A sample should be taken from inflammatory exudate.
- Make the myringotomy slightly larger if tube insertion is planned.

16

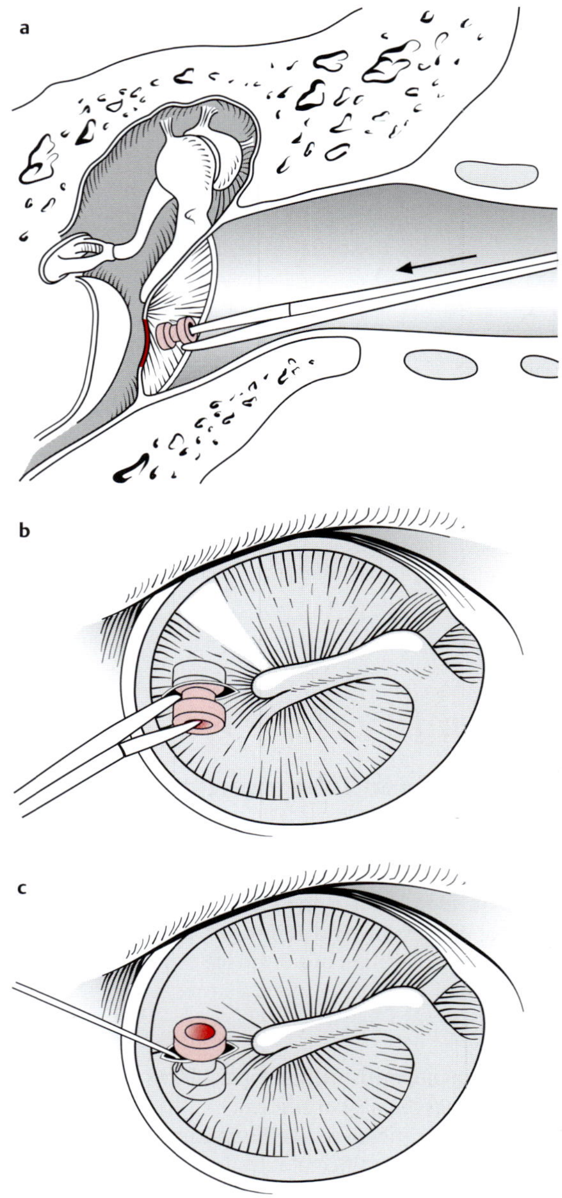

Fig. 16.5a–c Myringotomy with tube insertion.
a The grommet is introduced into the ear with a microforceps.
b The leading edge of the inner flange is slipped beneath the edge of the myringotomy.
c The rest of the inner flange is pushed through the incision with a small hook.

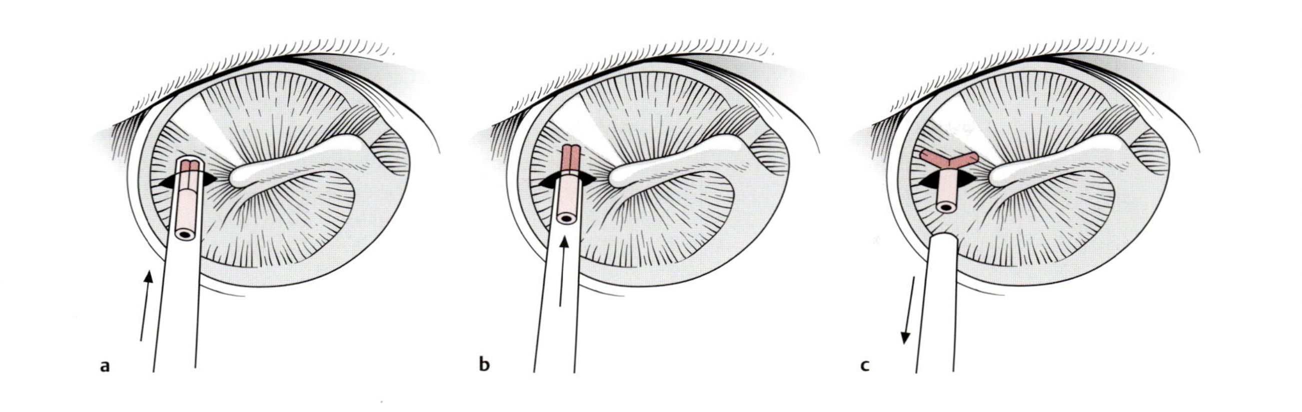

Fig. 16.6a–c T-tube with applicator.
The tube is introduced into the middle ear with the applicator. When the tube is released, the T-shaped tabs expand to hold the tube in place while the applicator is carefully withdrawn.

! Risks and Complications

- Persistent tympanic membrane perforation, recurrent otorrhea, cholesteatoma formation (indication for subsequent tympanoplasty).
- Infection or rejection of the drainage tube (if persistent, the tube should be removed).
- Vascular puncture (jugular bulb, internal carotid artery).
- Ossicular chain injury with conductive hearing loss.
- Inner ear damage, tinnitus.
- Slippage of the tube into the middle ear cavity (removed by tympanoscopy).

Postoperative Care

- Water should be kept out of the ear canal.
- The tube should remain in place for 3–12 months. If spontaneous expulsion does not occur, the tube is removed under the microscope by pulling on the stem or grasping the pull string with a small forceps. (Usually this can be done without anesthesia, even in children.)

Alternatives

Laser myringotomy, electrosurgical myringotomy (thermoparacentesis with a cautery needle, usually remains patent for 4 weeks).

Splinting a Tympanic Membrane Perforation

Surgical Principle

The infolded edges of the tympanic membrane perforation are everted and held in place with a splint.

Indications

Fresh, gaping tympanic membrane perforations with inverted edges up to 1 week after the injury.

Contraindications

- Fresh welding splatter injury.
- Acute infection with otorrhea.
- Ossicular chain defects or large perforations with tissue loss (tympanoplasty is indicated).
- Small slitlike perforations (tend to heal well spontaneously).

Specific Points Regarding Informed Consent

- Persistent perforation, conductive hearing loss.
- Possible need for secondary tympanoplasty.
- Inner ear damage, tinnitus—may be pre-existing due to original trauma (presurgical audiogram required).
- Traumatic cholesteatoma.
- Transient vertigo or facial nerve paralysis due to local anesthetic.

Anesthesia

Local or general anesthesia. Topical anesthesia may be adequate in some cases.

Surgical Technique

- **Positioning.** In some cases the sitting position may be used with the upper body tilted back and the head immobilized (assistant). Otherwise (especially with general anesthesia) the patient is positioned supine with the head turned to the side and immobilized on a headrest or ring.
- **Approach.** Transcanal. An endaural auxiliary incision is occasionally necessary.

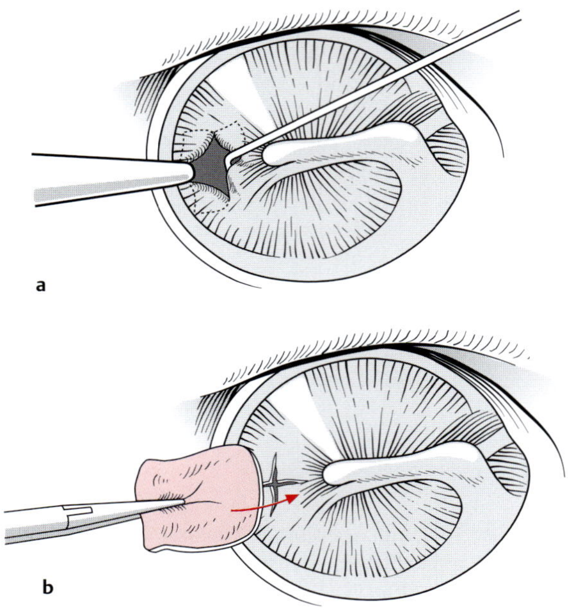

Fig. 16.7a, b Splinting a tympanic membrane perforation.
a Infolded edges are everted with a small hook and microsuction tip.
b The everted edges are splinted with a Silastic strip.

- The infolded edges of the tympanic membrane perforation can be everted with a small 90° hook. Longer, deeply inverted membrane tags can be retrieved from the middle ear cleft with a microsuction tube (**Fig. 16.7a**).
- A silastic patch is placed over the reduced perforation, or a small perforation can be covered, e.g., with a paper splint that will adhere to the edges of the tear (**Fig. 16.7b**).
- The ear canal is packed with foam (e.g., Gelfoam) or ointment-impregnated strips.

Rules, Tips, and Tricks
- All squamous epithelium must be everted from the middle ear cavity.
- Edges that fall back into the middle ear cavity can be supported with a small piece of Gelfoam introduced into the middle ear.
- Irrigation and suction will often reopen wound edges that have been fixed by clotting.

! Risks and Complications
- Persistent perforation, recurrent otorrhea, cholesteatoma formation (indication for subsequent tympanoplasty).
- Inner ear damage, tinnitus.
- Transient vertigo or facial nerve paralysis due to local anesthetic.

Postoperative Care

Perioperative antibiotics. The patient is told to avoid nose blowing up to 1 week after the surgery. Packing remains in place for 2–3 weeks.

17 Surgical Approaches, Harvesting Grafts, and Implants

Surgical Approaches

The transcanal (endomeatal) approach to the tympanic membrane without incising the ear canal is adequate for myringotomies, tube insertions, and splinting tympanic membrane perforations. More extensive procedures require an endaural or postauricular approach to provide better visibility and access.

Endaural Approach

Surgical Principle

Extended approach to the external ear canal, tympanic membrane, and middle ear by making an incision between the tragus and root of the helix. The endaural incision is also called the Heermann incision.

Indications

- Exostosis.
- Circumscribed tumors of the ear canal.
- Foreign body extraction.
- Stapes surgery.
- Surgical correction of minor malformations.
- Tympanoscopy and second-look procedures.
- Tympanoplasty without an extensive mastoidectomy.

Contraindications

- Mastoidectomy in patients with extensive pneumatization (relative), otogenic complications, or petrous bone fractures.
- Tympanoplasty for large cholesteatoma or poor visualization of lesions in the anterosuperior and inferior quadrants of a narrow, sharply angled ear canal (relative, depending on the surgeon's experience).

Anesthesia

Local anesthesia or general endotracheal anesthesia.

Surgical Technique

Positioning. The patient is positioned supine on the operating table with the head turned to the side and immobilized on a headrest or ring.

Exposure. The auricle is pulled upward and backward by an assistant. The meatal entrance is spread open with a nasal speculum.

Incision. The first incision, made with a No. 10 or 15 blade, extends outward from the approximate center of the bony roof of the ear canal, initially keeping the blade in contact with the bone. It then follows the fissure between the tragal cartilage and root of the helix, which is easily visualized by adjusting the speculum tension, and runs parallel to the anterior helical rim. It may be only ca. 1 cm long (e.g., for stapes surgery) or may extend past the root of the helix, depending on the necessary degree of exposure.

Temporalis fascia. When the incision reaches the end of the bony ear canal, it becomes more superficial and divides just the skin past that point, leaving the temporalis fascia and underlying muscle intact (**Fig. 17.1**). Next, the subcutaneous tissue and remaining connective tissue strands over the temporalis fascia and helix are mobilized by a combination of sharp and blunt dissection with a scissors, periosteal elevator, or scalpel.

Meatal incision. The second, circumferential incision is made to the bone with a No.15 blade or round incision knife ca. 1 cm medial to the opening of the ear canal. It starts at the 6 o'clock position on the canal floor and circles upward to the 12 o'clock position on the posterior wall of the canal, where it meets the first incision at a right angle.

Flap dissection. The triangular flap formed by the incisions is reflected laterally over the suprameatal spine with a periosteal elevator, keeping the blade in contact with the bone (**Fig. 17.2**). The self-retaining retractor blades are placed anteriorly and posteriorly, and if necessary a second endaural retractor can be placed at right angles to the first.

Tympanomeatal flap. A tympanomeatal flap is outlined by making additional incisions toward the tympanic membrane at the 5 o'clock and 11 o'clock positions in the right ear or the 1 and 7 o'clock positions in the left ear (**Fig. 17.3**; see Rules, Tips, and Tricks below).

> **Rules, Tips, and Tricks**
> - Do not incise the helical cartilage or temporalis fascia.
> - Place the incision just anterior to the auricle to avoid damaging the superficial temporal artery and extensions from the superficial branch of the facial nerve.

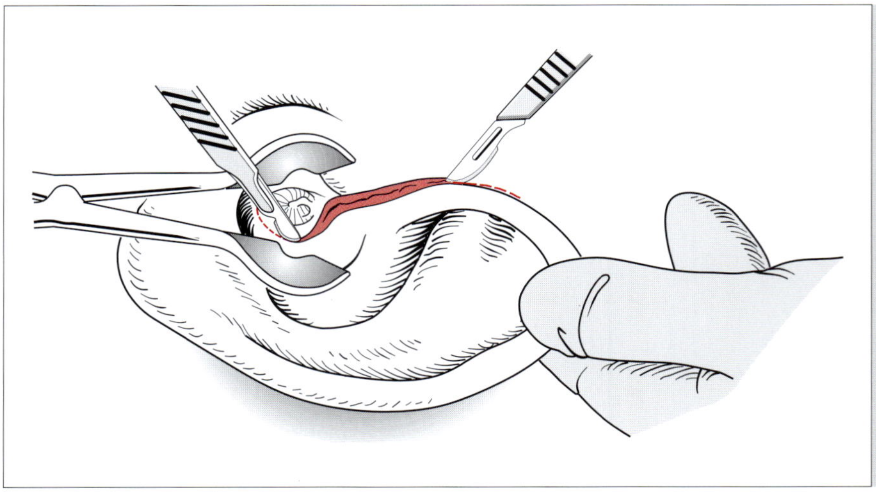

Fig. 17.1 Endaural approach.
The surgical site is exposed by inserting a speculum and pulling the auricle upward and backward. The first incision starts in the roof of the ear canal and runs outward, parallel to the root of the helix. The second, circumferential incision is made in the bony posterior wall of the ear canal ca. 1 cm from the meatal entrance.

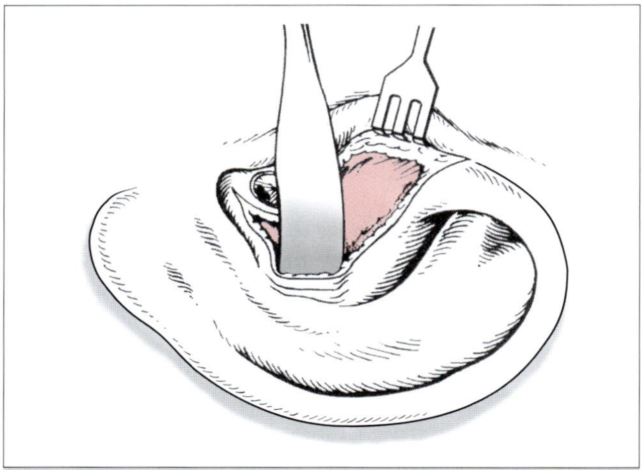

Fig. 17.2 Endaural approach.
The posterior wall flap is mobilized over the suprameatal spine with a periosteal elevator.

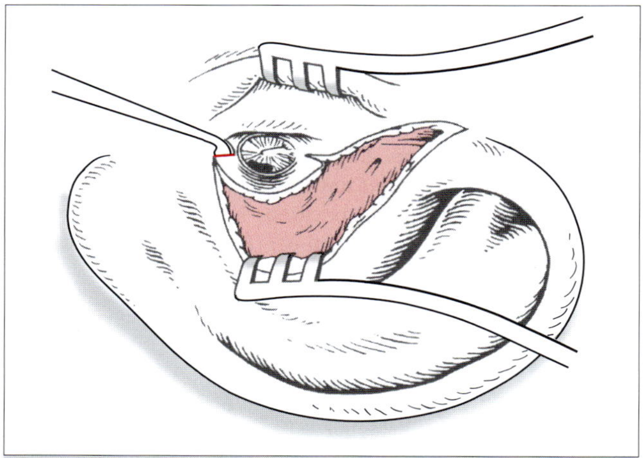

Fig. 17.3 Endaural approach.
The tympanomeatal flap is created by making additional incisions at the 5 and 11 o'clock positions in the ear canal.

- A narrow bony meatal entrance can be enlarged with a grinder or conical burr to create a funnel-shaped cavity.
- If a bony overhang in the anterior canal wall is obscuring the anterior quadrants, it can be taken down with a diamond burr. First a U-shaped flap based on the tympanic membrane is cut over the prominence, dissected with a round knife to the tympanic membrane annulus, and reflected onto the drum. The prominence is then burred down, and the flap is returned.
- The distance of the circumferential incision from the tympanic annulus, and thus the length of the tympanomeatal flap, is variable. A longer (more laterally placed) flap incision is useful in cholesteatoma surgery for covering the bone defect in the posterior canal wall. A shorter flap (closer to the tympanic membrane) is better for a stapedectomy as it provides more space within the ear canal.
- If broad exposure of the mastoid is required, the skin incision can be extended upward and backward around the root of the helix into the postauricular sulcus. Before the incision is extended, the retractors should be loosened so that the cut can be continued in a straight line.

! Risks and Complications
- Auricular perichondritis.
- Injury of the parotid capsule.
- Postoperative hemorrhage due to temporal artery injury.
- Special procedures are available for managing other complications.

Postauricular Approach

Surgical Principle

A posterior incision is made around the root of the auricle, and the entrance to the ear canal is exposed. For a tympanoplasty, the ear canal is opened medial to the suprameatal spine. For a mastoidectomy, the periosteum over the mastoid cortex is divided and reflected from the bone.

Indications

- Tympanoplasty.
- Cholesteatoma removal.
- Antrotomy.
- Mastoidectomy, including treatment of otogenic complications.
- Saccotomy.
- Facial nerve decompression.
- Translabyrinthine approach to the internal auditory canal.
- Cochlear implant (modified approach, see Chapter 23).
- Implantable hearing aids.
- Glomus tympanicum tumors.
- Obliteration of a radical cavity.

Contraindications

None.

Anesthesia

Local anesthesia or general endotracheal anesthesia.

Surgical Technique

Skin incision. The auricle is pulled forward with the left hand (for a right-handed surgeon). The incision is made several millimeters behind the postauricular sulcus, extending from the root of the auricle to the level of the earlobe base and dividing both the skin and subcutaneous tissue. A mastoidectomy incision starts just behind the auricle and extends down to the level of the mastoid tip, curving away from the postauricular sulcus as it descends (**Fig. 17.4**). While the auricle is pulled forward and laterally, the tense connective tissue and the retroauricularis muscle are divided semisharply with a scalpel or by scissor-spreading and -cutting dissection to their junction with the cutaneous ear canal, which is easily identified by applying digital counterpressure from the auricle. The exposure is continued superiorly to the temporalis fascia.

Suprameatal spine. A semicircular incision is made around the ear canal and ca. 5 mm away from it, keeping the blade in contact with the bone. The periosteum over the mastoid cortex is incised at a right angle to that incision, and the soft tissues are reflected with a periosteal elevator (**Fig. 17.5a**). At this point the posterolateral circumference of the ear canal can be isolated and the suprameatal spine exposed.

Palva flap. The Palva flap is a large posterior flap based on the auricle (**Fig. 17.5b**). It is useful for cavity obliteration.

Meatoplasty. The posterior wall of the cutaneous ear canal is incised from the 6 o'clock to 12 o'clock position, placing the incision 0.5–1 cm medial to the lateral boundary of the bony ear canal (not used for mastoidectomy alone). The roof of the ear canal is then incised laterally to the cartilage with a No. 15 blade (**Fig. 17.6**), and the meatoplasty flap is reflected upward and secured beneath the retractor blade (**Fig. 17.7**). A second

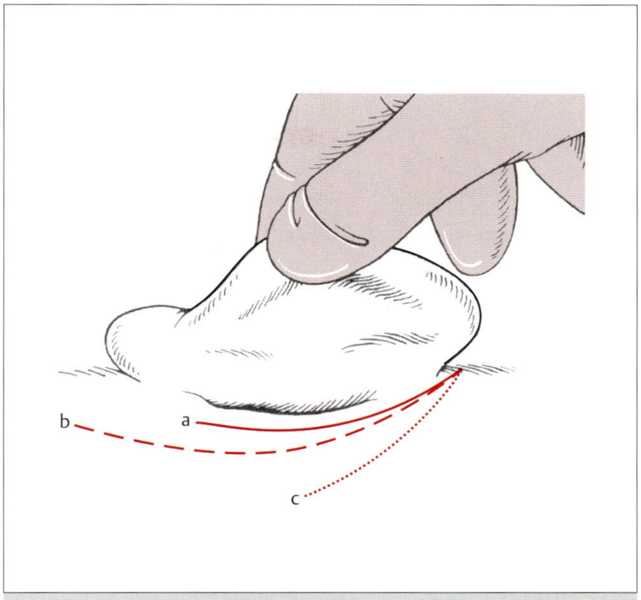

Fig. 17.4 Postauricular approach.
The incision for a tympanoplasty is placed several millimeters behind the postauricular sulcus (a). A mastoidectomy incision runs from the postauricular sulcus to the tip of the mastoid (b). A posterosuperior oblique incision is used for performing an antrotomy in infants (c).

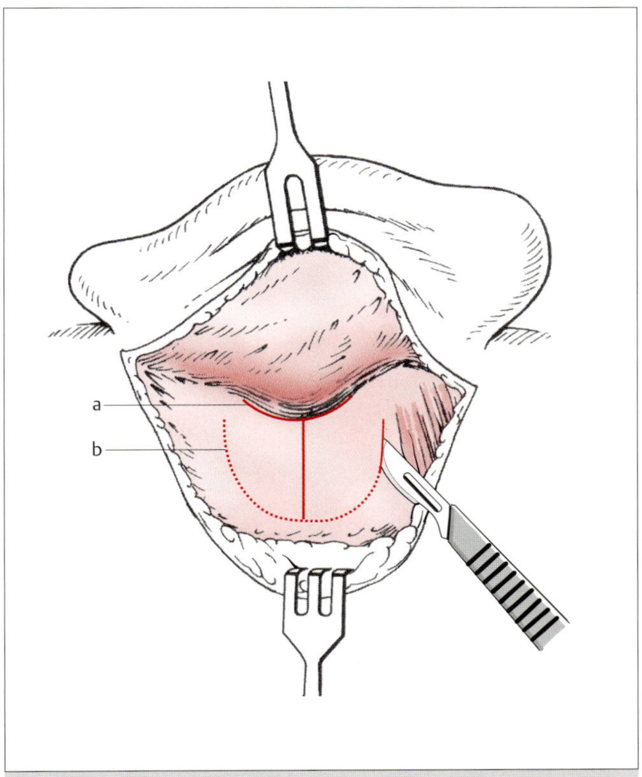

Fig. 17.5a, b Postauricular approach.
A posterior incision is made around the meatal entrance, and a perpendicular extension is made through the periosteum (a). A Palva flap (b) is outlined.

17

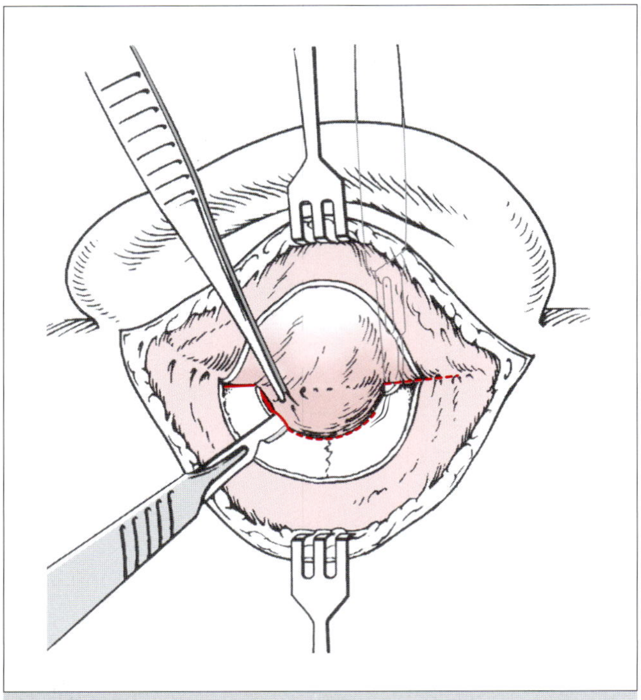

Fig. 17.6 Postauricular approach.
The isolated "tube" of the ear canal is incised over its posterior circumference, and the roof of the canal is incised.

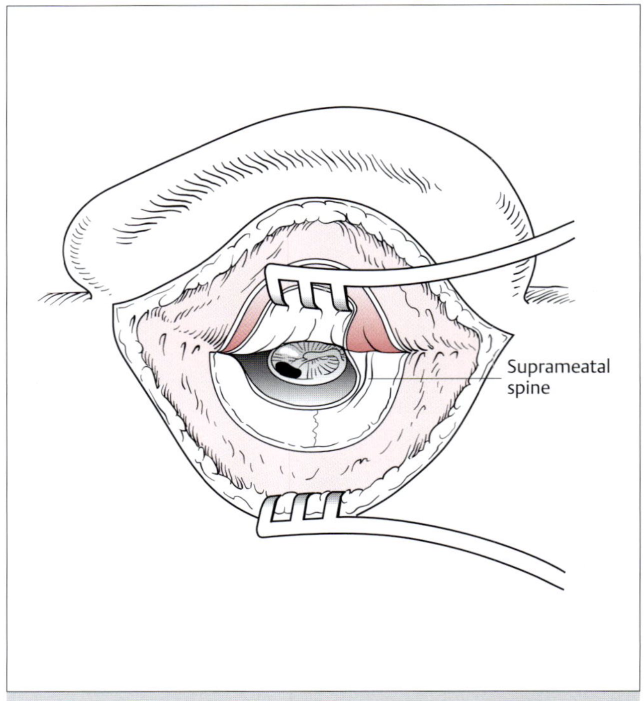

Fig. 17.7 Postauricular approach.
The meatoplasty flap is reflected laterally to expose the tympanic membrane.

retractor can be placed at right angles to the first to establish a postauricular-transcanal approach.

Enlarging the ear canal. A narrow bony ear canal can be enlarged with a burr to create a funnel-shaped cavity.

Rules, Tips, and Tricks

- Always establish sufficient access with optimum exposure.
- Any reconstructive measures should be planned preoperatively so that the incisions can be modified as needed (e. g., a Palva flap).
- The posterior aspect of the ear canal should be isolated only to the necessary extent as the remaining attachments will facilitate the incision.
- The incision around the roof of the ear canal should not cut the temporalis muscle, as this is likely to cause heavy bleeding.
- A superior oblique incision that does not expose the entire mastoid region is preferred in infants, because the facial nerve and stylomastoid foramen still occupy a far lateral position and the mastoid is still poorly developed.

! Risks and Complications

- Auricular perichondritis.
- Injury to the parotid capsule.
- Special procedures are available for managing other complications.

Alternatives

If the surgery is limited to a mastoidectomy and a tympanoplasty is not proposed, the periosteum over the mastoid cortex can be opened with an H-shaped incision and the bone exposed to the suprameatal spine, superiorly to the temporal line, and back to the posterior limit of the mastoid. The sternocleidomastoid muscle is released from the mastoid tip by a combination of blunt and sharp dissection with a periosteal knife.

Instead of a Palva flap, cavity reduction can also be accomplished with a connective tissue-periosteal flap based superiorly in the area of the temporalis muscle. It is best to divide and reflect just the skin initially and then deepen the flap through the subcutaneous connective tissue. After skirting the ear canal, the incision extends to the level of the mastoid tip and turns back upward on the posterior surface of the mastoid. The flap is raised with a periosteal knife and elevator and reflected superiorly.

Harvesting Graft Material

Autologous fascia, perichondrium, and cartilage are the principal graft materials available for repairing a tympanic membrane perforation. Graft selection depends on the size and location of the perforation, the quality of middle ear ventilation, and the workability of the graft material.

Fascia

Surgical Principle

A sufficiently large piece of temporalis fascia is exposed and dissected free. Temporalis fascia is easy to harvest, but it is more difficult to inset than perichondrium because of its poor shape stability in an undried condition.

Indications

Repair of small to medium-sized defects. Can also be used to cover cartilage palisades.

Contraindications

None.

Surgical Technique

Exposure. Starting from the access incision (endaural above the intercartilaginous incision, postauricular above the ear canal), the temporalis fascia is mobilized with a periosteal elevator and scissors. Exposure is increased with a small three-pronged retractor (**Fig. 17.8**).

Dissection. An incision at the inferior border is bluntly undermined by scissor-spreading dissection or with a periosteal elevator (**Fig. 17.9**). A patch of the desired size is outlined (remember to allow for shrinkage). Adherent fat is removed with a pointed scissors, and the graft is stored in a moist covered dish.

Alternative. Fascia can be smoothed with a fascial press and dried. The graft is easier to cut and underlay in this dried condition.

Perichondrium

Surgical Principle

A sufficiently large piece of perichondrium is dissected from the tragus or from the posterior surface of the conchal cartilage. Perichondrial grafts have a slightly better survival rate than fascial grafts and are easier to work with, even in infection-prone ears. Generally, however, they can be used only on medium-sized perforations because of their limited size, and they are more difficult to harvest than fascia.

Indications

Closure of small to medium-sized tympanic membrane defects.

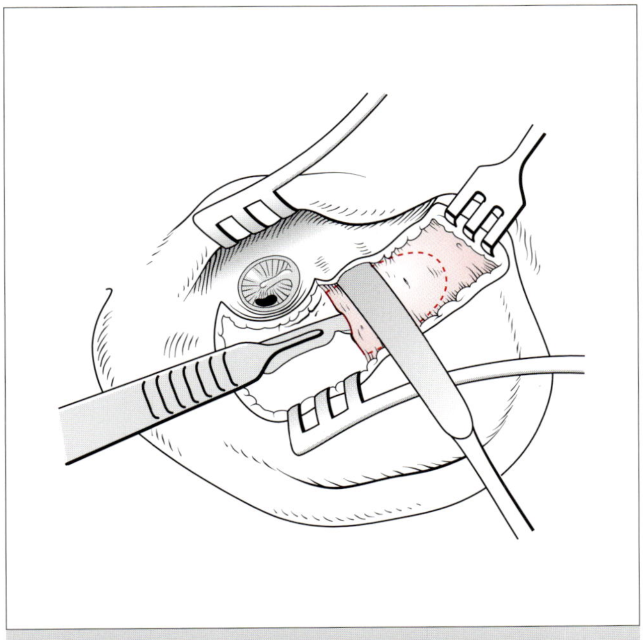

Fig. 17.8 Harvesting fascia through an endaural incision. The temporalis fascia is exposed with a periosteal elevator.

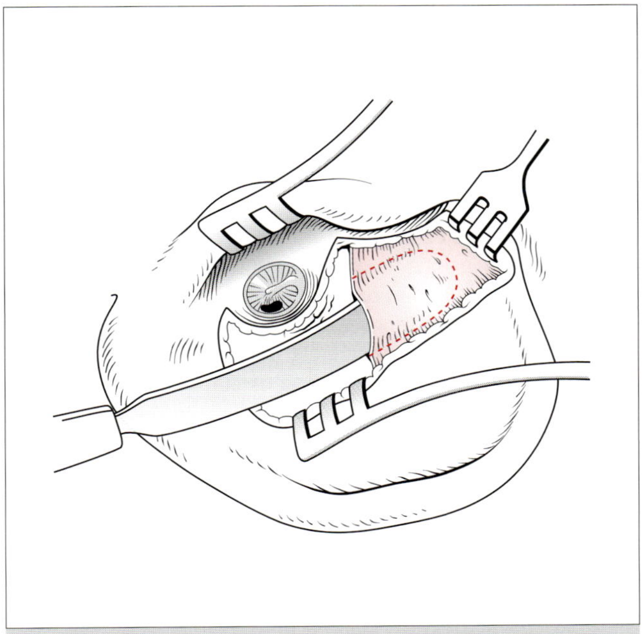

Fig. 17.9 Harvesting fascia through an endaural incision. The fascia is undermined and the graft is outlined.

Contraindications

None.

Surgical Technique

Tragus

Incision. A transverse skin incision 1–1.5 cm long skirts the ear canal ca. 5 mm below and parallel to the superior border of the tragus (**Fig. 17.10a**). The upper wound margin is retracted with a two-pronged hook.

Exposure. The cartilage surface on the meatal side is exposed by a combination of sharp and spreading dissection with a Freer elevator and dissecting scissors. The perichondrium is incised and bluntly elevated with a closed pointed scissors (**Fig. 17.10b**).

Harvesting the graft. A perichondrial graft of the desired size is harvested. If a larger flap is needed, the tragal cartilage can be exposed on the anterior and posterior sides and harvested toward the tympanic membrane after making another transverse incision. The perichondrium is incised at its border and dissected in continuity from its posterior to anterior surface (**Fig. 17.10c**). Afterward the cartilage itself is reimplanted into the pouch.

Concha

Incision. Postauricular approach.

Exposure. The soft tissue on the posterior side of the concha is elevated and the perichondrium is exposed by cutting and spreading with the scissors (**Fig. 17.11**). A finger is placed in the conchal bowl to help with plane orientation.

Harvesting the graft. The perichondrium is incised to the desired size and bluntly elevated (cutting and spreading with a pointed scissors, periosteal elevator).

Cartilage

Surgical Principle

Cartilage is harvested from the tragus or concha (e.g., from the cymba conchae) using the same technique as for perichondrium. Cartilage is easy to handle, maintains its shape, has good mechanical strength, and tends to heal well even in infection-prone ears. It is more difficult to handle than perichondrium during transplantation, however. It may be used in the form of a palisade, plate, disk, or perichondrium–cartilage composite graft.

Indications

- Defects of any size and location. Cartilage is particularly useful for repairing subtotal defects, defects associated with impaired middle ear ventilation, retraction pockets, and recurrent perforations.
- Coverage of implants.
- Reconstruction of the posterior canal wall.
- Cavity obliteration.

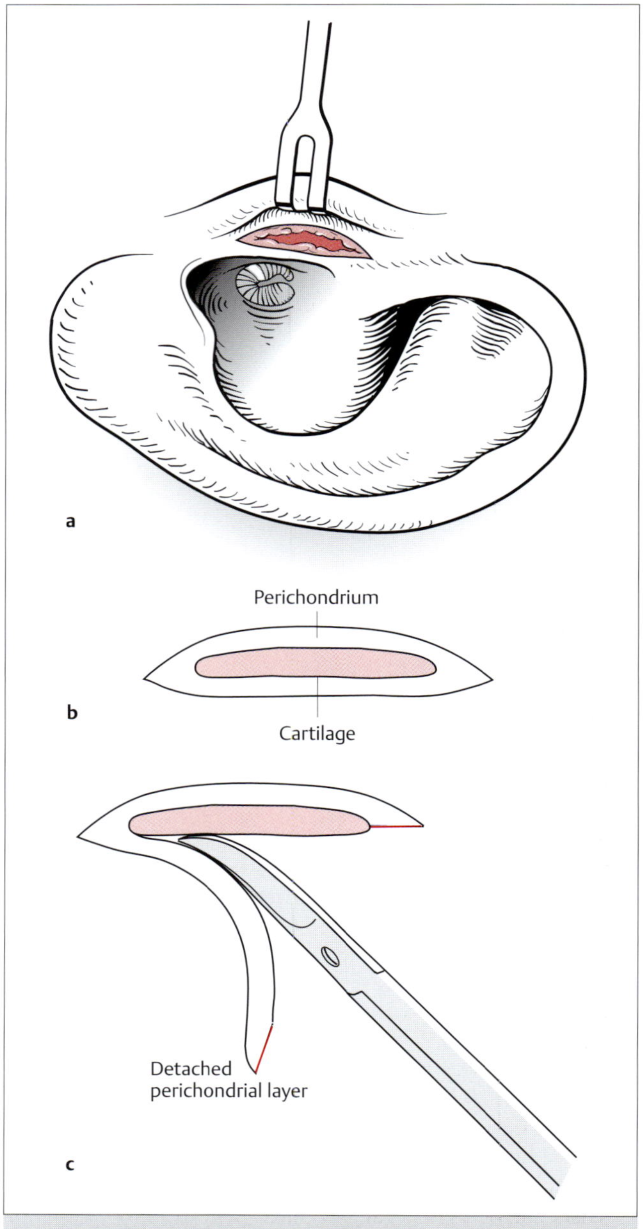

Fig. 17.10a–c Harvesting perichondrium or cartilage from the tragus.
a Incision.
b Cross-sectional view of the cartilage.
c Dissection of the perichondrium. If necessary, the anterior layer of perichondrium can be harvested in continuity with the posterior layer to obtain a larger graft.

Contraindications

None.

Surgical Technique

Incision. Cartilage is exposed by the same approach as used for harvesting perichondrium. The anterior cartilage surface of the tragus is additionally exposed, leaving the perichondrium on

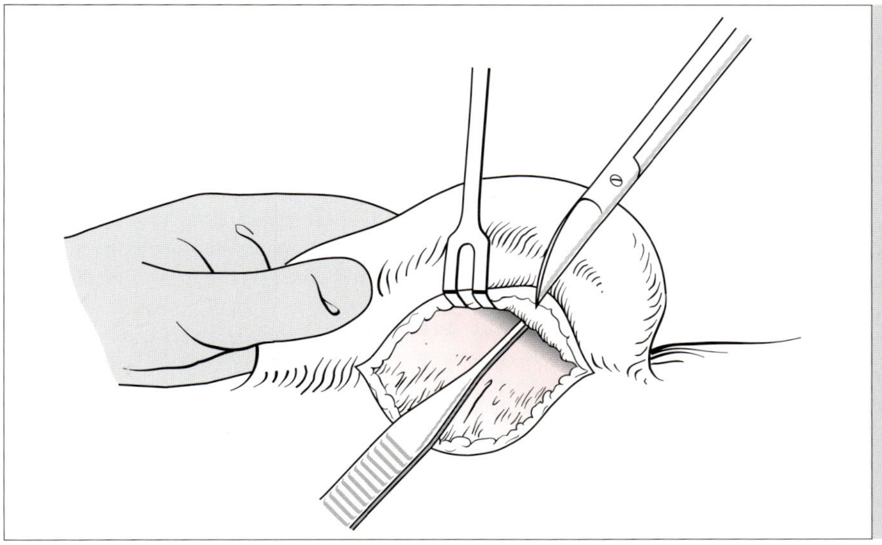

Fig. 17.11 Harvesting perichondrium and cartilage from the auricular concha.

the cartilage. This is done by deepening the transverse skin incision through the cartilage and leaving the tragal dome intact to preserve the outer contour.

Harvesting the graft. The exposed cartilage is outlined to the desired graft size and removed, leaving the tragus with an outer supporting framework if required. Hemostasis must be meticulous.

When conchal cartilage has been harvested, the concha is packed with ointment-impregnated strips for 3–5 days to prevent othematoma.

Cartilage Preparation

Palisades. The harvested cartilage and perichondrium is cross-cut into strips ca. 0.2 mm thick with a scalpel or cartilage slicer (e.g., Kurz). These struts are trimmed to the desired length when they are implanted.

Plates. Can be used as full-thickness slabs or cut into slices 0.1–1.0 mm thick, depending on the necessary mechanical strength.

Disk. Can be used in full or reduced thickness for placement between the head of an ossicular prosthesis and the tympanic membrane.

Perichondrium–cartilage composite graft. Particularly useful for subtotal defects. Usually the cartilage is harvested larger than the requisite graft size and is thinned on one side only, leaving the perichondrium intact on the other side. A cartilage ring at least 3–4 mm wide is cut from the thinned side with a scalpel or round incision knife, elevated from the opposite perichondrium, and discarded (**Fig. 17.12**). This leaves a central cartilage disk adherent to the perichondrium, which can then be divided for easier use or incised to accommodate the manubrium of the malleus. The graft is placed with the cartilage toward the middle ear cavity and the perichondrium applied to the lower part of the tympanic membrane.

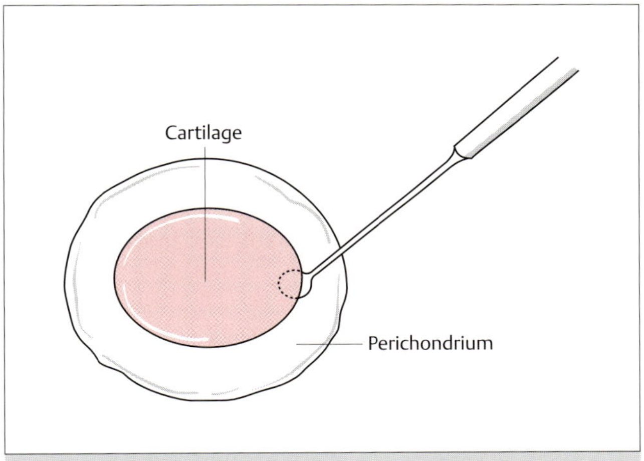

Fig. 17.12 Harvesting perichondrium and cartilage. A composite island graft is created by separating a cartilage ring from the underlying perichondrium.

> **! Risks and Complications of Harvesting Cartilage and Perichondrium**
> - Auricular perichondritis.
> - Injury to the parotid capsule.
> - Alteration of tragal contours.
> - Distortion of the cartilaginous ear canal due to scarring.

Implants

Autologous malleus and incus grafts are still considered biologically optimum materials for reconstructing ossicular discontinuities, although their long-term stability has been called into question. The use of ossicles from cholesteatoma ears has also been questioned, and the use of ossicular allografts is considered obsolete because of the potential for infection.

Numerous synthetic implant materials (ceramics, plastics, bone cement, metals) have been investigated in recent years for their mechanical properties, biocompatibility, biostability, clinical results, and custom-fitting capabilities. Studies have shown that no single material is best for all applications, although titanium has become the dominant material in reconstructive middle ear surgery because it is lighter and stiffer than gold, is resilient, can be custom-fitted, is very biocompatible, and has good sound-conduction properties based in part on new designs with a clip mechanism and a slender shape that permit visual inspection of the coupling site.

Ossicular prostheses are available for partial or total replacement of the ossicular chain (PORP = partial ossicular chain replacement prosthesis, TORP = total ossicular chain replacement prosthesis).

Ceramic prostheses (aluminum oxide ceramic, glass ceramic, hydroxyapatite) can be custom-shaped with a diamond burr. Tricalcium phosphate ceramic is used for cavity obliteration.

Teflon and other plastics have a place in stapes surgery, including use as piston coatings for metal prostheses.

Metals: Although titanium is the overall material of choice, gold and platinum implants are also still used in stapes surgery, for example.

Rules, Tips, and Tricks

- A cartilage disk can be interposed between the head of an ossicular allograft and the tympanic membrane.
- The prosthesis should be very accurately sized for length. It should be long enough to tent the tympanic membrane slightly without exerting too much pressure on the stapes or footplate.
- An interposed cartilage disk on the head of a prosthesis should not come into contact with the bony framework (poor sound conduction due to fixation).
- The chorda (if present) can be used to stabilize the prosthesis.
- A TORP can be further stabilized on the footplate by placing a thin cartilage plate across the base of the stapes arch with a central perforation to accommodate the prosthesis.

! Risks and Complications

- Extrusion of the implant.
- Absorption of the implant.
- Tilting and dislocation of the implant.
- Bony fixation of the implant.
- Footplate perforation or rupture of the annular ligament.

18 Tympanoplasty

Surgical Principle

- Tympanoplasty encompasses a range of surgical measures to improve hearing and eradicate disease in patients with chronic otitis media, tympanic membrane perforation, or ossicular discontinuity.
- The tympanic membrane can be reconstructed with fascia, perichondrium, or cartilage. The ossicular chain can be reconstructed with autologous or synthetic material. This chapter reviews the basic techniques involved in reconstructing the tympanic membrane and ossicular chain and eradicating disease in the middle ear cavity or mastoid.
- The classic Wullstein classification of tympanoplasties is expanded by adding two subgroups to the type III reconstruction: A, in which the stapes is present, and B, in which only the footplate is present.

Indications

- Dry or wet, central or peripheral tympanic membrane perforation with or without an ossicular discontinuity, possibly after prior surgery for inflammatory middle ear disease.
- Adhesive processes, tympanosclerosis, sequelae to a petrous bone fracture or middle ear trauma, suspected ossicular discontinuity following an old antrotomy.
- Candidates for an ossicular reconstruction should have an air-bone gap of at least 20 dB and acceptable inner ear function.

Contraindications

- Deafness in the opposite ear (relative).
- Limited capacity for follow-up care, as in small children (relative).
- Poor inner ear function (drainage only).
- Otogenic complications (relative, may necessitate a two-stage procedure).
- Simultaneous tympanoplasty in both ears (a 3-month interval should elapse between the two procedures).
- Very severe otorrhea and otitis externa (relative).

Specific Points Regarding Informed Consent

- Lack of hearing improvement, exacerbation of hearing loss, or deafness (may be delayed due to implant problems).
- Tinnitus.
- Vertigo.
- Altered taste sensation (chorda tympani).
- Recurrent perforation, graft rejection, otorrhea, cholesteatoma formation, reoperation, second-look procedure.
- Intracranial complications.
- Heavy scarring of the incision and auricle, keloid formation.
- Neuralgiform pain.
- Facial nerve injury.
- Patients may be told to avoid diving or flying for a certain period.

Surgical Principle

- PT, PTT, platelet count, simple blood count.
- Complete audiometry, test for spontaneous nystagmus and fistula symptoms, Schüller radiograph, high-resolution CT if required.
- Perioperative antibiotics may be indicated.

Special Instruments

- Otomicroscope
- Small drill, variable speed to 40 000 rpm, with an angled handpiece; drill bits and burrs of varying size, shape (round, cylindrical, pear-shaped), and finish (diamond, hard metal).
- Set of round incision knifes, small hooks, needles, curettes (House), antrum hooks, Rosen elevator.
- Assorted otologic microforceps (e.g., Heermann), cup microforceps, malleus head punch, middle ear scissors, Weingartner grasping forceps.
- Suction tips, microsuction tips, suction-irrigators.
- Bipolar coagulation.
- Manual and self-retaining retractors (Plester, Helms).

Anesthesia

Local or general anesthesia.

Reconstruction of the Tympanic Membrane

Type I Tympanoplasty

Surgical Technique

Positioning. The patient is positioned supine with the head turned to the side and immobilized on a headrest or ring.

Approach. Endaural or postauricular (Chapter 17). The graft is harvested, and the plane of the tympanic membrane is adequately exposed with self-retaining retractors. If necessary, the entrance to the ear canal can be enlarged with a burr.

Recipient bed. The margins of the perforation are freshened by cutting around them with a sickle knife held at an oblique angle to the tympanic membrane. A microforceps grips the resected tissue with the margins under tension (**Fig. 18.1a, b**).

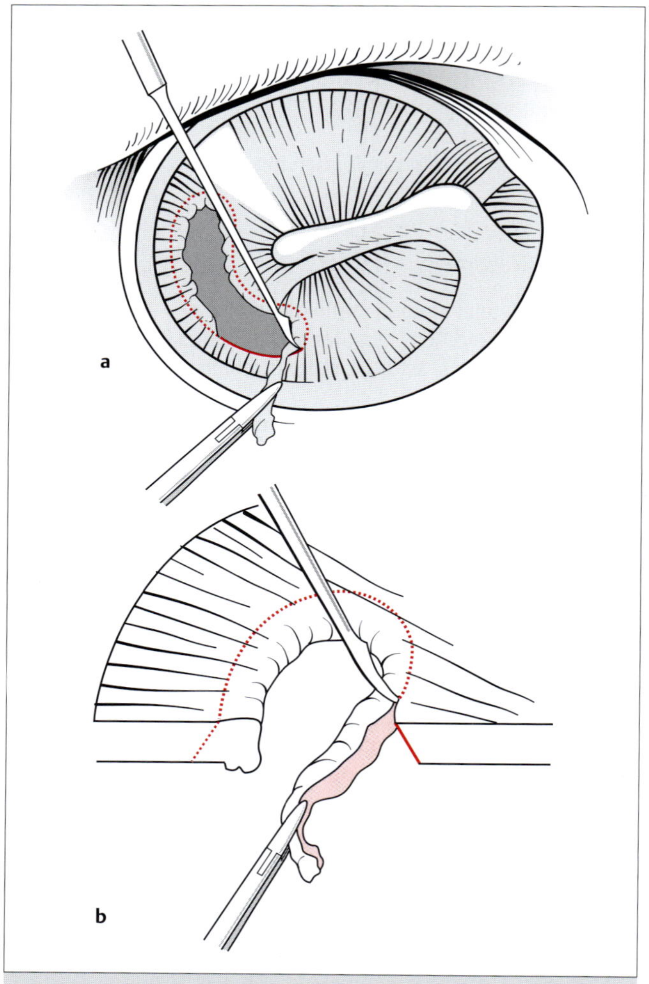

Fig. 18.1a, b Tympanoplasty.
a The margins of the tympanic membrane perforation are freshened with a sickle knife while a microforceps keeps the margins tense.
b The knife is angled relative to the plane of the tympanic membrane.

This step is always completed before the tympanic annulus is separated from the sulcus.

Tympanomeatal flap. The tympanomeatal flap is outlined with a straight round knife. Cuts are made at the 11 and 5 o'clock positions in the right ear and at 1 and 7 o'clock in the left ear (see **Fig 17.3** and **Fig. 18.2**; see also Chapter 17). The meatal flap is elevated toward the tympanic membrane from the bone with an angled round incision knife, aided by a suction tip (**Fig. 18.3**).

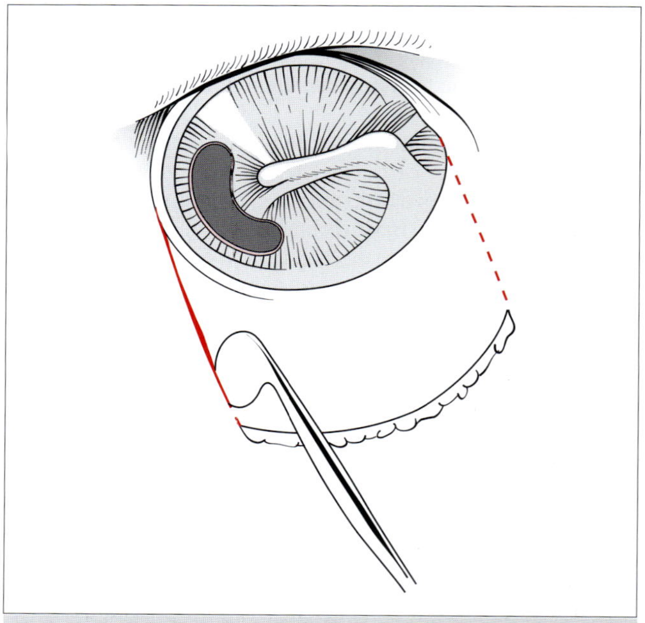

Fig. 18.2 Tympanoplasty.
Outlining the tympanomeatal flap.

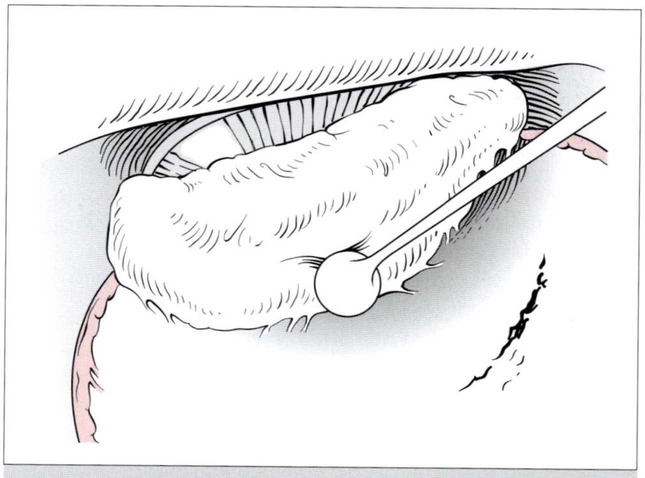

Fig. 18.3 Tympanoplasty.
The tympanomeatal flap is elevated from the bone.

Opening the middle ear cavity. The middle ear cavity is opened in the posterosuperior quadrant, where the annulus is easier to detach from the sulcus. As the tympanomeatal flap is raised, the thin mucoperiosteum becomes tense and can be divided without damaging the chorda tympani. The annulus fibrosus is dissected from the sulcus below the attachment of the chorda tympani, using first a sickle knife and then a round incision knife. The mobilized tympanomeatal flap is reflected forward (**Fig. 18.4**).

Evaluation of the ossicular chain. The bony posterolateral attic wall (area that can be under-run with a round knife) is taken down with the House curette—after first thinning it with a diamond burr if necessary—until the long process of the incus, the stapes, and the tympanic facial nerve segment can be identified (**Fig. 18.5**). At this point the manubrium of the malleus is probed very gently with a needle to assess the continuity and mobility of the ossicular chain.

Graft selection. The graft (fascia, perichondrium, or cartilage) is sized so that it will safely overlap the perforation on all sides and extend slightly onto the posterior canal wall (to allow for shrinkage; see Chapter 17).

Graft placement. The graft is introduced into the middle ear cavity with a needle and suction tip, allowing approximately 3 mm of overlap between the graft and perforation margins. The graft may be placed medial to the manubrium and is held in place by adhesion (underlay technique, **Fig. 18.6**). Later the posterior portion of the graft will be below the tympanomeatal flap and will slightly overlap the bony posterior wall of the ear canal.

Rules, Tips, and Tricks

- Graft overlap of the perforation margins should be sufficient to allow for graft shrinkage, and adequate contact should be established between the graft and manubrium.
- Avoid lateralization of the tympanic membrane.
- Placing gelatin sponge in the middle ear to support the graft should be done very sparingly, if at all, because of the risk of scar adhesions.
- The postauricular approach is better for very anterior perforations. A somewhat larger tympanomeatal flap is raised, extending to ca. 2 o'clock in the right ear and 10 o'clock in the left ear, to facilitate anterior pull-through of the graft.

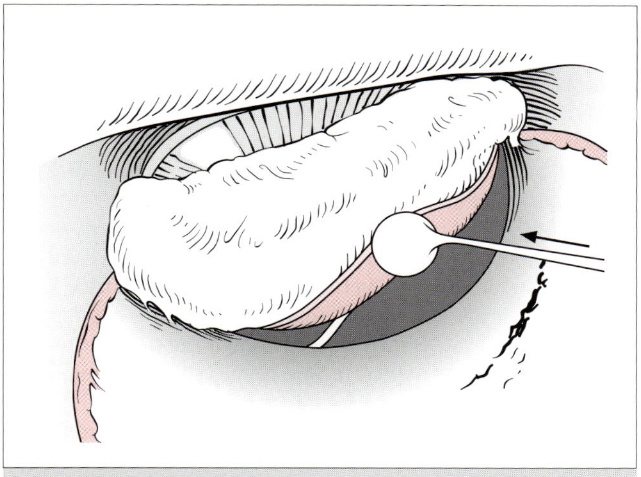

Fig. 18.4 Tympanoplasty.
The middle ear cavity is opened in the posterosuperior quadrant. The mucoperiosteum is divided while the chorda tympani is preserved.

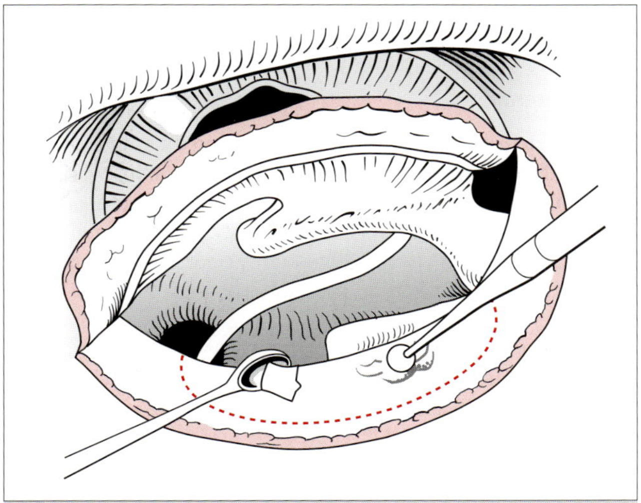

Fig. 18.5 Tympanoplasty.
The posterolateral attic wall is taken down so that the ossicular chain can be assessed.

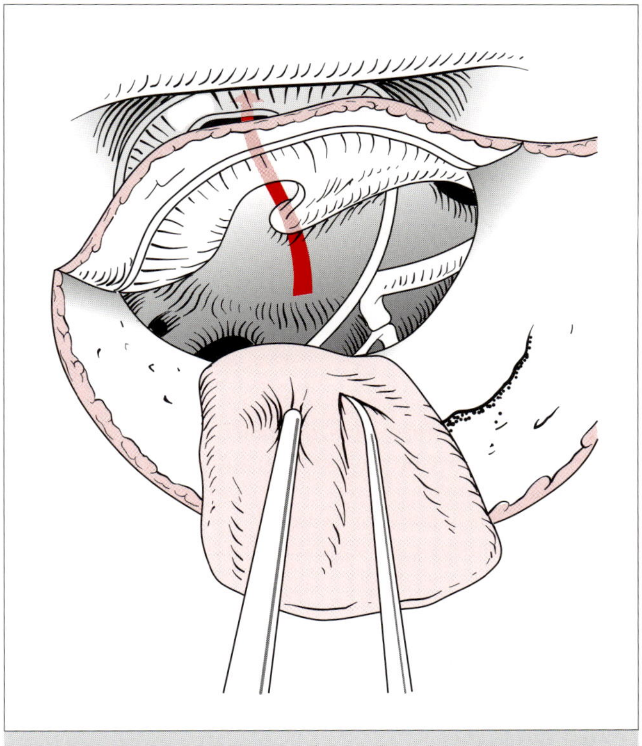

Fig. 18.6 Tympanoplasty.
The graft is placed behind the tympanic membrane and medial to the manubrium (underlay technique).

18

- Scar adhesions or mucosal folds that obstruct ventilation should be divided.
- Broad adhesions with the promontory wall or ossicular chain should be widely cleared while preserving the mucoperiosteum. The cartilage palisade technique is used for tympanic membrane reconstruction.
- Nitrous oxide administration should be discontinued during graft placement as it may cause the graft to separate from the perforation.

Returning the flap. The tympanomeatal flap is returned to its original position with meticulous reapproximation of the flap margins. Rounded silastic strips (**Fig. 18.7**) are placed into the ear canal to cover the junction of the replaced meatoplasty and tympanomeatal flap while also supporting the graft from the lateral side (**Fig. 18.8**).

Wound closure. The ear canal is packed with antibiotic-impregnated gelatin sponge and short, superficial strips. The wound is closed in layers.

! Risks and Complications

- Iatrogenic cholesteatoma (flap cholesteatoma caused, for example, by incomplete detachment of the annulus from the sulcus).
- Auricular perichondritis, distortion due to scarring.
- Conductive hearing loss due to ossicular dislocation or poor vibration characteristics of the graft.
- Facial paralysis may be harmless and transient due to local anesthesia. Otherwise, immediate facial nerve reconstruction is required.
- Sensorineural hearing loss, tinnitus, vestibular nerve damage (e.g., due to manipulation of the ossicular chain, contact with drill, suction or drilling noise).
- Recurrent perforation, otorrhea, graft rejection.
- Altered taste sensation due to chorda tympani lesion.
- Excessive scarring, keloid formation, neuralgiform pain.
- Meatal stenosis, epithelial defects.
- Wound infection.

Postoperative Care

- Perioperative antibiotics.
- Patients with postoperative infection or poor wound healing should receive broad-spectrum antibiotics until culture results are known.
- Packing is left in place for 3 weeks.
- Valsalva maneuvers are started on the first postoperative day.
- See Chapter 14 for details.

18

Alternatives

Closure Technique

Modified underlay technique. With a lack of residual anterior membrane, the graft can be delivered to the repair site using a pull-through technique. The anterior annulus is undermined to the bone at one or two points with a sickle knife, and one end of the graft is pulled through the tunnel to the plane of the tympanic membrane with a tiny hook or suction tip (**Fig. 18.9**). If an adequate margin is present, the same technique can be used on the anterior pars tensa without undermining the annulus.

Onlay technique. The epithelium is elevated from the tympanic membrane surface along with the manubrium and returned after the graft has been placed on the tunica propria. The margins of the perforation are freshened, and the tympanomeatal flap is dissected with an angled round knife over the firmly adherent posteroinferior annulus onto the tunica propria. In this way the tympanic membrane epidermis can be developed anteriorly in continuity with the tympanomeatal flap. It is dissected from the manubrium and short process with a sickle knife.

There is a risk that a flap cholesteatoma may form as a result of residual squamous epithelium, and blunting of the tympanomeatal angle may occur. Advantages are a more stable anterior graft placement and a normal volume of the middle ear cavity.

Myringoplasty. *Special type of type I tympanoplasty:* The tympanic membrane is closed with an underlay technique without evaluating the ossicular chain and without mobilizing the posterior annulus (prerequisites are a healthy tympanic membrane and middle ear and no conductive impairment). Generally this procedure involves an endaural approach with an autologous graft, freshening the perforation with a sickle knife, and removing the rim of loose epithelium with a cup forceps. A small fascial graft is introduced through the perforation and approximated to the medial surface of the tympanic membrane with a needle and suction tip.

Reperforations. *Small reperforations:* With a dry middle ear, the margins of the perforation are freshened with a sickle knife and the epithelial rim is removed. A pressed, postauricular fat-connective tissue graft is passed through the perforation with a needle, approximated with a microsuction tip, and covered laterally with silastic film.

Larger reperforations require a repeat tympanoplasty, which is done after sequelae and swelling from the initial procedure have subsided.

Graft Materials

Perichondrium. This material is best suited for small to medium-sized tympanic membrane defects that are susceptible to infection. It is similar to fascia in its workability and handling.

Cartilage. Cartilage is preferred for reconstructing subtotal defects, closing defects associated with poor ventilation or retraction pockets, recurrent perforations, and infection-prone ears.

The palisade technique is particularly useful for very anterior defects without adequate margins, impaired eustachian tube ventilation, and adhesive processes.

Cartilage–perichondrium composite grafts with a cartilage disk are excellent for reconstructing subtotal defects or old welding spatter injuries. The central cartilage disk (see Chapter 17, p. 365) is placed with its perichondrial side against the tympanic membrane. It can also be incised for easier application, or a portion may be excised to accommodate the (de-epithelial-

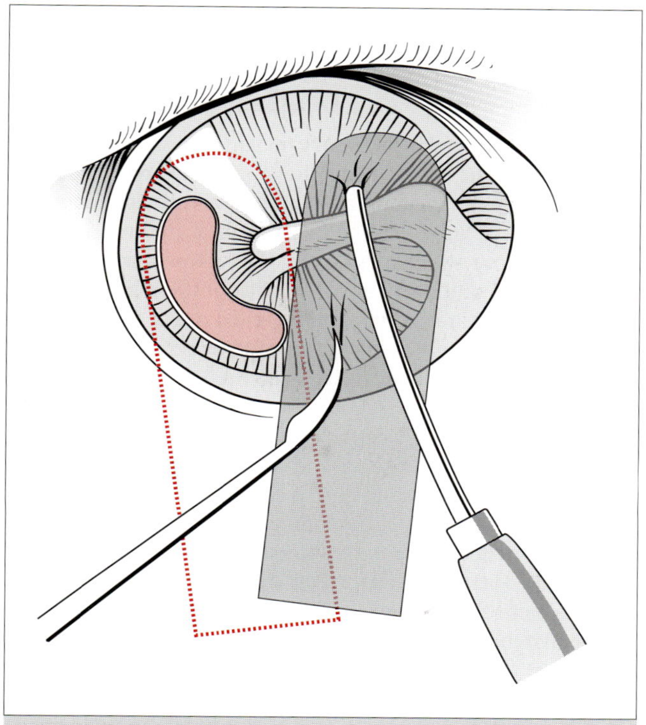

Fig. 18.7 Tympanoplasty.
Inserting the silastic film.

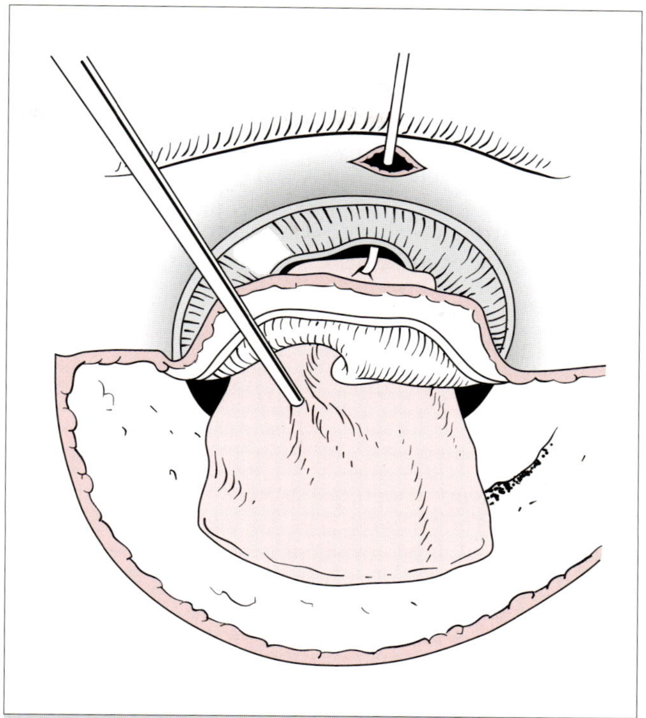

Fig. 18.9 Tympanoplasty.
Modified underlay technique for a deficient anterior recipient bed. The graft is grasped at one end and pulled into place.

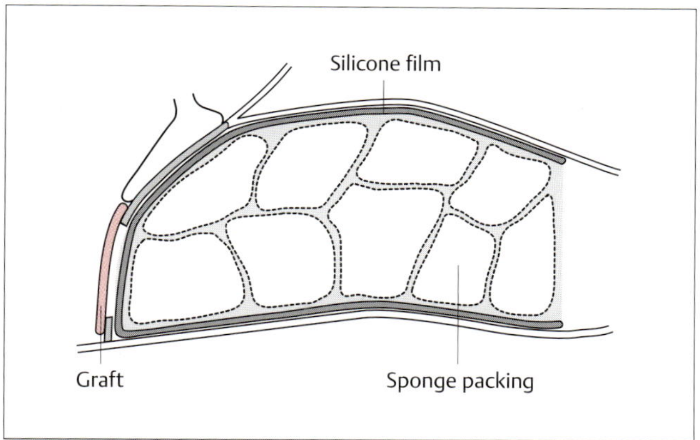

Fig. 18.8 Tympanoplasty.
Longitudinal section of the ear canal shows the graft position, gelatin sponge packing, and silastic film.

ized) manubrium ("under-overlay" technique). A pure cartilage disk graft is worked and used in much the same way.

Palisades. Approximately six precut cartilage struts (see Chapter 17, p. 365) are wedged into place beneath the tympanic membrane from one side of the perforation to the other, all directed parallel to the manubrium. They are shortened according to their position so that their intrinsic tension creates a slight bow (**Fig. 18.10a, b**). The struts are covered laterally with perichondrium or fascia.

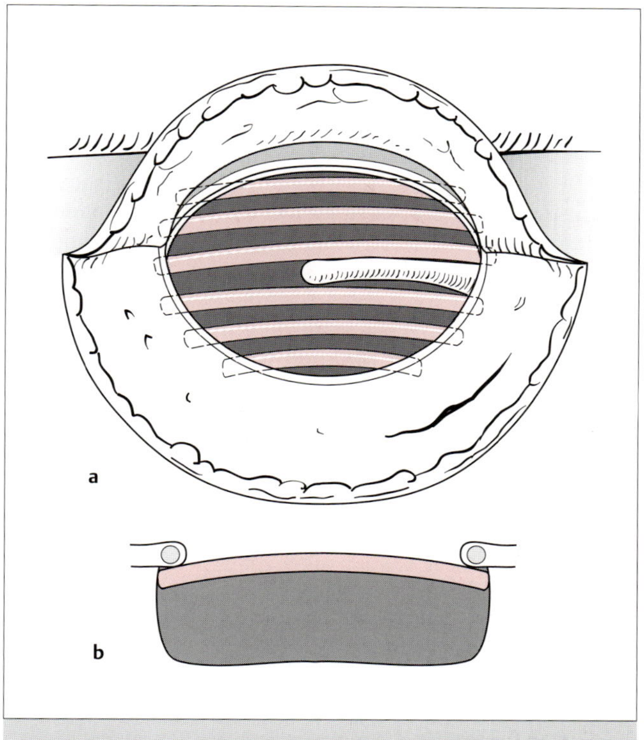

Fig. 18.10a, b Tympanoplasty. Palisade technique.
a The palisades are placed parallel to the manubrium.
b They are wedged into a slightly bowed position within the middle ear cavity.

18

Ossicular Chain Reconstruction

An ossicular chain reconstruction follows evaluation of the ossicular chain and the eradication of middle ear disease. It is done after the tympanic membrane graft has been placed and before the tympanomeatal flap is replaced to close the middle ear cavity.

The reconstructive measures vary according to the location and extent of the ossicular defect.

Lenticular Process Defect (Type II Tympanoplasty)

Surgical Technique

A defect in the lenticular process or incudostapedial joint is reconstructed and bridged with glass ionomer cement. While still malleable, a small bead of cement is placed on the head (capitulum) of the stapes and shaped with a round knife or Rosen elevator to form a connection with the incus. This process can be repeated if necessary during the several minutes it takes for the cement to harden. Before the cement is applied, the oval and round windows should be protected from accidental contact (e.g., covered with Gelfoam).

Alternative

Conversion to a type IIIA tympanoplasty by interposition (see below).

Incus Defect or Loss (Type IIIA Tympanoplasty)

Surgical Principle

The defect is bridged with a partial ossicular chain replacement prosthesis (PORP) (stapes elevation) consisting of autologous ossicles or synthetic material (preferably a titanium implant, see Chapter 17).

Incus-to-Stapes or Malleus-to-Stapes Reconstruction

Indications

- Ossicular discontinuity in which the stapes is intact and the body of the incus or malleus head shows no abnormalities.
- Isolated idiopathic fixation of the malleus head (where mobilization would risk reankylosis).

Contraindications

Osteitic or cholesteatomatous involvement of the ossicles that are needed for autologous replacement.

Surgical Technique

Removal. The ossicular chain is evaluated, and somewhat more of the lateral attic wall is taken down. A needle or 90° hook is passed up into the incudomalleolar joint and rotated about its axis to separate the joint. The incus is dislocated with the 90° hook. To remove the malleus head, the lateral attic wall must be taken down anteriorly until the neck of the malleus can be seen. While the chorda tympani is pulled down from the cutting plane, a malleus head nipper is placed on the malleus neck under vision. The malleus head is removed and retrieved with a needle (**Fig. 18.11**).

Grinding the graft. The incus or malleus head is held with a grasping forceps. The short and long processes of the incus are ground with a diamond burr. A socket for the stapes head is ground into the stump of the long process or into the cut surface of the malleus head with a fine diamond burr (**Figs. 18.12** and **18.13**). The size of the socket should only slightly exceed the diameter of the stapes head.

Reconstruction. Following placement of the tympanic membrane graft, the head of the malleus or body of the incus is gripped on its rounded surface with a microsuction tip and advanced to the stapes head. It is held at a slight angle to the suction axis so that its relation to the stapes head can be seen. A needle is used to seat the socket precisely on the capitulum and align the graft over the stapes, at which point the suction is released. The graft can be further stabilized by placing it against the chorda tympani (**Fig. 18.14**).

Generally the incus is braced against the side of the manubrium. This position can be stabilized by burring a notch into the short process for articulation with the manubrium (**Fig. 18.15**).

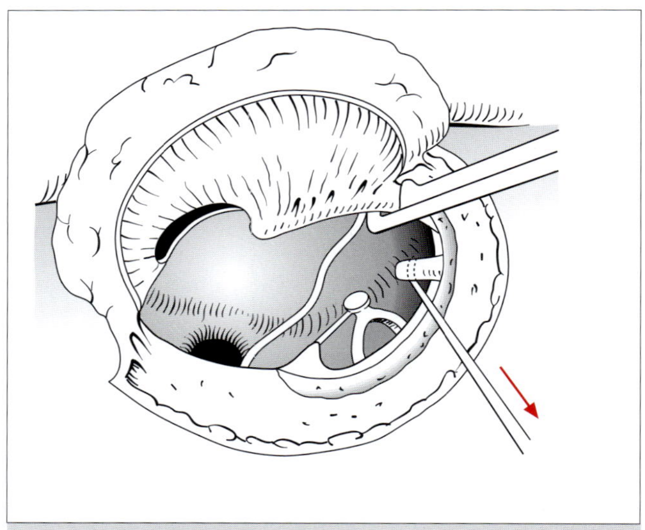

Fig. 18.11 Tympanoplasty.
The body of the incus is removed with a 90° hook. The head of the malleus is removed from the malleus neck with a nipper while the chorda tympani is retracted downward.

18

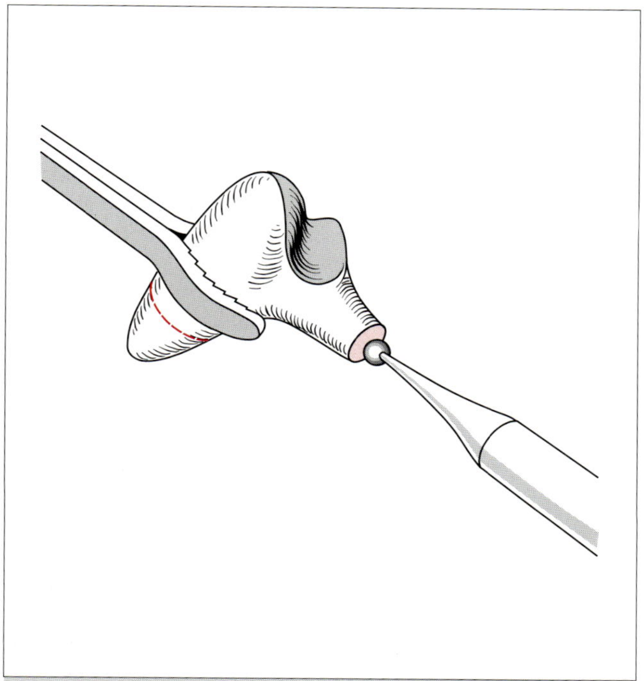

Fig. 18.12 Tympanoplasty.
Grinding the incus.

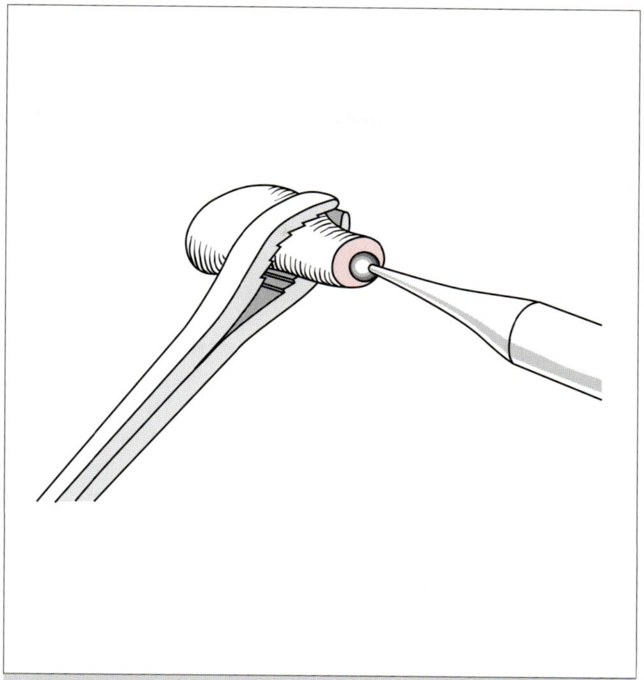

Fig. 18.13 Tympanoplasty.
A socket is drilled in the resected malleus head to receive the head of the stapes.

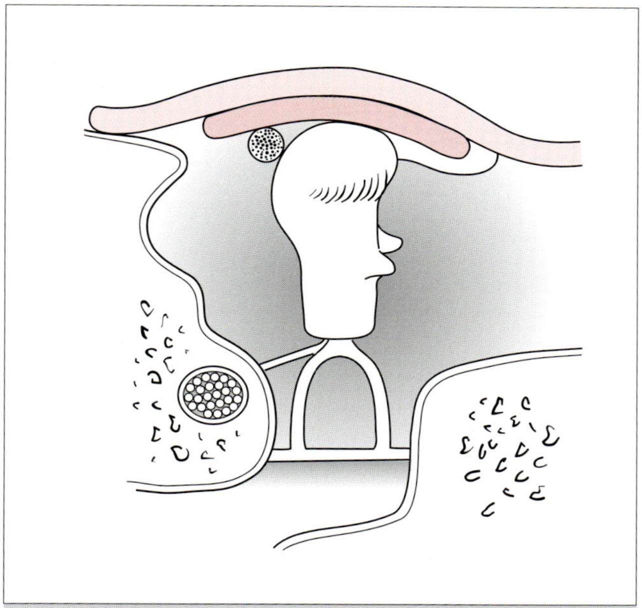

Fig. 18.14 Tympanoplasty.
The malleus head is positioned on top of the stapes. It is apposed to the chorda tympani for added stability. A cartilage cap can be interposed if the manubrium is absent.

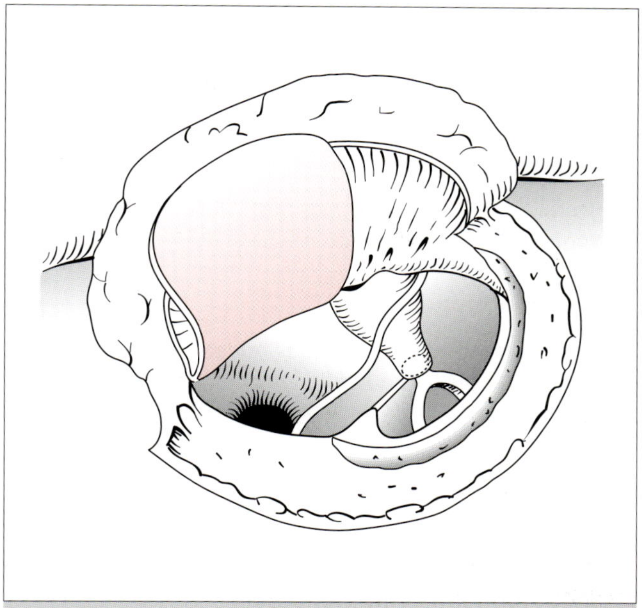

Fig. 18.15 Tympanoplasty.
The incus is positioned on the stapes and apposed to the manubrium.

Titanium Partial Ossicular Chain Replacement Prosthesis (PORP)

Indications

Ossicular discontinuity with an intact stapes, especially when the incus and malleus head are absent. Also appropriate for adhesive processes.

Surgical Technique

The correct length of the prosthesis is determined. The sized implant is advanced to the stapes with a microforceps or suction tip, and the foot of the prosthesis is placed onto the stapes head. It may be necessary to crimp the bell of the prosthesis over the capitulum, depending on the implant design, but it is better to use an implant with self-retaining spring tabs. The head plate of the prosthesis is braced against the manubrium, if this structure is present and has not been medialized. A cartilage cap slightly larger than the head plate should always be interposed between the manubrium and prosthesis (**Fig. 18.16a, b**).

Alternatives

- The defect can be bridged with a ceramic prosthesis.
- If the distance between the manubrium and stapes head is relatively short and the manubrium is not medialized, a ceramic prosthesis can be interposed that bears a socket for the stapes head and a notch for the manubrium.
- A malleostapediopexy, in which a wire is looped around the partially undermined manubrium and extends to the stapes head, is rarely performed today because the manipulations may dislocate the stapes.

Stapes Defect

Isolated Stapes Defect

Incudopalatinopexy

An absent stapes superstructure is bridged with a wire prosthesis that is looped around the long process of the incus and engages against a connective tissue graft on the footplate.

Combined Stapes Defect

Total Ossicular Chain Replacement Prosthesis (TORP) (Type IIIB Tympanoplasty)

18

Indications

Ossicular discontinuity with absence of the incus and stapes arch or the entire ossicular chain.

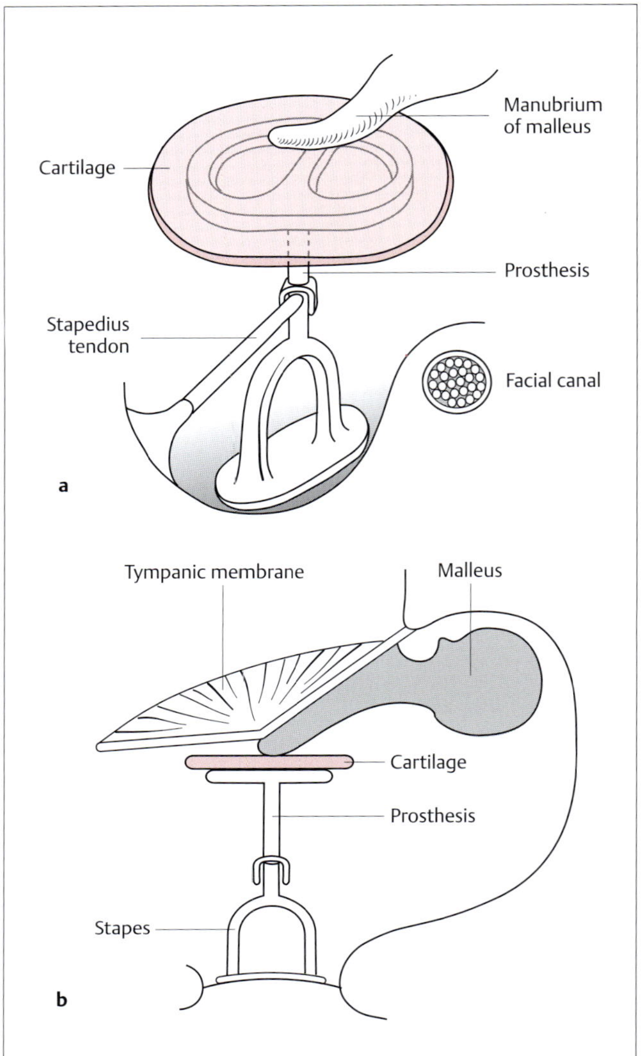

Fig. 18.16a, b Tympanoplasty.
Ossicular chain reconstruction with a titanium PORP.
a The prosthesis is placed between the manubrium and stapes head. A cartilage cap overlaps the head plate of the prosthesis on all sides.
b Sectional view.

Surgical Technique

Titanium implants are preferred. The necessary implant length is measured and sized. Ideally the implant should be just long enough to tent the tympanic membrane slightly without exerting too much pressure on the footplate. The TORP is positioned on the footplate (**Fig. 18.17a, b**). It can be stabilized by wedging a small cartilage plate between the crural stumps, the plate bearing a central socket for the foot of the TORP. When a fascial graft is used, a cartilage disk is interposed between the head plate of the prosthesis and the tympanic membrane remnant. When a cartilage–perichondrium composite graft is used, it is sufficient to have full contact between the cartilage and the head plate of the prosthesis. If the manubrium is present, the head plate should be braced against the side of the manubrium

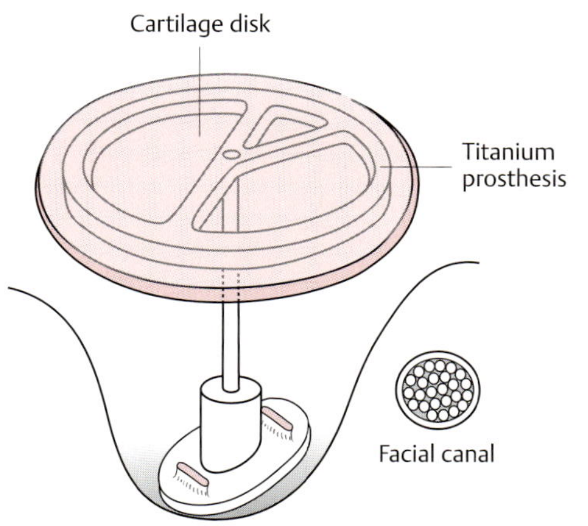

a

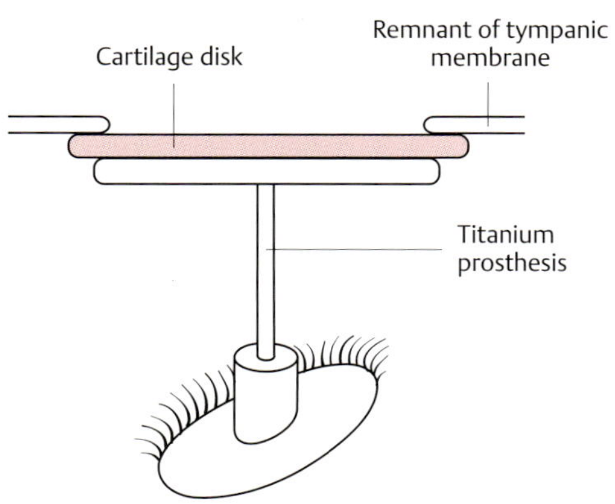

b

Fig. 18.17a, b Tympanoplasty.
Ossicular chain reconstruction with a titanium TORP.
a The prosthesis is seated in the oval window niche.
b Sectional view.

or placed beneath it. If this tilts the prosthesis shaft by more than 45°, however, the TORP should be placed directly beneath the tympanic membrane graft without having this contact.

Rules, Tips, and Tricks

- The PORP or TORP reconstruction should be long enough to slightly tent the tympanic membrane or graft.
- When a synthetic prosthesis is used or an autologous graft is used with an absent manubrium, a cartilage plate or disk should be interposed between the head plate of the prosthesis and the tympanic membrane to prevent extrusion. This cartilage should not have any bony contact, however; otherwise it might become fixed to the bone.
- The chorda tympani (if present) should be placed against the head plate of the prosthesis or stapes elevation for stability.
- After the tympanomeatal flap has been returned, it should be slightly lifted again with the needle and suction tip to assess the position of the implant and its contact with the tympanic membrane. The head plate of the prosthesis should not have any contact with the bony frame (fixation).
- If a revision seems likely, consider using a titanium implant as it allows for optimum fixation between the autologous incus or malleus head and the stapes.
- Consider also that bone resorption may compromise the long-term results of autologous reconstructions, although the early results are usually better than with synthetic materials.

Alternatives

Type IV Tympanoplasty

Surgical principle. The round window niche is aerated via the eustachian tube while the epithelialized oval window is directly exposed to sound from the ear canal. The best audiometric result that can be obtained with this procedure is an air–bone gap of ca. 30 dB.

Indications. Absence of the ossicles, eustachian tube dysfunction, and shallow middle ear cavity. A type IV tympanoplasty is sometimes performed when the squamous epithelium of a cholesteatoma has not been completely removed from the oval window niche, or after previous radical otologic surgery.

Technique. A strip of silastic film folded lengthwise into a tube is placed between the eustachian tube and round window beneath the edge of the tympanic membrane remnant. A fascia graft is incised in trapdoor fashion and placed over the film and beneath the edge of the tympanic membrane. It spares the oval window niche, lying against the wall of the middle ear cavity medially and toward the attic. The tympanomeatal flap is laid over the graft. If the oval window niche no longer contains squamous epithelium, it is lined with some thin split-thickness skin (**Fig. 18.18a, b**).

Malleoplatinopexy

If the malleus is intact but the incus and stapes are missing, a wire prosthesis is looped around the partially undermined manubrium and is placed against a connective-tissue pad in the oval window niche (**Fig. 18.19**).

Malleovestibulopexy

With an ankylosed footplate, usually in the setting of tympanosclerosis with a fixed stapes, a two-stage procedure is performed in which the malleus head is resected, then the footplate is perforated by a stapedotomy (see Chapter 21), and a prosthesis (e.g., platinum band, Teflon piston) is hooked over the partially undermined manubrium. The piston is inserted into the perforation.

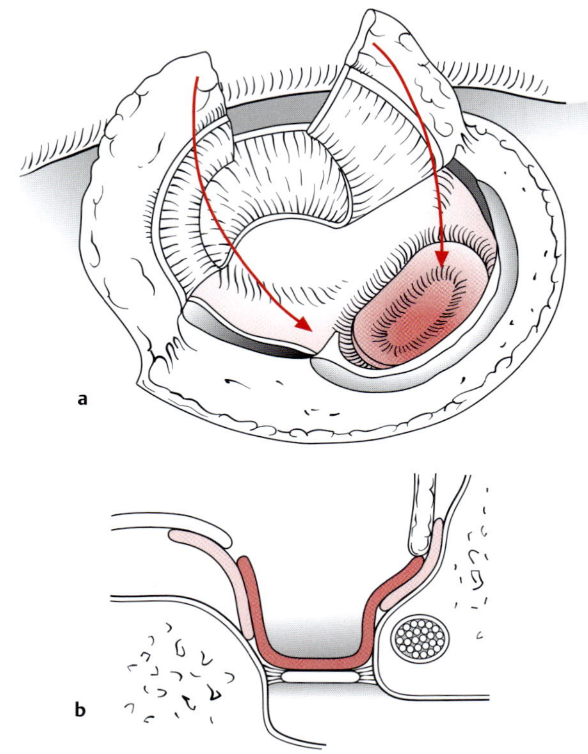

Fig. 18.18a, b Type IV tympanoplasty.
a The fascial graft and oval window niche viewed from above. The oval window niche is covered with a thin split-thickness skin graft.
b Sectional view with the grafts in place.

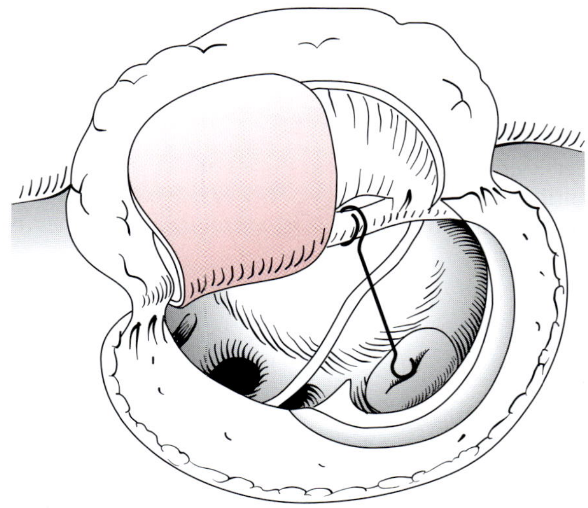

Fig. 18.19 Tympanoplasty.
Malleoplatinopexy with a wire prosthesis placed between the manubrium and footplate.

Eradication of Middle Ear Disease

Tympanosclerosis

Surgical Technique

Plaques are removed from the tympanic membrane with a sickle knife, needle, 90° hook, and cup forceps to restore membrane vibration. The surgeon proceeds much more cautiously in the middle ear cavity and especially in the oval window niche after taking down the lateral attic wall. Special care is taken about the facial nerve canal, and under no circumstances should the oval window be opened. The removal of tympanosclerosis should proceed in layers. If the stapes is mobile, the fixed incus is removed. The malleus head is resected, placed upon the capitulum for stapes elevation, and the perforation is underlaid with a graft (type IIIA tympanoplasty).

If the stapes footplate is also fixed by tympanosclerosis, stapes elevation is withheld initially, and malleovestibulopexy (see above) is performed in a second session 6–12 months later. This technique has an unfavorable audiologic prognosis, and there is a significant risk of postoperative deafness.

Granulating Process in Chronic Suppurative Otitis Media

Surgical Technique

While polyps are consistently removed as a rule, the removal of granulations from the middle ear cavity and ossicular chain with a cup forceps should be done sparingly only at sites where significant ventilation problems may occur, as good spontaneous regression tends to occur after tympanoplasty. Heavy bleeding is prevented by irrigation with naphazoline or dilute suprarenin solution. This also aids identification at critical sites such as the ossicular chain and chordofacial angle (caution: exposed facial nerve).

Otorrhea in Chronic Suppurative Otitis Media

Inspection of the Antrum

Surgical Principle

The antrum is opened by drilling a hole in the posterosuperior canal wall to assess the need for an antrotomy or mastoidectomy.

Indications

- Persistent otorrhea in chronic otitis media despite previous antibiotic therapy.
- Significant granulating process extending at least into the aditus.

Surgical Technique

After dissections in the middle ear have been completed and the lateral attic wall has been adequately taken down (facial nerve clearly visible), the posterior canal wall is drilled out at a corresponding site ca. 5–10 mm lateral to the tympanic annulus. This cavity is deepened with a diamond burr parallel to the presumed course of the skull base while preserving a bony bridge over the posterior attic, until only a thin, translucent bony layer remains over the antrum (**Fig. 18.20**). This final layer is removed with a curette. After the antrum has been inspected, the drill hole is plugged with connective tissue.

> **!** **Risks and Complications**
> - Dural injury (in patients with a low dura).
> - Facial nerve injury.
> - Incus dislocation or damage from the drill.

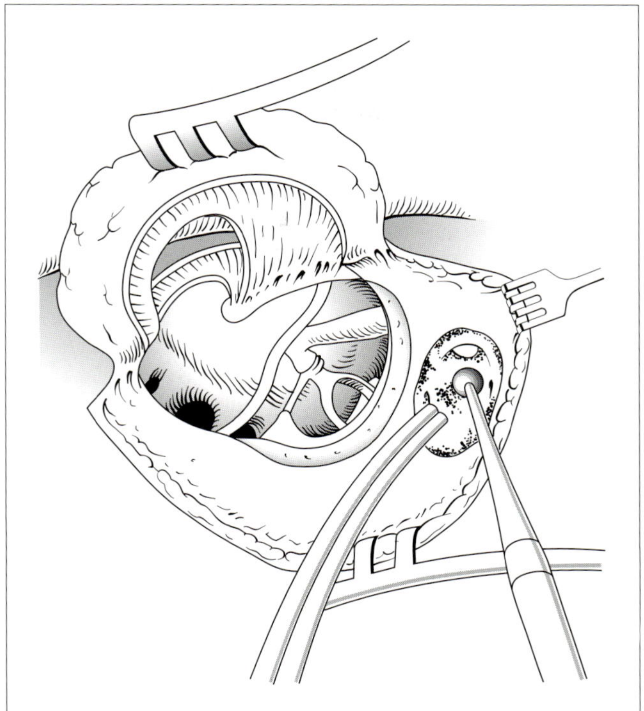

Fig. 18.20 Tympanoplasty.
Inspection of the antrum. Once the incus and facial nerve have been be positively identified in the middle ear cavity, the air cells over the posterosuperior canal roof are opened parallel to the skull base with a diamond burr.

Antrotomy or Mastoidectomy from the Mastoid Cortex during Tympanoplasty

Indications

- Tendency for massive granulation tissue formation.
- Obstruction of the antrum.
- Alternative to more technically demanding transcanal inspection of the antrum for equivocal mastoid findings.

Surgical Technique

See Chapter 19. The extent of the antrotomy/mastoidectomy is determined by actual findings. The air cells are exenterated only to the extent that significant pathology is found. The antrum must be aerated, however, and so occasionally the lateral attic wall over the incus must be carefully removed from the antrum using a House curette (**Fig. 18.21**).

A drain may be placed for several days postoperatively if drainage is copious. The surgery concludes by re-approximating the raised periosteal flap to the corresponding portion of the ear canal.

Cholesteatoma

Surgical Principle

Surgery involves the exposure and complete removal of cholesteatoma in the middle ear and mastoid, tracing the growth direction of the mass from the tympanic perforation. A simultaneous effort is made to improve hearing by tympanoplasty, prevent recurrence of the cholesteatoma, and facilitate postoperative care.

Techniques

Open or canal-wall-down technique (synonyms: radical mastoid cavity, radical cavity, atticoantrotomy, atticotomy). The cholesteatoma is removed by taking down part or all of the posterior canal wall and/or lateral attic wall. If this is followed by cavity obliteration, then (by definition) only cavity reduction by lowering the external soft tissues after removal of the mastoid tip still qualifies as an open technique. Cavity obliteration with a Palva flap or cartilage grafts is considered a secondary closed technique. Often this distinction is made intraoperatively after the cholesteatoma has been fully exposed and the size of the "radical cavity" can be assessed.

The advantages of the canal-wall-down technique over the intact-wall approach (below) are that it allows for more confident cholesteatoma removal and more reliable follow-up, and often simplifies the removal of recurrent disease. Disadvantages are more difficult postoperative care and occasional otorrhea.

Closed or intact-canal-wall technique (synonyms: anterior–posterior approach, posterior approach, atticotomy with reconstruction). The cholesteatoma is removed while preserving or reconstructing the posterior canal wall and/or lateral attic wall.

Advantages are the preservation of normal meatal function and easier follow-up care. One disadvantage is a higher recurrence rate. The posterior technique is also considered a technically demanding procedure.

For practical reasons and to simplify nomenclature, we will refer to atticoantrotomy (= radical operation) and atticotomy as the open technique, and the techniques involving canal wall reconstruction or cavity obliteration will then be presented as alternatives.

The anterior–posterior approach with primary preservation of the posterior canal wall represents the closed technique.

Atticoantrotomy (Radical Operation, Open Technique, Canal-Wall-Down Technique)

Indications

- Extensive cholesteatoma associated with poor or moderate mastoid pneumatization.
- Narrow mastoid due to an anterior sinus position or low dura.
- Complications of cholesteatoma (sinus thrombosis, meningitis).
- Cholesteatoma in children.

Surgical Technique

Approach. The postauricular approach is preferred for larger cholesteatomas, but the endaural approach can be used. If a Palva flap or periosteal-connective tissue flap will be used for cavity obliteration, it is precut at this time (see **Fig. 17.5b**).

Meatoplasty (see **Figs. 17.6** and **17.7**). The self-retaining retractors are inserted and also serve to hold back the triangular meatal flap. The entrance to the bony ear canal is enlarged with a grinder or large burr.

Tympanomeatal flap. The tympanomeatal flap is outlined with a straight round incision knife, making incisions at the 11 and 5 o'clock positions in the right ear and at 1 and 7 o'clock in the left ear (see **Fig. 17.3** and **Fig. 18.2**; see also Chapter 17). One option is to temporarily remove the meatal portion of the flap to protect it from inadvertent damage by the drill, and reimplant it later. It can be removed by making a circumferential incision just lateral to the tympanic membrane with an angled round incision knife and temporarily storing the excised flap in NaCl solution.

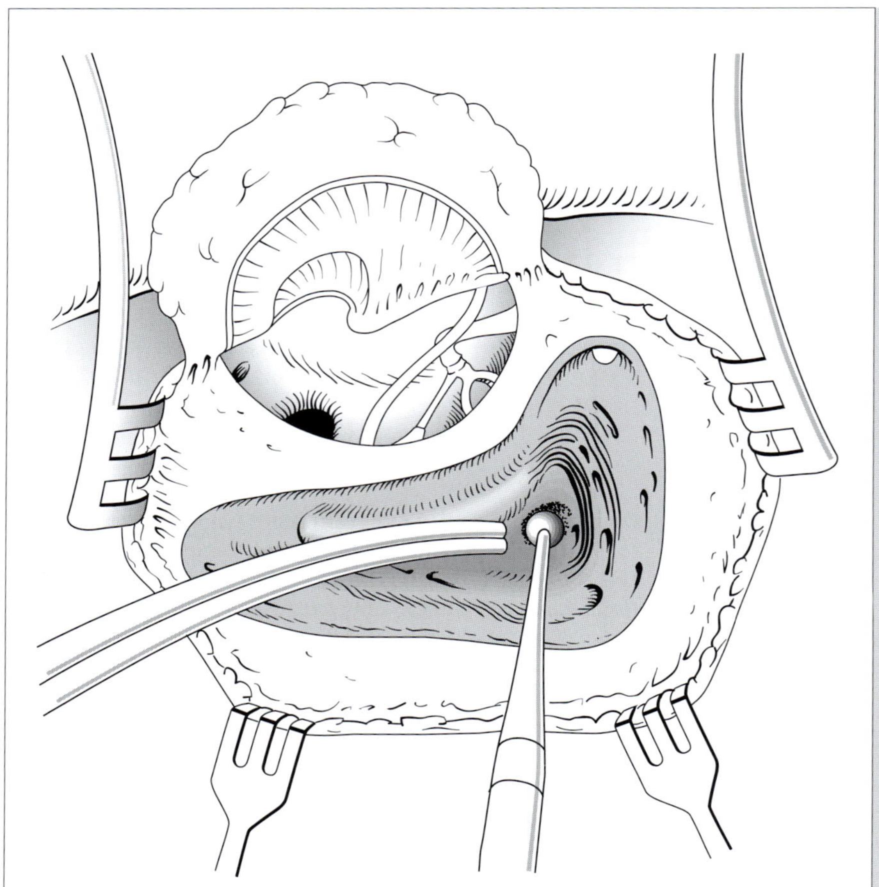

Fig. 18.21 Tympanoplasty with mastoidectomy.
The air cells are drilled out from the mastoid cortex, and tympanoplasty is performed through the ear canal.

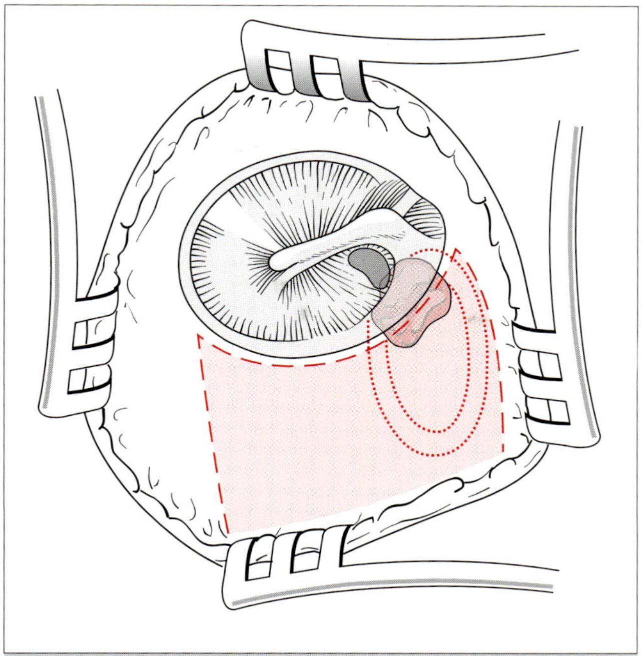

Fig. 18.22 Atticoantrotomy.
The cholesteatoma sac is traced from the perforation toward the antrum. The removable portion of the tympanomeatal flap is indicated by shading.

Exposure. The cholesteatoma sac is traced from the peripheral defect. Exposure is aided by widely thinning the canal bone over the attic and toward the antrum with a burr to eliminate overhangs (**Fig. 18.22**). A diamond burr is used when working near the attic. The thin layer remaining over the cholesteatoma is progressively removed from the edge of the perforation with a House curette. The overlying mastoid bone is continuously removed until the end of the cholesteatoma sac is exposed (**Fig. 18.23**). The facial nerve is identified by elevating the tympanic membrane from the sulcus in the posterosuperior quadrant. At this point the removable portion of the overhang at the junction of the lateral attic wall with the posterior canal wall is easily accessed from below with a House curette.

Dissection. The fully exposed cholesteatoma sac is bluntly mobilized from the periphery with a Rosen elevator or antrum hook. First, however, the middle ear cavity must be inspected to assess the relation of the cholesteatoma to the ossicular chain. A small cholesteatoma that loosely abuts the ossicular chain from the lateral side can be carefully separated from the ossicles.

Oval window niche. If the ossicular chain is encased or eroded, the cholesteatoma sac is incised, debris is aspirated from the sac, and the contents of the oval window niche are carefully probed with a needle. An intact but encased ossicular chain is opened by inserting a medium-sized 90° hook into the incudostapedial joint. The incus is dislocated upward and, if necessary, removed (**Fig. 18.24**). Often at this stage the course of the facial nerve can be indirectly identified below the cho-

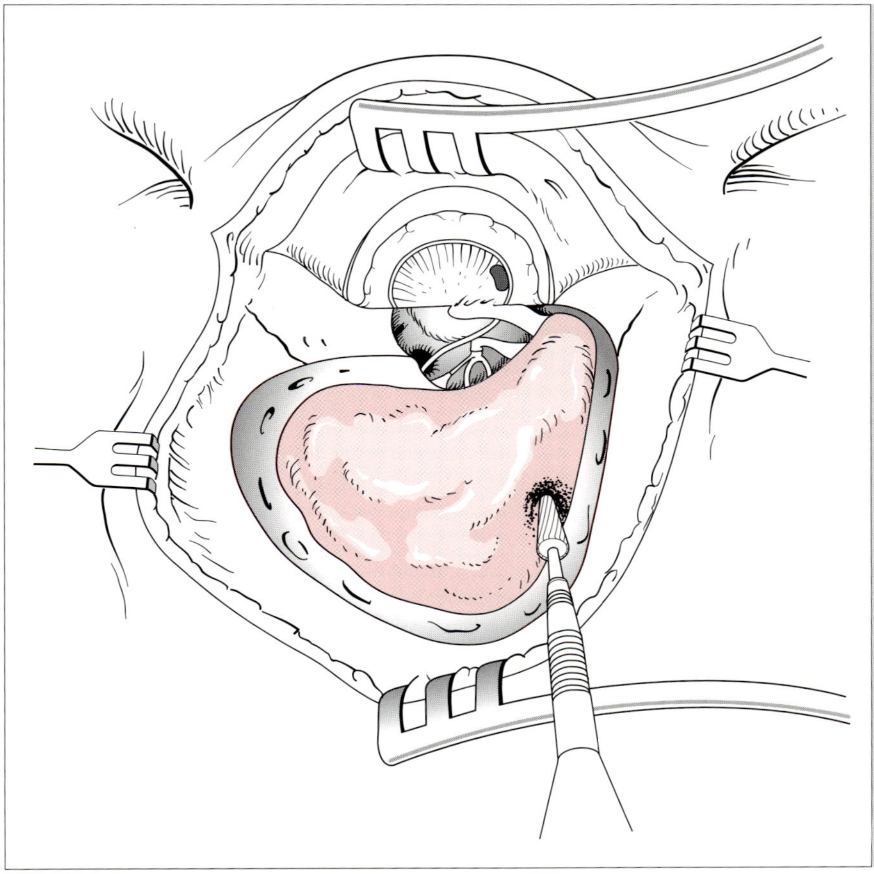

Fig. 18.23 Atticoantrotomy.
The bone over the cholesteatoma is removed. The mass is clearly visible in the mastoid and attic.

18

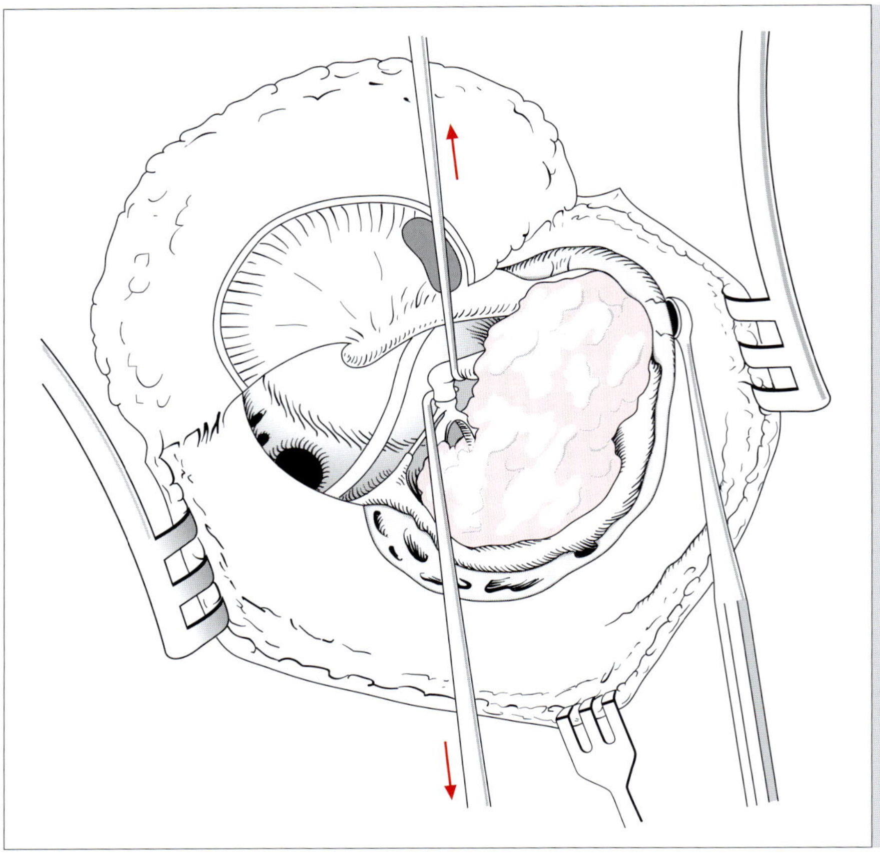

Fig. 18.24 Atticoantrotomy.
Opening the ossicular chain. The incudostapedial joint is separated and dislocated with a 90° hook.

lesteatoma matrix. Material is dissected from the oval window niche and stapes with a sickle knife or needle and microsuction tip, preferably in continuity, while working parallel to the course of the stapedius tendon.

Attic. The malleus head must be resected in most cases (see above). When the bone has been removed to the tegmen tympani, the entire epitympanum can be accessed from below. It is often necessary to divide the tensor fold and tensor tendon. While dissecting the medial attic wall, the surgeon probes for any dehiscence in the bony facial canal.

Semicircular canal. The cholesteatoma sac, which has been mobilized from the sides and debulked by incision and aspiration, is carefully dissected from the bone over the horizontal semicircular canal under high magnification, working from the mastoid toward the attic and using slow, gentle pushing movements of a sickle knife or Rosen elevator.

Labyrinthine fistula. A labyrinthine fistula appears as a dark feature visible beneath the cholesteatoma matrix. The matrix is carefully dissected from around the edges while leaving the fistula alone (**Fig. 18.25**). The fistula is then sealed with bone dust and covered with fascia or perichondrium. Fistula granulations or cholesteatoma that have invaded the semicircular canal must be removed. Starting from the fistula, the changes are traced into healthy tissue while drilling open or removing the bony fistula margins with a diamond burr and House curette, and the cavity is obliterated with bone dust. This treatment is often followed by labyrinthine dysfunction.

Facial nerve. In dissections around the facial canal, it is important to identify a landmark such as the cochleariform process, pyramidal eminence, or horizontal semicircular canal. The overlying matrix is probed to check for dehiscence of the bony canal.

Sinus tympani. A cholesteatoma in the hypotympanum and sinus tympani should be removed in continuity whenever possible by broad, blunt dissection of the matrix. With a very deep sinus tympani, the overhang in the posterior canal wall should also be burred down. To protect the facial nerve, it may be necessary to identify the nerve by locating the sinochordal angle.

Dura. Cholesteatoma and any granulations are dissected from an exposed area of dura. The bone defect can be carefully enlarged about its circumference with a diamond burr and House curette to find healthy dura for establishing the correct plane. A larger bone defect is subsequently closed with a cartilage disk inserted between the bone and dura.

Sinus. Granulations and matrix should also be dissected from the sinus while enlarging the bone defect. Sinus aspiration may be necessary in the presence of inflammatory changes.

Petrous apex. Cholesteatomas may develop extensions to the petrous apex, which appear anterior to the semicircular canal/facial nerve genu or between the semicircular canals. If the extension is not too deep, it can be removed with a needle and sickle knife after drilling open the access site slightly with a

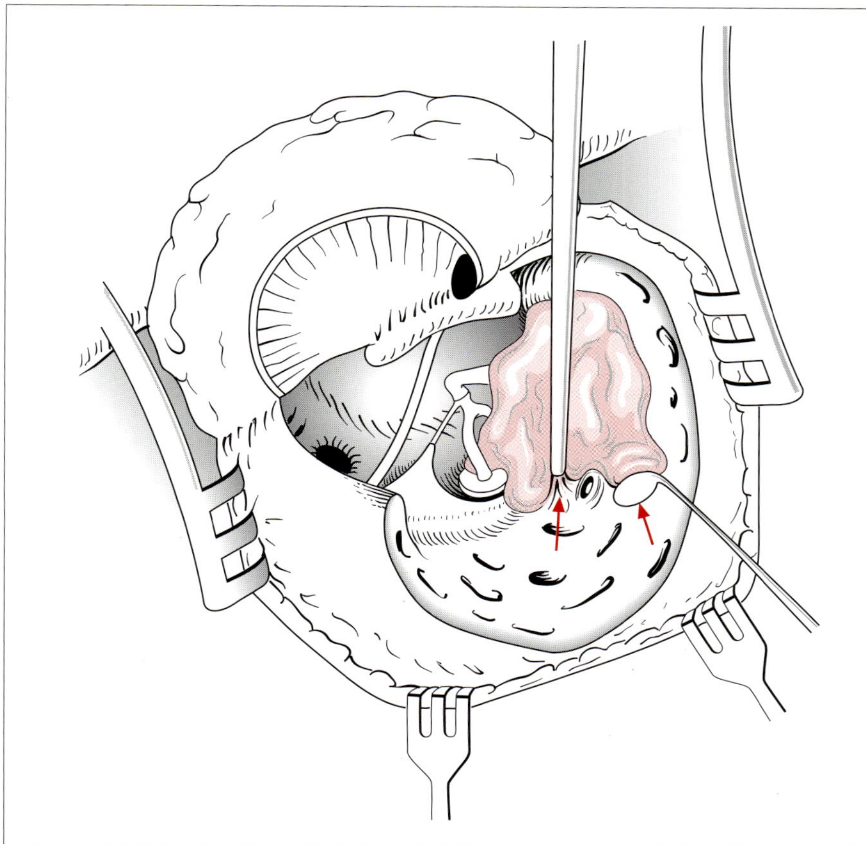

Fig. 18.25 Atticoantrotomy.
A labyrinthine fistula is carefully dissected parallel to the fistula site. The epithelium is indirectly mobilized.

burr. More extensive involvement may require a transtemporal or translabyrinthine approach.

Smoothing the cavity. The surgical cavity is smoothed with a large diamond burr. When a radial cavity is created, the facial ridge, the part of the posterior canal wall covering the facial nerve, must be taken down to the level of the nerve, first using a Rosen burr and then a diamond burr when working closer to the nerve. The aim is to create a smooth transition from the floor of the cavity to the floor of the ear canal. Bony overhangs in the epitympanum and other sharp edges should be smoothed.

Tympanoplasty. The ossicular chain is generally reconstructed with a type IIIA or IIIB procedure, or occasionally a type IV (pp. 372ff and 375f). Because the lateral attic wall is absent, the tympanic membrane is braced against the medial attic wall, resulting in a shallow middle ear cavity. If the tympanic membrane remnant is large enough, it is placed more deeply to engage against the medial attic wall. Approximately 5 mm from the tympanic annulus, a circumferential incision is made from the roof to the center of the anterior canal wall, and this tympanomeatal flap (including the annulus) is disengaged from the sulcus (**Fig. 18.26**). The tensor tendon must also be divided before the tympanic membrane is lowered.

With a larger tympanic membrane defect, the drum is reconstructed with cartilage palisades or perichondrium. A groove for the palisades can be drilled into the posterior canal wall to stabilize the cartilage struts.

Graft placement is described under Type IV Tympanoplasty (p. 375f).

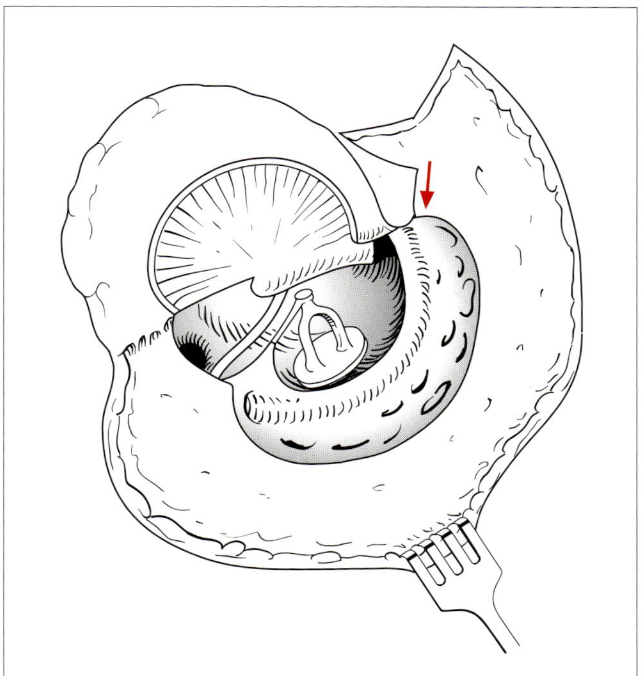

Fig. 18.26 Atticoantrotomy.
The tympanic membrane is placed more deeply against the medial attic wall, resulting in a shallow middle ear cleft. The arrow indicates the direction of the advancement along the anterior canal wall.

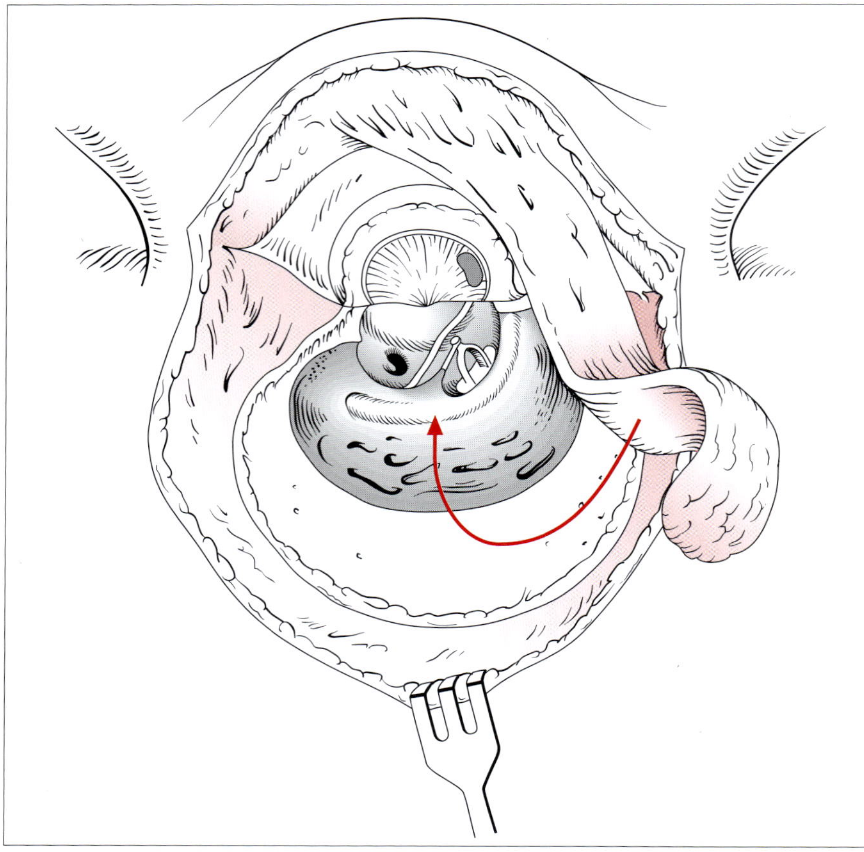

Fig. 18.27 Atticoantrotomy.
Cavity obliteration with a Palva flap.

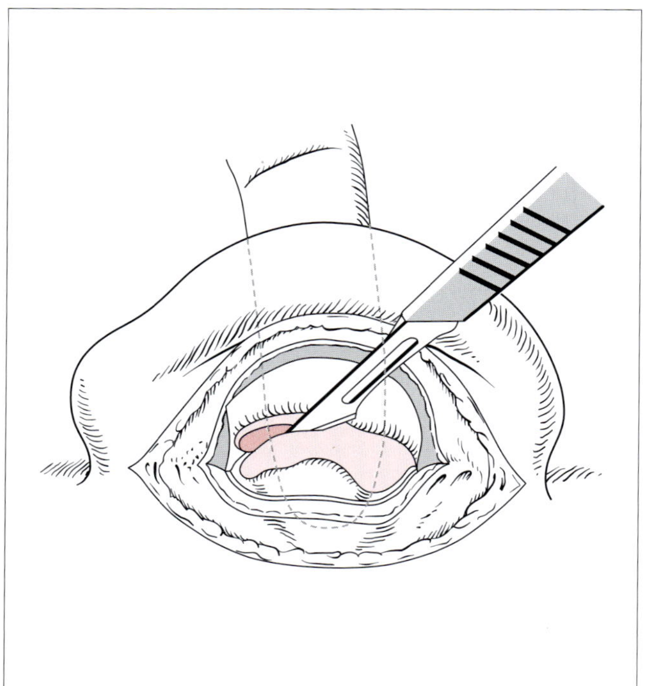

Fig. 18.28 Atticoantrotomy.
Meatoplasty. The conchal cartilage at the meatal entrance is resected against counterpressure from the index finger.

Cavity obliteration. *Large radical cavity:* The sternocleidomastoid muscle is released from its insertion, and the mastoid tip is removed to the bony sinus plate. The posterior canal wall is taken down to the level of the facial nerve, and the posterior edge of the cavity is taken down to sinus level. This allows the external soft tissues to sag inward, obliterating the lower portion of the cavity.

A *medium-sized cavity* is partially obliterated by swinging a Palva flap into the bowl (**Fig. 18.27**). Bone chips can additionally be placed behind the flap.

Relatively small cavities that communicate with the ear canal usually do not require obliteration.

Meatoplasty. To obtain sufficient enlargement of the meatal entrance, a fairly generous amount of cartilage is excised about the entrance from the posterior side of the concha. The index finger is placed anteriorly to palpate the incision and stabilize the cartilage (**Fig. 18.28**). The meatal skin incision is then extended outward to enlarge the cutaneous entrance as well. The meatal entrance is fixed posteriorly to the connective tissue with two subcutaneous sutures. Finally, the meatal flap and the removed tympanomeatal flap are returned to their original position, and the ear canal is lined with silicone strips.

Rules, Tips, and Tricks

- Whenever possible, remove the cholesteatoma in continuity to avoid leaving small remnants.

18

- Remove all cholesteatoma matrix before proceeding with tympanoplastic measures. If this is uncertain, a second-look operation should be scheduled 1 year later.
- Remove troublesome overhangs to improve visibility. The cavity should be ground smooth, taking particular care to create a smooth transition with the canal floor. Cavity obliteration is necessary to prevent a siphoning effect below the level of the ear canal.
- Remove all matrix including the vascular perimatrix.
- Evaluate the condition of the ossicular chain before manipulating the ossicles. The chain should be opened if necessary.
- Use higher magnification when working on a labyrinthine fistula, the dura, the facial nerve, or in the oval window niche.
- Identify landmarks prior to facial nerve dissection.
- If the matrix cannot be confidently separated from the chorda tympani, the chorda may be resected if absolutely necessary.

! Risks and Complications

- Usual risks of tympanoplasty (see p. 370).
- Recurrent cholesteatoma.
- Labyrinthine fistulas greatly increase the risk of deafness and vertigo.
- A relatively large defect in the bony skull base may predispose to a dural prolapse or subarachnoid cyst with extension into the mastoid cavity or ear canal.

Alternatives

- **Reconstruction of the posterior canal wall with a cartilage plate.** After the dissections have been completed, a cartilage graft is placed under moderate tension between the roof of the cavity and the facial ridge. Grooves are drilled at both bony contact points to keep the plate in a slightly curved position. A clear pathway must be left for air to pass through the middle ear from the eustachian tube to the mastoid (**Fig. 18.29**). At all other sites the cartilage plate should be well apposed to surrounding tissues; any gaps can be closed with cartilage strips. The cartilage plate is covered by the replaced tympanomeatal flap and also by the meatal flap from above.
- **Atticoantrotomy** with temporary resection of the bony posterior canal wall (Feldmann) and **osteoplastic tympanotomy** (Wullstein) are not described further owing to their technical challenges and because they exceed our present scope.

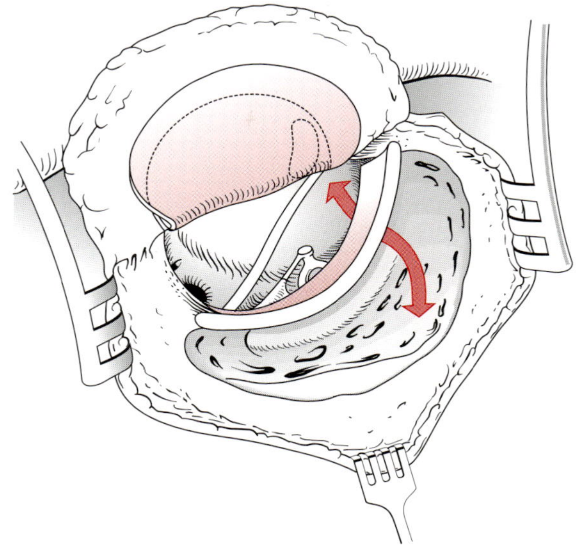

Fig. 18.29 Atticoantrotomy.
The posterior canal wall is reconstructed with a cartilage graft. Grooves are drilled in the recipient bone bed to allow for graft placement under tension.

Atticotomy

Indications

Cholesteatoma confined to the attic and originating from shrapnel perforation or a retraction pocket.

Surgical Technique

Approach. Endaural or postauricular. Graft material is harvested and a meatoplasty is performed (see Chapter 17; see **Figs. 17.6** and **17.7**). Self-retaining retractors are inserted. The bony entrance to the ear canal is enlarged to a funnel-shaped opening with a large burr or grinder.

Tympanomeatal flap. The tympanomeatal flap is outlined with a straight round knife by making incisions at 11 and 5 o'clock in the right ear and at 1 and 7 o'clock in the left ear (see **Fig. 17.3** and **Fig. 18.2**; see Chapter 17). The meatal portion of the flap is temporarily removed by making a circumferential incision just lateral to the tympanic membrane. It is stored for later reimplantation.

Dissection. Starting from the perforation, the canal bone over the attic is thinned with a burr and then a House curette, and the lateral attic wall is taken down to the border of the cholesteatoma sac or to the tegmen tympani (**Fig. 18.30**).

Cholesteatoma removal. A small cholesteatoma that is only loosely apposed to the ossicular chain can be separated from the chain in continuity and removed.

Ossicular chain dissection. Involvement of the ossicular chain may necessitate resection of the malleus head or extraction of the incus (see above). After the tympanic membrane has been freed from the sulcus in the posterosuperior quadrant and the attic wall has been taken down over the oval window niche,

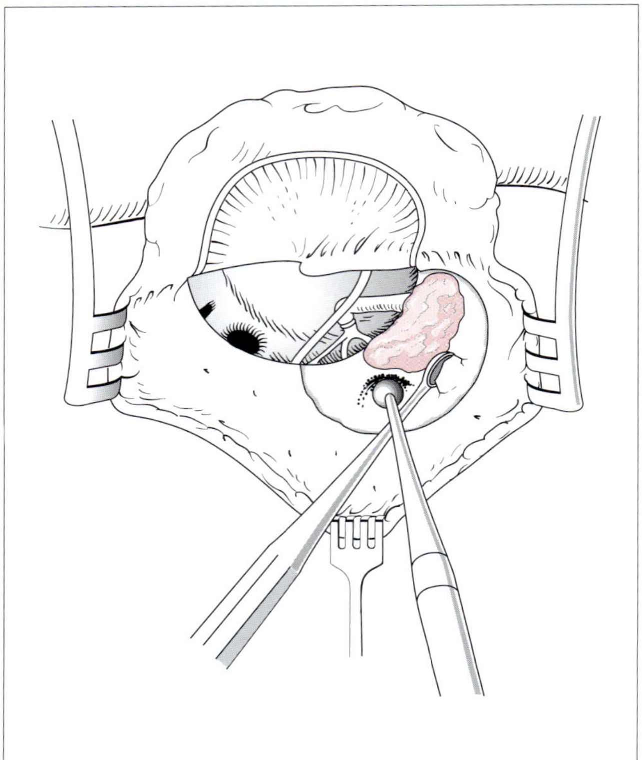

Fig. 18.30 Atticotomy.
Starting from the defect, the bone over the attic is progressively removed.

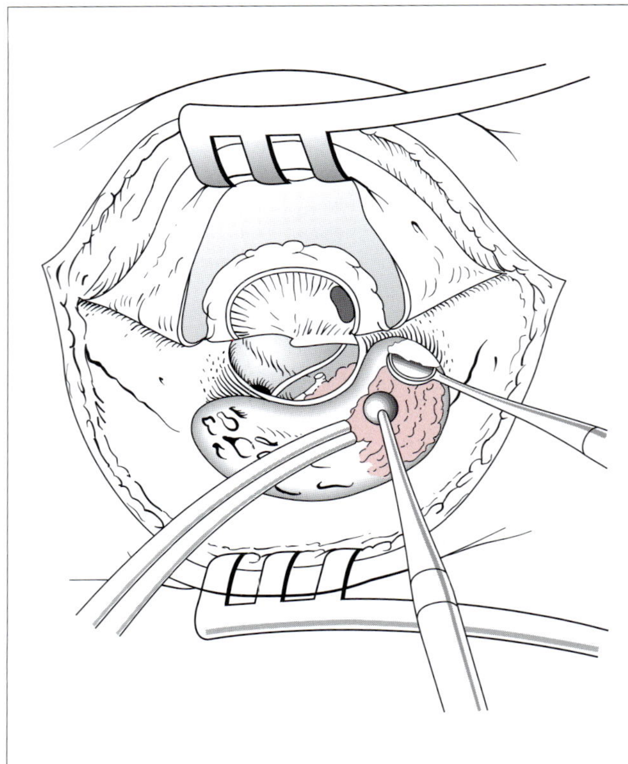

Fig. 18.31 Anterior–posterior approach.
The last bony layer covering the antrum is removed with a curette. The depth of the antrum is estimated in relation to the plane of the tympanic membrane.

the incudostapedial joint is separated and the incus is extracted with a medium-sized 90° hook.

Attic dissection. All of the matrix is removed in continuity with the ossicular chain remnants, and the tensor fold is divided to improve postoperative aeration (closed technique). Another option is to leave behind the medial matrix for later epithelialization of the attic (open technique).

Ossicular chain reconstruction. Standard tympanoplasty rules are followed in reconstructing the ossicular chain.

Defect reconstruction. *Closed technique* (with good eustachian tube function): A cartilage–perichondrium composite graft is placed against the tympanic membrane margin using an underlay technique. Its cartilage component covers the attic defect while the rest of the perichondrium is in contact with the bone of the ear canal. The meatal flap is reimplanted. The rest of the procedure follows standard tympanoplasty technique.

18

Open technique: In cases where medial matrix has been left behind, the aditus ad antrum is covered with perichondrium or fascia to establish contact with the tympanic membrane in the posterior quadrant. The tympanic membrane itself is set more deeply to establish contact with the attic. Approximately 5 mm from the annulus, a circumferential incision is made from the roof to the center of the anterior canal wall, and this tympanomeatal flap is separated from the sulcus along with the annulus (**Fig. 18.26**). The tensor tendon is divided so that the tympanic membrane can be lowered. This results in a shallow middle ear cavity with a communication between the attic and ear canal.

Anterior–Posterior Approach, Closed Technique

Surgical Principle

Combined cholesteatoma removal through the ear canal and mastoid with preservation of the posterior canal wall. The chordofacial angle and the attic are broadly opened from the mastoid.

Indication

Cholesteatoma extending into or past the antrum with a well-pneumatized mastoid.

Contraindications

- Very limited anatomic access in the mastoid process.
- Anterior sinus position.

Anesthesia

General or local anesthesia.

Surgical Technique

Approach. Postauricular approach with broad exposure of the mastoid cortex.

Harvesting graft material (see Chapter 17). An incision is made around the ear canal, and the periosteum over the mastoid cortex is incised at a right angle to the canal incision. The periosteum is mobilized with a periosteal elevator (see **Fig. 17.5a**).

Meatoplasty (see Chapter 17, **Fig. 17.6**). The cutaneous ear canal is incised to a depth of 1 cm along its posterior circumference, turning the incision outward to the cartilage at the roof of the canal. The meatal flap is held back with the self-retaining retractor (see **Fig. 17.7**). Another retractor is used to maintain mastoid exposure. The bony meatal entrance is widened with a large burr.

Tympanomeatal flap. The tympanomeatal flap is cut (see **Fig. 17.3** and **Fig. 18.2**) and elevated toward the tympanic membrane (see **Fig. 18.3**).

Mastoidectomy. Starting from the mastoid cortex as described in Chapter 19, the cell system is drilled open toward the antrum using the suprameatal spine and temporal line as landmarks. The zygomatic cells are opened along with the mastoid cells (so that the final layer over the attic can be removed through the antrum with a curette), but the mastoid is excavated only to the degree necessary to expose and dissect the cholesteatoma. The posterior canal wall is not thinned too much initially. A diamond burr is used near the antrum, whose depth is estimated by noting the position of the tympanic membrane in the ear canal. The final bony layer is removed with a curette to avoid breaching the cholesteatoma sac (**Fig. 18.31**). Initially the sac is exposed posteriorly and superiorly, after first identifying the middle cranial fossa and sinus plate as anatomic landmarks.

Opening the middle ear cavity. The tympanic membrane is separated from the sulcus posterosuperiorly, and the lateral attic wall is taken down above the oval window niche. If space is very limited, the posterior canal wall can be drilled open slightly from the meatal side, but the remaining wall must be thick enough to prevent necrosis. The cholesteatoma sac is bluntly separated from the lateral attic wall under the bony bridge with an angled round incision knife.

Two-cavity approach. Using the short crus of the incus or the horizontal semicircular canal for orientation, the chordofacial angle is drilled open through the mastoid cavity with a diamond burr, which is directed parallel to the presumed course of the facial nerve (**Fig. 18.32**). Even when working upward, the surgeon keeps a safe distance from the facial nerve and removes the thinned bony overhangs with a curette. When the lumen of the middle ear is reached, the cholesteatoma is bluntly dis-

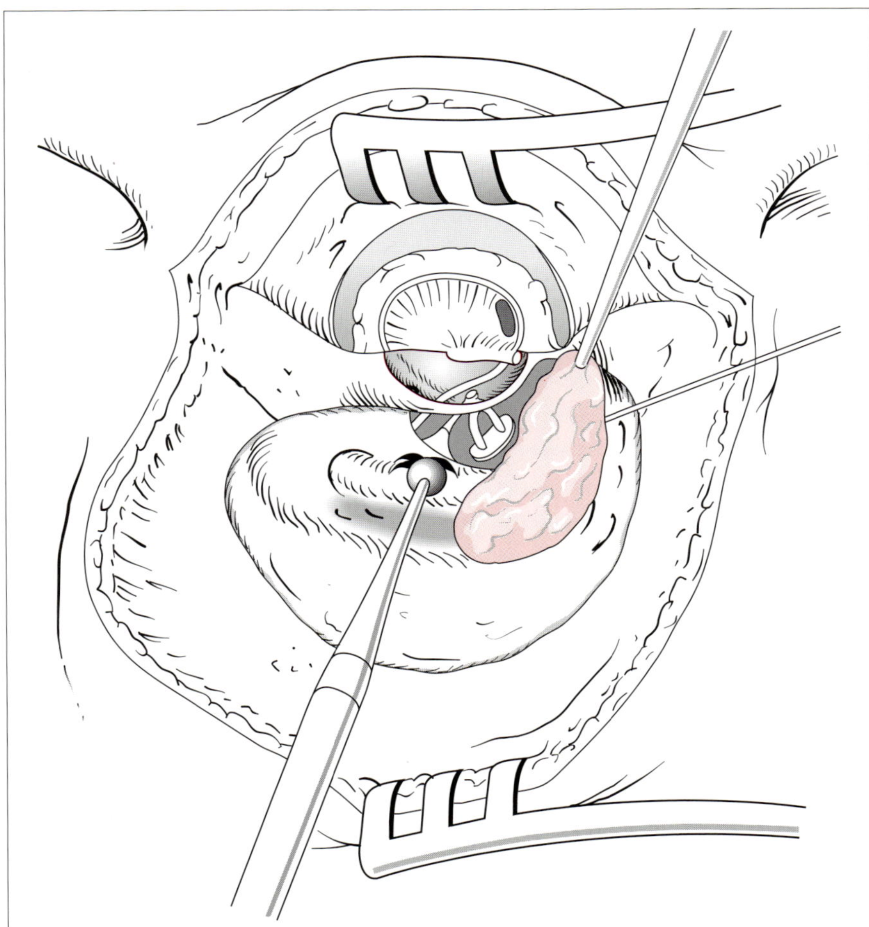

Fig. 18.32 Anterior–posterior approach. The chordofacial angle is drilled open prior to mobilizing the cholesteatoma sac.

18

sected from its walls. The ossicular chain and facial nerve are identified. This may require incision of the cholesteatoma sac. If the ossicular chain is intact, the incudostapedial joint is disarticulated with a 90° hook.

Mobilization of the cholesteatoma. Further mobilization of the cholesteatoma is done alternately from the anterior and posterior sides. Critical sites are the passageway beneath the lateral attic wall in the area of the chordofacial angle, the anterior attic, and the hypotympanum. It may be necessary to extract the incus, resect the malleus head, and aspirate the cholesteatoma sac before it can be delivered from the middle ear. An effort is always made to avoid tearing the matrix, for only an in-continuity dissection will allow the cholesteatoma to be removed completely using the two-cavity approach.

Reconstruction. Tympanic membrane closure and ossicular chain reconstruction require no specialized techniques and follow the standard rules of tympanoplasty. The connective tissue is sutured to the periosteum at the meatal entrance.

Rules, Tips, and Tricks

A second-look operation is performed in 1–2 years to exclude residual cholesteatoma.

! Risks and Complications

- Increased risk of facial nerve injury.
- Residual cholesteatoma is more common than with an open technique.
- Additional risks are listed on page 370.

18

19 Surgery of the Mastoid Process

Mastoidectomy

Surgical Principle

- The air cells of the mastoid process are exenterated from the mastoid cortex while preserving the posterior wall of the ear canal.
- The skull base is skeletonized to the middle and posterior cranial fossae, the sigmoid sinus is skeletonized, and sufficient antral patency is established.

Indications

- Mastoiditis and its complications.
- Cholesteatoma.
- Cholesterol granuloma.
- Granulating mastoiditis in chronic mesotympanic otitis media.
- Chronic otitis media with effusion.
- Access for facial nerve decompression, translabyrinthine neurectomy or acoustic neuroma excision, saccotomy, cochlear implant, partially implantable hearing aids.

Contraindications

- General medical condition (relative).
- Relative: absence of mastoid pneumatization, complete eburnation, extreme anterior position of the sigmoid sinus.

Specific Points Regarding Informed Consent

- Deafness, hearing loss due to inner ear pathology or ossicular discontinuity.
- Tinnitus.
- Vertigo.
- Altered taste sensation (chorda tympani).
- Facial nerve injury.
- Heavy scarring of the incision and auricle, keloid formation.
- Neuralgiform pain.
- Dural injury with meningitis, brain abscess.
- Sinus injury with hemorrhage.
- Postauricular contraction or fistula formation.
- Stenosis of the ear canal.

Surgical Principle

Schüller radiograph, blood count, ESR; high-resolution CT if required.

Special Instruments

Suction irrigator or combined drilling and irrigation system, antrum hook, House curette.

Anesthesia

General anesthesia. Local anesthesia is also an option.

Surgical Technique

Positioning. The patient is positioned supine on the operating table with the head turned to the side and immobilized on a headrest or ring.

Approach. Postauricular skin incision (see Chapter 17, **Fig. 17.4**). The incision is extended to the mastoid tip. The entire mastoid process is exposed, and the self-retaining retractors are inserted.

Exposure. The periosteum is opened with an H-shaped incision (**Fig. 19.1**). It is widely reflected from the mastoid cortex with a periosteal elevator from the temporal line to the mastoid tip and from the suprameatal spine to the posterior border of the mastoid. The sternocleidomastoid muscle is released from its insertion with a periosteal knife (**Fig. 19.2**).

Opening the bone. The mastoid cortex is initially opened between the suprameatal spine and temporal line with a large cutting burr, which is applied to the bone in long strokes directed parallel to the temporal line (**Fig. 19.3**). The boundary of the middle cranial fossa is exposed. The opening is saucerized and deepened with a conical burr.

Locating the antrum. The antrum is approached obliquely upward along the base of the middle cranial fossa and the posterosuperior wall of the ear canal using a burr and a curette. The latter instrument is particularly useful in well-pneumatized bone.

Identification. The antrum presents as a cavity of variable size and is identified by the bright, shiny, hard bone of the horizontal semicircular canal, which lies behind the short crus of the incus. The antrum must be differentiated from the large surrounding air cells. Orientation is aided by probing with an

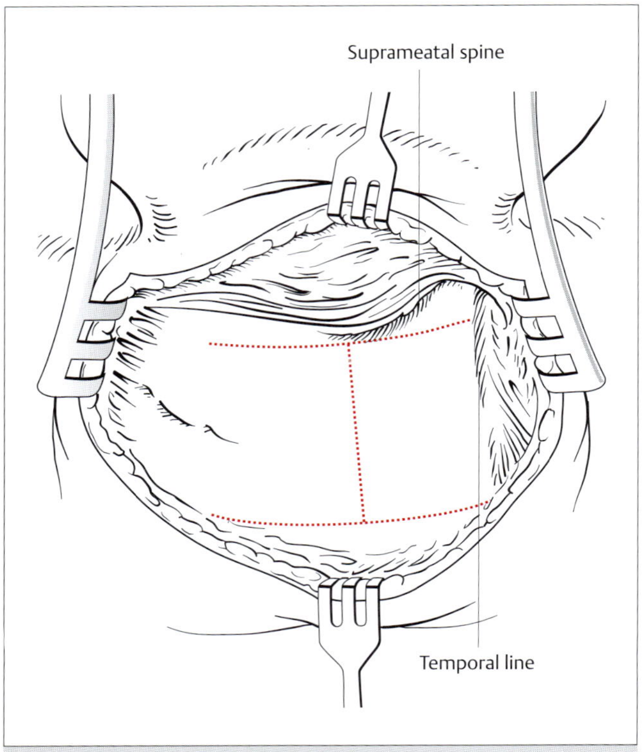

Fig. 19.1 Mastoidectomy.
The periosteum over the mastoid cortex is opened with an H-shaped incision.

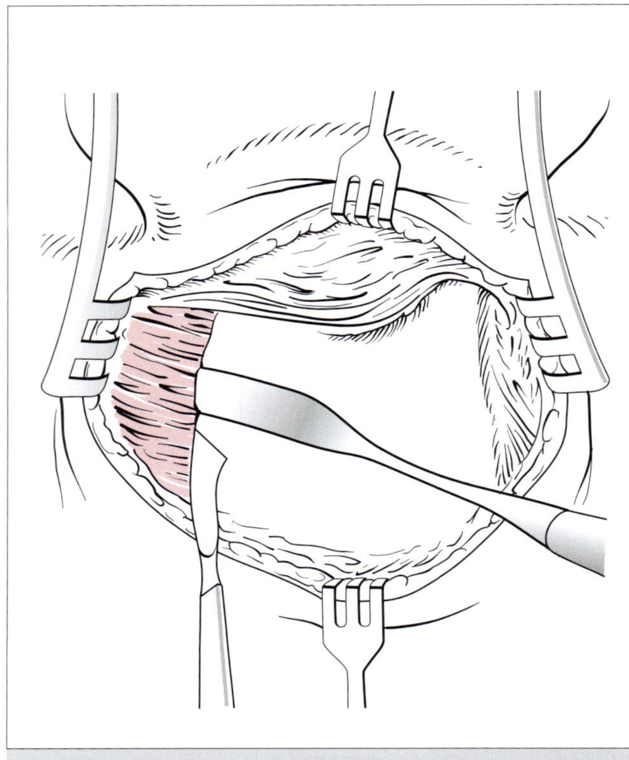

Fig. 19.2 Mastoidectomy.
The mastoid cortex is exposed. The sternocleidomastoid muscle is released with a periosteal knife.

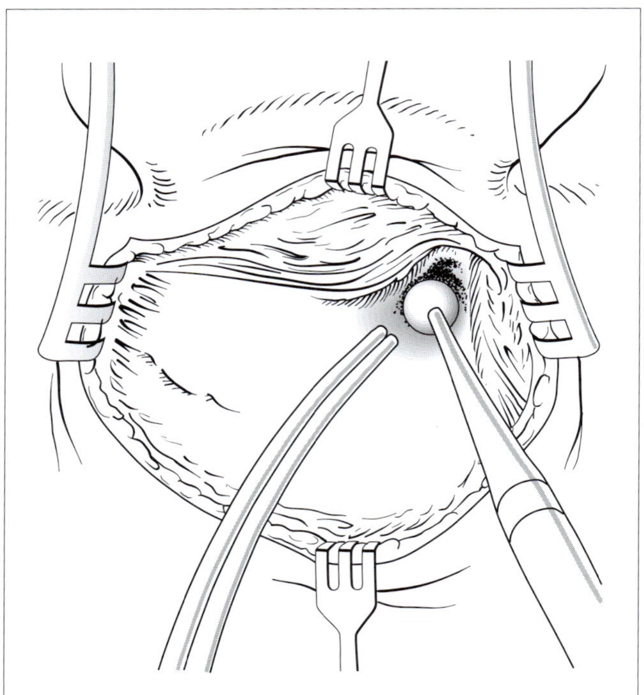

Fig. 19.3 Mastoidectomy.
The cortex between the suprameatal spine and temporal line is opened with a large cutting burr.

19

antrum hook. If a Körner septum (hard, thick bony plate lateral to the antrum) is blocking direct access and limits the depth of the exposure, it should be burred down from the posterior side.

Enlarging the aditus. The aditus ad antrum is enlarged with the House curette and, if necessary, small diamond burrs while scrupulously avoiding any contact between the drill and the ossicular chain. The aditus is enlarged until the incudomalleolar joint is visible in the epitympanum.

Mastoidectomy. Next, the air cells are exenterated with a large cutting burr, first working posteriorly into the sinodural angle and Citelli cell and then widely skeletonizing the sinus plate with a large diamond burr while also removing the retrosinus cells (**Fig. 19.4**).

It may also be necessary to drill anteriorly into the zygomatic cells, depending on the indication. The Trautmann triangle located behind the posterior semicircular canal should be exposed as well. The perifacial air cells are opened after removing the cells on the posterior canal wall. This is done only with the diamond burr and curette, working strictly parallel to the course of the facial nerve. When this step has been completed, the mastoid tip is also drilled out.

Dura and sinus exposure. If it is suspected that inflammatory changes have spread to the sinus and dura, both structures should be exposed and inspected even in the absence of a visible breach. After the sinus and dura have been skeletonized, the bone covering these structures is thinned further at a circumscribed site, and the thin bony plate is gently broken inward

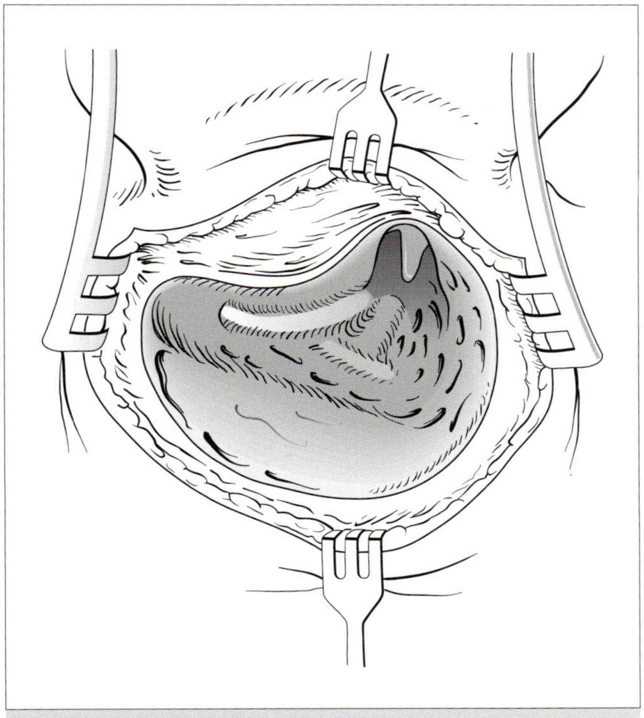

Fig. 19.4 Mastoidectomy.
The semicircular canal and body of the incus are visible in the antrum and aditus ad antrum. The middle cranial fossa, sigmoid sinus, and facial canal are skeletonized.

and elevated with a round incision knife. If the dura or sinus has already been exposed spontaneously, granulations will generally be found on the exposed area. The eroded bony margins are extended—thinned with a diamond burr and the remaining shell elevated with an angled round incision knife—until normal dura or sinus wall is encountered. From there the granulations are elevated in the proper plane with the angled round knife and removed with a cup forceps. Additional steps (sinus aspiration, dissection of the dura) may be necessary and are described below under Treatment of Otogenic Complications.

Concluding the operation. Remaining overhangs are smoothed with a large diamond burr, and all bone dust is carefully removed by irrigation. A drainage tube is inserted and brought out the lower end of the wound. The periosteum is reapproximated with sutures, and the meatal entrance is fixed posteriorly. The wound is closed in layers. The ear canal is packed if it has been opened or mobilized.

Rules, Tips, and Tricks

- The extent of air-cell removal is variable, depending on the findings. The dura and sinus should always be evaluated, however, when dealing with mastoiditis and its complications. Clinical findings may require exposing the air cells at the root of the zygomatic arch.
- Take tissue samples for histology and microbiology.
- Establish sufficient antral patency.
- Use curettes in the vicinity of the ossicular chain; never touch it with a rotating burr.
- A myringotomy or tympanostomy tube may also be necessary, depending on the findings.
- Remove granulations and polyps only under vision and after identifying the malleus head and incus. If bleeding obscures vision, control it by local application of Privine drops or dilute suprarenin solution.
- When skeletonizing the facial nerve with a diamond burr, work strictly parallel to the course of the nerve and only after identifying the horizontal semicircular canal as a landmark.
- Use the largest possible diameter of cutting burr or diamond burr, generally applied in a linear, stroking pattern over a broad area. Apply the burr with minimal pressure and use a high rotation speed except in certain situations (e. g., hemostasis, occasionally at critical structures). Use copious irrigation with a large suction tip.
- If a subperiosteal abscess has eroded through the bone, use that site to gain access to the air-cell system.
- A Schüller radiograph can disclose an anterior position of the sigmoid sinus or a low position of the dura. This will eliminate the element of surprise during surgery, making it easier to avoid these structures.

! Risks and Complications

- Facial paralysis (requires early facial nerve reconstruction).
- Incus dislocation (hearing loss, deafness, tinnitus, vertigo); two-stage tympanoplasty may be necessary due to possible inner ear damage.
- Dural injury (seal with fibrin-coated collagen or with a fascial patch tucked between the bone and dura).
- Sinus injury (seal with fibrin-coated collagen or a muscle patch; pack off a large tear; see Sinus Thrombosis below.
- Opening a semicircular canal (seal the opening with bone dust and fibrin glue; give antibiotics and corticosteroids).
- Postauricular fistula.
- Meatal stenosis.

Postoperative Care

- Antibiotic therapy (may be changed on the basis of smear results).
- Flush the drain daily with 0.9 % NaCl until the return is clear, then remove.
- Sutures are removed on the seventh postoperative day.

Bezold Mastoiditis

Bezold mastoiditis is a condition in which a gravitation abscess forms due to pus tracking from the mastoid tip into the upper sternocleidomastoid muscle and upper posterior neck muscles. The patient assumes a typical cocked head position, and any head movements are extremely painful.

Surgical Principle

Mastoidectomy is performed with removal of the mastoid tip. The upper vascular sheath is exposed and the abscess is drained.

Indication

Any suspicion of a gravitation abscess in mastoiditis.

Surgical Technique

Skin incision. The skin incision is extended from the mastoid to the superior half of the sternocleidomastoid muscle.

Mastoidectomy. Complete exenteration of the air-cell system. The bony shell of the mastoid tip is removed with a Luer rongeur or burr.

Abscess drainage. The anterior border of the sternocleidomastoid muscle and the vascular sheath are exposed. The compartments are bluntly spread open. Drains are placed in the mastoid and abscess cavity and brought out of the lower end of the wound.

Wound closure. The wound is closed in layers, a dressing is applied, and packing is placed in the ear canal.

Antrotomy

Surgical Principle

The antrum and aditus are widely opened from the mastoid cortex to improve aeration while leaving the posterior wall of the ear canal intact. Only a portion of the air-cell system is exenterated. A continuum exists from antrotomy to mastoidectomy, depending on the findings.

Indications

- Mastoid evaluation in the setting of a tympanoplasty for chronic mesotympanic otitis media with significant drainage.
- Persistent otitis media with effusion.

Surgical Technique

Same as mastoidectomy, but does not include exenterating the air-cell system to the sinodural angle or drilling out the perisinus cells. In most cases the perifacial cells and mastoid tip are also left alone.

Antrotomy in Infants

Surgical Principle

Exposure and removal of osteitic and osteomyelitic changes in the antrum and periantral region.

Indications

Antritis in infants that is overt (postauricular redness, swelling, or fluctuation) or occult (often associated with failure to thrive and an otherwise unexplained elevation of ESR).

Specific Points Regarding Informed Consent

See under Mastoidectomy, page 387.

Anesthesia

General anesthesia.

Surgical Technique

Incision. The skin incision is made ca. 0.5 cm behind the postauricular sulcus and extends obliquely backward onto the mastoid, which is weakly developed at this age.

Exposure. The delicate periosteum is incised and reflected until the temporal line and suprameatal spine can be seen. The meatal tube should not be isolated or mobilized. The anterior border of the mastoid should also be respected because the facial nerve is very superficial in that area.

Identifying the antrum. If there is no spontaneous erosion from a subperiosteal abscess and no increased bleeding points in the bone to point the way, the antrum is exposed by drilling open the cortex between the suprameatal spine and temporal line. It occupies a relatively cranial site and is very superficial because the air-cell system is still poorly developed in infants (**Fig. 19.5**). The incus is exposed and the aditus ad antrum is enlarged.

Air-cell removal. Additional cell removal should be done with a curette or with a diamond burr, which is directed paral-

19

lel to vulnerable structures and is applied to the bone with very little pressure.

Dissection. After the overhangs have been smoothed, granulations are carefully removed. The incus should never be dislocated. Erosions to the middle cranial fossa or sinus are enlarged, and the granulations are exposed to healthy dura or sinus wall. They are elevated at that location with an angled round incision knife and removed with a cup forceps. Sinus aspiration, if necessary, is described below.

Concluding the operation. A drainage tube is inserted and brought out of the lower end of the wound. The incisions are closed in layers. Packing is placed into the meatal entrance.

Rules, Tips, and Tricks

- The meatal tube should not be mobilized, because of the subsequent risk of stenosis.
- Because the mastoid is still poorly developed at this young age, exposure of the mastoid cortex should be done sparingly. The mastoid should not be exposed anteriorly past the suprameatal spine and should be exposed inferiorly only to the level of the meatal floor (the facial nerve runs very laterally within the mastoid and is very superficial outside the mastoid).
- Expose the dura and sinus if erosive or osteitic changes are found in the bone or if there is clinical evidence of an otogenic complication.
- Spontaneous perforation by a subperiosteal abscess can be used to gain surgical access to the mastoid.
- Because the air-cell system may be very friable, instruments should be used with very little force to avoid inadvertent nerve injury due to slippage.
- When heavy granulations are present, probe with an antrum hook for orientation. Be careful not to dislocate the incus, which can be safely manipulated only with a rotary motion toward the tegmen.

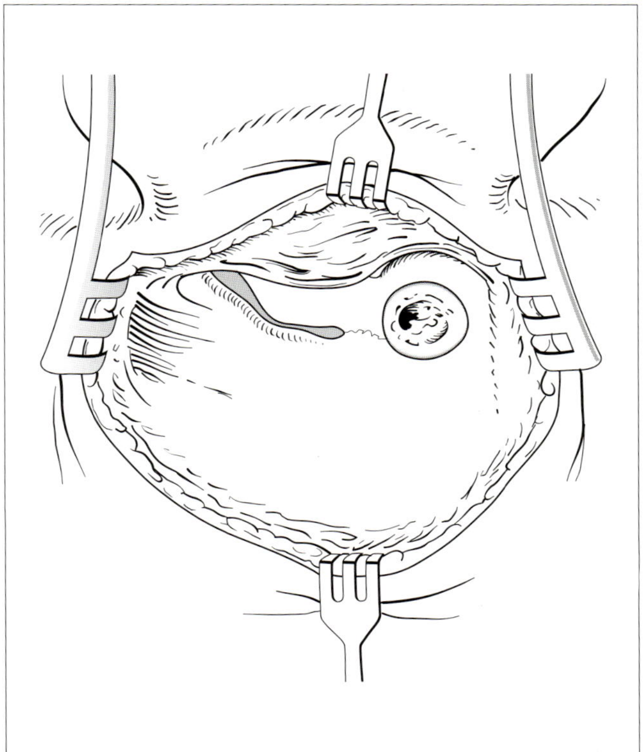

Fig. 19.5 Antrotomy in an infant.
The antrum at this age is superficial and extends far cephalad. Key landmarks are the suprameatal spine and temporal line, as in adults.

! Risks and Postoperative care
See under Mastoidectomy above.

Treatment of Otogenic Complications

Sinus Thrombosis

Surgical Principle

Eliminate the primary focus by mastoidectomy or by an atticoantrotomy if the thrombosis has resulted from cholesteatoma. Thrombosis is confirmed by needle aspiration of the sinus. Thrombus is removed from the venous sinus to prevent further progression. Jugular vein ligation in the neck may be necessary if the thrombosis is shedding septic emboli.

Indications

Any suspicion of sinus thrombosis. Besides the classic fulminating, septic clinical picture, which may be associated with meningitis symptoms and signs of distant septic metastasis from mastoiditis or cholesteatoma, there may also be bland, asymptomatic forms whose manifestations are often masked by antibiotic therapy.

Specific Points Regarding Informed Consent

- See Tympanoplasty in Chapter 18 (p. 367) and Mastoidectomy in this chapter (p. 387).
- Disclose the severity and risks posed by the thrombosis; multiorgan involvement.
- CNS complications, cranial nerve deficits.
- Jugular vein ligation in the neck (see Chapter 9, surgical treatment of tonsillogenic cellulitis and tonsillogenic sepsis).

Operative Planning

Clinically suspicious cases should be investigated by MRI, CT, high-resolution CT, and if necessary by a neurologic examination and medical evaluation.

Anesthesia

General anesthesia.

Surgical Technique

Mastoid surgery. A complete mastoidectomy is performed through a postauricular approach, or an atticoantrotomy in cholesteatoma patients, with the exenteration of all accessible air cells including retrosinus cells.

Skeletonization. The sinus is skeletonized distally from the sinodural angle, and the remaining sinus plate is thinned with a large diamond burr.

Exposure. If the sinus plate has already been perforated, usually by a perisinus abscess, the defect is enlarged with a curette or sinus punch. The extent of bone removal depends on the extent of visible changes and deposits that are found on the sinus wall, which normally presents a smooth, bluish appearance. The exposure may extend from the transverse sinus to the second genu in front of the jugular bulb. If spontaneous perforation has not occurred, the thin bony shell is carefully fractured inward with a round incision knife, which is also used to elevate the fragments from the site until the sinus wall can be adequately assessed and, if necessary, aspirated with a needle.

Dissection. The easiest technique is to start at a site where the sinus wall is still normal and elevate the granulations and thick fibrinous deposits with a round incision knife until the sinus wall is exposed. If the sinus wall has a smooth, bluish appearance, no further measures are necessary.

Needle aspiration. If wall changes are found and it is not immediately evident that thrombosis is present, needle aspiration should be performed. The course of the sinus must be positively identified to avoid inadvertent puncture of the dura. Antiseptic is applied to the selected site with a small sponge stick, and a needle mounted on a syringe is introduced into the sinus at a tangential angle, directing the needle axis along the sinus axis while drawing back the plunger (**Fig. 19.6**). If sufficient blood is aspirated, the puncture site can be resealed with a muscle patch and the procedure may be concluded. Many cases of bland, nonpurulent thrombosis with no clinical evidence of sepsis and no definite signs of perisinus inflammation are managed conservatively with massive antibiotic coverage.

Thrombus extraction. If purulent thrombosis is found, the sinus wall is incised longitudinally with a sickle knife. Thrombus and purulent necrotic material are suctioned from the vessel. This is continued into the transverse sinus as long as inflammatory necrotic material is obtained. Nowadays the jugular bulb itself is not evacuated. If bleeding occurs after thrombus extraction, the sinus is packed off with a collagen fleece sponge or "Heidelberg pack" (Spongostan or gelatin sponge wrapped with oxycellulose) tucked between the bony sinus shell and the sinus wall (**Fig. 19.7**).

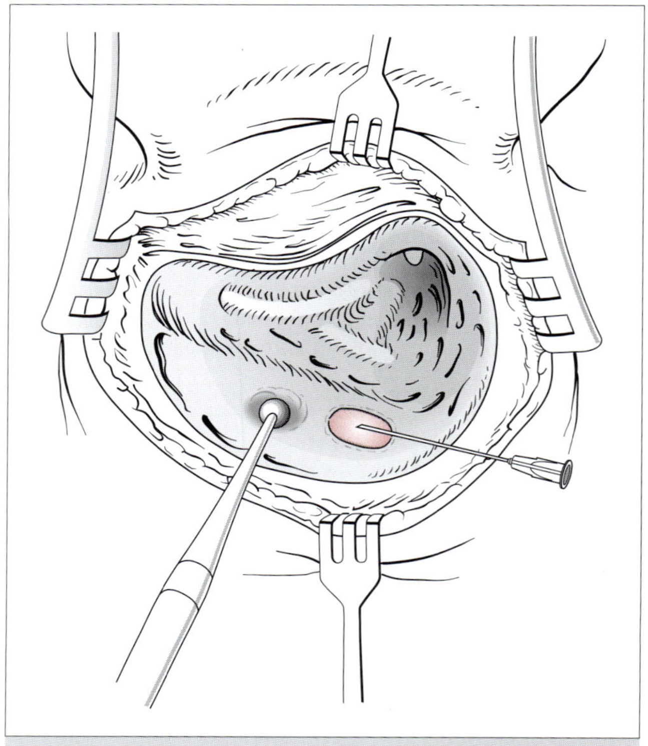

Fig. 19.6 Sinus thrombosis.
The sinus plate is skeletonized with a diamond burr. The aspirating needle is introduced tangentially along the sinus axis.

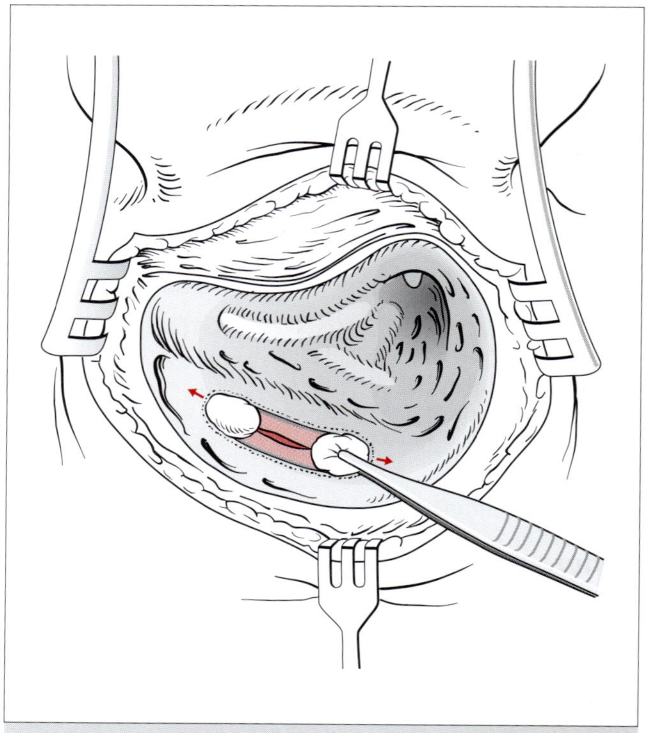

Fig. 19.7 Sinus thrombosis.
The sinus is packed off with collagen fleece sponges tucked between the bony sinus shell and vessel wall.

19

Wound closure. The wound is closed in layers over a drainage tube that is brought out of the lower end of the wound.

Jugular vein ligation. Jugular vein ligation in the neck is indicated for a purulent sinus thrombus that is associated with clinical manifestations of sepsis (see Chapter 9).

Rules, Tips, and Tricks

- When the sinus has been opened, mechanical positive-pressure ventilation should be maintained to prevent air embolism.
- Positive identification of the sinus is aided by exposing a long sinus segment and, if necessary, by also exposing the adjacent dura.
- If the mastoid extends far posteriorly and is very well pneumatized, extend the postauricular incision to a T-shaped incision (auxiliary limb 3 cm toward the occiput).
- Often the sinus wall is markedly thickened due to perisinus inflammation, and a needle inserted at a tangential angle may take a few moments to aspirate intraluminal blood. Do not discontinue the puncture too soon.
- Separate the sinus wall from the bone and have packing material ready before incising the sinus wall so that profuse bleeding can be quickly attended to.

! Risks and Complications

- See Tympanoplasty in Chapter 18 (p. 367) and Mastoidectomy in this chapter (p. 387).
- Septic metastases in multiple organs, multiorgan failure.
- CNS complications such as meningitis, brain abscess, spread of sinus thrombosis, increased intracranial pressure, cranial nerve deficits (IX–XII).
- Complications of jugular vein ligation in the neck (see Chapter 9, surgical treatment of tonsillogenic cellulitis and tonsillogenic sepsis).

Postoperative Care

- Heparinization only in consultation with a neurologist.
- CT/MRI follow-up, neurologic follow-ups.
- The drain is removed when fluid drainage stops.
- High-dose antibiotic therapy, changed as needed based on sensitivity results.
- The condition of the patient may necessitate intensive care.

Epidural Abscess, Meningitis

Surgical Principle

Eliminate the primary focus by mastoidectomy or by an atticoantrotomy if the condition has resulted from cholesteatoma. The epidural abscess is drained, and the dura is exposed at the portal of entry.

Indication

Any suspicion of otogenic meningitis or epidural abscess formation.

Specific Points Regarding Informed Consent

- See Tympanoplasty in Chapter 18 (p. 367) and Mastoidectomy in this chapter (p. 387).
- Disclose the severity and risks posed by the disease.
- CNS complications.

Operative Planning

Exclusion of brain abscess by MRI, CT, high-resolution CT, and if necessary by neurologic examination.

Anesthesia

General anesthesia.

Surgical Technique

Mastoid surgery. A complete mastoidectomy is performed through a postauricular approach, or an atticoantrotomy in cholesteatoma patients, with the exenteration of all accessible air cells.

Skeletonization. The bony base of the middle and posterior cranial fossae is exposed with cutting burrs, switching finally to a large diamond burr. The sinus is skeletonized distally from the sinodural angle.

Exposure. Spread to the dura is traced by enlarging the bone defect with a diamond burr and round incision knife until a full circumference of normal dura has been exposed. In the absence of a spontaneous perforation, the bony base is still thinned with a burr and carefully broken inward and dissected with an angled round incision knife to expose the dura. The exposed dura is lifted slightly about its circumference to check for more peripheral pathologic changes.

Dissection. Epidural granulations and thick fibrinous deposits are separated from normal-appearing peripheral areas with the round incision knife. If the dura appears smooth with a grayish-white sheen, no further measures are necessary.

Abscess drainage. Epidural abscesses will naturally drain following the steps described above. If a bulge in the dura is seen after granulations are removed, a subdural abscess should be suspected. Generally this collection can be aspirated with a needle introduced at a tangential angle. Nowadays it would be appropriate to discuss further management with a neurosurgeon.

Wound closure. The wound is closed in layers over a drain that is brought out at the lower end of the wound. With large defects in the bony base of the middle cranial fossa, a cartilage plate can be placed into the bone defect to prevent dural prolapse, although it should be considered whether drainage takes precedence.

Postoperative Care

- See postoperative details in Chapter 14.
- CT/MRI follow-up, neurologic follow-ups.
- The drain is removed when fluid drainage stops.
- High-dose antibiotic therapy, changed as needed based on sensitivity results.

! Risks and Complications

- See Tympanoplasty in Chapter 18 (p. 367) and Mastoidectomy in this chapter (p. 387).
- CNS complications such as meningitis and brain abscess.
- A relatively large defect in the bony skull base may predispose to a dural prolapse or subarachnoid cyst with extension into the mastoid cavity or ear canal.

20 Surgery of the Middle Ear and Facial Nerve after Trauma

Middle Ear Trauma

Injuries of the Tympanic Membrane and Ossicular Chain

Tympanoplastic principles are followed (see Chapter 18, p. 367ff). The possibility of dural or cerebral prolapse through fractures in the roof of the ear canal or tegmen should always be considered.

Rupture of the Round or Oval Window

Surgical Principle

A fistula in the round or oval window is exposed and covered with connective tissue via tympanoscopy.

Indications

Acute, usually fluctuating hearing loss, often with vertigo and tinnitus after trauma or a massive rise of intracranial pressure (e.g., exertion during heavy lifting).

Specific Points Regarding Informed Consent

- See Stapedectomy in Chapter 21 (p. 399).
- Emphasize the uncertain prognosis for residual hearing and vertigo.

Surgical Technique

Incision. Endaural as in stapes surgery (Chapter 21, p. 399).

Window exposure. The posterolateral attic wall is taken down with a House curette until the pyramidal process can be seen. The bony overhang over the hypotympanum is also taken down slightly. The overhanging upper border usually prevents a direct view of the round window itself and can be carefully burred down (**Fig. 20.1**).

Window inspection. Using high magnification, the surgeon looks for a tear in the annular ligament, a footplate fracture, or a window rupture. The stapes is gently rocked with a needle (alternating pressure test) to check for perilymph leakage from the round or oval window niche.

Fistula repair. A perilymphatic fistula is covered with connective tissue. A ruptured round window is closed by placing fibrin-coated connective tissue into the niche.

Rules, Tips, and Tricks

- Slight dislocations of the footplate should be carefully reduced and connective tissue packed around the footplate. Massive dislocations or displaced footplate fractures are an indication for stapedectomy.
- The round window is often veiled by delicate mucous membranes that prevent the direct visualization of a rupture. Leakage of perilymph in response to the alternating pressure test confirms a window rupture.

Postoperative Care

- Stennert infusion protocol (starting with 1 g hydrocortisone).
- Avoid straining or other acts that could raise the intracranial pressure.

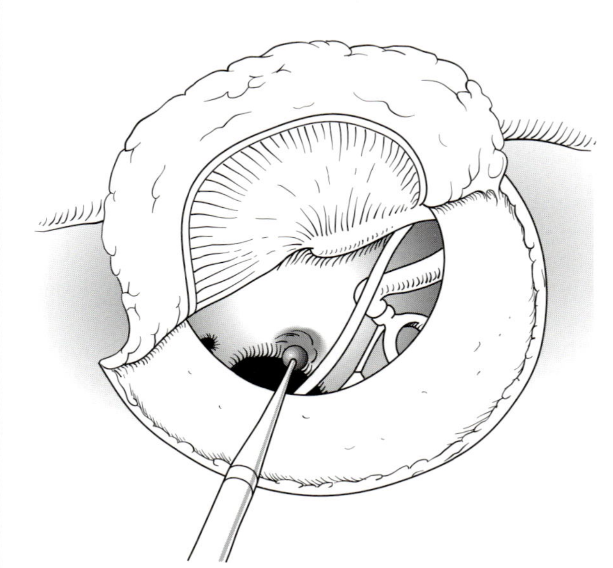

Fig. 20.1 Window rupture.
The overhang over the round window is removed with a burr.

Otorrhea of Cerebrospinal Fluid

Surgical Principle

Fracture lines are exposed by performing a mastoidectomy and, if necessary, opening the tympanic spaces. The fracture is traced to the dural tear, which is identified and closed with fascia, perichondrium, or fibrin-coated collagen fleece.

Indications

- Persistent (approx. 8 days) CSF leak following trauma or surgery.
- Traumatic CSF leak in a patient with pre-existing chronic otitis media (immediate action required).
- Spontaneous CSF leak in chronic otitis media.

Contraindications

- Grave prognosis due to intracranial trauma or multiple injuries.
- Spontaneous closure.

Specific Points Regarding Informed Consent

Same as for a mastoidectomy (Chapter 19, p. 387).

- Persistent CSF leak. Emphasize the possible need for reoperation or extending to a transtemporal or translabyrinthine approach (deafness, vertigo).
- Increased risk of meningitis and brain abscess.
- Sinus hemorrhage.

Operative Planning

High-resolution CT.

Anesthesia

General anesthesia.

Surgical Technique

Exposure. A complete postauricular mastoidectomy is performed, which includes exposure of the attic over the aditus (see Chapter 19, p. 387ff). If the CSF leak is located in the tegmen tympani, the middle ear cavity is also opened through a transmeatal approach (see Chapter 18, p. 368 ff).

Locating the dural leak. The fracture line in the skull base is traced to the dural tear by elevating the bone fragments with a round incision knife and thinning or enlarging the fracture margins with a diamond burr. The edges of the dural tear must be completely exposed on all sides.

Dural closure. After the dura has been adequately separated from the surrounding bony margin, the fibrin-coated graft is tucked between the bone and dura with a generous overlap. A needle, round incision knife, antrum hook, and Rosen elevator are useful instruments for positioning the graft.

Opening the ossicular chain. If the dural tear is located in the tegmen tympani, it will be necessary to open the ossicular chain (Chapter 18, p. 379f) unless the fracture has already disrupted the chain.

Wound closure. Same as in mastoidectomy.

Rules, Tips, and Tricks

- The full extent of the fistula must be exposed and inspected.
- Watertight closure of the fistula is essential.
- If a small CSF fistula cannot be located initially, the intrathecal injection of 1:1 fluorescein dye diluted with 0.9 % NaCl will make it easier to identify the leak. This requires the use of a special blue filter on the otomicroscope. Because intrathecal fluorescein is not an approved use, special informed consent is required for this application.
- If the position or extent of the petrous apex does not permit adequate exposure and secure closure of the dural tear, a transtemporal or translabyrinthine approach is required. This cannot always be determined preoperatively, even with high-resolution CT scans.
- Larger bone defects are backed with cartilage (to prevent meningocephalocele). Extensive bone defects may require coverage with a ceramic plate.
- A profuse CSF leak that hampers graft placement may be staunched by elevating the patient's upper body and head. A more reliable solution is lumbar drainage, which may be continued if necessary during the initial postoperative days.

! Risks and Complications

- Same as in mastoidectomy (see Chapter 19, p. 389).
- Special risks are facial paralysis, meningitis, brain abscess, and sinus hemorrhage.

Postoperative care

- Antibiotic coverage is continued for several days.
- Lumbar drainage may be required.

Tympanic and Mastoid Facial Nerve Surgery

Surgical Principle

Exposure of the tympanic and mastoid segments of the facial nerve through a transmastoid approach with incision of the nerve sheath, removal of a bone fragment, or facial nerve grafting.

Indications

- Early traumatic facial paralysis involving the tympanic or mastoid segment of the facial nerve based on electrophysiologic testing.
- Late facial paralysis without nerve regeneration where the fracture line involves the tympanic or mastoid segment.
- Relative indication: idiopathic facial palsy with an unfavorable course (EMG).
- Facial paralysis in chronic otitis media.

Contraindications

- General medical condition.
- Late paralysis with EMG signs of regeneration.

Specific Points Regarding Informed Consent

- Same as mastoidectomy (see Chapter 19, p. 387).
- Possible need to harvest a graft from the great auricular nerve or sural nerve, auxiliary incision, sensory deficits.
- Long recovery period, uncertain prognosis, partial recovery/residual paralysis, mass movements.
- It may be necessary to open the ossicular chain or proceed with tympanoplasty.

Operative Planning

High-resolution CT scans. Some cases may require MRI or EMG and other electrophysiologic tests.

Anesthesia

General anesthesia.

Surgical Technique

Approach. Postauricular incision and complete mastoidectomy with exposure of the antrum, short crus of the incus, and horizontal semicircular canal. Skeletonize the base of the middle cranial fossa and sinus plate, thin the posterior canal wall, and exenterate the cells of the mastoid tip.

Identification. Starting from the incudal fossa (at the short crus of the incus), the facial recess is drilled open between the chorda tympani and facial nerve, and the bony fallopian canal is identified under high magnification in front of the semicircular canal and below the tip of the short process of the incus.

Defining the course of the facial nerve. The further course of the facial nerve is now skeletonized down from the oval window niche to the stylomastoid foramen with a diamond burr, working with broad strokes parallel to the nerve, until the epineurium is visible through the thinned bone. The chordofacial angle is completely exposed. The ossicular chain is also visible at this point, and the nerve can be evaluated in its passage below the ossicular chain as far as the geniculate ganglion. The bone covering the nerve is so thin in this area that it does not require thinning with a burr.

Exposure. The last bony layer is opened with an elevator, excavator, or round incision knife (**Fig. 20.2**). If the tympanic segment also must be exposed, especially with a low dura, consider opening the ossicular chain (see Chapter 18, p. 379f) and then performing a tympanoplasty to avoid damaging the chain.

Dissection. Bone fragments and impaled splinters are removed. If nerve continuity is disrupted, the ragged stumps should be trimmed smooth with a neurectomy scissors. A short dehiscence can be bridged by rerouting the nerve from its canal and performing an end-to-end anastomosis. A longer defect is repaired by interposing a graft from the great auricular nerve. Because the graft fits snugly within the bony canal, it is usually unnecessary to fix it with sutures or fibrin glue (suture technique, see Chapter 13, p. 306). The repair site is covered with fascia or collagen fleece.

Wound closure. Same as in mastoidectomy.

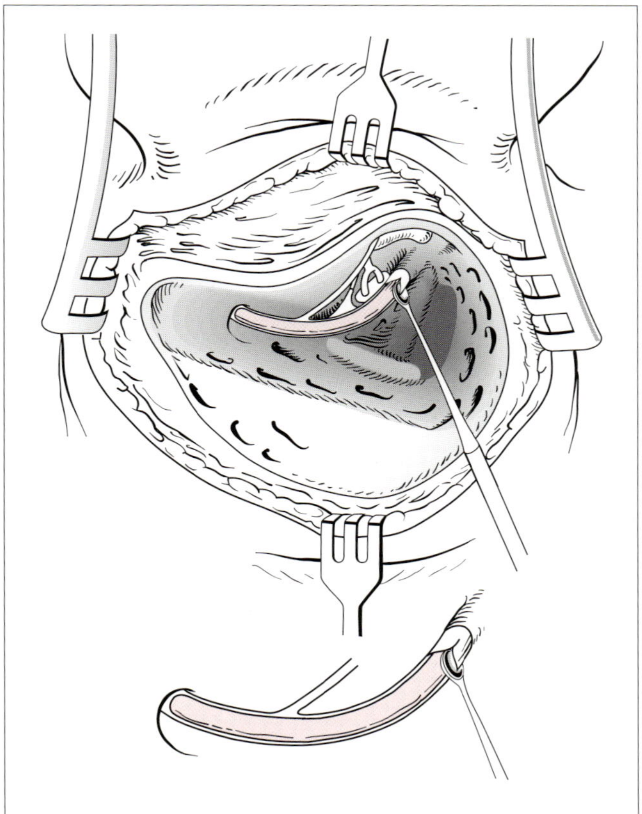

Fig. 20.2 Facial nerve surgery.
The nerve is exposed in the chordofacial angle, and the last bony layer is removed with an elevator.

Rules, Tips, and Tricks

- Identify anatomic landmarks before locating the nerve. (Anatomy may be altered after trauma.)
- Use only a diamond burr, House curette, or elevator when working close to the facial nerve. Irrigate copiously to prevent thermal injury.
- The facial nerve runs anterior to the horizontal semicircular canal at the level of the canal. Because of the tangential view angle at this site, the semicircular canal partially hides the nerve from view. In exposing the nerve, then, always drill in front of the semicircular canal; do not drill into the apex of the canal.
- Potentially troublesome bleeding from fracture lines is controlled by pressing bone wax into the bleeding site.

Risks and Complications

- Same as in mastoidectomy (see Chapter 19, p. 389).
- Erosion of the horizontal semicircular canal during tangential drilling of the fallopian canal at the second genu.
- Ossicular dislocation.
- Dural injury, especially in patients with fracture-related dural or cerebral prolapse.

Postoperative Care

- Same as in mastoidectomy (Chapter 19, p. 389).
- Stennert infusion protocol.
- Watch-glass dressing.
- Mimetic muscle exercises should be started when initial signs of regeneration appear (twitching, initial voluntary motor activity).

21 Stapes Surgery

Stapedectomy

Surgical Principle

Restore sound conduction in stapes ankylosis by partial removal of the posterior third of the footplate (stapedectomy) or occasionally the entire footplate, or by making a small perforation 0.6–0.8 mm in diameter (stapedotomy) or inserting a stapes prosthesis.

Indications

- More than a 20-dB air–bone gap (allowing for the Carhart notch) in suspected otosclerosis, negative Rinne. With bilateral otosclerosis, the ear with poorer hearing should be operated first.
- Impaired sound conduction in the oval window due to tympanosclerosis or sclerosis of the annular ligament.
- Minor malformation.

Contraindications

- Air–bone gap too small.
- Insufficient cochlear reserve, provided a gain in discrimination cannot achieve hearing aid fitness (relative contraindication).
- Pregnancy (after 4 months).
- Deafness in the opposite ear (relative contraindication).
- Inflammatory changes in the ear canal or middle ear.
- Simultaneous stapes surgery in both ears (operations should be scheduled at least 3–6 months apart).

Specific Points Regarding Informed Consent

- Deafness (approx. 1 % risk), lack of hearing improvement, deterioration of hearing—may be delayed due to slippage or loosening of the prosthesis, or may result from further progression of otosclerosis.
- New tinnitus or worsening of preexisting tinnitus. No more than 50 % of patients show improvement of preexisting tinnitus.
- Vertigo, usually in the immediate postoperative period or first few days, but may persist in rare cases (piston too long, part of the footplate sunken into the vestibule).
- Altered taste sensation (chorda tympani).
- Reoperation.
- Intracranial complications.
- Heavy scarring of the incision and auricle, keloid formation.
- Neuralgiform pain.
- Facial nerve injury.

Operative Planning

Complete audiometry, test for spontaneous nystagmus, Schüller and Stenvers radiographic views. Perioperative antibiotics if necessary.

Special Instruments

See under Tympanoplasty in Chapter 18 (p. 367). Also, reinforced 90° hook, very fine Fisch or Plester footplate hooks, perforator, McGee crimper, stapes prosthesis, measuring instrument (gauge). Some techniques require a microdrill (Skeeter) or laser (CO_2 or Er:YAG).

Anesthesia

Local anesthesia is advantageous as it allows for intraoperative auditory testing, and any vertigo due to an oversized prosthesis can be quickly detected and corrected. General anesthesia may also be used.

Surgical Technique

Positioning. The patient is positioned supine on the operating table with the head turned to the side and immobilized on a headrest or ring.

Exposure. Endaural incision (see Chapter 17, p. 359f) with a No.15 blade. The initial 1-cm incision is made laterally from the center of the bony roof of the ear canal through the intercartilaginous fissure and parallel to the anterior helical rim. The second incision is made circumferentially from the 6 o'clock to the 12 o'clock position about 0.5 cm inside the bony meatal entrance. The two incisions form a triangular flap that is raised, reflected outward, and secured with the self-retaining retractor. Small pieces of connective tissue are harvested from the endaural incision.

With a large ear canal, it may be possible to omit the meatal flap or even use a pure endomeatal (transcanal) approach without an endaural auxiliary incision (this requires a self-retaining aural speculum and angled instruments). The tympanomeatal flap is outlined by making additional incisions toward the tympanic membrane at 5 and 11 o'clock in the right ear or 1 and 7 o'clock in the left ear (see **Fig. 17.3**). The flap is elevated to the annulus with an angled round incision knife.

Opening the middle ear cavity. The annulus is elevated in the posterosuperior quadrant, and the middle ear cavity is entered by dividing the thin, tense mucoperiosteum with a sickle knife while sparing the chorda tympani. The tympanomeatal flap is further mobilized and reflected (**Fig. 21.1**).

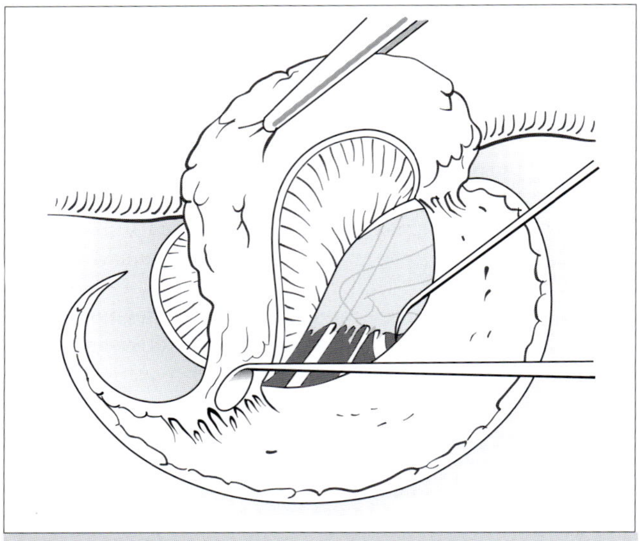

Fig. 21.1 Stapedectomy.
The tympanomeatal flap is developed and the mucoperiosteum is divided to enter the middle ear cavity.

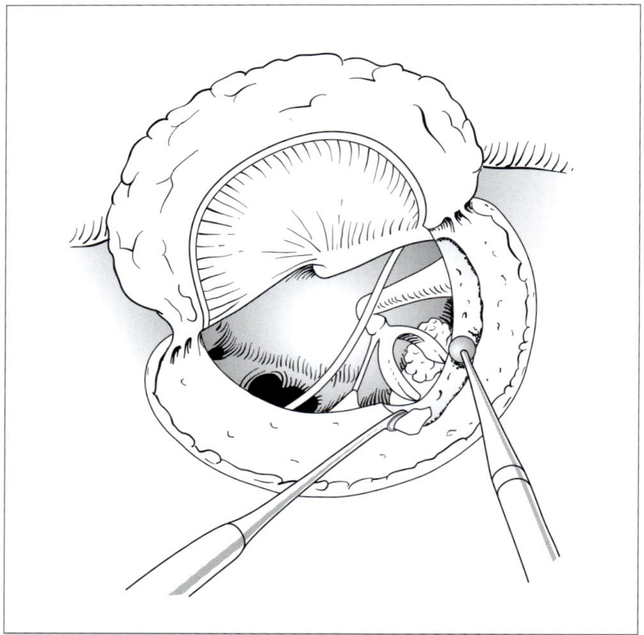

Fig. 21.2 Stapedectomy.
The oval window niche is exposed with a House curette. The exposure may be aided with a diamond burr.

Exposure of the oval window niche. The lateral attic wall is taken down with a House curette to expose the pyramidal eminence and facial nerve over the oval window niche (**Fig. 21.2**). The long process of the incus is gently probed with a needle or microhook; concomitant movement of the manubrium rules out malleus fixation. Stapes fixation is easily recognized by moving the incus from side to side.

Stapes dissection. The distance from the incus to the footplate (measured distance + 0.2–0.3 mm = necessary length of prosthesis) is measured with a gauge (**Fig. 21.3**). The incudostapedial joint is separated with a medium-sized 90° hook, and the stapedius tendon is divided with the sickle knife (**Fig. 21.4**).

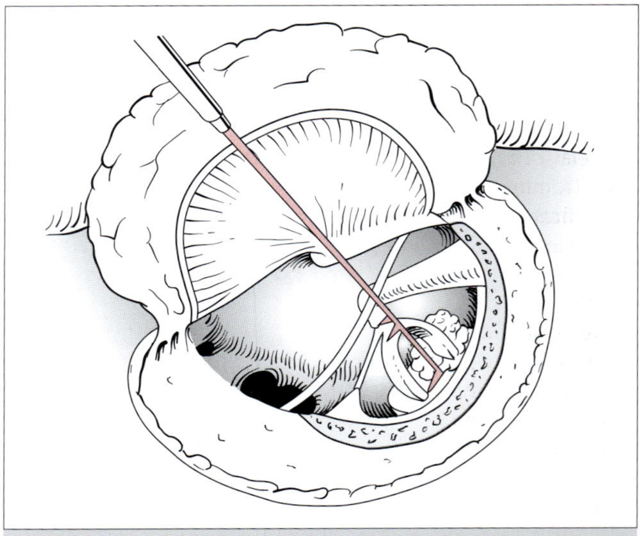

Fig. 21.3 Stapedectomy.
The distance from incus to footplate is measured with a gauge.

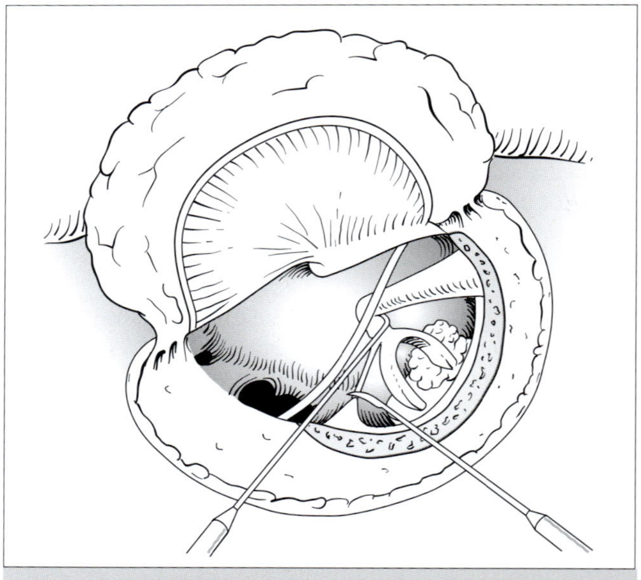

Fig. 21.4 Stapedectomy.
The incudostapedial joint is separated with a 90 ° hook, and the stapedius tendon is divided.

First the posterior and then the anterior stapes crus is fractured with a medium-sized 90° or 45° hook that is applied close to the footplate and is twisted slightly toward the promontory to shear off each crus at its base (**Fig. 21.5**). The stapes arch is extracted with a microforceps (**Fig. 21.6**).

Opening the vestibule. The mucosa surrounding the footplate is scored and divided with a slightly curved needle. The mucosa may then be separated from the footplate, although this is not essential (fragments may remain attached to the mucosa during footplate extraction). Working under high magnification, the surgeon perforates the footplate at the junction of the middle and posterior thirds with the perforator, which is applied to the footplate with a slight twisting motion (**Fig. 21.7**). The hand should be securely braced to avoid exerting too much pressure.

Footplate extraction. The footplate (if still intact) is now split apart with fine 45° or 90° hooks inserted into the perforation. The posterior third of the footplate or the fragments are first elevated with a 45° hook and then extracted with a 90° hook (reinforced Fisch or Plester hook or pick, **Fig. 21.8**). High magnification is still used at this stage to avoid penetrating too deeply into the vestibule. Under no circumstances should these manipulations cause mobile portions of the footplate to sink into the vestibule.

Reconstruction. The stapes prosthesis (e.g., platinum band–Teflon or titanium model, properly sized, average length 4.5 mm, piston diameter 0.4–0.8 mm) is grasped with a fine alligator forceps and held so that the long axis of the prosthesis is at a slight angle to the forceps axis (**Fig. 21.9**). The eyelet of the prosthesis is threaded over the long process of the incus. The lower end of the piston should project only ca. 0.2–0.3 mm into the vestibule. The position of the prosthesis can still be adjusted at this stage with the 90° hook. When the piston is perfectly positioned, the eyelet is crimped onto the long process of the incus with a McGee forceps (**Fig. 21.10**), and the placement is again checked for accuracy. The small pieces of connective tissue harvested at the start of the operation are packed around the piston to seal the window (**Fig. 21.11**).

Concluding the operation. Blood clots are suctioned from the hypotympanum, and the tympanomeatal and meatal flaps are returned to their original positions. The ear canal is lined with silicone film and packed with ointment-impregnated strips. The wound is closed and a dressing is applied.

Special Intraoperative Situations

Premature Separation of the Footplate ("Floating" Footplate)

If the footplate is generally mobile during manipulations before the perforation has been made, the surgeon should attempt to separate the annular ligament at a small site with a needle, working toward the promontory, or drill a small hole directly adjacent to the annular ligament with a very fine, low-speed diamond burr to create a site where a hook can be passed beneath the footplate to elevate it. The oval window is then covered with a small piece of connective tissue that overlaps the window on all sides, creating a foundation on which the prosthesis is placed. With proper facilities, a better option is to convert to a laser stapedotomy, in which even a floating footplate can be perforated using a noncontact laser technique.

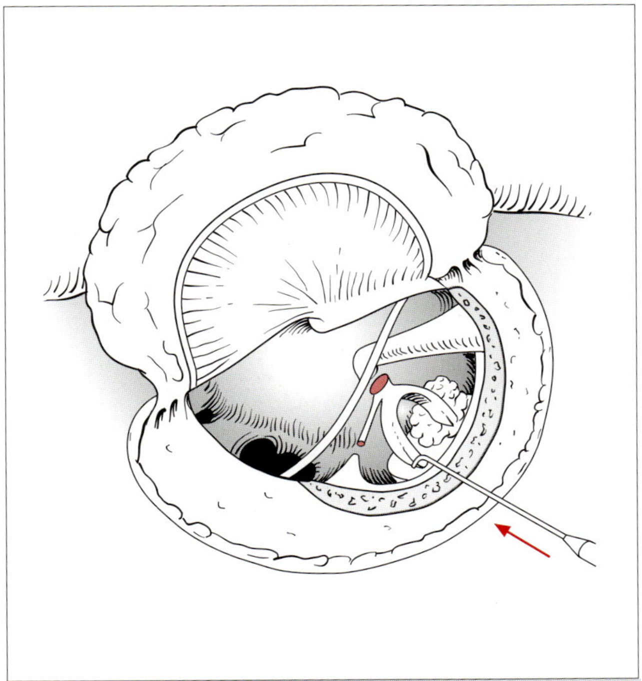

Fig. 21.5 Stapedectomy.
The stapes crura are fractured with the 90° hook.

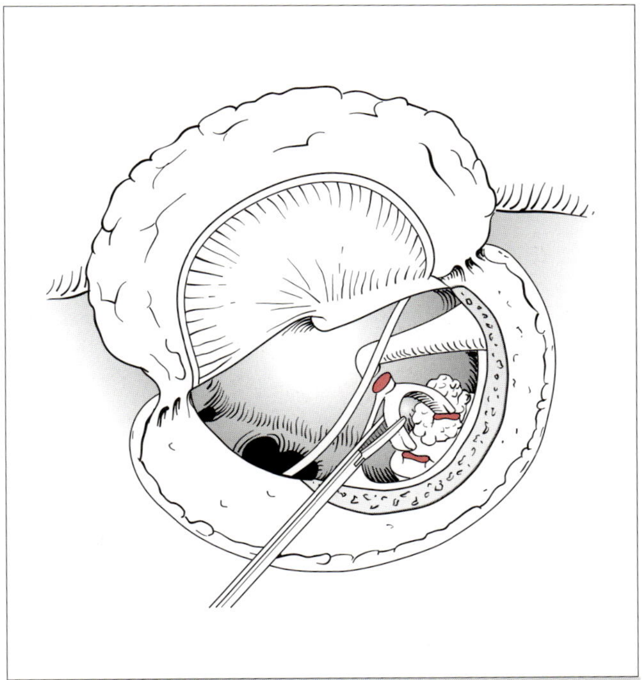

Fig. 21.6 Stapedectomy.
Extraction of the stapes arch.

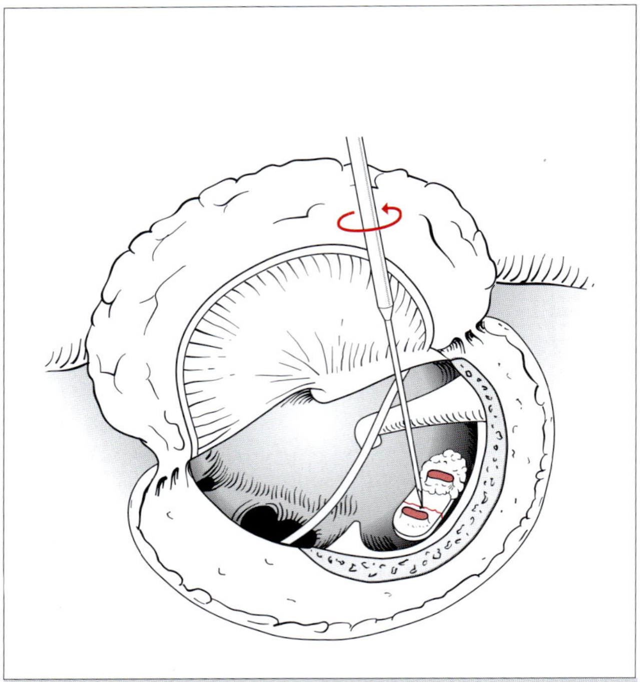

Fig. 21.7 Stapedectomy.
Perforation of the footplate.

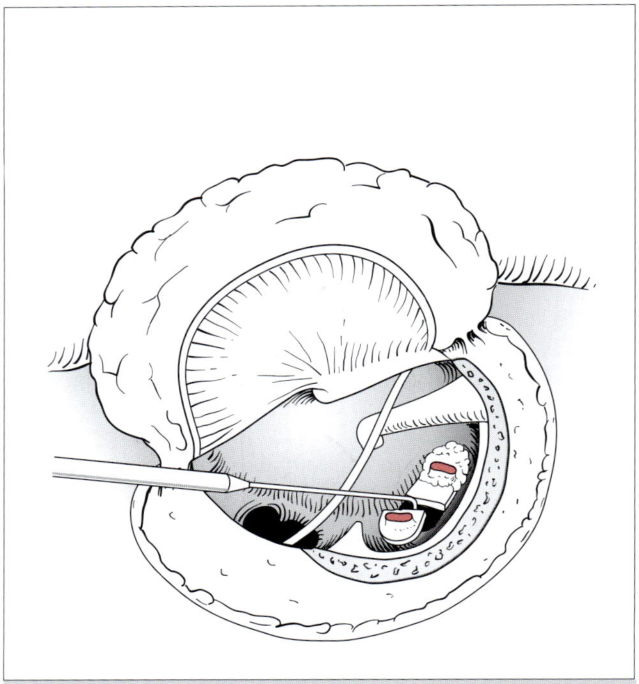

Fig. 21.8 Stapedectomy.
The posterior third of the footplate is extracted with the 90° hook.

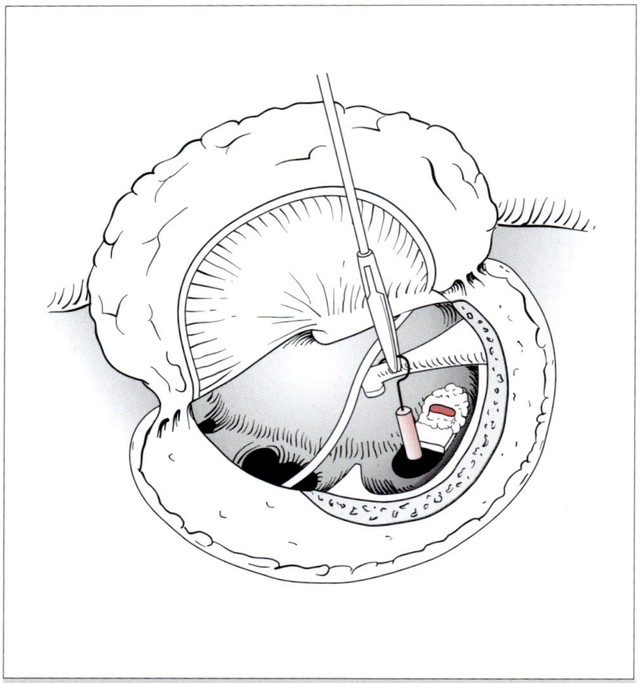

Fig. 21.9 Stapedectomy.
The prosthesis is introduced with a small alligator forceps. The prosthesis is held at a slight angle to the forceps axis.

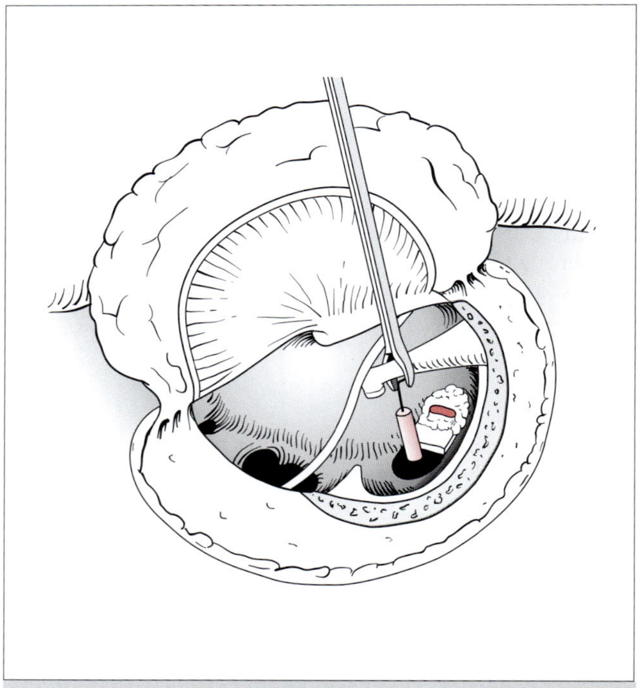

Fig. 21.10 Stapedectomy.
The eyelet of the stapes prosthesis is slid over the long process of the incus and crimped into place with McGee forceps.

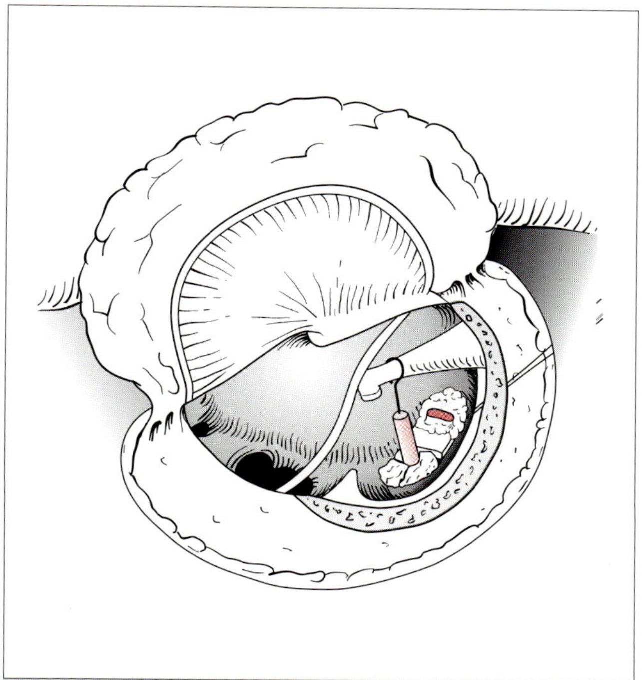

Fig. 21.11 Stapedectomy.
Connective tissue is packed around the piston to seal the vestibule.

Perilymphatic Gusher

If cerebrospinal fluid (CSF) gushes from the opened vestibule because of a wide communication between the CSF space and perilymphatic space, the procedure should be halted at once. The head and upper body are elevated to lower the CSF pressure. The oval window niche is sealed with connective tissue or fibrin-coated collagen that extends to the long process of the incus. Lumbar puncture can be done for additional decompression. In a laser stapedotomy, it may be possible to seal the leak by inserting the piston and covering the site with fat or connective tissue during lumbar drainage of CSF. When this is successful, the procedure can be concluded in the usual way.

Overhanging Facial Nerve

A facial nerve that dangles into the niche, usually exposed, or a vascular anomaly can make it impossible to dissect in the niche without jeopardizing the facial nerve. Although it is possible in principle to drill a hole in the promontory and insert a piston, treatment with a hearing aid provides a risk-free alternative.

Obliterative and Very Advanced Otosclerosis

If stapedectomy cannot be performed because the perforator will not penetrate the otosclerotic niche, a recommended alternative is stapedotomy with a Skeeter drill or laser. A hole is carefully drilled through the footplate with a 0.6-mm burr on a Skeeter microdrill operating at low speed. The upper part of the opening is then widened with a 1-mm diamond burr to prevent the piston jamming in the long, narrow hole.

Rules, Tips, and Tricks

- Use cautious movements and atraumatic technique when working in the oval window niche and vestibule.
- Always work with optimum vision, especially in the oval window niche.
- Establish a bloodless field before opening the vestibule.
- Match the length of the prosthesis to the size of the defect.
- Always perforate the footplate before extracting it.
- When working on the footplate, use the smallest possible microsuction tips and never apply suction directly to the vestibule. Use a low suction setting.
- Visualization of the oval window niche can often be improved by slightly adjusting the patient's head position relative to the surgeon. An overhanging promontory wall can be taken down with a low-speed diamond burr. This should be done carefully because of the risk of opening the cochlea.
- The surgeon's arm and hand should be securely braced during all critical manipulations.
- Always use the House curette with a "twisting and pulling-out" motion.
- Avoid trauma to the chorda tympani. It can be displaced anteriorly from the niche to improve visualization. The bony canal of the chorda tympani can be removed to ca. 3 mm with the House curette to minimize traction.
- Several drops of 1:100 000 suprarenin solution can be placed in the oval window niche shortly before dissection of the footplate to control bleeding.
- Optimum coupling of the prosthesis to the long process of the incus is important for a satisfactory hearing result (too loose: deficient sound conduction; too tight: eventual necrosis). Coupling of the prosthesis can be significantly improved by using pistons with a clip mechanism (see different types shown in **Fig. 21.12**).

! Risks and Complications

- Vertigo may occur if portions of the footplate sink into the vestibule or the prosthesis is too long (revision indicated). Surgical trauma may also cause postoperative vertigo.
- Intraoperative sensorineural hearing loss or deafness. Hearing loss that starts on the second or third postoperative day and progresses rapidly to deafness, usually accompanied by nystagmus, is suspicious for early granuloma formation in the oval window niche. (Treat with high-dose corticosteroids, Stenvers infusion protocol, and intravenous antibiotics. If symptoms do not improve within 24 hours, revise by removing the prosthesis, connective tissue, and granulations without entering the vestibule. Then cover the oval window niche with fascia.)
- Perilymphatic fistula (fluctuating hearing loss, vertigo, tinnitus). Revision is indicated.
- Slippage of the prosthesis on the long process of the incus, necrosis of the long process. Revision is indicated.
- Facial paralysis.

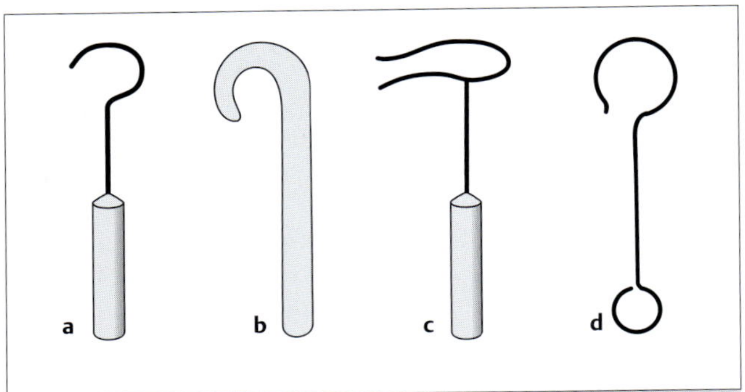

Fig. 21.12a–d Stapedectomy.
Different types of stapes prosthesis.

Postoperative Care

- Bed rest on the day of the operation.
- Continue perioperative antibiotics only with a complicated course.
- Treat as needed with an antivertiginous drug.
- No nose blowing for 8 days. Keep water out of the ear for 8 weeks.
- Daily Weber test (tuning-fork lateralization).
- Check daily for spontaneous nystagmus.

Stapedotomy

Surgical Principle

Restore sound conduction in stapes ankylosis by making a small hole in the footplate 0.4–0.8 mm in diameter with a perforator or Skeeter microdrill and inserting a stapes prosthesis. This procedure is less traumatizing than a partial or complete footplate extraction.

Surgical Technique

Exposure, opening the middle ear cavity, and exposing the oval window niche. Same as in stapedectomy.

Footplate perforation. The stapes superstructure may be left intact if space permits—otherwise it is removed using standard technique. The footplate is pierced with a perforator using a slight twisting motion, and the perforation is enlarged with the next larger size of perforator or pick to ca. 0.4–0.7 mm, depending on the piston diameter (test with sizer). Another option is to perforate the footplate with a Skeeter microdrill operating at low speed.

Reconstruction. The sized prosthesis is introduced and slid onto the long process of the incus. The piston is placed into the vestibule, inserting it no deeper than 0.2–0.3 mm. Its 0.4- to 0.6-mm diameter should just allow it move freely within the drill hole. It is coupled to the long process of the incus with a crimper or clip mechanism. Then the stapes superstructure, which has been supporting the stapes, is disengaged and removed as in a stapedectomy. Two or three small pieces of fat or connective tissue are packed around the vestibule to seal it. The remaining steps are the same as in a stapedectomy.

Laser Stapedotomy

Surgical Principle

The laser assists in removal of the stapes superstructure, and the footplate is perforated entirely with noncontact laser pulses. No portion of the footplate is extracted. The rest of the procedure is the same as in a stapedectomy.

A CO_2 or Er:YAG laser is coupled to the operating microscope. Argon laser energy is delivered through flexible fibers controlled with a micromanipulator system.

Surgical Technique

Opening the ossicular chain. The approach is the same as in a stapedectomy. The incudostapedial joint is still disengaged with a conventional 90° hook. Next, the laser is used to lyse the stapedius tendon and then divide the posterior crus of the stapes close to the footplate. The anterior crus can be fractured with a hook, or it may be blindly divided with an argon laser beam before extracting the stapes arch with a small forceps.

Perforation. A perforation 0.5–0.7 mm in diameter is created in the posterior portion of the footplate with 6–12 overlapping laser bursts (**Fig. 21.13**).

Reconstruction. A piston 0.4–0.6 mm in diameter is introduced using standard stapedotomy technique.

Laser energy parameters. The energy parameters depend on the laser technique and application site. The settings recommended for CO_2 lasers range roughly from 2 to 6 W with a 0.05-second pulse length. Argon lasers are operated at approximately 2 W with a 0.1-second pulse length. The exact settings will depend on the specific situation.

! Laser Risks in the Ear

- Temperature elevation in the inner ear, especially with an argon laser. Reportedly, the development of a micro-handpiece has minimized this problem.
- Opinions differ on the potential for inner ear injury due to shock-wave generation by a Er:YAG laser.
- Risk of collateral injury (to the facial nerve) by a CO_2 laser because of a discrepancy between the aiming beam and the surgical beam (structures at risk are covered with moist gelatin sponge).

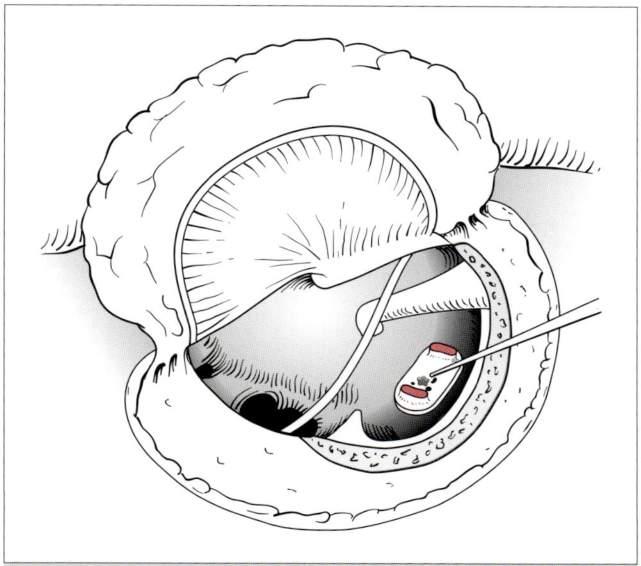

Fig. 21.13 Stapedotomy.
The footplate is perforated in a rosette pattern with multiple laser bursts.

- Loss of perilymph from the vestibule: halt further laser application until the vestibule refills with fluid (to prevent direct exposure of inner ear structures to the beam).

Tympanoscopy

Provisional opening of the middle ear cavity due to suspected otosclerosis or ossicular chain defect.

The steps are like those in a stapedectomy including exposure of the ossicular chain in the oval window niche. This may be followed by a tympanoplasty and stapedectomy, depending on the findings, or the procedure may be discontinued at this point.

Stapes Revision

Surgical Principle

Attempted correction of recurrent conductive hearing loss or vertigo after previous stapes surgery, repeating the steps of the initial procedure but being extremely careful with manipulations about the niche and vestibule.

Indications

Recurrence of conductive hearing loss:

- Dislocation of the prosthesis on the incus or in the vestibule.
- Necrosis of the long process of the incus.
- Recurrent sclerosis or fibrosis of the oval window.
- Loosening of the prosthesis with tension phenomenon (brief hearing improvement after a Valsalva maneuver).

Fluctuating or rapidly progressive hearing loss, vertigo, new tinnitus:

- Perilymphatic fistula.
- Prosthesis too long.
- Early granuloma.

Specific Points Regarding Informed Consent

Standard disclosures for stapes surgery, plus the following:

- Risk of no hearing improvement or further hearing loss, significantly increased risk of deafness (10% or more).
- New tinnitus or worsening of pre-existing tinnitus.
- Vertigo: new, persistent, or increased.

Surgical Technique

The steps are the same as in a stapedectomy including ossicular exposure in the oval window niche. Local anesthesia is preferred as it allows intraoperative feedback on vertigo and hearing.

Exploration. Exploratory steps include inspection of the ossicular chain, testing ossicular mobility with a needle probe, and testing the stapes with alternating pressure. The findings will then dictate the rest of the procedure.

Prosthetic loosening. Crimp the eyelet more tightly onto the incus.

Incus necrosis. Replace the piston. With a stapedotomy, carefully remove the old piston. With a stapedectomy, it is better to cut the piston off and leave it alone. Create a new footplate perforation with a Skeeter drill or laser. Reinsert a piston of the proper shape and length for the revision.

Piston too long. Replace as above, but with a shorter piston. Usually it is unnecessary to make a new perforation.

Window closure. Create a new perforation with a Skeeter drill or laser. Dissect extremely carefully due to possible adhesions with the saccule and utricle.

Perilymphatic fistula. Seal the fistula with connective tissue.

Rules, Tips, and Tricks

- Given the high risk of deafness on reopening the vestibule, consider a hearing aid as a possible alternative. The hearing aid may be fitted primarily or after tympanoscopic evaluation.
- Revision procedures require considerable experience on the part of the surgeon. It is best to refer the patient to a specialized center.

22 Surgical Treatment of Vertigo

F. Hoppe

Gentamicin Therapy

Surgical Principle

Ablation of the labyrinth in a patient with paroxysmal vertigo (e.g., Ménière disease) by the intratympanic administration of gentamicin.

Indication

Paroxysmal vertigo refractory to conservative therapy in Ménière disease with endolymphatic hydrops.

Contraindications

- Gentamicin allergy.
- Severe bilateral sensorineural hearing loss (relative).

Specific Points Regarding Informed Consent

- Same as for myringotomy (see Chapter 16, p. 355).
- Persistence of vertigo attacks, possible constant vertigo in many patients (postablation dizziness is rapidly compensated in most cases). Up to 80% chance of improving complaints, but long-term relapse may occur.
- Hearing loss does not improve and may worsen. Risk of deafness is up to 5% in patients with significant pre-existing sensorineural hearing loss, otherwise lower.
- Tinnitus is usually unchanged.

Operative Planning

Plan for local anesthesia. Position the patient as for a tympanoplasty (see Chapter 18, p. 367).

Special Instruments

Sickle knife, 1-mL syringe with a 0.1-mL scale, angled needle or 1.0-mm attachment on suction tip.

Surgical Technique

Positioning. Same as for a tympanoplasty or mastoidectomy.

A small radial incision is made in the *anterosuperior quadrant* of the tympanic membrane. A total of 0.3 mL (= 12 mg) gentamicin is slowly instilled into the middle ear cleft. The patient lies still for approximately 30 minutes with the head turned 45° to the side (otosurgical position).

> **! Risks and Complications**
> Additional hearing loss or deafness, tinnitus, constant vertigo.

Postoperative Care

The procedure may be repeated on days 8 and 15. Inner ear function should be monitored. If threshold decline is noted, discontinue gentamicin therapy.

Alternatives

Besides the "titrated" interval application described here, there are other protocols that involve the microcatheter-assisted administration of gentamicin continuously or on several consecutive days.

Saccotomy

Surgical Principle

The endolymphatic sac is decompressed or opened through a mastoidectomy approach while preserving the labyrinth, facial nerve, and sigmoid sinus.

Indication

Vertigo refractory to conservative therapy in Ménière disease with endolymphatic hydrops.

Contraindications

No special contraindications.

Specific Points Regarding Informed Consent

- Same as for mastoidectomy (see Chapter 19, p. 387).
- Vertigo may persist.
- Approximately 70–75 % chance of improving complaints.
- Risk of deafness is up to 5 % in patients with significant preexisting sensorineural hearing loss.

Operative Planning

Mastoidectomy, postauricular approach.

Special Instruments or Implants

Silicone triangle.

Anesthesia

Local or general anesthesia.

Surgical Technique

Positioning. Same as for tympanoplasty and mastoidectomy.

Approach. Complete postauricular mastoidectomy.

Exposure of the semicircular canals. The lateral semicircular canal is identified as a landmark. The posterior semicircular canal is then identified posterior, perpendicular and slightly medial to the lateral canal, and its apex is exposed. The bone over the apex of the posterior semicircular canal, and if necessary the lateral canal, is thinned longitudinally with a diamond burr until the blue line can be seen.

Tracing the blue line. The blue line of the posterior semicircular canal is traced down toward the floor of the ear canal. Given the proximity of the facial nerve, it is a good precaution to identify its mastoid segment at this stage.

Exposure. Drilling with the diamond burr is continued to expose the Trautmann triangle posterior to the posterior semicircular canal. The endolymphatic sac and duct are found in the lower portion of the triangle (**Fig. 22.1**).

Saccotomy. The endolymphatic sac is incised (**Fig. 22.2**), and a silicone triangle is inserted into its lumen (**Fig. 22.3**). The postauricular wound is closed, and a dressing is applied.

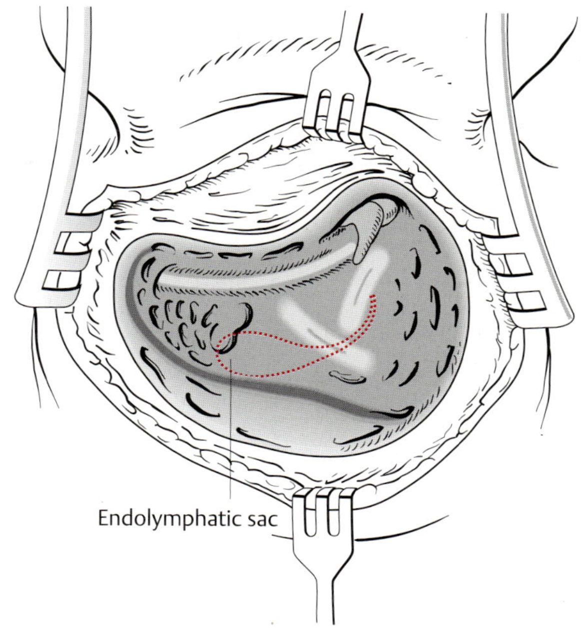

Fig. 22.1 Saccotomy.
The endolymphatic sac is exposed in the lower portion of the Trautmann triangle after first identifying the lateral and posterior semicircular canals and the facial nerve.

Rules, Tips, and Tricks

The posterior semicircular canal (blue line) and mastoid segment of the facial nerve must be positively identified.

! Risks and Complications

- Drilling injury to the facial nerve during dissection of the endolymphatic sac.
- Drilling injury to the semicircular canal.
- Opening the sigmoid sinus.
- Incision of the dura (duplication of the dura) with a cerebrospinal fluid fistula due to misidentification of the dura as the endolymphatic sac.

Postoperative Care

- Daily tuning-fork test of hearing. Bone conduction may also be tested.
- Daily nystagmus testing.

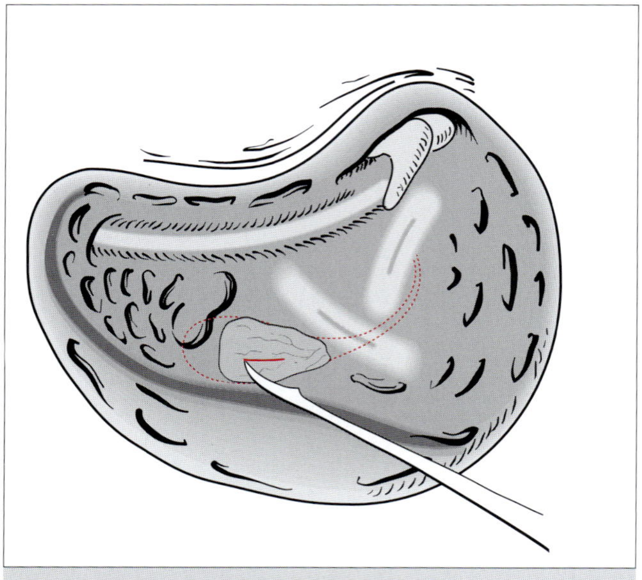

Fig. 22.2 Saccotomy.
The endolymphatic sac is opened with a sickle knife.

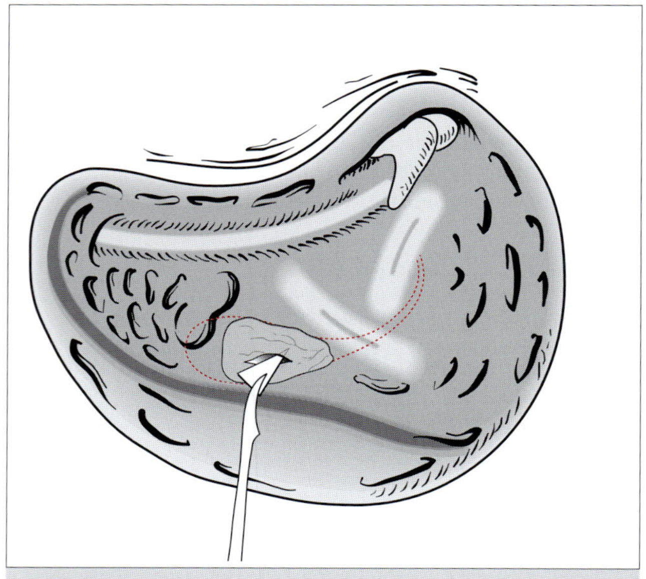

Fig. 22.3 Saccotomy.
A silicone triangle is placed into the sac for drainage.

Alternatives

- Gentamicin therapy (see above).
- Transtemporal neurectomy in hearing patients, translabyrinthine neurectomy in deaf patients.
- Labyrinthectomy with instillation of ototoxic agents into the opened and exenterated labyrinth.

23 Surgical Implantation of Hearing Aids

F. Hoppe

Given our limited scope, this chapter offers only a brief overview of implantable hearing aids. This type of surgery is usually reserved for specialized centers.

Bone-Anchored Hearing Aids (BAHA)

Surgical Principle

Sound is transmitted to the inner ear by bone conduction through an osseointegrated titanium post in the temporal squama, which is connected directly to an external hearing aid with an electromagnetic transducer.

Indications

- Inoperable congenital aural atresia.
- Conductive hearing loss with intractable otorrhea in the setting of chronic otitis media.
- Sensorineural hearing loss in a patient with persistent otitis externa.

Surgical Technique

The surgery is usually performed under local anesthesia. A titanium post is implanted into a hole 3–4 mm deep that has been drilled into the temporal squama. The surrounding scalp is thinned and depilated. The procedure may be performed in one or two stages. In a two-stage procedure, a titanium abutment is screwed onto the post after a healing period of 8–12 weeks, and the sound processor is attached to the abutment.

Partially Implantable Hearing Aids

Surgical Principle

Sound is transmitted directly to an intact, mobile ossicular chain by an electromagnetic vibrator. The amplifier is implanted in a postauricular bone bed, and the receiver is worn externally behind the ear. Three different systems are currently available on the market.

Indications

Sensorineural hearing loss not correctible with conventional hearing aids (e.g., severe recurrent otitis externa, anatomic obstacles to wearing a hearing aid in the ear canal). Different indications apply to different implants, depending on the level of inner ear function.

Surgical Technique

A vibrator (active or passive) is coupled to the ossicular chain (long process of the incus, body of incus) through a mastoidectomy. The chordofacial angle may also be drilled open.

The amplifier is implanted in a postauricular bone bed.

Cochlear Implant

Surgical Principle

A multichannel electrode is positioned into the cochlea through a mastoidectomy, and a processor is implanted behind the ear.

Indications

Congenital or acquired bilateral deafness in cases where the auditory nerve is responsive to electrical stimulation (promontory test) and the inner ear is anatomically normal. Cochlear implantation can be done in patients as young as 4 months of age.

Contraindications

- Auditory nerve unresponsive to electrical stimulation.
- Cerebral malformations (relative).

Specific Points Regarding Informed Consent

Same as in mastoidectomy. There is also a future risk of potentially fatal meningitis from the spread of labyrinthitis. This risk is highest in children, given their greater susceptibility to serous and suppurative forms of otitis.

The patient or caregiver should be informed about postoperative care requirements.

Operative Planning

Postauricular incision with a special extension for implanting the processor.

Special Instruments

- Dummy processor, dummy electrode.
- Implant.
- Clip may be needed for attaching the electrode.

Anesthesia

General anesthesia. Local anesthesia is also an option.

Surgical Technique

- Retroauricular flap incision (**Fig. 23.1**).
- The skin flap (ca. 0.5 cm thick) is raised.
- The temporalis muscle is incised and reflected.
- A bed for the processor (dummy) is drilled into the bone.
- A broad mastoidectomy is performed.
- The short crus of the incus is exposed.
- The horizontal semicircular canal is identified.
- The facial nerve and chorda tympani are identified.
- The chordofacial angle is drilled open (**Fig. 23.2**).
- The incudostapedial joint and round window are visualized.

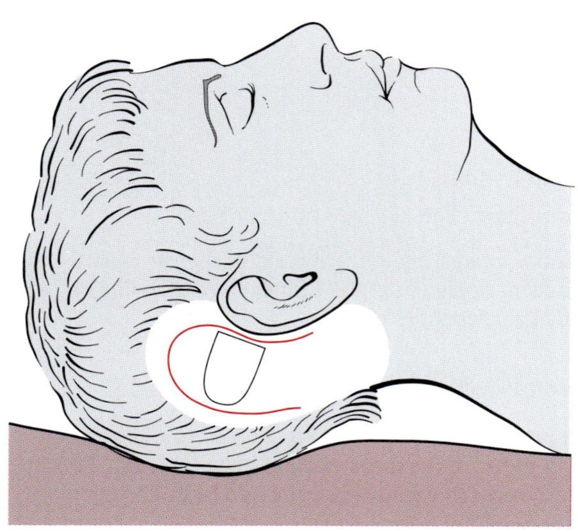

Fig. 23.1 Cochlear implant.
Skin incision.

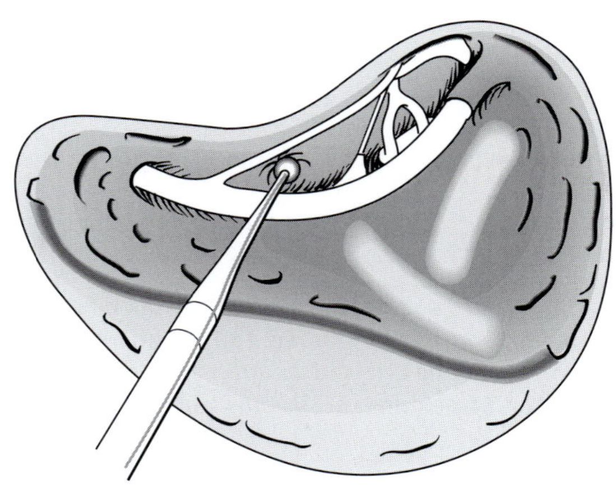

Fig. 23.2 Cochlear implant.
The chordofacial angle is drilled open.

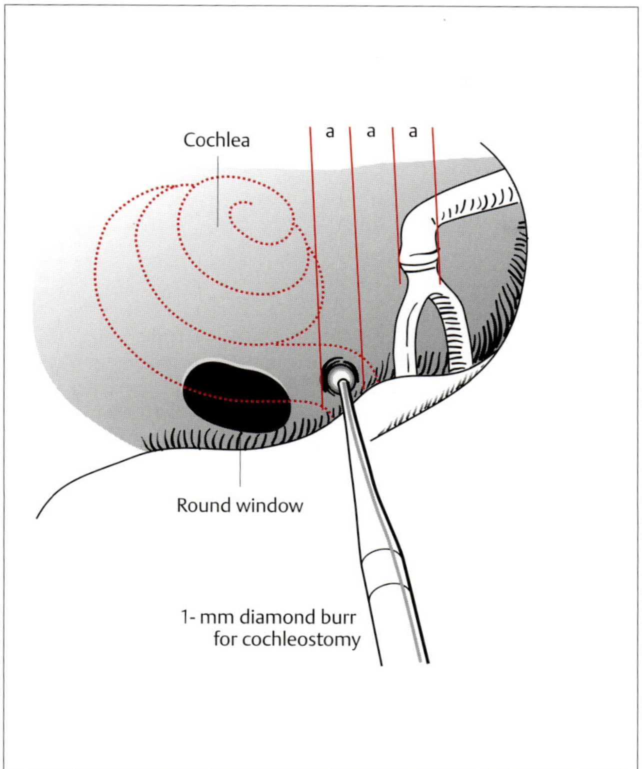

Fig. 23.3 Cochlear implant.
The cochlea is opened with a 0.8-mm burr between the incudostapedial joint and round window (twice the width of the stapes head (**a**), projected from the joint onto the promontory).

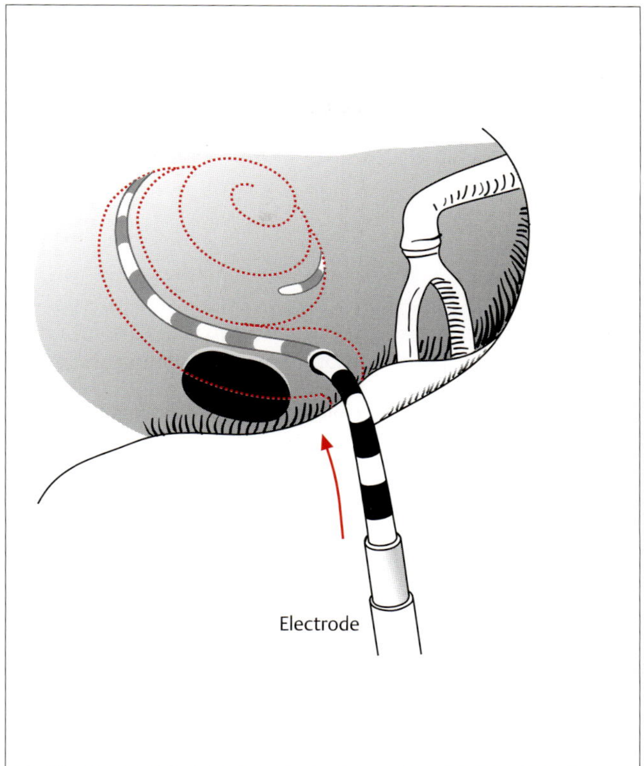

Fig. 23.4 Cochlear implant.
The electrode is inserted into the cochlea.

- The cochlea is opened with an 0.8-mm burr between the incudostapedial joint and round window (twice the width of the capitulum projected onto the promontory, **Fig. 23.3**).
- The dummy electrode is inserted (2.5 cochlear turns).
- The processor is implanted in the bone bed.
- The electrode is gently inserted into the cochlea (**Fig. 23.4**).
- The neutral electrode is inserted beneath the periosteum above the ear.
- The wound is carefully closed to prevent hematoma formation.
- A foam pressure dressing is applied.

Rules, Tips, and Tricks

- All landmarks should be positively identified.
- Prevent postauricular hematoma formation.
- Apply rigorous patient selection criteria.

! Risks and Complications

Facial nerve injury.

Postoperative Care

- Continue the pressure dressing for 5 days.
- Remove the sutures on the 10th postoperative day.
- Schedule an initial fitting at 4–6 weeks.

Bibliography

Abbé R. A new plastic operation for the relief of deformity due to double harelip. Med Rec 1898;53:477

Al-Sebeih K, Manoukian J. Systemic steroids for the management of obstructive subglottic hemangioma. J Otolaryngol 2000;29(6):361–366

Ambrosch P, Kron M, Steiner W. Carbon dioxide laser microsurgery for early supraglottic carcinoma. Ann Otol Rhinol Laryngol 1998;107(8):680–688

Anderson JR. A reasoned approach to nasal base surgery. Arch Otolaryngol 1984;110(6):349–358

Anderson JR, Ries WR. Rhinoplasty: Emphasizing the External Approach. New York: Thieme-Stratton; 1986

Arden RL, Nawroz-Danish M, Yoo GH, Meleca RJ, Burgio DL. Nasal alar reconstruction: a critical analysis using melolabial island and paramedian forehead flaps. Laryngoscope 1999;109(3):376–382

Ariyan S. The pectoralis major myocutaneous flap. A versatile flap for reconstruction in the head and neck. Plast Reconstr Surg 1979;63(1):73–81

Avelar JM, Psillakis JM, Viterbo F. Use of large composite grafts in the reconstruction of deformities of the nose and ear. Br J Plast Surg 1984;37(1):55–60

Bailey M, Hoeve H, Monnier P. Paediatric laryngotracheal stenosis: a consensus paper from three European centres. Eur Arch Otorhinolaryngol 2003;260(3):118–123

Bakamjian VY. The deltopectoral skin flap in head and neck surgery. In: Conley J, Dickinson JT. Plastic and Reconstructive Surgery of the Head and Neck. Stuttgart, New York; Thieme; 1972

Baudet J. La reimplantation du pavillon de l'òreille mutilé. La Nouvelle Presse Medicale 1972;5:344

Becker DG, McLaughlin RB Jr, Loevner LA, Mang A. The lateral osteotomy in rhinoplasty: clinical and radiographic rationale for osteotome selection. Plast Reconstr Surg 2000;105(5):1806–1816, discussion 1817–1819

Bergler W. Laser in der Mundhöhle und im Oropharynx. LaryngoRhinoOtol. Stuttgart: Thieme; 2003;82 Supplement 1:77–88

Bergler W, Huber K, Hammerschmitt N, Hölzl M, Hörmann K. Tonsillectomy with the argon-plasma-coagulation-raspatorium – a prospective randomized single-blinded study. [Article in German] HNO 2000;48(2):135–141

Bewarder F, Pirsig W. Long-term results of submucous septal resection (author's transl). [Article in German] Laryngol Rhinol Otol (Stuttg) 1978;57(10):922–930

Beyer-Machule CK. Plastische Chirurgie der Lider. Stuttgart: Enke; 1982

Beyer-Machule CK, von Noorden CK. Lider, Orbita, äußere Augenmuskeln. In: Heilmann K, Paton D. Atlas der ophthalmologischen Operationen, Bd I. Stuttgart: Thieme; 1985

Bhanot S, Alex JC, Lowlicht RA, Ross DA, Sasaki CT. The efficacy of resorbable plates in head and neck reconstruction. Laryngoscope 2002;112(5):890–898

Bielamowicz S, Stager SV, Badillo A, Godlewski A. Unilateral versus bilateral injections of botulinum toxin in patients with adductor spasmodic dysphonia. J Voice 2002;16(1):117–123

Birck HG, Parrish RT. The movable stent in choanal atresia. Laryngoscope 1986;96(2):135–139

Blitzer A, Brin MF, Stewart CF. Botulinum toxin management of spasmodic dysphonia (laryngeal dystonia): a 12-year experience in more than 900 patients. Laryngoscope 1998;108(10):1435–1441

Borges AF, Alexander JE. Relaxed skin tension lines, Z-plasties on scars, and fusiform excision of lesions. Br J Plast Surg 1962;15:242–254

Brent B. The correction of mi-rotia with autogenous cartilage grafts: I. The classic deformity? Plast Reconstr Surg 1980;66(1):1–12

Brent B. The correction of microtia with autogenous cartilage grafts: II. Atypical and complex deformities. Plast Reconstr Surg 1980;66(1):13–21

Bruintjes TD, van Olphen AF, Hillen B. Review of the functional anatomy of the cartilages and muscles of the nose. Rhinology 1996;34(2):66–74

Burget GC, Menick FJ. Aesthetic Reconstruction of the Nose. St. Louis: Mosby Year Book; 1994;57–91

Burget GC, Menick FJ. Aesthetic restoration of one-half the upper lip. Plast Reconstr Surg 1986;78(5):583–593

Byrd HS, Salomon J, Flood J. Correction of the crooked nose. Plast Reconstr Surg 1998;102(6):2148–2157

Calhoun KH, Seikaly H, Quinn FB. Teaching paradigm for decision making in facial skin defect reconstructions. Arch Otolaryngol Head Neck Surg 1998;124(1):60–66

Chatrath P, Black M, Jani P, Albert DM, Bailey CM. A review of the current management of infantile subglottic haemangioma, including a comparison of CO(2) laser therapy versus tracheostomy. Int J Pediatr Otorhinolaryngol 2002;64(2):143–157

Chongchet V. A method of antihelix reconstruction. Br J Plast Surg 1963;16:268–272

Clodius L. Die Praxis der Chirurgie der Narben. Chir Prax 1973;17:455

Cole P. Biophysics of nasal airflow: a review. Am J Rhinol 2000;14(4):245–249

Cole P. The four components of the nasal valve. Am J Rhinol 2003;17(2):107–110

Constantian MB. Four common anatomic variants that predispose to unfavourable rhinoplasty results: a study based on 150 consecutive secondary rhinoplastics. Plast Reconstr Surg 2000;105:316–33

Constantinidis J, Federspil P, Iro H. Functional and esthetically oriented reconstruction of lip defects. [Article in German] HNO 2000;48(7):517–526

Converse JM, Wood-Smith D. Technical details in the surgical correction of the lop ear deformity. Plast Reconstr Surg 1963;31:118–128

Cottle MH, Loring RM, Fischer GG, Gaynon IE. The maxilla-premaxilla approach to extensive nasal septum surgery. AMA Arch Otolaryngol 1958;68(3):301–313

Daniel RK. Rhinoplasty: a simplified, three-stitch, open tip suture technique. Part I: primary rhinoplasty. Plast Reconstr Surg 1999;103(5):1491–1502

Daniel RK. Rhinoplasty: a simplified, three-stitch, open tip suture technique. Part II: secondary rhinoplasty. Plast Reconstr Surg 1999;103(5):1503–1512

Davis J. Aesthetic and Reconstructive Otoplasty. Berlin: Springer; 1986

Davis RK, Hayes JK. Management of supraglottic cancer: selected endoscopic laser resection and postoperative irradiation. Adv Otorhinolaryngol 1995;49:231–236
Davis RK. Endoscopic surgical management of glottic laryngeal cancer. Otolaryngol Clin North Am 1997;30(1):79–86
de Mello-Filho FV, Carrau RL. The management of laryngeal fractures using internal fixation. Laryngoscope 2000;110(12):2143–2146
Dedo HH, Yu KC. CO(2) laser treatment in 244 patients with respiratory papillomas. Laryngoscope 2001;111(9):1639–1644
Deitmer T. Tonsillektomie. Indikationen und Ausführung heute. In: Ganz OH, Iro H (eds). HNO-Praxis Heute. Berlin–Heidelberg: Springer; 2000
Dennis DP, Kashima H. Carbon dioxide laser posterior cordectomy for treatment of bilateral vocal cord paralysis. Ann Otol Rhinol Laryngol 1989;98(12 Pt 1):930–934
Denoyelle F, Mondain M, Gresillon N, Roger G, Chaudre F, Garabedian EN. Failures and complications of supraglottoplasty in children. Arch Otolaryngol Head Neck Surg 2003;129(10):1077–1080, discussion 1080
Derkay CS. Recurrent respiratory papillomatosis. Laryngoscope 2001;111(1):57–69
van Dishoeck EA, Lashley FON. Closure of a septal perforation by means of an obturator. Rhinology 1975;13(1):33–37
Draf W. Eingriffe am intracraniellen N. facialis bis zum Foramen stylomastoideum. In: Naumann HH. Kopf und Halschirurgie. Vol 2. 2nd ed. Stuttgart: Thieme; 1996
Dufourmentel C, Mouly R. Chirurgie plastique. Paris: Flammarion; 1959
Dünne AA, Folz BJ, Kuropkat C, Werner JA. Extent of surgical intervention in case of N0 neck in head and neck cancer patients: an analysis of data collection of 39 hospitals. Eur Arch Otorhinolaryngol 2004;261(6):295–303
Dyer WK II, Yune ME. Structural grafting in rhinoplasty. Facial Plast Surg 1997;13(4):269–277
Eckel HE, Sittel C. Bilateral recurrent laryngeal nerve paralysis. [Article in German] HNO 2001;49(3):166–179
Eckel HE, Volling P, Pototschnig C, Zorowka P, Thumfart W. Transoral laser resection with staged discontinuous neck dissection for oral cavity and oropharynx squamous cell carcinoma. Laryngoscope 1995;105(1):53–60
Eckel HE. Local recurrences following transoral laser surgery for early glottic carcinoma: frequency, management, and outcome. Ann Otol Rhinol Laryngol 2001;110(1):7–15
Eitschberger E, Merklein C, Masing H, Pesch HJ. Deviations of septum cartilage after unilateral separation of Mucoperichondrium in rabbits (author's transl). [Article in German] Arch Otorhinolaryngol 1980;228(2):135–148
El Hakim H, Waddell AN, Crysdale WS. Observations on the early results of treatment of recurrent respiratory papillomatosis using cidofovir. J Otolaryngol 2002;31(6):333–335
Esser JFS. Die Rotation der Wange und allgemeine Bemerkungen bei chirurgischer Gesichtsplastik. Leipzig: Vogel; 1928
Estlander JA. Méthode d'autoplastie de la joue ou d'une levre par un lumbeau emprunt l'autre levre. Rev Mens Med Chir 1877;1:344
Ey W. Errors in and dangers of surgical therapy of anatomical and functional changes of the anterior septum. [Article in German] Z Laryngol Rhinol Otol 1969;48(1):38–43
Feuerstein SS, Krespi YP, Sachdev RK. Transnasal correction of choanal atresia. Head Neck Surg 1980;3(2):97–104
Fisch U, Dillier N. Technique and long-term results of stapedotomy. [Article in German] HNO 1987;35(6):252–254
Fisch U. Tympanoplasty, Mastoidectomy and Stapes Surgery. 2nd ed. New York: Thieme; 1994
Foda HMT, Magdy EA. Combining rhinoplasty with septal perforation repair. Facial Plast Surg 2006;22(4):281–288
Ford CN. Serial excision and advancement flaps in the management of facial lesions. Otolaryngol Head Neck Surg 1983;91(2):156–164
Friedrich G. Titanium vocal fold medializing implant: introducing a novel implant system for external vocal fold medialization. Ann Otol Rhinol Laryngol 1999;108(1):79–86
Friedrich G, Mausser G, Nemeth E. Development of a jet tracheoscope. Value and possible uses in superimposed high frequency jet ventilation in endoscopic surgery of the respiratory tract. [Article in German] HNO 2002;50(8):719–726
Fritsch MH. Incisionless otoplasty. Facial Plast Surg 2004;20(4):267–270
Fritzmeier F, Draf W. Surgical treatment of benign and malignant lip tumors. [Article in German] HNO 1982;30(9):326–332
Furnas DW. Correction of prominent ears by conchamastoid sutures. Plast Reconstr Surg 1968;42(3):189–193
Gallivan GJ. Bilateral vocal fold posterior glottic/subglottic stenotic web resected with contact tip Nd-YAG laser. J Voice 2002;16(3):415–421
Gammert C, Masing H, Eitschberger E. Die plastisch-chirurgische Versorgung von Septumabszessen. In: Probst J. 15. Jahrestagung der Deutschen Gesellschaft für Plastische und Wiederherstellungschirurgie. Berlin: Springer; 1980:198–200
Kastenbauer ER. Special methods of reconstructive surgery in the facial region (author's transl). [Article in German] Arch Otorhinolaryngol 1977;216(1):123–250
Gersuny R. Über einige kosmetische Operationen. Wien Med Wochenschr. 1903;48:2253–2257
Gibson T, Davis WB. The distortion of autogenous cartilage grafts: Its cause and prevention. Br J Plast Surg 1958;10:257–274
Giudice M, Piazza C, Foccoli P, Toninelli C, Cavaliere S, Peretti G. Idiopathic subglottic stenosis: management by endoscopic and open-neck surgery in a series of 30 patients. Eur Arch Otorhinolaryngol 2003;260(5):235–238
Grabb WC, Myers MB. Skin Flaps. Boston: Little Brown; 1975
Grevers B. Aktuelle Aspekte zu Klinik, Diagnostik und Therapie entzündlicher Erkrankungen der Mundhöhle, des Oropharynx und der Speicheldrüsen. In: Verhandlungsbericht 1997. D. Ges. für HNO-Heilk., Kopf- und Halschirurgie. Springer; 1997:1–46
Gruber RP, Friedman GD. Suture algorithm for the broad or bulbous nasal tip. Plast Reconstr Surg 2002;110(7):1752–1764, discussion 1765–1768
Guyuron B, Uzzo CD, Scull H. A practical classification of septonasal deviation and an effective guide to septal surgery. Plast Reconstr Surg 1999;104(7):2202–2209, discussion 2210–2212
Haas E. On the reconstruction of nose defects. [Article in German] Z Laryngol Rhinol Otol 1968;47(4):251–264
Habler O. Procedure for reduction of allotransfusion in operative medicine. [Article in German] HNO 2003;51(1):8–11
Hall WJ, Watanabe T, Kenan PD, Baylin G. Transseptal repair of unilateral choanal atresia. Arch Otolaryngol 1982;108(10):659–661
Hartnick CJ, Hartley BE, Lacy PD, et al. Topical mitomycin application after laryngotracheal reconstruction: a randomized, double-blind, placebo-controlled trial. Arch Otolaryngol Head Neck Surg 2001;127(10):1260–1264
Häusler R, Schär PJ, Pratisto H, Weber HP, Frenz M. Advantages and dangers of erbium laser application in stapedotomy. Acta Otolaryngol 1999;119(2):207–213
Häusler R. Fortschritte in der Stapeschirurgie. LaryngoRhino-Otol. Stuttgart: Thieme; 2000;79, Supplement 2:95–139
Heermann J. Auricular cartilage palisade tympano-, epitympano-, antrum- and mastoid-plasties. Clin Otolaryngol Allied Sci 1978;3(4):443–446
Heumann H, Reimann B, Stelzner J, Lange-Stumpf U, Kretz FJ. Using the laryngeal mask in adenotomy and tonsillectomy in children. [Article in German] HNO 2001;49(8):664–669
Helling K, Abrams J, Bertram WK, Hohner S, Scherer H. Laser tonsillectomy in tonsillar hyperplasia of early childhood. [Article in German] HNO 2002;50(5):470–478
Helms J. Chirurgie an Labyrinth und innerem Gehörgang. In: Naumann HH. Kopf und Halschirurgie. Vol 2, 2nd ed. Stuttgart: Thieme; 1996.

Helms J. Sanierende und rekonstruktive Operationen an Gehörgang, Mittelohr und Felsenbein. In: Naumann HH. Kopf und Halschirurgie. Vol 2, 2nd ed. Stuttgart: Thieme; 1996

Herbert DC. A subcutaneous pedicled cheek flap for reconstruction of alar defects. Br J Plast Surg 1978;31(2):79–92

Hertig P. A new technique for the plastic reconstruction of the lower lip. [Article in French] Pract Otorhinolaryngol (Basel) 1965;27:157–166

Hewell TS, Tardy ME. Nasal tip refinement—reliable approaches and sculpture. Facial Plast Surg 1984;1:87–124

Hildmann H, Sudhoff H, Jahnke K. Grundzüge einer differenzierten Cholesteatomchirurgie. Laryngorhinotology 2000;79(Suppl 2):S73–S94

Holmström H. Clinical and pathologic features of maxillonasal dysplasia (Binder's syndrome): significance of the prenasal fossa on etiology. Plast Reconstr Surg 1986;78(5):559–567

Hörmann K, Hirth K, Maurer JT. Surgical therapy of sleep-related respiratory disorders. [Article in German] HNO 1999;47(4):226–235

Huizing EH. Long term results of reconstruction of the septum in the acute phase of a septal abscess in children. Rhinology 1984;22(1):55–63

Huizing EH, de Groot JAM. Functional reconstructive nasal surgery. Stuttgart: Thieme; 2003

Hüttenbrink KB. Zur Rekonstruktion des Schallleitungsapparates unter biomechanischen Gesichtspunkten. Laryngorhinootologie 2000;79(Suppl 2):S23–S51

Imre J. Lidplastik und plastische Operationen anderer Weichteile des Gesichts. Budapest: Studium-Verlag; 1928.

Isshiki N, Haji T, Yamamoto Y, Mahieu HF. Thyroplasty for adductor spasmodic dysphonia: further experiences. Laryngoscope 2001;111(4 Pt 1):615–621

Jansen C. The combined approach for tympanoplasty (report on 10 years' experience). J Laryngol Otol 1968;82(9):779–793

Johns M. Chirurgie der Speicheldrüsen. In: Naumann HH, Helms J, Herberhold C, et al. Kopf- und Hals-Chirurgie. Stuttgart: Thieme; 1995; Vol 1/II:809–30

Jovanovic S. Lasers in otology. [Article in German] Laryngorhinootologie 2003;82(Suppl 1):S21–S53

Jovanovic S, Schönfeld U. Application of the CO2 laser in stapedotomy. Adv Otorhinolaryngol 1995;49:95–100

Kastenbauer ER. Special methods of reconstructive surgery in the facial region (author's transl). [Article in German] Arch Otorhinolaryngol 1977;216(1):123–250

Kazanjian VH. The repair of nasal defects with the median forehead flap. Surg Gynecol Obstet 1946;83:37

Killian G. Die submucöse Fensterresektion der Nasenscheidewand. Arch Laryng Rhino 1904;16:362–387

Kleinsasser O. Mikrolaryngoskopie und endolaryngeale Mikrochirurgie. Technik und typische Befunde. Stuttgart: Schattauer; 1968

Kleinschmidt S. Methods and techniques of anesthesia for securing the airway in ENT medical interventions. [Article in German] HNO 2002;50(10):901–905

Kleinschmidt S, Plinkert PK, Fuchs-Buder T, Seyfert UT. Haemostatic disorders in ENT patients. Part 2: Pathophysiology, diagnostics, clinical feature and therapy. [Article in German] HNO 2003;51(3):251–265, quiz 265–266

Koltai PJ. Starplasty: a new technique of pediatric tracheotomy. Arch Otolaryngol Head Neck Surg 1998;124(10):1105–1111

König F. Zur Deckung von Defekten der Nasenflügel. Berl KlinWschr. 1902;7:137

Kreibig G. Vereinfachte Operationsmethoden zum Ersatz der Augenlider. Klein Mbl Augenheilk; 1950

Laccourreye H, Laccourreye O, Weinstein GS, Menard M, Brasnu D. Supracricoid laryngectomy with cricohyoidoepiglottopexy: a partial laryngeal procedure for glottic carcinoma. Ann Otol Rhinol Laryngol 1990;99(6 Pt 1):421–426

Laccourreye O, Laccourreye L, Muscatello L, Périé S, Weinstein G, Brasnu D. Local failure after supracricoid partial laryngectomy: symptoms, management, and outcome. Laryngoscope 1998;108(3):339–344

Laccourreye O, Laccourreye L, Garcia D, Gutierrez-Fonseca R, Brasnu D, Weinstein G. Vertical partial laryngectomy versus supracricoid partial laryngectomy for selected carcinomas of the true vocal cord classified as T2N0. Ann Otol Rhinol Laryngol 2000;109(10 Pt 1):965–971

Laccourreye O, Papon JF, Kania R, Crevier-Buchman L, Brasnu D, Hans S. Intracordal injection of autologous fat in patients with unilateral laryngeal nerve paralysis: long-term results from the patient's perspective. Laryngoscope 2003;113(3):541–545

Lange G. The intratympanic treatment of Menière's disease with ototoxic antibiotics. A follow-up study of 55 cases (author's transl). [Article in German] Laryngol Rhinol Otol (Stuttg) 1977;56(5):409–414

Leuwer R. Hearing disorder. Mechanical management of hearing loss: conventional and implantable hearing aids. [Article in German] Laryngorhinootologie 2005;84(Suppl 1):S51–S59

Lichtenberger G, Toohill RJ. Endo-extralaryngeal suture technique for endoscopic lateralization of paralyzed vocal cords. Oper Tech Otolaryngol–Head Neck Surg 1998;9:166–171

Limberg A. Plastic interchange of triangular flaps. Odont Stomat 1928;2:74

Lippert BM, Teymoortash A, Folz BJ, Werner JA. Wound healing after laser treatment of oral and oropharyngeal cancer. Lasers Med Sci 2003;18(1):36–42

Loke D, Ghosh S, Panarese A, Bull PD. Endoscopic division of the ary-epiglottic folds in severe laryngomalacia. Int J Pediatr Otorhinolaryngol 2001;60(1):59–63

Luckett WH. A new operation for prominent ears based on the anatomy of the deformity. Surg Gynecol Obstet 1910;10:635–637

Luckhaupt H. Tonsillektomie, Adenotomie, Paukenergüsse. In: Hildmann H, Koch U (eds). Hals-Nasen-Ohren-Chirurgie im Kindes- und Jugendalter. Verhandlungsbericht 1999. Berlin, Heidelberg, New York, Tokyo: Springer; 1999

Luckhaupt H. Tonsillektomie, Adenotomie, Paukenergüsse. In: Verhandlungsbericht Dt. Gesellsch. f. Hals-Nasen-Ohrenheilkunde. Referate Hildmann H, Koch U (Hrsg). Berlin, Heidelberg: Springer; 1999

Mahieu HF, Dikkers FG. Indirect microlaryngostroboscopic surgery. Arch Otolaryngol Head Neck Surg 1992;118(1):21–24

Majer EH, Rieder W. Technic of laryngectomy permitting the conservation of respiratory permeability (cricohyoidopexy). [Article in German] Ann Otolaryngol Chir Cervicofac 1959;76:677–681

Maran AGD, Lund VJ. Clinical Rhinology. Stuttgart: Thieme; 1990

Masing H, Steiner W. Treatment of choanal atresia. [Article in German] Laryngol Rhinol Otol (Stuttg) 1984;63(4):181–183

McFarlane RM, Heagy FC, Radin S, Aust JC, Wermuth RE. A study of the delay phenomenon in experimental pedicle flaps. Plast Reconstr Surg 1965;35:245–262

Meyer R. Rekonstruktion der Nasenflügel mit zusammengesetzten Ohrmuschel-Transplantaten. Mschr Ohrenheilk. 1955;89:27

Milton SH. The effects of "delay" on the survival of experimental pedicled skin flaps. Br J Plast Surg 1969;22(3):244–252

Mlynski G, Löw J. Die Rhinoresistometrie – eine Weiterentwicklung der Rhinomanometrie. Laryngorhinootologie 1993;72:608–610

Monnier P. Acquired laryngotracheal stenosis in childhood. Dilatation or resection? [Article in German] HNO 1999;47(5):451–453

Monnier P, Lang F, Savary M. Partial cricotracheal resection for severe pediatric subglottic stenosis: update of the Lausanne experience. Ann Otol Rhinol Laryngol 1998;107(11 Pt 1):961–968

Mowlavi A, Masouem S, Kalkanis J, Guyuron B. Septal cartilage defined: implications for nasal dynamics and rhinoplasty. Plast Reconstr Surg 2006;117(7):2171–2174

Müller J. Hearing disorder. Mechanical management of hearing loss: cochlear implants and brain stem implants—current developments in the last 10 years. [Article in German] Laryngorhinootologie 2005;84(Suppl 1):S60–S69

Murakami WT, Wong LW, Davidson TM. Applications of the biomechanical behavior of cartilage to nasal septoplastic surgery. Laryngoscope 1982;92(3):300–309

Mustarde JC. The correction of prominent ears using simple mattress sutures. Br J Plast Surg 1963;16:170–178

Myer CM III, O'Connor DM, Cotton RT. Proposed grading system for subglottic stenosis based on endotracheal tube sizes. Ann Otol Rhinol Laryngol 1994;103(4 Pt 1):319–323

Naumann HH, Wilmes E. Operationen bei Stapesankylose. In Naumann HH. Kopf- und Halschirurgie. Vol 2, 2nd ed. 1996

Nockemann PF. Die chirurgische Naht. Stuttgart: Thieme; 1980

Nolst-Trenite GJ. Rhinoplasty. The Hague: Kugler Publications; 1993

van Olphen A. Complications of pyramid surgery. Facial Plast Surg 1997;13(1):15–23

Olze H, Gerhardt HJ, Kaschke O. Long-term results after modified Réthi-plasty in childhood. [Article in German] Laryngorhinootologie 1998;77(7):371–375

Papel ID, Nachlas NE. Facial Plastic and Reconstructive Surgery. St. Louis, Baltimore: Mosby Year Book; 1992

Parell GJ, Becker GD. The tension nose. Facial Plast Surg 1984:1:81–86

Pascher W, Dzirsk B. The treatment of dislocation of the arytenoid cartilage by mobilization in indirect microlaryngoscopy. [Article in German] Vestn Otorinolaringol 1996;6(6):27–29

Piquet JJ, Chevalier D. Subtotal laryngectomy with crico-hyoido-epiglotto-pexy for the treatment of extended glottic carcinomas. Am J Surg 1991;162(4):357–361

Pitanguy I, Salgado F, Radwanski HN, Bushkin SC. The surgical importance of the dermocartilaginous ligament of the nose. Plast Reconstr Surg 1995;95(5):790–794

Plester D, Hildmann H, Steinbach E. Atlas der Ohrchirurgie. Stuttgart: Kohlhammer; 1989

Powell N, Humphreys B. Proportions of the Aesthetic Face. New York; Thieme-Stratton; 1984

Price JC, Davis RK. The deltopectoral flap v the pectoralis major myocutaneous flap. Which one? Arch Otolaryngol 1984;110(1):35–40

Réthi A. On scarred stenoses of the larynx. [Article in German] Monatsschr Ohrenheilkd Laryngorhinol 1967;101(3):101–105

Rettinger G. Current aspects of septorhinoplasty [Article in German]. Otorhinolaryngol Nova 1992;2:70–79

Rettinger G. Epistaxis. In: Kastenbauer E, et al. (eds). Oto-Rhino-Laryngologie in Klinik und Praxis, Vol 2. Stuttgart: Thieme; 1992:363–68

Rettinger G. Three-step reconstruction of saddle nose deformities. In: Nolst-Trenite GJ. Rhinoplasty. The Hague: Kugler; 1993:191–200

Rettinger G, Masing H. Nasal splinting with thermoplastic material. [Article in German] HNO 1980;28(9):320

Rettinger G, Masing H, Heinl W. Management of septal perforations by rotationplasty of the septal mucosa. [Article in German] HNO 1986;34(11):461–466

Robbins KT, Clayman G, Levine PA, et al; American Head and Neck Society; American Academy of Otolaryngology--Head and Neck Surgery. Neck dissection classification update: revisions proposed by the American Head and Neck Society and the American Academy of Otolaryngology-Head and Neck Surgery. Arch Otolaryngol Head Neck Surg 2002;128(7):751–758

Robbins KT, Davidson W, Peters LJ, Goepfert H. Conservation surgery for T2 and T3 carcinomas of the supraglottic larynx. Arch Otolaryngol Head Neck Surg 1988;114(4):421–426

Ross R, Fisher JC, Ninnemann JL. Hauttransplantationen. Stuttgart, New York: Thieme; 1989

Rudert H. Laminotomy after Réthi. Report of treatment of 8 stenoses and 3 atresias of the larynx (author's transl). [Article in German] Laryngol Rhinol Otol (Stuttg) 1976;55(2):138–144

Rudert HH, Werner JA, Höft S. Transoral carbon dioxide laser resection of supraglottic carcinoma. Ann Otol Rhinol Laryngol 1999;108(9):819–827

Sasaki CT, Marotta JC, Lowlicht RA, Ross DA, Johnson M. Efficacy of resorbable plates for reduction and stabilization of laryngeal fractures. Ann Otol Rhinol Laryngol 2003;112(9 Pt 1):745–750

Scheithauer MO, Rettinger G. Compromised protective function of facial skin. Surgical treatment of compromised facial skin function. [Article in German] Laryngorhinootologie 2005;84(Suppl 1):S233–S247

Schmoldt U, Hildmann H, Servatius K. Submucous turbinate resection. [Article in German] Laryngol Rhinol Otol (Stuttg) 1985;64(7):328–330

Schneider B, Denk DM, Bigenzahn W. Functional results after external vocal fold medialization thyroplasty with the titanium vocal fold medialization implant. Laryngoscope 2003;113(4):628–634

Schönweiler R, Zwirner P. Dosierung von Botulinumtoxin Typ B bei spasmodischer Dysphonie vom Adduktortyp. HNO 2005;53:166–173

Schröder U, Jungehülsing M, Klussmann JP, Eckel HE. [Cricohyoidopexy (CHP) and Cricohyoidoepiglottopexy (CHEP). Indication, complications, functional und oncological results]. HNO 2003;51(1):38–45

Schultz-Coulon HJ, Laubert A. Laryngotracheoplasty in early childhood. [Article in German] HNO 1988;36(1):1–12

Schultz-Coulon HJ. Three-layer repair of nasoseptal defects. Otolaryngol Head Neck Surg 2005;132(2):213–218

Sesterhenn AM, Dünne AA, Braulke D, Lippert BM, Folz BJ, Werner JA. Value of endotracheal tube safety in laryngeal laser surgery. Lasers Surg Med 2003;32(5):384–390

Sesterhenn AM, Wagner HJ, Alfke H, Werner JA, Lippert BM. Treatment of benign tracheal stenosis utilizing self-expanding nitinol stents. Cardiovasc Intervent Radiol 2004;27(4):355–360

Sewell DA. Supracricoid partial laryngectomy with cricohyoidopexy. Op Tech Otol Head Surg. 2003;14:27–33

Sherris DA, Kern EB. The versatile autogenous rib graft in septorhinoplasty. Am J Rhinol 1998;12(3):221–227

Spector JE, Werkhaven JA, Spector NC, et al. Preservation of function and histologic appearance in the injured glottis with topical mitomycin-C. Laryngoscope 1999;109(7 Pt 1):1125–1129

Staindl O. Therapy of saddle nose. [Article in German] Laryngol Rhinol Otol (Stuttg) 1983;62(8):348–355

Staindl O, Chmelizek-Feurstein C. Scars and scar revision. [Article in German] HNO 1983;31(6):183–192

Steiner W. Results of curative laser microsurgery of laryngeal carcinomas. Am J Otolaryngol 1993;14(2):116–121

Steiner W, Ambrosch P. Endoscopic laser surgery of the upper aerodigestive tract. With special emphasis on tumor surgery. Stuttgart: Thieme; 2000

Fischer M, Frerich R, Schrader M. Long-term results of radium contact irradiation of laryngeal carcinoma and their relevance in modern therapeutical regimens. [Article in German] Laryngorhinootologie 2001; 80(3, Supplement 1)156–160

Stenstroem SJ. A "natural" technique for correction of congenitally prominent ears. Plast Reconstr Surg 1963;32:509–518

Stoll W, Nieschalk M. Congenital abnormalities of the prenasal space: glioma, fistulas and epidermoid cysts. [Article in German] Laryngorhinootologie 1996;75(12):739–744

Strutz J. Chirurgische Therapie der Hör- und Gleichgewichtsorgane, Mittelohr. In: Strutz J, Mann W. Praxis der HNO-Heilkunde, Kopf- und Halschirurgie. Stuttgart: Thieme; 2001

Sulsenti G. Chirurgia Funzionale ed Esthetica del Naso. Milano: Ghedini Editore; 1994

Tanzer R. Congenital deformities. In: Converse JM. Reconstr Plast Surg 2. Vol 3. Philadelphia: Saunders; 1977

Thomas JR, Roller J. Cutaneous facial surgery. Stuttgart: Thieme; 1992

Tolsdorff P. Das Seromukotympanon. Heutige Vorstellungen zu Genese und Therapie. HNO-Praxis Heute. 1993;13:1–34

Toriumi DM, Josen J, Weinberger M, Tardy ME Jr. Use of alar batten grafts for correction of nasal valve collapse. Arch Otolaryngol Head Neck Surg 1997;123(8):802–808

Tos M. Manual of Middle Ear Surgery. Vol 1–4. Stuttgart, New York: Thieme; 1993–1999
Verse T, Pirsig W. Indications for performing uvulopalatopharyngoplasty and laser-assisted uvulopalatopharyngoplasty. [Article in German] HNO 1998;46(5):553–561
Verwoerd CDA, Verwoerd-Verhoef HL. Rhinosurgery in children. In: Nolst-Trenite GJ. Rhinoplasty. The Hague: Kugler Publications; 1993: 201–209
Walther LE. Dysequilibrium. Restorative management in dysequilibrium. [Article in German] Laryngorhinootologie 2005;84(Suppl 1):S70–S91
Webster CC, Davidson TM, Smith RC. Broken line scar revision. Clin Plast Surg 1977;4(2):263–274
Webster RC, Smith RC, Smith KF, Barrera A, Hamdan US. Local flaps for the middle third of the face. Facial Plast Surg 1984;1(1):1–30
Weerda H. Der "bilobed-flap" in der Kopf- und Halschirurgie. Arch Otorhinolaryngol 1978;219:181–190
Weerda H. The trauma of the auricle (author's transl). [Article in German] HNO 1980;28(7):209–217
Weerda H. Special techniques in the reconstruction of cheek and lip defects (author's transl). [Article in German] Laryngol Rhinol Otol (Stuttg) 1980;59(10):630–640
Weerda H. Reconstruction of the lower lip. [Article in German] Laryngol Rhinol Otol (Stuttg) 1983;62(1):23–28
Weerda H. Classification of congenital deformities of the auricle. Facial Plast Surg 1988;5(5):385–388
Weerda H. Embryology and structural anatomy of the external ear. Facial Plast Surg 1988;5:85–91
Weerda H. Chirurgie der Ohrmuschel. Stuttgart: Thieme; 2004
Weerda H, Siegert R. Complications of otoplasty and their treatment. [Article in German] Laryngorhinootologie 1994;73(7):394–399
Weinstein GS, Laccourreye O, Ruiz C, Dooley P, Chalian A, Mirza N. Larynx preservation with supracricoid partial laryngectomy with cricohyoidoepiglottopexy. Correlation of videostroboscopic findings and voice parameters. Ann Otol Rhinol Laryngol 2002;111(1):1–7
Weisberger EC, Hanke W. Reconstruction of full-thickness defects of the cheek. Arch Otolaryngol 1983;109(3):190–194
Werner JA, Lippert BM. Lateral fixation of the vocal cord instead of tracheotomy in acute bilateral vocal cord paralysis. [Article in German] Dtsch Med Wochenschr 2002;127(17):917–922
Werner JA, Dünne AA, Lippert BM. Indications for neck operation in undiagnosed lymph node metastases. 2. Neck dissection in the clinical N0 neck. [Article in German] HNO 2002;50(4):370–378, quiz 378–379
Werner JA, Dünne AA, Lippert BM. Indications for neck operation in undetected lymph node metastases. 1: Basic principles of lymphogenic metastatic behavior of otorhinolaryngology cancers. [Article in German] HNO 2002;50(3):253–262, quiz 262–263
Werner JA, Dünne AA, Myers JN. Functional anatomy of the lymphatic drainage system of the upper aerodigestive tract and its role in metastasis of squamous cell carcinoma. Head Neck 2003;25(4):322–332
Werner JA, Dünne AA, Folz BJ, Lippert BM. Transoral laser microsurgery in carcinomas of the oral cavity, pharynx, and larynx. Cancer Control 2002;9(5):379–386
Werner JA, Dünne AA, Folz BJ, Lippert BM. Laser surgery for T2 glottic carcinoma. Otorhinolaryngol Nova. 2003;12:36–41
Werner JA, Lippert BM, Dünne AA, Ankermann T, Folz BJ, Seyberth H. Epiglottopexy for the treatment of severe laryngomalacia. Eur Arch Otorhinolaryngol 2002;259(9):459–464
Wigand ME. Restitutional surgery of the ear and temporal bone. Stuttgart, NewYork: Thieme; 2001
Wilhelm T, Weber BP. Perioperative prevention of thromboembolism in ENT medicine. [Article in German] HNO 1996;44(1):31–32
Wilhelmi BJ, Blackwell SJ, Phillips LG. Langer's lines: to use or not to use. Plast Reconstr Surg 1999;104(1):208–214
Wullstein HL, Wullstein SR. Tympanoplastik: osteoplastische Tympanotomie. Stuttgart: Thieme; 1986
Yellin SA. Aesthetics for the next millennium. Facial Plast Surg 1997;13(4):231–239
Zahnert T. Hearing disorder. Surgical management. [Article in German] Laryngorhinootologie 2005;84(Suppl 1):S37–S50
Zeitels SM, Davis RK. Endoscopic laser management of supraglottic cancer. Am J Otolaryngol 1995;16(1):2–11
Zeitels SM, Healy GB. Laryngology and phonosurgery. N Engl J Med 2003;349(9):882–892
Zenk J, Iro H. Die Sialolithiasis und deren Behandlung. Laryngorhinootologie 2001;80(Suppl 1):S115–S136
Zisser G. Primärrekonstruktive Eingriffe zum Lippenersatz nach Exzision bösartiger Tumoren. Acta Chir Austriaca 1974;6:49

B

Index

Page references in *italic* type refer to illustrations.

D

E

F

T

U

V

W

Y

Z